LARGE ANIMAL CLINICAL PROCEDURES
for VETERINARY TECHNICIANS

LARGE ANIMAL CLINICAL PROCEDURES
for VETERINARY TECHNICIANS

ELIZABETH A. HANIE, DVM, MS
FORMER DEPARTMENT CHAIR
VETERINARY MEDICAL TECHNOLOGY PROGRAM
GASTON COLLEGE, DALLAS, NORTH CAROLINA

With **711** *illustrations, including* **560** *in full color*

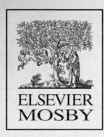

ELSEVIER
MOSBY

ELSEVIER
MOSBY

11830 Westline Industrial Drive
St. Louis, Missouri 63146

LARGE ANIMAL CLINICAL PROCEDURES   ISBN 0-323-02855-1
FOR VETERINARY TECHNICIANS
Copyright © 2006 by Mosby, Inc.

NOTICE

Knowledge and best practice in this field are constantly changing. As new research and
experience broaden our knowledge, changes in practice, treatment and drug therapy may
become necessary or appropriate. Readers are advised to check the most current information
provided (i) on procedures featured or (ii) by the manufacturer of each product to be
administered, to verify the recommended dose or formula, the method and duration of
administration, and contraindications. It is the responsibility of the practitioner, relying on
their own experience and knowledge of the patient, to make diagnoses, to determine dosages
and the best treatment for each individual patient, and to take all appropriate safety
precautions. To the fullest extent of the law, neither the Publisher nor the Author assumes
any liability for any injury and/or damage to persons or property arising out or related to
any use of the material contained in this book.

Library of Congress Cataloging-in-Publication Data

Hanie, Elizabeth A.
  Large animal clinical procedures for veterinary technicians / Elizabeth A. Hanie.
    p. cm.
  Includes bibliographical references and index.
  ISBN 0-323-02855-1 (pbk.)
 1.   Veterinary medicine. 2.   Animal health technicians. I.   Title.
 SF745.H33 2006
 636.089--dc22

2005040696

Publishing Director: Linda Duncan
Managing Editor: Teri Merchant
Publishing Services Manager: Patricia Tannian
Project Manager: Kristine Feeherty
Designer: Amy Buxton

Working together to grow
libraries in developing countries

www.elsevier.com | www.bookaid.org | www.sabre.org

ELSEVIER   BOOK AID International   Sabre Foundation

Printed in China

Last digit is the print number: 9 8 7 6 5 4 3 2 1

With love to the memory of my grandfather, **T. FOLEY TREADWAY, JR.,** who taught me the value of an education, the wisdom of principles applied with compassion, and the absolute necessity of a sense of humor;

And to my grandmother, **EUGENIA E. TREADWAY,** the family's "steel magnolia," whose grace and generous spirit have been an inspiration to us all.

Preface

This book was born partially out of frustration. When searching for teaching materials on large animal topics while teaching in the Veterinary Medical Technology Program at Gaston College, I became aware of several things. There are many thorough, well-written texts on in-depth topics such as nutrition, pharmacology, anesthesiology, and radiology. However, general and practical information on large animal clinical techniques and procedures is often spread among multiple references, and the information on large animals often seems to take a backseat to small animal topics. This book does not attempt to replace the excellent in-depth references that are available, nor is it intended to be a comprehensive textbook of large animal nutrition, pharmacology, anesthesiology, husbandry, breeds, and diseases. Rather, it is intended to be a clinically oriented reference that will help the veterinary technician become a strong contributor to the large animal veterinary health care team. It is assumed that the reader has had basic courses or instruction in breeds, husbandry, nutrition, and other subjects taught in an AVMA-accredited veterinary technology program.

Education for veterinary technicians should be much more than just a "how to put Tab A into Slot B" endeavor. Good technicians can put Tab A into Slot B with proper technique. A great technician, however, not only puts Tab A into Slot B but also wants to know *why* there is a Tab A and exactly what Slot B is for. Over the years of working with many technicians in both academic and private practice settings, I have found that this desire to know *why* seems to make certain technicians stand out among their peers. To that end, I have tried to provide some background and explanation on the procedures so that the technician can have a better understanding of the art and science of large animal veterinary practice.

ELIZABETH A. HANIE

Acknowledgments

I would like to recognize **the many veterinary technicians** with whom I have had the privilege of working with over the years, often in some difficult and challenging situations; I couldn't have done it without you!

Many thanks **to the clinicians and staff at the Marion duPont Scott Equine Medical Center (1988-1991)** for help and guidance during my equine surgical residency.

Thanks to **Dr. Susan L. White, DVM, MS, DACVIM,** an excellent clinician and an inspiration to me while I was a student at the University of Georgia.

Thank you, **Betty D. Jones, RN, Department Chair of Medical Assisting and Phlebotomy at Gaston College,** for being such a wonderful mentor and friend.

Many thanks to **Kathy J. Neunzig, RVT,** for sharing professionalism, knowledge, and horsemanship with the students in large animal labs; your assistance was invaluable.

Thanks to **Robin F. Bynum, RVT, Lacey S. Wright, RVT,** and **Robin's horses, Princess and Carolina Babe,** for being such good sports and great subjects for the photographs.

Thank you, **Teri Merchant** and the staff at Elsevier for being so patient and helpful through this experience.

Thanks **to family and friends** for all of your encouragement and support during this project.

And, of course, **thanks to the students in the Veterinary Medical Technology Program at Gaston College from 1995 to 2003;** I assure you that the learning was a two-way street. Thanks to all of you for *my* education.

Contents

part I

EQUINE CLINICAL PROCEDURES

Hospital/Clinic Procedures in Equine Practice

Large animals present unique circumstances and challenges for their examination and treatment. The size of these animals generally presents difficulties with their transportation, so most large animal work is performed on the farm. This type of large animal practice, in which the veterinarian takes the necessary supplies and equipment to the farm and performs the diagnostic and treatment procedures there, is called *ambulatory practice* or *field service*. Mobile veterinary units may be homemade or purchased from companies that specialize in their design. The unit may range from simple storage bins to large fiberglass units with refrigerators, running hot/cold water, and storage space for supplies and equipment. These units may be adapted to cars, vans, or trucks (Fig. 1-1). The mobile

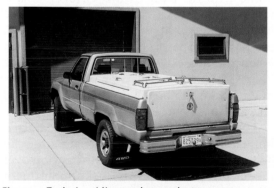

Fig. 1-1. Typical mobile veterinary unit. (From McCurnin DM, Lukens RL: Veterinary practice management. In McCurnin DM, Bassert JM, editors: *Clinical textbook for veterinary technicians*, ed 6, St Louis, 2006, Saunders.)

unit should be treated as a mobile medical facility and stocked and maintained as such. Inventory should be taken at least daily, and items restocked as necessary. Cleanliness and disinfection of the mobile unit should be routinely performed for sanitation and to maintain acceptable appearance to clients. Dirty facilities, whether buildings or vehicles, may give the impression that the veterinarian has disregard for sanitation or is simply too lazy to maintain his or her equipment. Technicians are often responsible for maintaining cleanliness and inventory for the mobile unit.

Many large animal clinics and hospitals are available nationwide, but special transportation in trailers or livestock vans is required to reach these "haul-in" facilities. Transportation of large animals may be problematic. Not all large animal owners own a trailer or livestock van; therefore transportation must be arranged through a friend or professional livestock transportation company. There may be a significant amount of time required to arrange for an animal's transportation, and in some parts of the country the nearest large animal hospital may be several hours away. When dealing with an emergency case where assessment and treatment are urgent, the time delay related to finding transportation, loading, and driving the animal to the hospital can have devastating consequences.

Many large animals are raised for commercial production of meat, milk, hair, skin, organs, or other products. The actual dollar value of many of these animals depends on their ability to generate these products and produce offspring. It is an unfortunate fact of life that the amount of money available for health care and veterinary medicine is often limited by the animal's production value. Most farmers provide what they can for diagnosis and treatment of their livestock, but the monetary value of the animal may fall far short of what is required for its medical or surgical treatment. It is disheartening to tell a farmer that surgery for a cow's broken leg is possible but may cost several thousand dollars, knowing that the realistic value of the cow may only be $400. In addition to maintaining the farm and the other animals on the farm, the farmer must provide for his or her family, too, and at some point these economic considerations must enter the decision-making process.

The monetary value of horses is usually considerably more than that of production livestock (at least in the mind of the owner!). Emotional attachment often plays a role in the owner's decision to finance a horse's treatment. Also, many horses are accustomed to being handled and transported, making transportation to a hospital more practical than that of other large animals. Finally, there are more equine haul-in facilities than there are for other large animal species. Therefore horses are generally more likely than livestock to be evaluated and treated at large animal clinics.

Because of cost and practicality, not all sick large animals have the luxury of going to a hospital or clinic. Improvising examinations and treatments on the farm are often required and can present challenging situations, many of which can have completely successful outcomes. Accurate assessment of the facilities, personnel, and costs involved is important when planning to treat sick animals on the farm. These same factors must be considered in the hospital environment, too.

The following principles of facility care and maintenance apply to large animal hospitals and clinics, but most can be adapted to care for animals at their home farms with a little imagination and planning.

ADMISSIONS/MEDICAL RECORDS

Horses usually arrive at the clinic accompanied by their owners, although sometimes horses' trainers or agents travel with the horse instead. In the case of professional transportation companies, the owner/agent rarely travels with the horse and the van driver may be the only person arriving with the horse. Therefore determining who is actually accompanying the horse and who is in charge of the decision-making processes for the horse is important. Depending on the circumstance, the owner, trainer, or agent for the horse may be responsible for the decisions; determine who this person is and obtain his or her contact information (e.g., phone numbers). Treatment is often delayed until permission can be obtained from the owner or agent, so accurate information is essential, especially in emergency cases.

Most horses are transported with protective gear such as leg wraps, head bumpers, or blankets. Much of this gear is not necessary during the hospital stay and should be sent home with the owner/transporter. If this is not possible, place these items in a plastic bag or storage bin and mark it clearly with the horse's name so that it can be returned when the horse is discharged. Loss of these items, although usually not very expensive, might make the hospital seem disorganized and is poor client "PR."

The medical record should be started immediately when the horse arrives; time can be saved by filling out basic information over the telephone when the horse's appointment is made by the owner/agent or referring veterinarian. The basic information should include patient signalment and billing information (Fig. 1-2). A treatment authorization

**ADMISSION
INFORMATION**

OWNER INFORMATION

Last Name _____

First Name _____

Farm Name _____

Address _____

City _____ State _____ Zip _____

SSN _____

Home Phone (_____) _____

Work Phone (_____) _____ Ext. _____

Co-Owner's Name _____

Home Phone (_____) _____

Work Phone (_____) _____ Ext. _____

AGENT/TRAINER INFORMATION

Last Name _____

First Name _____ Middle _____

Address _____

City _____ State _____ Zip _____

Phone _____

REFERRING VETERINARIAN

Name _____

Practice Name _____

Address _____

City _____ State _____ Zip _____

Phone (_____) _____

APPT. DATE: _____

Time: _____ AM   PM

To Be Admitted _____

CLINICIAN _____

MEDICAL RECORD #_____ _____ _____

NEW ACCOUNT? ☐ Yes   ☐ No

BILLING ADDRESS (if different)

Name _____

Address _____

City _____ State _____ Zip _____

INSURANCE INFORMATION

Company Name _____

Policy # _____

Agent _____

Address _____

City _____ State _____ Zip _____

Phone (_____) _____

PATIENT INFORMATION

Previous Patient? ☐ Yes   ☐ No

Name _____

Age _____

Breed _____

Sex: ☐ Stallion   ☐ Mare   ☐ Gelding
      ☐ Filly   ☐ Colt

Color _____

Estimated Value _____

Special Problems: _____
_____

Reason for Visit: _____
_____
_____
_____

Information obtained from: ☐ Ref. Vet.   ☐ Owner   ☐ Agent

Ref. Vet. to call and confirm?   ☐ Yes _____ Date & Time

METHOD OF PAYMENT

☐ Cash   ☐ Check   ☐ MasterCard   ☐ Visa

PAYMENT IN FULL IS EXPECTED WHEN THE PATIENT IS DISCHARGED

Fig. 1-2. Sample admission form.

form is advisable, as is a cost estimate form. Cost estimates can help prevent misunderstandings with the owner/agent, especially when a complicated medical or surgical case is to be treated. The cost of diagnosis and treatment of large animals usually far exceeds the cost of comparable procedures in small animals, primarily because of the large bodyweight and number of staff required to care for large animals. For example, pharmacy charges for use of the *same* drug in a horse versus a large dog may be 10 to 25 times higher for *each* dose of the drug in the horse, due to bodyweight alone. Many hospitals also include a charge sheet in the medical record so that each procedure performed and related supplies can be tracked for billing purposes.

One aspect that is somewhat unique to the horse industry is the widespread use of insurance. Although small animal insurance is becoming more commonplace, equine insurance has existed for many years. Equine insurance has three common types. *Mortality insurance* covers the value of the horse in case of death; the insurance company pays the owner the estimated worth of the horse if it dies, though there may be exclusions for certain causes of death. Because of the potential for fraud, it is sometimes necessary to get permission from the insurance company before treatment and/or euthanasia are performed. *Surgical insurance* covers specific costs of surgery and hospitalization, with some limitations—similar to human health insurance policies. Permission from the insurance company must often be obtained before performing elective and some emergency surgeries. *Loss of use insurance* states specifically the intended use of the horse, and if the horse cannot perform its intended use because of illness/injury, the owner may be reimbursed. Insurance companies must often be included in the decision-making processes for the patient; therefore it is important to

obtain this information as part of the medical record.

If euthanasia is to be performed, a euthanasia consent form should be included. If the owner/agent is not available to sign the euthanasia form, permission may be verbally obtained over the phone. Facsimile (FAX) communications may also provide a means to obtain necessary signatures. Sometimes it is not immediately known whether euthanasia will be necessary, yet it may become necessary later for the clinician to euthanize the horse with little notice. For example, the horse's emergency condition may suddenly "crash and burn" and require immediate euthanasia to prevent suffering; the time delay involved in trying to contact the owner/agent may result in unnecessary suffering. In these cases, having the owner/agent sign a euthanasia consent form when the horse first arrives at the hospital allows the clinician to humanely euthanize the horse in a truly crisis situation, then contact the owner after dealing with the crisis.

A basic physical examination form or patient flow sheet should be included for all horses to record temperature, pulse, respiration, bowel movement/urination, and food/water consumption information (Fig. 1-3). The physical examination form may be expanded for critical cases into an intensive care form (Fig. 1-4). A treatment form is useful to record and plan diagnostics and treatments and should provide a place for the technician/clinician to initial each procedure as it is performed. A form to record client communications is very important for documentation—all client communications should be summarized; the time, date and method of communication recorded; and the form signed. Other parts of the medical record depend on the nature of the case and may include radiology, ultrasound, endoscopy and laboratory reports, surgical procedures, and other pertinent information.

PHYSICAL EXAM FORM

(1) General	(2) Integument	(3) Musc-Skel
☐ N ☐ ABN	☐ N ☐ ABN	☐ N ☐ ABN
(4) Circulatory	(5) Respiratory	(6) Digestive
☐ N ☐ ABN	☐ N ☐ ABN	☐ N ☐ ABN
(7) Genital-Urinary	(8) Eyes	(9) Ears
☐ N ☐ ABN	☐ N ☐ ABN	☐ N ☐ ABN
(10) Nervous	(11) Lymphatic	(12) Mucous-Membranes
☐ N ☐ ABN	☐ N ☐ ABN	☐ N ☐ ABN

T _____ P_____ R _____ WT _____

DESCRIBE ABNORMAL (use numbers above)

TEMPORARY PROBLEM LIST	Initial Plan	
(1)	Dx	Rx
(2)		
(3)		

STUDENT/TECH.   **CLINICIAN**

Fig. 1-3. Basic physical examination form.

INTENSIVE CARE FLOW SHEET

DATE: _____

TIME	0100	0200	0300	0400	0500	0600	0700	0800	0900	1000	1100	1200
ATTITUDE/ PAIN												
TEMP												
RESP RATE												
HEART RATE												
MUCOUS MEMBRANES												
INTESTINAL MOTILITY												
FECES/ URINE												
DIGITAL PULSE												
PCV TP												
GASTRIC REFLUX												
FLUID THERAPY												
TOTAL FLUID ADMINISTR'D												
MEDICATION												
APPETITE												
INITIALS												

COMMENTS:

Fig. 1-4. Intensive care examination form.

The medical record may be kept on a clipboard or in a binder and placed on the patient's stall door or kept in a central nursing station of the hospital. Patient confidentiality should be considered when choosing a location for the patient's medical record; procedures, medications, and diagnostic test results are not intended to be public information. If the hospital allows visitors, and most do, the reputation of a horse, trainer, or stable may be jeopardized if this private information becomes public. The medical record should be in a form that allows it to travel around the hospital with the horse for its various procedures but be accessed only by hospital personnel.

PATIENT IDENTIFICATION

Proper patient identification (ID) is essential; surgery and even euthanasia have been performed on the wrong horse because of inadequate or inaccurate ID. It is important not only to record a horse's markings in written form in the medical record but to have some method of identifying the horse's stall and the horse itself. Patients are described by sex, breed, age, coat color, and markings. Descriptions in the patient signalment of color and natural markings may not be enough to distinguish an individual horse; for example, a "bay horse with a white star" may describe several horses in a large hospital or stable. Therefore an effort must be made to identify each horse as specifically as possible.

Technicians should be familiar with the proper terms for horse sex and age (Box 1-1). Slight variations in these terms may exist among different breeds, geographical location, and common jargon.

Markings may be natural or artificial (manmade). The most common natural markings used for ID in horses are point markings, scars, and hair whorls. There are six "points"

BOX 1-1	Age/Sex Terminology for the Horse

Foal: Young horse, from birth to weaning (usually at 4 to 7 months old)
Weanling: Young horse, from weaning to first birthday
Yearling: 1 year to 1½ years
Long Yearling: 1½ years to second birthday
Colt: Intact male between 2 and 3 years old
Filly: Female between 2 and 3 years old
Stallion: Intact male after third birthday
Mare: Female after third birthday
Gelding: Castrated male of any age

on domestic animals: the four legs, the head, and the tail. Points are usually black or white and are described as such. In particular, white point markings are the most distinguishing (Fig. 1-5, *A* and *B*). Leg and face markings are often described subjectively; for example, what one person may call a "full sock" is a "low stocking" to another, and this may be problematic. There is no standard level at which a sock becomes a stocking, a coronet becomes a pastern, and so on. Similar confusion exists with facial markings (e.g., no standard landmarks for strictly defining strips, stripes, blazes). To minimize confusion, it is preferable to either use a diagram to draw and label the markings (Fig. 1-6) or use a camera to photograph the animal for definitive ID. Drawings should be as accurate as possible; for instance, stars are not always in a perfect diamond shape, though they are often drawn that way. Stars are usually irregular in shape; in addition, they may be located above, at, or below eye level. These details are important. Facial markings are often continuous; for instance, a star may be continuous with a strip or stripe. When describing continuous facial markings, use a dash between the markings (e.g., star-strip, star-strip-snip). Photographs are especially useful for breeds with complicated coat patterns

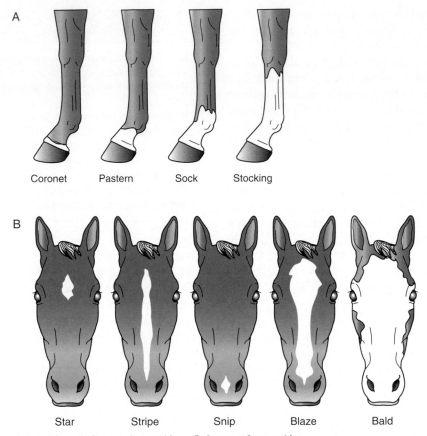

A

Coronet   Pastern   Sock   Stocking

B

Star   Stripe   Snip   Blaze   Bald

Fig. 1-5. White point markings. **A,** Common leg markings. **B,** Common face markings.

such as Paint Horses, Appaloosas, and Pintos, which are difficult to draw accurately.

If there are no markings on a leg or face, this should also be recorded for accuracy and to prevent fraudulent altering of medical records. Clearly indicate which body part lacks the markings and write "none" (e.g., left forelimb—none).

Coat color should always be recorded, though it is not a highly individual feature. Coat colors are not often distinguishing, especially among several breeds where there is little variation in coat color (e.g., most Standardbreds are bay). Additional confusion arises because there is no standard universal definition of coat colors. Each horse breed

registry defines its own acceptable and unacceptable coat colors and patterns, and these definitions may not be in agreement with other breeds. Foals present another challenge because a foal's coat color may be a different color from its eventual adult coat. The best example of this is the gray coat color; these horses are usually born black and lighten to gray with age, eventually progressing to white. For purposes of patient ID, record the coat color at the time of admission, not the anticipated adult color.

All horses have hair whorls (also known as swirls, cowlicks), which can be used for ID purposes (Fig. 1-7). Certain whorl locations are common to all horses, so whorls at these

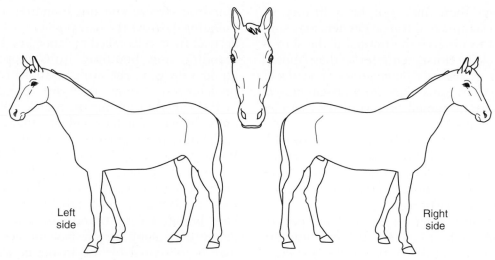

Fig. 1-6. Diagram to record leg and face markings.

Left side

Right side

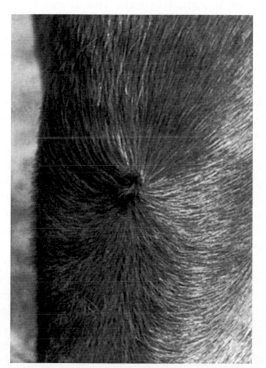

Fig. 1-7. Typical hair whorl found during clinical examination of a horse. (From Speirs VC: *Clinical examination of horses,* St Louis, 1997, Saunders.)

locations are not considered distinguishing features of an individual. Whorls on the flanks and over the trachea are common to all horses and seldom are helpful in definitive ID. However, some whorls occur at locations that are useful for ID. All horses have at least one whorl on the forehead between the eyes, but the whorl may be located above, below, or at the level of the eyes; the whorl may be right or left of midline, and some horses may have two or even three whorls in this area. When properly recorded, the forehead whorls are therefore useful. The other areas to check for distinguishing whorls are along the crest of the neck and along the jugular grooves. Do not assume that if there is a whorl on one side of the horse there will be a corresponding whorl on the other side. The standard written symbol for whorls is a simple "x" recorded on the horse's diagram or photo.

Muscle indentations above the jugular groove on the side of the neck are uncommonly seen. These indentations are readily seen and felt and are usually unilateral. They are generally assumed to result from trauma, although there may not be a history of known trauma to the area. Owners may simply fail to observe the trauma if the skin is not broken. Horsemen refer to these indentations as *wizard's thumbprints* or *warlock's thumbprints*. Since they are unusual, muscle indentations should be recorded as part of the patient ID.

Scars occur in two visible forms, those with hair and those without. Usually if a scar has hair, the hair will be white. Scars should be described by location, length, shape, and presence or absence of hair.

Chestnuts occur on the medial aspect of all limbs. Chestnuts are the evolutionary remnants of the digital pad of the first digit. They are small (1 to 3 cm), ovoid raised areas of cornified tissue proximal to the carpus on the forelimbs and at the level of the tarsus on the hindlimbs. They are seldom useful for ID purposes.

Although natural markings should always be recorded, many horses also have some form of permanent artificial ID that should be recorded in the medical record. Common forms of permanent artificial marking include lip tattoos, freeze brands, hot brands, and microchips. Lip tattoos are placed on the labial mucosa (inner lining) of the upper lip and are commonly used on racehorses. The tattoo is usually a combination of numbers and letters that identify the year of birth and the horse's registration number. Lip tattoos are usually applied to racehorses when they enter race training, most often as 2-year-olds.

Brands may be required by certain breed registries. Registries mandate the type, configuration, and location of the brand. Any owner, however, may brand an animal with a symbol of his or her choice where he or she prefers. Brands are usually placed on the side of the neck, over the triceps muscle on the forelimb, or on the hip/thigh area of the hindlimb. There are two types of branding—freeze and hot branding. Freeze branding destroys the hair pigment, which is derived from cells called melanocytes. Freeze branding uses branding irons dipped in liquid nitrogen. The iron is applied for a predetermined time necessary to kill the melanocytes but sparing the follicle cells that grow the hair. The hair will eventually grow back white (no pigment) in several months. White horses may be freeze branded, but the iron is applied longer to kill not only melanocytes but also the hair follicle so that there is no regrowth of hair; the result is a bald brand. Freeze brands are commonly placed high along the crest of the neck and may be obscured by the mane; be sure to look beneath the mane for freeze brands and other markings. Hot branding is considered by some to be more painful than freeze branding, which numbs the nerves within seconds of application of the freeze branding iron. However, many people who have performed hot brand procedures maintain that the discomfort of the horse is minimal during the procedure and is comparable to that produced by freeze branding. The goal of hot branding is to kill the hair follicles, producing a hairless scar.

Microchips can be inserted subcutaneously in horses and are usually placed in the neck area. Microchips are encoded for the individual horse and require a special sensor to scan the horse and read the ID code. This form of ID is gaining popularity in the horse world.

Age is best confirmed with registration papers if the horse has a breed registry. Many horses do not have breed registries, however, and their owners are relied upon for information on the horse's age. Examination of the teeth is a well-accepted method of aging horses but requires experience to be accurate. Teeth can be intentionally altered for deceptive purposes to make them appear younger, a practice known as *bishoping*.

Excellent references on aging the horse by dentition are available.*

It is common practice to place a stall card on each stall door for identification of the patient in the stall. The patient's signalment is usually recorded on the card; again, be sensitive to issues of confidentiality when displaying this information. The best way to identify a patient, however, is to place some form of ID directly *on* the patient; a patient ID tag can be made. (Small animal plastic ID collars are well-suited for this use.) Form the ID tag or band into a circle, and tape or braid it to the horse's mane, forelock, tail, or halter.

STALL/HOSPITAL MAINTENANCE AND CARE

In a clinical setting horses are housed primarily in stalls. Stalls should be cleaned daily to remove manure and wet spots (urine). There are two basic approaches to stall cleaning: (1) Remove only the soiled bedding and try to spare as much bedding as possible (picking) or (2) remove all bedding, soiled or not, down to the stall floor (stripping). Whether a stall is picked or stripped depends largely on the nature of the case and the habits of the horse. Some horses are very "neat," defecating and urinating in particular spots; these patients' stalls can be successfully picked for perhaps several days. At the other end of the spectrum are the "pigpens" of the horse world—there is no pattern to their defecations/urinations, and they may walk repeatedly through their eliminations, scattering feces and urine all over the stall. Picking will be difficult for these cases. Stalls of horses with diarrhea are also difficult to pick.

For cases that lend themselves to picking, the stall should be checked at least twice daily and picked as necessary. Wet urine spots

---

*American Association of Equine Practitioners: *Guide for determining the age of the horse,* Lexington, Ky, 2002, AAEP.

should be removed to the depth to which the urine has soaked. After removing the soiled bedding, replace as much bedding as was removed by picking. Horses that are active in their stalls may push bedding against the walls of the stall; be sure to spread this bedding back toward the center of the stall to create an even surface.

Stripping of bedding should occur at least every few days for any patient and more frequently if warranted by the nature of the case. After stripping the stall, the bedding must be completely replaced. This is obviously more expensive than picking and more time-consuming; therefore stripping should be done judiciously. Stripping should always be done after a patient is discharged, to allow for thorough stall cleaning and/or disinfection between patients.

When cleaning stalls, do not overlook the walls and ceiling. Cobwebs are common on stall ceilings and walls and should be removed regularly, as it reflects poorly on hospital cleanliness to have webs, dust, and other particulate matter on these surfaces.

Barn aisles shoud be swept at least once daily. Usually, two to three times daily is required to maintain cleanliness and neat appearance of the facility.

STALL FLOORING

There are two common types of stall floors: cement (concrete) and dirt/packed clay. Some older barns may have wood floors, but these are not often seen in a hospital setting. Each type of flooring has advantages and disadvantages.

Cement floors (and walls) are advantageous for hospital use because they can be disinfected and steam cleaned. Portable spray-type steam-cleaning machines can be taken from stall to stall to perform thorough cleansing of stalls between patients. This is especially valuable when the previous patient had a contagious disease. If steam cleaners are not used, disinfectants can be applied directly to the surface, scrubbed, and hosed. Dirt and wooden walls and floors are difficult to adequately disinfect with these procedures. The disadvantages of cement flooring are its expense to install; decreased patient comfort, especially for horses that lay down to sleep or are recumbent as a result of their disease; and sometimes compromised drainage. Proper contouring of the floor with a central drain is vital for drainage, and patient comfort can be improved with appropriately deep bedding for the case.

Rubber mats can be purchased and placed between the cement floor and the bedding layer. Some mats are solid rubber; others have a porous waffle-type construction to improve drainage. If solid mats are used, liquids cannot penetrate through the mats for drainage. Therefore moisture control must be provided by absorption into the bedding material. Obviously, absorbent bedding material should be used with solid mats. Rubber mats can greatly increase patient comfort, but they are expensive and difficult to maintain and thoroughly disinfect.

Dirt floors must be constructed properly to give acceptable drainage. Dirt floors have the obvious disadvantage of poor disinfection properties. If a contagious case is housed on a dirt floor, the stall may have to be isolated for days/weeks following dismissal of the contagious horse before another patient can be housed safely in the stall.

STALL BEDDING

Bedding material is placed on top of the stall floor to improve comfort and absorb urine and fecal liquids. The two most popular types of bedding material are wood shavings and grain (not pine) straw. Other types of bedding include sawdust, peat moss, and shredded paper. Each type of bedding has pros and cons.

Wood shavings are made from softwoods or hardwoods. Softwood shavings have good absorbency, often comparable to or better than straw. Shavings are generally less dusty than straw and are usually better tolerated by horses with respiratory allergies. Shavings may provide more of a cushion effect, which may benefit patients with sore feet or legs. However, wood shavings are more likely to get under bandages and casts and are more abrasive than straw. Wood bedding products are believed to harbor more gram-negative bacteria than straw, which may be an exposure concern for newborn foals. Therefore straw is preferred for foaling mares and young foals.

Sawdust is another wood product used for bedding. It can be unacceptably dusty, though, and the particles are small enough to be inhaled. Sawdust is poor bedding for foaling mares, young foals, and any horse with respiratory problems. Recumbent patients and foals may also be more prone to scratching their corneas on the particles when lying on their sides. (Young foals do not sleep standing as many adults do.)

Wood products, whether shavings or sawdust, must be free of black walnut (*Juglans nigra*) content. Black walnut causes acute laminitis (founder) in horses, though the exact route of toxin entry into the horse is not yet understood. When purchasing wood product bedding, ask the distributor to identify the types of wood in the product. Black walnut produces shavings and sawdust that are dark in color; however, other safe types of wood can produce similar dark colors. If dark shavings/sawdust particles are visible, avoid using the product unless the contents are known to be free of black walnut. Many distributors are not aware of black walnut's toxicity to horses.

Straw is usually oat or wheat straw. Oat straw is more absorbent than other straw types, though straw in general is not highly absorbent when compared with other types of bedding. Straw is naturally dusty, and dustiness will increase if the straw blades are chopped short. Straw is generally poor bedding for respiratory cases and gastrointestinal (GI) cases. Some horses will eat straw bedding; straw has little nutritional value for horses and may increase the likelihood of digestive problems if eaten in large quantities. It can be valuable to know if a horse has a tendency to eat its bedding or has a known sensitivity or allergy to certain types of bedding; this information should be obtained when the horse is admitted to the hospital, and the horse's bedding selected accordingly.

Peat moss is highly absorbent, and horses will not eat it. Peat moss is unlikely to harbor fungi and is not considered likely to contribute to respiratory conditions. Peat moss is cushiony when applied deeply and, combined with its absorbency, may be excellent bedding for recumbent ("downer") cases. Storage of peat moss should be in well-ventilated areas only.

Shredded paper products are highly absorbent bedding materials with little dust. Paper products are usually good products for respiratory allergies and other respiratory cases. Note, however, that newsprint can leave stains on the patient.

DAILY PATIENT CARE

All patient records should have a place to record food consumption, water consumption, bowel movement, and urination information. Even in the healthy horse, it is vital to monitor these parameters. When horses are moved to a clinic/hospital environment, they are typically stressed by the transportation and by being placed in an unfamiliar environment. The water and food sources are likely to be different from their home farm, and their intake may change and lead to GI problems. Equally important to the horse's "intake" is its "output"; defecations and urinations are important to note.

FEEDING PATIENTS

When the horse is admitted to the hospital, its at-home diet should be recorded. This information should include the type and amount of roughage (hay or grazing), concentrates (grains), and any supplements, as well as the normal feeding schedule. The at-home diet should be simulated as closely as possible in the hospital; radical changes in types and volumes of feed can cause GI problems.

Depending on the patient's disease, special feeding may be required. Sick horses are seldom fed concentrates because of increased concerns for developing GI problems. If it is difficult for the horse to chew or swallow, the food may need to be moistened or even made into a gruel. The clinician will prescribe any special diet for the patient.

Sometimes patients cannot be fed any food, and sometimes even water must be withheld for successful management of a particular disease. This is especially true with GI diseases. If these patients are depressed, they may not have an interest in food or water. However, some of these patients may have good appetites, and if food and/or water are withheld, they will eat or chew anything they can—bedding, wooden doors/walls, buckets, etc. Managing these horses may require placing a muzzle on them (Fig. 1-8). Muzzles are not always effective, since some horses can find inventive ways to eat around them, and some can get them off. If it is vital that the horse take nothing by mouth (NPO), it is better to remove all bedding and use rubber mats or inedible bedding such as peat moss.

Although it is a common procedure on horse farms, horses should not usually eat from the ground in a hospital setting. Manure and urine can contaminate the feed. Hay can be suspended in a hay net or placed in a hay rack; hay nets and slat-type hay racks should be higher than shoulder level to

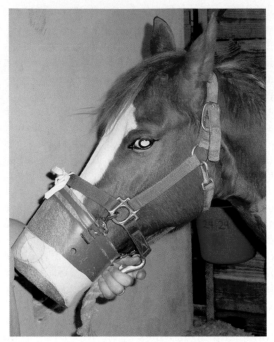

Fig. 1-8. Plastic bucket-style muzzle with clips to fasten to the halter. Note the addition of a string tie to the front of the halter nosepiece for extra security. Holes in the bottom of the muzzle allow access to water. (From French DD, Tully TN: Restraint and handling of animals. In McCurnin DM, Bassert JM: *Clinical textbook for veterinary technicians*, ed 6, St Louis, 2006, Saunders.)

prevent hooves from getting entangled in them if the horse paws with the front legs.

Horses should have access to supplemental salt and/or trace minerals. This may be provided in the form of loose salt or the more traditional block form (salt/mineral brick or "lick"). It is unnecessary to give each patient a full block; the blocks can be divided with a hammer or small saw for short-stay patients. Discard salt licks between patients as part of thorough stall cleaning.

Record the types and amount of feed offered to the horse, as well as what the horse actually eats. Some horses may eat their hay but refuse their grain or vice versa.

Some may eat fresh grass if it is available but refuse hay. Some may eat only a portion of what is put in the stall. What the horse eats *and* does not eat can be important information for the clinician.

WATERING PATIENTS

Water provision is a vital part of horse care. Fresh water provided daily is an absolute necessity. Horses have a large daily water consumption, averaging 5 to 10 gallons per day for maintenance of their baseline physiological functions.

Water can be provided in the stall with either manual or automatic methods. Manual watering involves filling a water container, usually a bucket, with a water hose. Automatic watering uses commercial automatic waterers; these devices generally consist of a stainless steel bowl that replaces the water lost from the bowl back to a consistent level. Automatic waterers are convenient for human caretakers but are not always helpful in a hospital setting. Most horses do not have these devices on their home farm and therefore do not know how to use them. The waterers make a noise when they refill, which repels many horses. Automatic systems are difficult to disassemble for thorough disinfection. Perhaps the biggest drawback in a hospital setting is the inability to accurately track a patient's water intake. There is no convenient way to monitor the amount of water entering the bowl under normal circumstances over a given period of time.

Manual watering is therefore preferable in the large animal hospital. Standard water buckets hold 5 gallons; therefore some horses may require two 5-gallon buckets in their stalls. Water containers should be checked more than once a day and filled as necessary. The amount of water consumed by a horse is important information and should be recorded at each "bucket check." Horses may not drink adequate amounts of water in the hospital setting because of stress, illness, or a different taste of the water from what they are accustomed to on their home farm. Water consumption is particularly important to monitor in GI patients.

Since opinions of what a "full bucket" means may vary, it is useful to standardize a full bucket by marking the fill level with tape or a nontoxic paint mark. This will provide consistency by having all caretakers fill the bucket to the same level. When estimating the amount of water consumed by the horse at each bucket check, do not assume that the amount of water missing from the bucket has actually been consumed by the horse. Some horses play with their water buckets (with their mouths or by pawing with the forelimbs), spilling large quantities of water on the floor. Sick horses may also place their noses in their buckets and splash their water without actually drinking. Therefore it is wise to check the stall floor in the area of the bucket to see if most of the water has been spilled or if it has, in fact, been consumed by the horse. Record the approximate amount of water consumed, and refill the bucket to the fill line.

Some horses benefit from electrolyte water solutions. Electrolyte water is generally made by adding a commercially prepared electrolyte powder to a standard volume of water. Potassium chloride can be made with 6 to 10 g Lite salt/L water. Many horses will drink electrolyte water during hot weather to replace losses through sweat evaporation, and some simply seem to enjoy the alternative to plain water. Horses with diarrhea may also selectively drink electrolyte and bicarbonate solutions; bicarbonate water is made by adding 10 g baking soda/L water. Electrolyte water should never be used as the sole water source. Instead, it should be provided as a supplement to plain, fresh water.

Water buckets should generally be placed at or above shoulder level so that the horse's legs will not get caught in them.

Rubber buckets are easy to disinfect and last longer than metal buckets, which have a tendency to get crushed and may rust. In cold weather, water sources may freeze and the ice must either be physically broken and removed or prevented with commercially available electric water warming coils.

STALL/STABLE VENTILATION

Ventilation must be adequate not only in the barn aisles but also in individual stalls. Barn aisles are usually easy to ventilate by opening barn doors, but stalls are usually difficult to ventilate unless they have windows. Poorly ventilated stalls may benefit from stall fans, which may be easily provided by inexpensive floor fans hung outside the stall and above ground level by ropes or duct tape. Key issues with ventilation are preventing drafts and keeping dust levels to a minimum. Also, ammonia vapor is generated by urine in the stall. Ammonia is a respiratory irritant and may exacerbate respiratory diseases, especially in foals. Proper ventilation and stall cleaning to remove wet spots will minimize ammonia vapor.

GROOMING

The importance of daily grooming should not be overlooked. Grooming is not only essential for patient cleanliness but provides an opportunity to find developing or previously undetected problems. Swellings, lacerations, discharges, skin infections, and changes in attitude can all be observed during grooming.

Grooming should consist of the standard steps of curry combing, brushing, and hoof cleaning. The curry comb is the first step of grooming (Fig. 1-9, *A* and *B*). The curry comb is used on the fleshy (muscular) parts of the body only (i.e., not on the lower legs or face). It is used in a circular motion, firmly, to loosen deep-seated dirt and bring it to the surface, where it can be brushed off the horse. Brushes come in many varieties of bristle

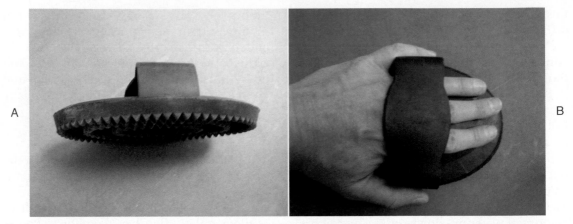

Fig. 1-9. Grooming using a curry comb. **A,** Curry comb. **B,** Holding the curry comb.

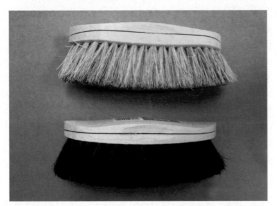

Fig. 1-10. Types of brushes. Stiff brush *(top)*, soft brush *(bottom)*.

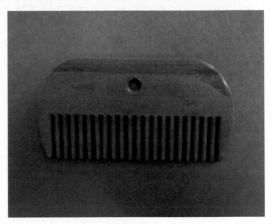

Fig. 1-11. Metal mane/tail comb.

stiffness and bristle materials (Fig. 1-10); in general, stiff bristles should be used only on fleshy parts of the body. Soft bristles may be used anywhere on the body, with special care on the face. Brushing should be done with short strokes, flicking the brush up and away from the coat at the end of the stroke. Flicking the brush kicks dirt particles off the horse, which is the purpose of brushing. Brushing is always done in the direction of the lay of the hair.

A towel may be used after brushing to remove any leftover surface debris. Moist towels can also be used to clean eye and nose discharges and the perineal region. The forelock, mane, and tail hairs are combed with a plastic or metal mane/tail comb (Fig. 1-11). Do not try to pass the comb through large amounts of hair at once—separate the hairs into small sections and comb each section individually.

Hoof cleaning is done with a hoof pick and brush. Several designs of picks and combs are available (Fig. 1-12). The hoof must be elevated to clean the bottom of the hoof; it is critical to clean this surface. The most common deficiency of hoof cleaning is failing to clean the recesses of the bottom of the hoof completely. The lateral sulci of the frog and the central sulcus of the frog are recesses of the hoof that should be thoroughly picked to help prevent bacterial and

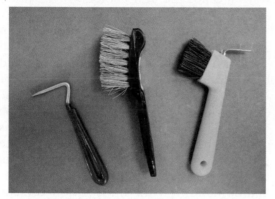

Fig. 1-12. Plain hoof pick, hoof brush, and combination hoof pick/brush.

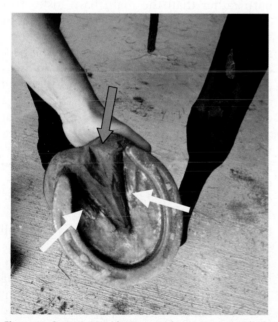

Fig. 1-13. Central sulcus *(green arrow)* and lateral sulci *(white arrows)* of the frog.

fungal infections (Fig. 1-13). Most people do not realize that the horse does not feel routine hoof picking unless trauma or infection has exposed sensitive tissue. Therefore the tendency is to pick so lightly that the cleaning is not effective. Unless sensitive tissue is exposed, use firm pressure on the hoof pick and brush.

Patient cleanliness may affect the patient's sense of well-being. Many horses are accustomed to grooming and enjoy it. Patient cleanliness also has a tremendous impression on the client. When clients visit their horse, and when they pick up their horse at the end of hospitalization, the patient should be "spotless." The veterinarian's and hospital's reputation rely on keeping patients and their surroundings clean.

SPECIAL CASES

Two types of cases require special considerations: contagious cases and recumbent ("downer") patients.

ISOLATION OF CONTAGIOUS CASES

Contagious equine diseases may affect a variety of body systems, but the majority of cases of concern in a hospital setting will affect the respiratory or GI tracts. Respiratory diseases are usually spread by direct contact with respiratory secretions; the secretions may be spread directly by coughing, sneezing, or nose-to-nose contact or indirectly by carrying secretions from infected horses to uninfected horses on clothing, equipment, hands, and so on. It has been estimated that coughing horses can propel respiratory droplets as far as 30 yards! One infected horse can rapidly spread its respiratory disease throughout a barn.

Infectious GI diseases are typically those that cause diarrhea. Horses with diarrhea can produce gallons of fecal water in a 24-hour period, and the excrement commonly contains an astounding number of infectious organisms. Like respiratory diseases, the GI infectious organisms may spread by direct or indirect contact. In most equine hospitals, diarrhea is so potentially contagious that any horse with loose or diarrheic stool is treated as contagious until proven otherwise.

Adding to the dilemma of contagious disease is the fact that horses may begin to shed the infectious organisms before they become overtly ill, and sometimes shedding may occur in the complete absence of clinical signs ("carrier" animals). This is especially true of *Salmonella* sp. GI infections.

The ramifications of an infectious disease outbreak in a hospital setting cannot be overemphasized. When otherwise healthy horses, hospitalized for routine procedures, become sick with a contagious disease while under the care of the hospital (or shortly after their discharge from the hospital), it can be a public relations disaster. *Salmonella* in particular is associated with a negative connotation among equine owners; this disease is difficult to eliminate from a barn, has many strains that are highly resistant to current antibiotic therapy, and has a well-known carrier state in horses. Owners are aware of these facts, and word will spread throughout a horse community if a hospital fails to successfully contain a case of *Salmonella*. Therefore it is best to overreact to a potentially contagious disease rather than underestimate the potential for spread of the disease to other horses in the hospital. Confirmed and potentially contagious cases should be isolated from the general hospital population.

Many hospitals have stalls that are reserved for use only by contagious cases. Larger facilities may even have barns dedicated to this purpose. In facilities where there is no dedicated isolation area, isolation can still be accomplished with a little improvisation. If there is no separate building available for isolation, the horse should ideally be placed in an area of the barn where there is minimal "traffic flow." This area will usually be a stall in an outer corner of the facility versus a centrally located stall. Isolation stalls should have flooring and walls that can be reliably disinfected; dirt floors and wooden walls are not the best choices for isolation areas.

Once a stall is identified as housing an isolation case, it should be clearly marked "isolation" and an isolation protocol should be instituted. When setting aside a stall for isolation, it is advisable *not* to post specific disease diagnostics where they can be viewed by the public; the patient's diagnosis or suspected diagnosis is privileged, private information and is potentially damaging to the hospital and the sick horse's owner and home farm if the information is made public.

The ideal isolation stall has an entrance that is open to the outside perimeter of the barn rather than the main barn aisle. This allows the horse to enter and exit without walking down the main aisle and also allows staff to clean the stall without carrying bedding and excrement through the main areas of the barn, where contamination could occur. Ideally an isolation stall also has a clearly defined "hot zone" around it; the hot zone is an area that no one should enter without permission or without proper personal protective gear. The hot zone can be defined with tape or paint on the barn floor or even hay bales stacked to restrict traffic around the stall. The stall can be further isolated by hanging sheets or blankets on all stall walls if the walls are not solid.

An isolation protocol should be established in every hospital, clearly identifying all aspects of handling a contagious or potentially contagious case. The protocol should identify criteria for what constitutes an isolation case, how the case will be isolated, and how the case will be handled after it is isolated. The isolation protocol should be specific and strictly enforced.

Because many diseases may be transferred indirectly on fomites, isolation cases should have stall cleaning implements and grooming tools dedicated to that single patient. These items should be kept in the "hot zone" and not travel to any area of the hospital where uninfected horses are housed or walked. Also, examination tools such as stethoscopes, thermometers, syringes, adhesive tape, and the like should either be dedicated to the isolation case or disinfected before being used on another patient. The cardinal rule is that *anything that enters the isolation hot zone does not leave the hot zone until it is disinfected.*

Many facilities find it helpful to put a treatment cart or shelving in the hot zone that contains the commonly used items for the case. This might include items such as grooming tools, syringes and needles, rectal sleeves, medications, thermometer, stethoscope, latex gloves, alcohol, Betadine solutions, and lead ropes. These items are disinfected or discarded after conclusion of the isolation case.

In addition to dedicated supplies for the patient, there must be established protocol for personal protective apparel for any staff handling the case. Some cases may be so potentially contagious that only certain staff will be designated each day to work with the case; a common example of this would be preventing staff who work with foals or immunocompromised patients from entering any isolation hot zones, because the threat of transmitting microbes to neonates is an unnecessary risk. Another consideration is that some infectious diseases are zoonotic, placing staff at risk for contracting the disease. Personal protection cannot be overemphasized.

Contagious microbes will be present on the stall floor. Therefore special attention

should be paid to footwear and preventing the spread of microbes through the hospital on shoes or boots. There are several approaches to footwear protection in the hot zone. Anyone entering the hot zone may remove his or her shoes and wear rubber boots (or slip them on over the shoes) upon entering the hot zone and then step in a disinfecting solution designed for dipping/scrubbing the boots upon entering *and* exiting the area ("foot bath"). Another approach is to provide disposable foot covers to pull over the shoes or boots. Disposable foot covers are made of plastic or surgical drape-type material and are readily available through medical supply companies.

Employees' hands should be protected with disposable examination gloves or rectal sleeves. If clothing needs to be protected, disposable or reusable surgical gowns can be placed in the hot zone for staff use. Some diseases may warrant donning protective caps and surgical masks. The isolation protocol should specifically identify the personal protective measures to be taken. Regardless of the protective clothing worn, hands should always be washed immediately after any contact with isolation equipment or patients; this is for protection of other patients *and* the technician. Hand washing between patients is good practice even when working with noncontagious animals in any hospital or clinic setting.

Patients should not leave the isolation area until discharged to go home or until the isolation conditions are resolved. Occasionally the patient's disease may require surgery, radiology, or other diagnostics that can only be provided in certain areas of the hospital. If the patient must be taken to these areas, walking through main barn aisles should be avoided. The patient should be brushed thoroughly to remove loose debris, and the feet picked out. Just outside the stall, the hooves should be scrubbed thoroughly with a dilute bleach solution (1:64) (2 oz bleach/1 gal water). After completing the diagnostic or surgical procedure, disinfect all equipment and floors contacted by the isolated animal.

Often overlooked when planning for an isolation case is the disposal of trash. Large garbage bags should be available in the hot zone, and a protocol established for disposal of the bag once it is full. Bags should be tied shut before transporting them out of the isolation area. The trash should always be treated as potentially contagious material.

Traffic in and out of the hot zone should be limited. These areas should be entered only when necessary; the patient's medical treatments should be combined as best as possible with feeding, watering, and stall cleaning schedules. Limit not only the number of people handling the case but also the number of times that they handle the case. Likewise, the patient should be restricted from entering areas where healthy patients are kept. If the horse will be handwalked for exercise, use the back stall door or put the horse in a corner stall where it does not have to travel down barn aisles.

Diarrhea cases should not be fed off the ground, because it risks continual reinfection of the patient (most diarrheal diseases are transmitted by the fecal-oral route). Hay nets, hay racks, and feed buckets suspended above ground level are alternatives. Attention should also be paid to limiting contamination of the patient and stall by frequent cleaning, which will usually be necessary more than once a day. The patient's hindquarters should also be kept clean to minimize contamination and prevent scalding of the perineal area from diarrhea. Because horses with diarrhea can drench their tails with fecal water, thorough cleaning of soiled tails is important. However, tail bathing is time consuming and places staff at risk for personal contamination. A better approach is to prevent tail soiling by placing a tail bag on the patient. As soon as diarrhea is observed, the tail is washed with warm water and mild detergent. A tail bag is easily constructed from a rectal sleeve (see Chapter 6) to keep the tail free of diarrheic stool and should be changed every 24 to 48 hours.

Diarrhea will scald the skin of the perineum and hindlimbs. These areas should be cleaned as necessary with warm water and mild soap. Vigorous scrubbing should be avoided. Desitin ointment is helpful in preventing and treating skin scald in these areas, especially on foals.

After conclusion of a contagious case (dismissal or euthanasia), disinfection of all equipment, the stall, and hot zone must be done. Laundry (e.g., towels, blankets, gowns) should be shaken free of bedding while still in the stall and placed in a plastic bag that is tied or taped shut before being taken to the laundry room. Hot zone laundry should be washed separately with detergent and 1 cup of bleach. All other porous materials such as tape rolls, unopened syringes, needles, examination gloves, cotton swabs, and gauze should be discarded; there is no effective way to clean and disinfect these items. Thermometers should be stripped of any string or tape and wiped down with dilute bleach mixture (1 cup bleach/5 gal water). Items that will be reused, such as stomach tubes/pumps and stethoscopes, should be cleaned initially inside the hot zone, have dilute bleach mixture applied, and then sealed in plastic bags for transport to other areas of the hospital where they may be further disinfected or sterilized in gas or steam autoclaves.

Ideally the stall should be steam-cleaned, if the equipment is available. Otherwise, the stall can be scrubbed with an appropriate disinfectant; dilute household bleach is suitable for most contagious cases—2½ cups bleach/5 gal water. Apply the dilute bleach and allow it to air dry; do not rinse it. The stall ceiling, walls, doors, and floor should be cleaned; do not forget the outside surfaces of the stall walls and doors. Stall-cleaning implements, grooming tools, buckets, treatment cart, etc. should be soaked in the bleach mixture for at least 10 minutes and allowed to air dry; these items do not leave the hot zone until disinfection procedures are completed. Some facilities go through the entire disinfection procedure twice and may even culture the stall and implements before removing their hot zone status. Dilute bleach may not be appropriate for certain diseases; appropriate disinfectants for specific diseases can usually be identified by consulting reference texts or appropriate disease experts.

RECUMBENT CASES

Recumbent cases refers to horses that preferentially spend most of their time lying on the ground or are physically unable to stand because of their disease. The typical diseases responsible for recumbency usually produce severe musculoskeletal pain, profound weakness, or neurological dysfunction. Recumbent large animals present significant and sometimes unique problems; many of the same problems are seen in recumbent small animals, but the size of large animals increases the risk of problems and increases the difficulty in preventing and treating the complications when they occur.

Another factor to keep in mind when working with recumbent large animals is that the nature of the animal is to stand. Domestic large animals are species of prey, and survival instinct drives them to try to stand on their own legs. This instinct may lead to violent and persistent attempts to stand, although they may not succeed. These animals may do great damage to themselves and their surroundings during their struggle to stand, and personnel working with the case must be alert and cautious when working around them.

Recumbent cases require intensive care, typically round-the-clock devotion to the patient. When deciding whether to pursue care for the recumbent case, the facilities and staff available must be considered and realistically evaluated. The owner must be informed about the time requirements, labor requirements, and the costs related to providing round-the-clock care.

When managing a recumbent animal, the following complications must be anticipated and measures instituted to attempt to prevent them. Also realize that, despite making every attempt to prevent complications, complications may still occur even in well-managed cases. There are simply too many variables involved to make any preventive measure 100% effective.

Problems associated with recumbency include decubital ulcers, compartment syndrome, eye trauma, limb trauma, respiratory disease, bladder dysfunction, and GI dysfunction.

Decubital ulcers are commonly known as pressure sores (Fig. 1-14). When animals lay in

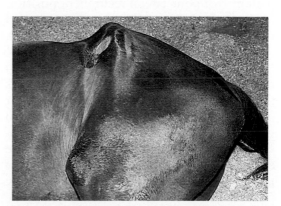

Fig. 1-14. Decubital ulceration (pressure sores) of the skin in a recumbent patient. (From Moore RM: Equine medical and surgical nursing. In McCurnin DM, Bassert JM: *Clinical textbook for veterinary technicians,* ed 5, St Louis, 2002, Saunders.)

one position for extended periods of time, circulation is compromised. Compromise to both arterial and venous blood supply may occur if the body weight of the animal exceeds the pressure inside these vessels. If the pressure outside the vessel (body weight) exceeds the pressure inside these vessels (blood pressure), collapse of the vessel will occur. Areas particularly prone to developing decubital ulcers are those with bony prominences; these areas lack fleshy muscle and skin, which cushion other areas and help prevent this complication. The areas most prone to developing decubital ulcers are therefore the tuber coxae (point of the hip), lateral prominences of the shoulder and hock, and the orbital/zygomatic arch area of the head.

Prevention of decubital ulcers is attempted through proper bedding and patient repositioning. Bedding for recumbent cases should be deep, yet not rigid enough to compromise the blood circulation. Deep layers of straw or shavings, thick foam pads, waterbed mattresses, and peat moss can all provide resilient bedding that applies fairly even pressure against the patient's body.

Repositioning typically means rolling the patient from one lateral recumbent position to the opposite recumbency (i.e., left lateral to right lateral recumbency, and vice versa). Rolling is ideally performed every 2 hours. Rolling large animals usually requires two to three people and may be dangerous unless the patient is completely paralyzed or unconscious. Patients with some ability to move their limbs may resist rolling by violent limb movements; personnel must use extreme care during the rolling procedure to prevent injury to themselves and the patient. Occasionally, in order to make the procedure safe for staff and patient, heavy sedation or anesthesia may be necessary.

Repositioning is best accomplished using a three-point system. Ropes are placed around the forelimb pasterns, the hindlimb pasterns, and the head/halter or neck. The ropes should be placed carefully, especially around the pasterns; a slip knot can be placed in the rope, which can be swung over the hoof and pastern from a safe distance. The person placing the rope should stand out of reach of the leg's range of motion to avoid being struck by the leg or hoof if the horse struggles. Once in place, a staff member should walk the rope around the horse's body and assume a position on the dorsal side of the patient. When the limb ropes have been secured, the head/neck rope can be secured. The head/neck rope should be long enough to avoid striking distance of the front hooves; grasping the halter with the hands is not advisable as a substitute for a head rope unless the horse is completely immobile. All personnel should be out of striking range of the legs (unless the horse is completely immobile) before the actual rolling procedure begins. All of the ropes are then drawn taut and, on verbal cue, the horse is rolled over into the opposite recumbency. Bedding and padding should then be rearranged as necessary to cushion the animal in its new position.

Compartment syndrome is not uncommon in recumbent large animals, regardless of the cause of recumbency. Recumbent animals of all species are susceptible to compartment syndrome, but the heavy bodyweight of large animals exacerbates the problem. Muscle compartments refer to the fact that some muscles in the body are encased in a dense connective tissue called fascia, which has little elasticity. Compartment syndrome is caused by the collapse of vessels inside a muscle compartment, due to the heavy body weight of the animal pressing down on the compartment's blood and lymphatic vessels. Collapse of vessels eventually compromises nutrition and waste elimination for the muscle and nerve cells inside the compartment, resulting in various degrees of muscle and nerve dysfunction. In recumbent animals, rolling and proper bedding are the primary methods of attempted prevention. Compartment syndrome is a significant problem in anesthetized animals and is discussed in more detail in Chapter 8.

Eye trauma is a consideration in recumbent large animals due to the position of their eyes. The eyes are wide set in large animals; this is typical anatomy in animals that are preyed upon. Wide-set eyes allow a larger, wider field of vision that may let the animal see predators more readily. However, when the eyes are located laterally on the head, they are exposed to trauma more so than eyes placed in a more median position. When animals with lateral or bits lay in lateral recumbency, the head basically rests on the orbit and eye. The eye will therefore be resting on the bedding material and susceptible to trauma unless protective measures are applied. The most common eye trauma is corneal ulceration from abrasions from the bedding. Corneal ulcers are recognized by the classic signs of tearing and blepharospasm (squinting) and are confirmed by fluorescein staining of the cornea. (See Chapter 11.) Prevention is attempted through use of nonabrasive materials in the head area such as smooth pads or cloth to cover abrasive surfaces and possibly protective headgear such as eye cups or helmets. Also, a small inflated 12-inch tire inner tube can be placed underneath the eye area to lift it off the ground surface.

Leg trauma may occur if the recumbent animal is not completely paralyzed and is capable of leg motion. These animals may try repeatedly and unsuccessfully to rise, since their natural instinct is to try to stand. These unsuccessful attempts can lead to significant musculoskeletal trauma, especially from thrashing of the legs. Recumbent animals should have leg protection provided by leg bandages, and bandages should generally be applied to all four limbs. If possible, horseshoes should be removed from recumbent horses to minimize trauma if the horse strikes itself (or personnel) with its hooves.

Recumbent patients are at increased risk for developing respiratory problems. The risk often relates to the patient's primary disease and is probably increased by gravity-induced congestion of the "down" (lower) lung. Regular rolling of the patient is helpful in reducing the risk of pleuritis and pneumonia associated with recumbency.

Bladder and rectum evacuation may be issues in recumbent patients, especially in neurological cases where the bladder and rectum may not be capable of normal emptying. Abnormal emptying usually relates to the muscular sphincters that control emptying of the bladder and/or rectum and falls into one of two categories: (1) sphincters that are too tight and therefore prevent normal emptying and (2) sphincters that are too relaxed and cannot retain the contents of the storage organs. Even if neurological and sphincter function is normal, recognize that some animals will not void while lying down; they may only void if assisted to stand or elevated in a body sling to a standing position.

In order to aid fecal voiding, the diet (if the patient can eat) should be highly digestible and as moist as possible. Warm mashes and fresh grass are good choices for most patients. Fecal output should be monitored, and, if insufficient, regular rectal evacuation (at least twice daily) will be required using a gloved hand and liberal lubrication. If the anal sphincter is lax or if the patient has diarrhea, fecal material will flow freely from the anus. Fecal water and urine can cause skin scald, which is irritation and inflammation of the skin. Recumbent patients should have the perineal area cleaned often and may benefit from application of ointments such as Desitin to the perineum and inner thigh regions. Bedding in the hindquarter area should be checked often and changed as necessary.

Bladder management of recumbent patients is critical to prevent pressure damage to the urinary tract and urinary tract infections. Unlike small animals, manual expression of the bladder is not possible externally and may only occasionally be accomplished internally through rectal palpation. However, bladder expression via the rectum risks perforating the rectal wall—generally avoid it except in select cases.

When the bladder sphincter cannot contract fully, urine may dribble out of the bladder, sometimes almost continuously. Although the obvious external problems in this situation will be urine scald and wet bedding, remember that internally the bladder is distended with stagnant urine and is susceptible to infection (bacterial cystitis). When the bladder sphincter cannot relax, urine accumulates and distends the bladder, leading to multiple problems including rupture of the bladder or ureters from the high internal pressures. In these cases the clinician must provide an exit for the urine, and in large animals this means bladder catheterization. Catheters may be either indwelling (Foley) or intermittently inserted (mare or stallion urinary catheter) several times a day. Catheterization of any type greatly increases the risk of bladder infection, and catheterized animals often receive prophylactic antibiotics while being treated. Great attention to sterile technique should be followed during bladder catheterization. (See Chapter 5.)

Some cases may be capable of standing with the assistance of ropes or slings. Slings are only useful for patients who have some limb control; they are intended to assist, not substitute for, the ability to stand. When completely immobile patients are placed in a sling, they will simply slump and have difficulty breathing; they may even slide out of some slings. Assisted standing should be performed as often as is reasonable, given the patient's disease and staff/equipment available. Many patients will eat, defecate, and urinate only when standing. Cleaning/grooming, physical examination, and some treatments are easier to perform when the patient is standing.

If the patient is capable of oral intake, food and/or fresh water may be offered. The patient's disease will dictate whether this is possible or even advisable. When oral intake is offered, the patient should be in sternal recumbency to minimize the risk of aspiration of material into the lungs. Hay bales or supporting pads may be used to hold the patient in sternal recumbency, since many recumbent cases cannot hold themselves in this position. If food or water is to be given via nasogastric tube, keep the horse in sternal recumbency if possible for the intubation procedure.

DISINFECTION AFTER PATIENT DISMISSAL

Following a patient's release, either due to successful treatment or perhaps loss of the patient through death, the patient's stall, grooming tools, and medical equipment/supplies should be cleaned and disinfected before being used on another patient. The stall should be stripped of food and bedding, and the stall walls, ceiling, and floor cleaned thoroughly. The level of disinfection depends on whether the case had a contagious disease and the nature of the contagious disease, if present. In most cases dilute bleach (1 cup household bleach/5 gal water) is an economical and effective disinfectant. Some disease organisms may require stronger bleach solutions (1 part bleach to 10 parts water), or special commercially prepared disinfectants such as quaternary ammonium compounds, phenolic compounds, or iodophors. Isopropyl alcohol may be adequate for some pieces of medical equipment such as stethoscopes when the patient had no known contagious condition.

Before applying any disinfectant, all organic matter (e.g., blood, discharges, excrement, bedding) should be removed. Quaternary ammoniums and bleach are inactivated by organic matter. Phenols and iodophors are considered to have some activity in the presence of organic matter, but activity will become less reliable with increasing amounts of debris. Organic matter can be removed by scrubbing with brushes and brooms or by using a portable steam cleaner if available. Brushes, mops, and brooms can be used to apply the disinfectant solution to the stall surfaces. Dilute bleach can be allowed to air dry on the treated surfaces.

Stall-cleaning tools and grooming tools should ideally be disinfected after use on any patient, although this can sometimes be omitted if the case was not contagious. Avoid transporting these items through uncontaminated areas of the hospital until they have been disinfected.

Water/feed buckets and pans should always be cleaned and disinfected between patients, regardless of case history. Buckets and pans should be scrubbed with brushes and soaked for at least 10 minutes in diluted bleach. Buckets should be rinsed thoroughly with water before using them on the next patient. Hay nets can be disinfected by soaking them in dilute bleach.

Well-managed hospitals have an established protocol for disinfection that covers both noninfectious and infectious case situations. When in doubt about the case's diagnosis, it is best to assume contagion and disinfect accordingly. Some facilities will perform microbial cultures on the stall after disinfection procedures and will not let another case into the stall until culture results are negative for infectious organisms.

SUGGESTED READING

McCurnin DM, Bassert JM: *Clinical textbook for veterinary technicians*, ed 5, St Louis, 2002, Saunders.

Sirois M: *Principles and practice of veterinary technology*, ed 2, St Louis, 2004, Mosby.

Speirs VC: *Clinical examination of horses*, St Louis, 1997, Saunders.

2

History and Basic Physical Examination of Horses

When a patient is presented for evaluation, a database that will become part of the medical record is generated. The minimum database for any patient includes the history and physical examination. This database may be expanded to include laboratory tests, diagnostic imaging, special examinations of body systems, etc.

The history and physical examination are the most important part of the database and serve as the starting point for identifying the patient's problems. "Problems" are any conditions that require medical or surgical treatment *or* that compromise the quality of life. Most clinicians use a problem-oriented approach to diagnosis and treatment; this provides a logical method to work through the simplest to the most complicated medical and surgical cases. A thorough history and a complete physical examination are essential for successful problem solving.

HISTORY

There are several approaches available for taking a patient's history. If owners are allowed to give the history without any guidance, they typically provide a rambling discourse that leaves out essential information, fails to follow a timeline, and includes unnecessary information. Some experienced horsemen provide an excellent history with little coaching, but most owners do not know how to give a concise, useful summary of their horse's condition. Approaches to history-taking range from letting an owner talk without any guidance to the "inquisition" approach where the history-taker asks specific questions. Some clients may need these extremes, but most respond best to the middle-of-the-road approach of "coaching." In the coaching approach, the person taking the history lets the owner tell his or her story but asks specific questions along the way to guide the owner and ensure details are not missed. Most owners do not know what is significant information and what is not, so the history-taker must attempt to get the relevant information and prevent the owner from going off on a useless tangent. Owners also seldom appreciate the value of a timeline and tend to wander through the time sequence; the questioner must try to keep the information in a sequential format.

Once the history is obtained, it must be evaluated for accuracy. Some information may be difficult to evaluate, and some may be misleading. Some owners give false information to spare embarrassment; they do not want to appear ignorant or admit they may have made a mistake.

History-taking should be tailored according to the patient's problems. For example, if a contagious disease is suspected, the patient's vaccination history, possible exposure to other infected animals, and health management practices of the farm should be investigated.

Another consideration is that many owners treat their animals before calling the veterinarian. This is fairly common in large animal practice, especially with production animals; economics often dictate whether the owner calls the veterinarian immediately or attempts to solve the problem independently. Owners may be reluctant to admit this information and may need to be asked specifically whether they have treated the animal and what they may have attempted for treatment.

PHYSICAL EXAMINATION

There are several types of physical examinations for equines. The *insurance examination* is required by the insurance company before a horse can receive insurance coverage. It may range from a basic examination to a thorough, in-depth examination; the type of insurance and the animal's value dictate the depth of examination required by the insurance company. The *prepurchase examination,* conducted before completing the sale of an animal, is a common procedure in equine practice. A seller and a buyer are identified, and the veterinarian performing the examination is presumed to be working in the buyer's best interest (the veterinarian is paid by the buyer). Like the insurance examination, the prepurchase examination is dictated by the intended use of the horse and its estimated value; it may be a simple physical examination or an in-depth examination including biopsies, blood samples, endoscopy, electrocardiogram/echocardiogram, and diagnostic imaging. Prepurchase examinations are often a source of lawsuits against the veterinarian, usually because of a misunderstanding of the purpose of the examination. Owners often believe that the examination is a guarantee for the future of the horse, yet the veterinarian has no crystal ball. Most veterinarians are keenly aware of this fact and go to great lengths to document the findings of prepurchase examinations

and not overstate their findings as predictions of future performance. The technician should understand the potentially sensitive nature of the insurance and prepurchase examination and help ensure accuracy and privacy of the results.

BASIC PHYSICAL EXAMINATION

The basic physical examination typically includes temperature/pulse/respiration (TPR), heart/lung auscultation, abdominal auscultation, hydration status, examination of mucous membranes, and height/weight measurement. More in-depth evaluations are covered under specific body systems.

After completing a physical examination of a patient, the technician may be in doubt as to whether certain findings are significant or concerning enough to warrant alerting the clinician in charge of the case. It is helpful to establish "when to call" guidelines as part of the patient's treatment orders. The clinician should establish ranges for examination parameters that need urgent attention, such as "if temperature >102.5°, call Dr." or "if heart rate >60 bpm, call Dr."

Body Temperature

Temperature is almost always taken rectally, using a standard mercury thermometer or a digital thermometer. Rarely, vaginal temperature may be used.

Although any thermometer may be used on large animals, special large animal thermometers are commonly available. Large animal thermometers are typically 5 inches long and have a thicker glass casing than regular thermometers (Fig. 2-1, *A*). In addition, they often include a ring top, which allows the user to attach a string (Fig. 2-1, *B*). Strings are helpful for two reasons: (1) aspiration of the thermometer into the rectum and (2) pushing the thermometer out of the rectum. Some horses pull the anus inward when the thermometer is in place; occasionally this

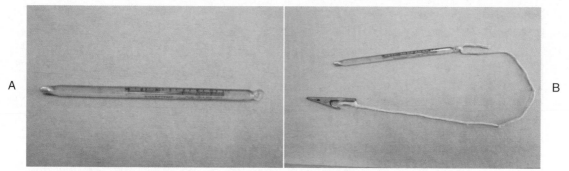

Fig. 2-1. **A**, Regular large animal thermometer. **B**, Ring-top thermometer with string and clip attached.

results in aspiration of the thermometer into the rectum. This is potentially serious if the thermometer breaks inside the rectum or if the horse strains to defecate; perforation of the rectum may occur and can be life threatening. The presence of the thermometer in the anus may also stimulate defecation; if this occurs, the thermometer passes out of the rectum and falls to the ground, often breaking. Broken thermometer glass can puncture hooves or skin or may be eaten as the horse browses for food. Because of these complications, it is common either to maintain a firm grip on the thermometer for the entire procedure or tie a string to the ring top and secure the string to the horse's tail hairs or hair coat (never the skin!) with a clothespin or alligator clamp. If the horse aspirates the thermometer, the string can be used to gently retrieve it or to follow the string manually into the rectum to retrieve it. If the horse pushes the thermometer out of the rectum, the secured string should prevent it from falling on the ground. Do not attach a piece of string longer than 12 inches; longer strings allow the thermometer to dangle on the legs, which causes some horses to kick.

Placing the rectal thermometer requires some tact. The thermometer should be lubricated with petroleum jelly, mineral oil,

water, or the time-honored method of spitting a small amount of saliva on the tip. Avoid dipping the thermometer in the horse's water bucket; this practice gives the impression of disregard for sanitary procedure. Even if the thermometer has been properly disinfected, owners view it as a piece of equipment that has been in other horses' rectums and has no place in their horse's water bucket.

To insert the thermometer, stand next to the horse's hindquarters, facing caudally (Fig. 2-2, *A*). Do not stand directly behind the horse. If the horse resists by kicking, the technician can stand behind a stall door or a stack of hay bales for protection. Grasp the tail near the base and elevate it or push it to the opposite side of the horse; it is not necessary to "crank" the tail to an extreme position—this only meets with resistance by the horse. Move the tail only enough to get clear entrance to the anus (Fig. 2-2, *B*). Some horses respond best to gently rubbing the perianal area before touching the anus with the thermometer; it is often good practice to let the horse know what is coming, rather than jamming the thermometer in the anus with no warning. The anal opening is identified either visually or by feel, and the thermometer gently inserted with a twisting motion (Fig. 2-2, *C*). If the

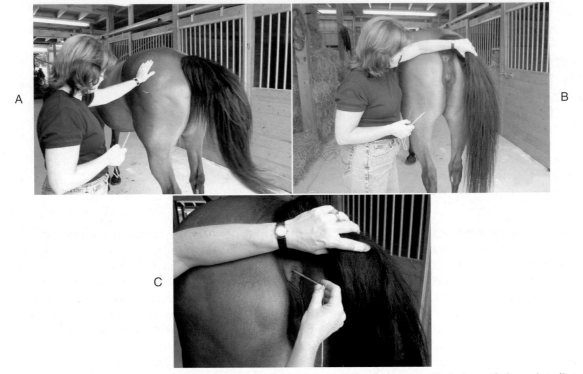

Fig. 2-2. **A,** When inserting rectal thermometer, stand facing caudally and maintain contact with the horse. **B,** Grasp the tail at the base and move it gently to the side. **C,** Insert the thermometer.

thermometer does not easily advance, *never* force it; the rectal wall may be perforated with very little force. If the horse strains in resistance, try distracting it by offering feed or having someone tap on the horse's forehead. The thermometer usually passes horizontally, but some horses require tipping the thermometer slightly upward (dorsally).

The thermometer should be advanced several inches into the rectum, then either handheld or clipped to the tail hairs (Fig. 2-3, *A*) or coat hairs (Fig 2-3, *B*). It should be left in place for at least 60 seconds (mercury type) or until the audible/visual signal is heard or seen (digital type).

Normal temperature varies by age, breed, and environment of the animal. Body temperature is typically lowest in the morning. Normal rectal temperature of the adult horse at rest is 99° F to 101.5° F. From 101.5° F to 102° F is the "gray zone"; this may be normal for some individuals, especially in hot weather. Above 102°F is always suspicious, except following physical exercise, which can easily temporarily elevate temperature to this level and above.

Other circumstances may influence temperature. Large breeds and draft horses tend to have low rectal temperatures. Neonatal foals may lack some ability to generate body heat and often have low body

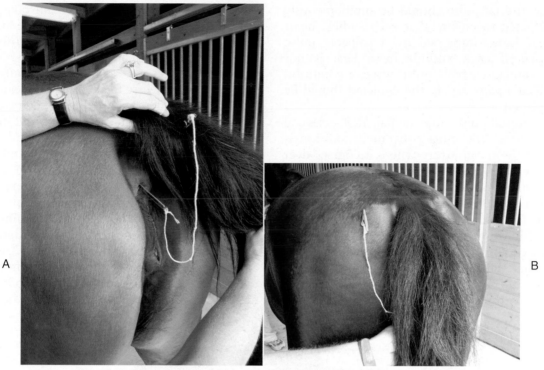

Fig. 2-3. A, The thermometer has been inserted and secured with the clip to the tail hairs. **B,** Thermometer secured to hair coat with the clip.

temperatures immediately after birth. Older foals may average approximately 1° F higher than adults for the first few days to weeks after birth.

Rectal procedures such as rectal examination may allow air to enter the rectum, leading to a balloon effect in which the rectum fills with air. This will falsely lower rectal temperature. Therefore temperature should be taken before any rectal procedure.

If the rectum contains feces, the thermometer tip may occasionally be inadvertently inserted into a fecal ball. This is the most common cause of unexpectedly low readings. If this occurs, the procedure should be repeated.

Pulse Rate/Heart Rate

The pulse rate is taken by palpation of arteries. Veins do not have palpable pulses because of the low blood pressures inside veins.

Strictly speaking, heart rate and pulse rate are not the same; heart rate refers to the number of heart beats/minute (bpm); pulse rate refers to the number of palpable arterial pulse waves/minute. In normal animals, heart rate and pulse rate are equal.

Auscultation of the heart is used properly for taking heart rate, not pulse rate. This is because some heart abnormalities may produce audible heart sounds that are not necessarily accompanied by an arterial pulse. For accuracy, if the heart is auscultated, the arterial pulse should be simultaneously palpated to ensure that each audible heart beat is accompanied by a palpable pulse wave. If each audible heart beat is not accompanied by a pulse wave, a condition called a *pulse deficit,* the clinician should be notified.

Arterial pulses may be palpated at several locations. The most convenient location is over the facial artery where it courses over the ventral aspect of the mandible, rostral to the origin of the masseter muscle (Fig. 2-4, *A*). Two or more fingers are lightly rolled back and forth across the mandible to identify the facial artery/facial vein bundle (Fig. 2-4, *B*). Once identified, the bundle is firmly pressed against the mandible to feel the arterial pulse (Fig. 2-4, *C*). If the bundle is pressed too tightly, the artery may be occluded and the

pulse not easily felt. A common mistake is not being patient when palpating large animal pulses; the heart rates are much lower than their small animal counterparts.

Other arteries are available for pulse-taking. The transverse facial artery is located in a horizontal depression about 1 inch caudal to the lateral canthus of the eye and just below the zygomatic arch (Fig. 2-5, *A* and *B*). The coccygeal artery supplies the tail and is located along the ventral midline of the tail (Fig. 2-5, *C*). The dorsal metatarsal artery is located between metatarsals 3 and 4 (cannon bone and lateral splint bone) on the hindlimbs (Fig. 2-5, *D*). The lateral and medial digital arteries can also be palpated where they course over the abaxial aspect of the proximal sesamoid bones of each leg, or just proximal to the collateral cartilages of each hoof

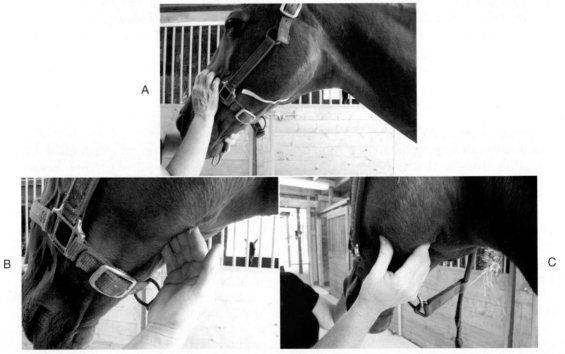

Fig. 2-4. Palpating arterial pulses. **A**, Location of the facial artery. **B**, Identify the facial artery along the medial aspect of the mandible. **C**, Press the vascular bundle against the medial aspect of the mandible.

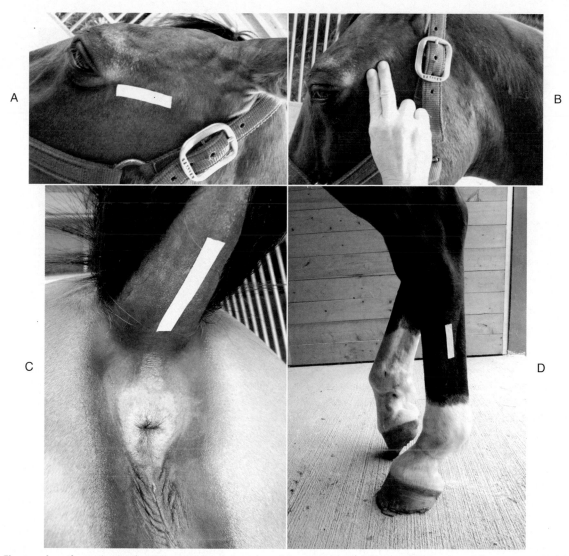

Fig. 2-5. Locating and palpating other arteries. **A,** Location of the transverse facial artery. **B,** Palpation of the transverse facial artery. **C,** Location of the coccygeal artery. **D,** Location of the dorsal metatarsal artery.

Continued.

(Fig. 2-5, *E, F,* and *G*). The carotid artery, like all arteries, has a pulse wave but is difficult to accurately palpate in large animals because of its deep position and is seldom useful for palpation.

The features of the pulse to be noted are rate and rhythm. The rate is recorded as number/minute. The pulse rate is normally 28 to 44 bpm in adult horses at rest. Immediately after birth, foals have a rate of 60 to 80 bpm. This climbs to 75 to 100 for the first week or two of life. This rate gradually declines toward the adult rate over the next several weeks to months. Athletically fit horses may normally have rates less than 28 bpm; 24 bpm is not uncommon in fit racehorses.

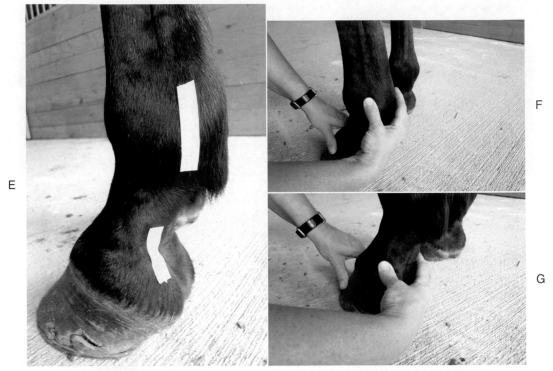

Fig. 2-5. cont'd E, Location of the lateral digital artery over the lateral proximal sesamoid bone and proximal to the lateral collateral cartilage. **F,** Palpation of the digital arteries over the proximal sesamoid bones. **G,** Palpation of the digital arteries proximal to the collateral cartilages.

Pulse rhythm is recorded as regular or irregular. Irregular rhythm likely indicates an arrhythmia of the heart. The most common irregularity of the pulse in horses is caused by a heart arrhythmia called second-degree atrioventricular (A-V) block. This arrhythmia is caused by failure of the electrical current generated by the atria to reach the ventricles; there is an intermittent "blockage" of current at the A-V node, which normally acts as an electrical gate between the atria and ventricles. This "blockage" results in dropped beats but usually in *a regular pattern.* Typically, the dropped beat occurs every third or fourth heartbeat and is readily identified by palpating the pulse. The regular rhythm is interrupted by a single "lost" (dropped) beat, with the "lost" beats occurring at regular intervals (beat-beat-beat-silence-beat-beat-beat-silence, etc.). Even though second-degree A-V block is usually a normal finding in horses, it should be noted in the medical record. Horses with this arrhythmia may have very low resting heart rates, less than 28 bpm. This arrhythmia is more common in fit horses and should disappear in any horse when the horse is exercised. It is believed to be caused by increased tone from the vagal nerve, part of the parasympathetic nervous system.

Pulse quality is often described as strong, bounding, weak, thready, or other nonspecific terms. Pulse quality is subjective; its usefulness depends on the experience of the person assessing the pulse and should not be overinterpreted.

Respiratory Rate

The number of respirations/minute can be counted several ways: (1) using a stethoscope to listen to air movement in the trachea or chest; (2) using a hand to feel movement of air in and out of a nostril; and (3) most commonly, simply counting chest excursions (rise and fall of the thoracic wall)/minute.

Respirations should be characterized by their effort and depth. Respiration may be described as shallow, deep, labored, gasping, and other nonspecific terms. Horses normally use a combination of thoracic and abdominal muscles to breathe; this is called costoabdominal breathing. Some painful conditions of the chest may lead to increased use of the abdominal muscles to breathe, referred to as an *increased abdominal component to the respiratory pattern.*

Normal horses cannot breathe through the mouth. If mouth-breathing is observed, it should be noted and brought to the attention of the clinician.

Respiratory noises are not uncommon in horses and may be significant. Noises may be characterized as wheezing, whistling, honking, snoring, fluttering, etc. Noises may be heard only at rest or perhaps only during exercise. It is important to note the horse's activity at the time the noise is heard. Equally important is to note whether the noise occurs during inspiration, expiration, or both.

The normal respiratory rate of an adult horse at rest is 6 to 12 breaths/minute. The rate is higher during hot weather or following physical activity. Foals have a high respiratory rate at birth due to the residual fluid in the lower airways. Newborn foals may have a respiratory rate from 80 to 90; this slows to 60 to 80 in the first 5 to 10 minutes after birth and gradually decreases to 20 to 40 for the first week or two of life.

Heart Auscultation

Horses are athletes; the heart of the average horse may be as large as a basketball. Auscultation may be done on the left or right side of the chest, though most of the heart valves and sounds are heard best from the left side. However, the right side should not be overlooked; some murmurs are audible only on the right side and will be missed if the horse is ausculted only from the left. Auscultation should be done in a quiet environment, perhaps requiring that the horse be taken to another area of the barn or hospital for ideal evaluation.

The landmarks for basic auscultation of the heart are the same on either side of the chest. The landmarks for dorsoventral position of the heart are the level of the shoulder joint for the heart base and the point of the elbow (olecranon) for the heart apex (Fig. 2-6). The craniocaudal position is defined by the caudal border of the triceps muscle, which roughly divides the heart into cranial and caudal halves. Using these landmarks, the position of the heart can be estimated.

Usually, the heart is best heard cranially to the caudal border of the triceps muscle. However, the triceps muscle is too thick to allow the heart sounds to be heard through it.

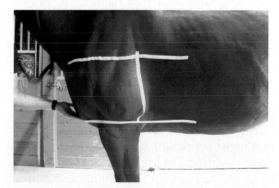

Fig. 2-6. Landmarks for the heart. The horizontal marks indicate the level of the shoulder and elbow joints. The vertical mark indicates the caudal border of the triceps muscle.

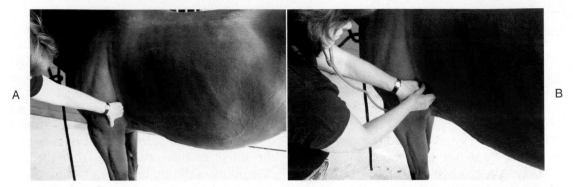

Fig. 2-7. Auscultating the heart. **A,** Gently lift the triceps muscle away from the chest wall. **B,** Place stethoscope against the chest wall, deep to the triceps muscle.

Therefore it is essential to place the head of the stethoscope directly against the chest wall but stay deep to the triceps muscle. This is easily accomplished by gently using a hand to lift the muscle slightly away from the chest wall before the stethoscope is positioned (Fig. 2-7, *A* and *B*). Another approach is to move the forelimb to a more forward position, as if the horse were taking a step forward, which moves the triceps cranially. However, many horses are reluctant to hold this position for any length of time.

The heart rate is counted as beats per minute. The cardiac sounds S_1 (lub) and S_2 (dub) are components of one heart beat. A common error, especially for those accustomed to small animal auscultation, is to count S_1 and S_2 as separate beats, essentially doubling the actual heart rate. The heart rate in large animals is slow, and the heart sounds are usually loud and distinct, leading to the possible confusion.

Auscultation is also used to detect abnormal heart sounds or murmurs. Murmurs are not uncommon in horses, though most murmurs are physiological, normal heart sounds and are simply the result of large volumes of blood moving at high speeds through the heart valves. Because of the large heart size,

these sounds are readily heard and are referred to as ejection murmurs. Ejection murmurs are commonly heard in horses and should disappear when the horse is exercised. True cardiac disease is unusual in horses but is usually accompanied by murmurs or other abnormal sounds. The clinician should be alerted whenever abnormal sounds are heard, as the sounds may need to be further characterized and investigated. Murmurs are assessed for loudness and also for when the murmur occurs in the cardiac cycle (systolic or diastolic). The horse may be exercised to see if the abnormal sound disappears, stays the same, or gets louder with exercise. Using these criteria, the clinician decides whether further diagnostic tests are warranted.

Lung Auscultation

Despite the large size of equine lungs, breath sounds may be difficult to hear. A quiet environment is important for an accurate evaluation.

The borders of the lung fields are the same for the right and left sides of the chest and are outlined in Fig. 2-8. The lung field basically consists of a cranioventral area and a caudodorsal area; part of the cranioventral field

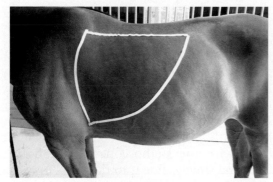

Fig. 2-8. Landmarks for the lung. Borders of the left lung field for auscultation.

is obscured by the shoulder musculature and cannot be heard. The stethoscope is placed in several locations within the lung field to listen to several breaths at each location (Fig. 2-9, *A* to *C*). Normally, air movement in and out of the airways should be heard and should not be accompanied by wheezing or gurgling, moist sounds. The clinician should be alerted if abnormal noises are heard. Equally significant may be the absence of breath sounds, which occurs in some respiratory diseases; the clinician should be alerted if this is detected.

Lung auscultation should *always* be performed on *both* sides of the chest. Respiratory diseases and other abnormalities do not necessarily affect both lungs and pleural cavities equally, and auscultation may be different over the right and left lungs.

Abdominal Auscultation

A stethoscope is used to listen to abdominal sounds, which are created by movements of the intestines. This is commonly referred to as *gastrointestinal motility* or *GI motility*. This is somewhat a misnomer because some sounds are generated by passive movement of gas and liquids in the intestines without actually being propelled by the intestinal musculature. Therefore it is not completely

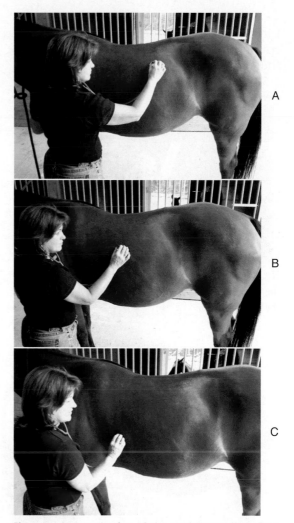

Fig. 2-9. **A,** Auscultation of the caudodorsal lung field. **B,** Auscultation of the midthorax. **C,** Auscultation of the cranioventral lung field.

accurate to assume that all intestinal sounds are due to functional intestines. This becomes important in the patient with GI disease; sick portions of intestine may have little or no purposeful motility, yet passive fluid and gas sounds may be heard. Experience is required to distinguish active from passive sounds.

Abdominal auscultation should be performed on both sides of the horse. The common site for auscultation is the *flank,* the area between the pelvis and the caudal

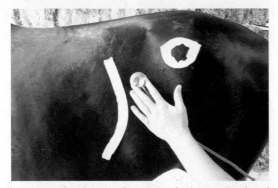

Fig. 2-10. Landmarks for abdominal auscultation in the flank area are the point of the hip (tuber coxae) and the last rib.

margin of the rib cage. The flank is normally slightly depressed. The point of the hip is the dorsal extent of the flank area (Fig. 2-10). The flank is only part of the total abdominal wall, and auscultation can be performed at any location on the abdominal wall. Horses may be sensitive in the flank and abdominal area, so these areas should be approached slowly and gently. A good approach is to place the hand with the stethoscope on the horse's back and slowly slide it to the flank or lower abdominal area.

A standard four-point auscultation is usually sufficient for most patients. The stethoscope is used to auscultate the upper flank and the lower flank on both sides of the abdomen. The four points are referred to as upper left, upper right, lower left, and lower right quadrants (Fig. 2-11, *A* to *D* and Box 2-1).

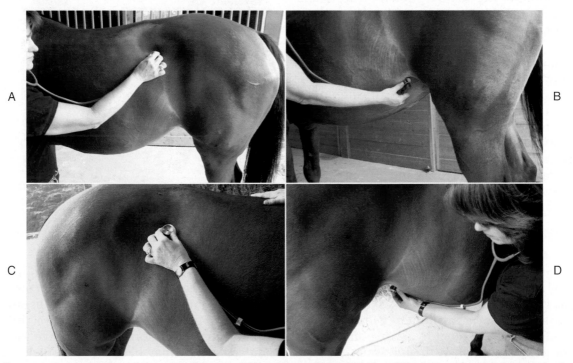

Fig. 2-11. **A,** Auscultation of the upper left abdominal quadrant. **B,** Auscultation of the lower left abdominal quadrant. **C,** Auscultation of the upper right upper abdominal quadrant. **D,** Auscultation of the lower right abdominal quadrant.

2-1   Four-Point Abdominal Auscultation

The four-point auscultation is recorded using a grid that identifies each abdominal quadrant as follows:

Upper Left Quadrant	Upper Right Quadrant
Lower Left Quadrant	Lower Right Quadrant

Results of the auscultation at each location are recorded as follows:
  0 = no motility heard
  +1 = hypomotility
  +2 = normal motility
  +3 = hypermotility

For example, a horse with hypomotility in the lower right quadrant and a normal number of borborygmi in all other quadrants would be recorded as follows:

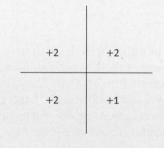

+2	+2
+2	+1

Intestinal motility sounds, also called *borborygmi,* have been described as sounding like thunder rumbling or an approaching freight train. These sounds are usually associated with coordinated, normal patterns of large intestinal motility. The number of borborygmi/minute are counted in each abdominal quadrant; the stethoscope should be left in place *at least 1 minute* at *each* of the four points to get an accurate count.

"Normal" motility is considered to be one to three borborygmi/minute in each abdominal quadrant. More than this is considered to be hypermotility, and less than this rate is considered to be hypomotility. Complete absence of borborygmus is equated with intestinal standstill, properly termed *ileus.* Ileus typically indicates serious intestinal disease and is often associated with increased morbidity and mortality. Remember, however, that gas and fluid "tinkling" sounds may *still be heard* in the patient with ileus. These are passive sounds and should *not* be confused with functional intestine.

Mucous Membranes

Mucous membranes are tissues that have the ability to make and secrete mucus. Mucous membranes' color is helpful for disease diagnosis. Several mucous membranes are readily visible to the examiner: the gums (gingiva) (Fig. 2-12, *A*), conjunctiva of the eye (Fig. 2-12, *B*), lining of the nostrils (Fig. 2-12, *C*), and inner surfaces of the vulva in females (Fig. 2-12, *D*). The inner surface of the ear pinna does not secrete mucus and is therefore not a mucous membrane, though it may be useful for detecting icterus and evidence of clotting disorders.

The mucous membrane color is usually light to dark pink (Fig. 2-13). The color may change with abnormalities of blood perfusion and oxygen content of the blood and other diseases. Cyanosis is a bluish tint that usually indicates extremely low oxygen content in the tissue. Brick red coloration indicates bacterial septicemia or septic shock, or both. Endotoxic shock in the horse has the unique characteristic of producing a purple gum line along the margins of the teeth; this is referred to as a *toxic line.* Yellowish coloring of the gums indicates icterus, usually relating to liver dysfunction or abnormal hemolysis of red blood cells. Pale mucous membranes may indicate anemia or poor perfusion; it should be noted that the gums

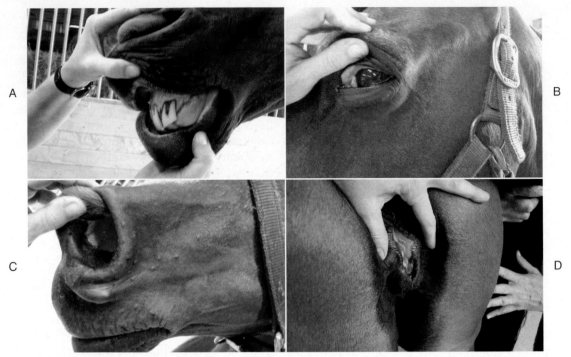

Fig. 2-12. Examination of mucous membranes. **A,** Examination of the gums. **B,** Examination of the conjunctiva. **C,** Examination of the mucosa of the nares. **D,** Examination of the vulva in the female.

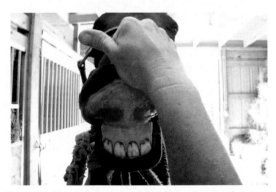

Fig. 2-13. Mucous membrane color. Normal gum color.

pinpoint hemorrhages less than 1 mm in diameter are called *petechial hemorrhages.* Hemorrhages 1 mm to 1 cm in diameter are called *ecchymotic hemorrhages.* Larger hemorrhages are referred to as *purpuric hemorrhages,* though these are rare on mucous membranes.

Mucous membranes are also assessed for moisture and are commonly described as moist, dry, tacky, or other subjective terms. This information is less useful than the color of the membranes.

Hydration Status

The hydration status of an animal is very important information. It may be measured with laboratory tests or estimated from the physical examination. Two main methods of assessing hydration of the animal on

of some horses are normally pale pink, and this does not indicate disease in these animals.

Clotting disorders may create reddish spotting of the mucous membranes. Small physical examination are the skin turgor test and the capillary refill time.

Skin turgor is also known as the *skin pinch test*. The loose skin over the lateral aspect of the neck is briefly and firmly pinched with the fingers and allowed to retract to its original position. In normally hydrated animals the skin will snap back to its original position in approximately 1 second or less. Dehydration (>5% dehydration) prolongs the response to longer than 1 second. Severely dehydrated animals may take 8 seconds or longer for the skin to retract. Skin turgor is less reliable in obese animals; fat in the cervical area may falsely improve the skin snap.

Capillary refill time (CRT) is assessed by pressing briefly but firmly on the gums with a fingertip to produce a "blanched" white spot (Fig. 2-14). The time for the original color to return to the blanched spot is counted in seconds. "Cranking" a horse's lips widely apart to access the gums is not necessary; the lips need only be elevated enough to see the gum line. Original color should return in less than 2.5 seconds. Dehydration and shock prolong the capillary refill time. Severe dehydration and severe shock may produce greatly prolonged CRT, from 5 to 8 seconds.

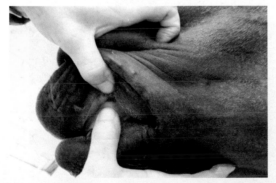

Fig. 2-14. Capillary refill time. Assessing capillary refill time.

Height/Weight Measurement

Height and weight measurement may serve different purposes. Height measurement may be required as part of the insurance and prepurchase examinations, for breed registration, and for entry into certain horse show classes. Weight measurement is usually used for calculating the proper dose of drugs and therapeutic substances and for formulating the animal's diet.

Height measurement may seem like a benign procedure to the novice horseman, but it can be a major issue for many horse owners. Registration of an individual into a particular breed may depend on the height of the adult animal; unregistered animals have little reproductive value. Competition at horse shows is another important area in which height may be a source of debate. Horse show classes are often divided into "pony classes" and "horse classes." A pony is defined as an individual measuring less than 14.2 hands at the withers. Pony classes are sometimes further divided into small and large pony classes. These divisions are based on height. Competition at some horse shows may be very keen, and owners of horses near the height limit of a particular class may even have the hoof length altered by trimming to meet the entrance requirements. Sometimes this trimming may be so extreme as to produce sore feet. Be aware that owners may try to apply extreme pressure on the official measurer to certify the height that they desire.

Height may be estimated roughly or measured precisely. Rough estimates may be made with a height/weight tape. This instrument is essentially a tape measure, marked in hands (1 hand = 4 inches). Height is ideally taken on a firm surface. The horse's head should not be elevated or lowered but should be in a horizontal position, paralleling the ground. The tape is secured on the ground with a foot just behind a forelimb (Fig. 2-15, *A*).

The tape is then stretched vertically to the withers, and the height read at the level of the most caudal mane hair or the highest point of the withers, according to the breed registry or competition rules (Fig. 2-15, *B*). The tape gives an approximation of the animal's height.

For precise determination of height, commercially made rigid measuring rulers are available. These rulers are made of metal and include carpenters' bubble levels to assure that the ruler is not tilted when the measurement is taken. Again, the animal should be on firm ground, the head and neck held level with the ground, and the measurement taken at the last mane hair or highest point of the withers, depending on the registry or rules of competition.

Weight may be roughly estimated with the height/weight tape or taken specifically with a livestock scale. The height/weight tape has one side calibrated for weight measurement; the weight tick marks are based on measurements at the girth of the horse. The tape is applied to encircle the horse at its girth, the area behind the withers just behind the forelimb (Fig. 2-16, *A* and *B*). The weight tape is formulated from logarithms of normal

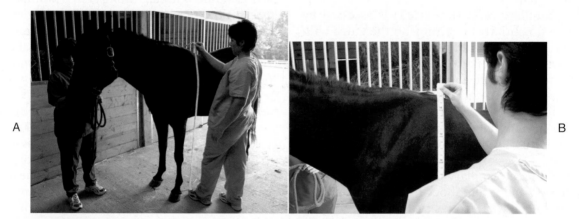

Fig. 2-15. Measuring height. **A,** Proper position for the height/weight tape for measuring height. **B,** Height is read at the highest point of the withers.

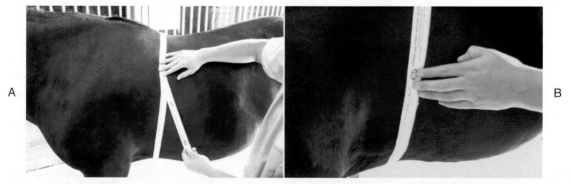

Fig. 2-16. Measuring weight. **A,** The weight tape is positioned around the thorax at the girth. **B,** Reading the weight tape.

animals and may be inaccurate for extremely thin or obese animals. The build of an animal may also affect the results. It should also be noted that height/weight tapes for cattle are not accurate for horses.

Precise weights for large animals may be obtained with livestock scales or digital livestock scales. Walk-over–style digital scales are popular at many hospitals and clinics and are replacing traditional livestock scales, which require adding lead weights to a balancing arm on the scale and are somewhat cumbersome to use.

SUGGESTED READING

Moore RM, Costa LRR: Equine medical and surgical nursing. In McCurnin DM, Bassert JM, editors: *Clinical textbook for veterinary technicians*, ed 5, St Louis, 2002, Saunders.

Speirs VC: *Clinical examination of horses*, St Louis, 1997, Saunders.

3

Physical Restraint of Horses

Restraint is the term used to imply control of an animal and may be necessary for medical and nonmedical procedures. The two types of animal restraint are physical restraint and chemical restraint. Sometimes both must be used to accomplish a procedure. *Physical restraint* refers to methods that are applied to the animal with or without use of special equipment. *Chemical restraint* refers to the use of pharmaceuticals to alter the animal's mental or physical abilities.

Restraint is more of an art than it is science. Skilled restrainers know the behavior and nature of the species they work with. This level of savvy takes time to acquire and is often best learned by watching experienced personnel. Good restraint involves understanding the natural instincts of the horse, being able to read an individual's temperament, and recognizing the extent of handling and training that an individual has (or has not) had. Several key points must be made regarding restraint of horses.

- Each animal is an individual, and each has a different background. A method of restraint that is totally effective for one horse may be completely ineffective for another. Avoid a cookie-cutter approach where all animals are treated similarly.
- Be flexible. When the selected method of restraint is not working, go to "plan B." Realize that you cannot force restraint on an animal that is intent on not accepting it, especially when the animal outweighs and outmuscles you many times over.

- In the world of nature animals are either predators or prey, and much of their behavior relates to this fact. Horses are prey. Their natural instinct when placed in a fearful situation is to run away. Sometimes this instinct is so strong that they will injure themselves in their effort to flee. Very few horses become aggressive in a fearful situation, but this does occur. Precautions must be taken with these individuals.
- Another strong natural instinct to remember is that horses are herd animals and often resist attempts to separate them from others in their group. Sometimes a buddy system approach—taking a second horse along—is helpful if the horse needs to be taken away from the group.
- Horses are naturally suspicious and respond best to a calm, deliberate approach. Using the voice and touch in a calm manner helps to gain their trust. Good horsemen typically maintain vocal *and* physical contact with the animals they are handling. Approaches are usually best made from the front end of the horse rather than from behind, and initial hand contact with the neck or withers makes a good introduction before moving on to other areas of the horse's body.
- Be careful when working in the horse's visual blind spots. Because of the location of their eyes, horses cannot see directly behind their hindquarters, directly in front of the tip of their nose, directly

between the eyes in the forehead area, and directly above the head between the ears. If you must work in these areas, avoid unannounced or rapid movements.

- Use the *least* amount of restraint necessary to do the job *safely* and do *not* apply it any longer than necessary.
- Horses are traditionally handled primarily from their left side (also called the *near side*). Unless the horse has not been handled, it will most likely be accustomed to a left-sided approach.
- The horse's head should always be attended. Control of the head usually enables control of the horse. For most procedures, the person "on the head" stands on the same side as the person performing the procedure and has the greatest responsibility for restraint of the animal and the safety of his or her coworker.
- *Never* stand directly in front or directly behind a horse during a procedure, unless protected by a barrier or mechanical device. Horses may strike with the front legs or kick with the hind legs in response to pain or fear. Horses may also throw their heads violently, causing injury. Even a normally "good horse" may display these responses when in pain or fear. Assume that all horses are capable of these responses when placed in certain situations.
- Take good care of your personal safety. Avoid getting into a position that you cannot leave quickly, such as stall corners or between the horse and a fence or wall. Also, do not be afraid to speak up if you are uncomfortable with a given situation or not up to the task. Your safety is of the utmost importance.
- The horse should be protected from dangers like sharp objects, hooks, buckets, loose boards, and light fixtures in case it rears, kicks, or throws its head or body. There is little point in risking serious lacerations or fractures from restraint for an otherwise simple procedure. Survey the area for potential hazards before beginning a procedure. The best prevention is to take the horse to an area without potential hazards or remove the hazards where possible.
- Patience is a virtue, and your virtue will be tested. Some procedures simply cannot be done safely on certain individuals in certain situations.

Be sure to plan ahead for the procedure. Few things are more frustrating than struggling to get a horse properly restrained, only to realize that a piece of equipment is out of reach or not working properly.

Another consideration is the possibility of professional liability lawsuits. The veterinarian is recognized legally as an expert and is responsible for anticipating the responses of his or her patients to veterinary procedures. Sometimes the veterinarian's choices of restraint may be influenced by this consideration and may even lead to refusal to perform certain procedures. The safety of the horse and the safety of the people handling the horse must be not only legal but ethical responsibilities.

Finally, realize that *any* form of restraint can become abusive. Applying a restraint method improperly or for too long can cross the line of humane restraint.

METHODS OF PHYSICAL RESTRAINT

HALTER AND LEAD ROPE

One of the most basic acts of horsemanship is placing a halter and lead rope (also called a *lead shank*) on a horse. It is also the first step in gaining control of a horse's head, which is the key to controlling the horse.

The horse should be approached from its left side; avoid standing directly in front of the horse. Usually, the halter is placed first, and then the lead rope is attached to the halter. Some horses need to have the lead rope placed around the neck first for initial control while the halter is being placed (Fig. 3-1, *A*). The halter has a small loop, which is placed around the nose, and a larger loop, which is placed over and behind the ears. Buckles or snaps are used to open and close the loops. As a courtesy to the horse, try not to drag the halter over the eyes and ears. Rather, spread the halter apart to avoid the eyes and lift or unbuckle the halter to avoid the ears. Once the halter is positioned and the buckles/snaps secured, the lead rope is attached (Fig. 3-1, *B* and *C*).

Once placed, the halter and lead rope may be used to lead the horse. The horse should not be led by grasping the halter; if the horse moves its head up or away, the operator may lose his or her grip, and if the horse bolts or runs, there is a risk of being dragged and seriously hurt (Fig. 3-2, *A*). Use the lead rope to lead the horse (Fig. 3-2, *B*). Hold the lead away from any buckles or chains, and *never* coil the lead around the fingers, hand, or arm (Fig. 3-2, *C* and *D*). If the horse bolts or runs, coiled rope may tighten around body parts; serious injury and death have resulted from this practice. Another practice to avoid is letting the lead rope drag on the ground; the horse may step on the rope, or the handler may become tangled in the rope, also resulting in injury.

To lead the horse, walk purposefully in the intended direction and do not look back at the horse. Some horses resent being held tightly by the lead rope, and giving it some slack may encourage it to follow the handler. Most horses respond best when the handler walks to the side of the head or neck.

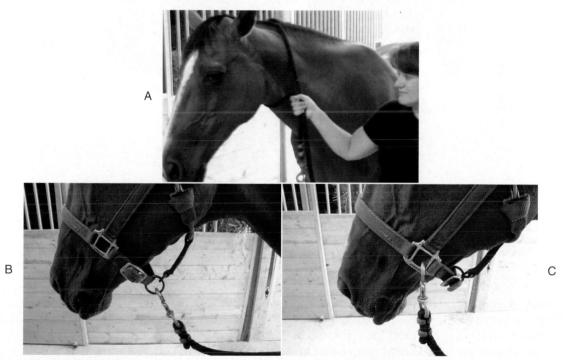

Fig. 3-1. Placing a halter and lead rope. **A,** Lead rope placed around the neck to get initial control of the horse. **B,** Attachment of the lead rope to the halter. **C,** Alternate attachment of lead rope to halter.

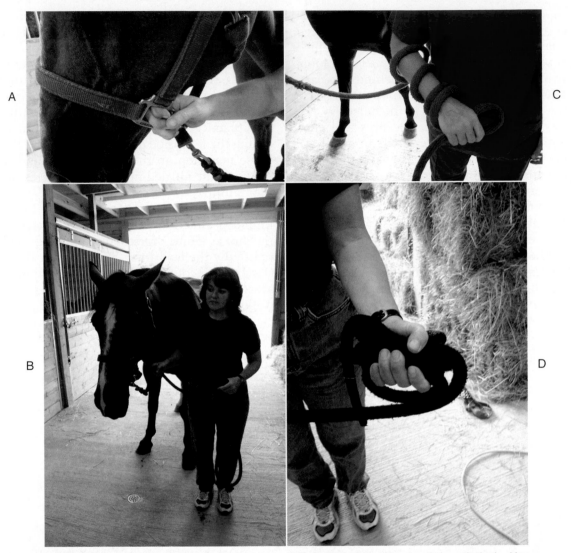

Fig. 3-2. Leading the horse using the halter and lead rope. **A,** Fingers should not be placed through the buckles or snaps of the halter. **B,** Proper hold of the lead rope. **C,** Improper coiling of lead rope around the arm. **D,** Improper coiling of lead rope around the hand.

Avoid walking far in front of the horse, where control of the horse is minimal.

When controlling the head for a procedure, the person on the head should realize that his or her first responsibility is his/her coworker's safety. If the horse becomes fractious, it is usually best to move the horse's hindquarters away from the clinician. This is done not by moving the hind end of the horse directly but by moving the head; the hindquarters usually move opposite to head movement. In other words, turning the head to the left usually results in the hindquarters moving to the right, and vice versa.

Lead ropes are made from many materials (e.g., nylon, leather, hemp, cotton) and have two basic designs: with or without a chain. Without a chain, the rope serves only as a lead, but the addition of a chain provides possibilities for several degrees of physical restraint. Note that using the chain portion of a lead to restrain foals as described later is *not* appropriate.

Chain shanks can be purchased with varying lengths of chain and thickness of the chain links. When a simple lead rope does not provide enough control, the chain portion of a chain shank can be placed over the nose or in the mouth for increasing restraint. In order to use the chain in this fashion, the halter must have side rings to slide the chain through and fasten the chain snap.

Placing the chain over the nose is a mild form of restraint. The chain is passed through the left ring of the nosepiece and over the nose to attach (1) to the right nosepiece ring (Fig. 3-3, *A*) or (2) through the right nosepiece ring and continuing to the right upper ring (Fig. 3-3, *B*) or (3) through the right nosepiece ring and continuing under the halter to attach to the large nosepiece ring between the mandibles (Fig. 3-3, *C*). Care should be taken to cross the chain over the halter noseband so that the noseband can act as a protective interface between the chain and the horse's skin (Fig. 3-3, *D*). A light, quick snap of the lead usually gets the horse's attention.

Placing the chain under the chin is not recommended—many horses will throw their heads or rear to avoid pressure from a chin shank, possibly causing injury to themselves (Fig. 3-4).

The chain can also be placed in the mouth as the next level of restraint. There are two basic positions for the chain. It can be positioned like a mouth bit, although the links of the chain tend to pinch the tongue and cheeks when pressure is applied, causing many horses to resist any pressure on the lead (Fig. 3-5). The chain can also be positioned to contact the gingiva above the upper incisors underneath the upper lip; this is called a *lip shank*. There is an acupressure point at this location on the gums, and constant pressure encourages release of natural endorphins in the brain, helping to calm the horse. The chain is passed through the left nosepiece ring, directly over the nose, and attached to the right nosepiece ring. The chain over the nose is slackened enough to allow the upper lip to be elevated, and the chain is placed carefully well above the incisors against the gums (Fig. 3-6, *A* to *E*). Gently take up the slack in the lead to obtain contact of the chain against the tissue. The lip shank is difficult to position, and once in place, constant pressure must be kept on the lead rope to keep the chain in position. A more recent modification of the lip shank is a commercial device that fits over the gums and behind the poll (another acupressure point) and is adjusted with small pulleys to the desired tension; instead of chain, nylon rope is used, making it less traumatic to the gums. Whenever a chain or any other device is placed in the mouth, it should *never* be snapped, jerked, or pulled on excessively; the tissues of the mouth are very sensitive, and it is easy to cross the line of humane restraint.

The lead rope can be used to tie the horse's head to a secure object, though this is rarely necessary and may have disastrous consequences if the horse panics and tries to run away. For most veterinary procedures, tying the horse does not justify the risks involved. If it is necessary to tie the head, use only a modified slip knot that can be released in an emergency (Fig. 3-7) and allow the horse enough slack to allow some movement of its head and neck. The less ability the horse has to move its head, the more

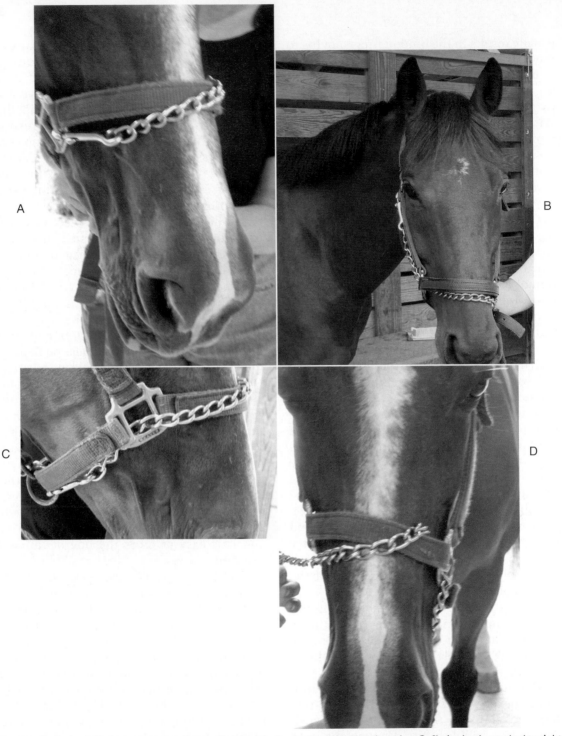

Fig. 3-3. Chain shank for increasing restraint. **A,** Chain shank attached to right nosepiece ring. **B,** Chain shank attached to right upper ring. **C,** Chain shank attached between the mandibles. **D,** The chain should cross the nosepiece to provide some protection for the horse. (**B** from McCurnin DM, Bassert JM: *Clinical textbook for veterinary technicians*, ed 6, St Louis, 2006, Saunders.)

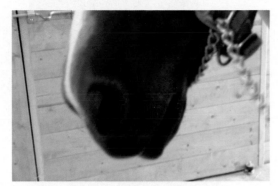

Fig. 3-4. Placement of chain shank under the chin.

likely it is to resist. Also, a horse should never be tied with a chain over its nose or in its mouth. *Never* leave a tied horse unattended. Be sure that whatever object the horse is tied to will not break and get dragged by the horse if the horse breaks free.

COVERING THE EYES
This is a time-honored method that can be applied to one or both eyes. Sometimes, when the horse cannot see the area being worked on, it will be submissive. Covering the eye on the same side as the procedure is the most common method but is often applied incorrectly. Placing the hand completely over the eye to force it shut is usually unnecessary and is often met with resistance (Fig. 3-8, *A*). All that is necessary is to block vision of the procedure, using an open hand like a curtain but allowing the horse to keep its eye open (Fig. 3-8, *B*).

Some horses respond favorably to blindfolding. These individuals and situations must be carefully selected, since not all horses accept a blindfold. Blindfolding is usually done by placing a towel over both eyes and tucking it underneath the halter. Blindfolds should be able to be removed easily if the horse panics, and the handler should have quick access to the blindfold if this occurs.

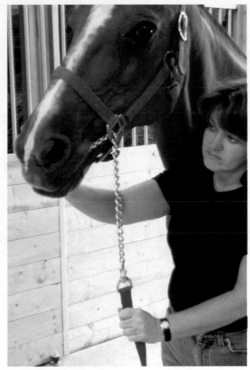

Fig. 3-5. Placement of the chain shank through the mouth.

ELEVATING A LEG
Elevating a leg is a mild form of restraint that is basically intended to discourage a horse from moving around or kicking, such as when trying to place leg bandages, taking radiographs, or clipping hair. It is not as useful for painful procedures but can be combined with other forms of restraint for increased effect. Elevating legs is also a common procedure for cleaning and examining the feet and legs.

Before elevating any leg, the horse should be standing "square," meaning that all four legs should be directly underneath the horse, with the weight evenly distributed. If a horse is standing with its legs sprawled or is balanced awkwardly, it is physically difficult for any horse to pick a leg up.

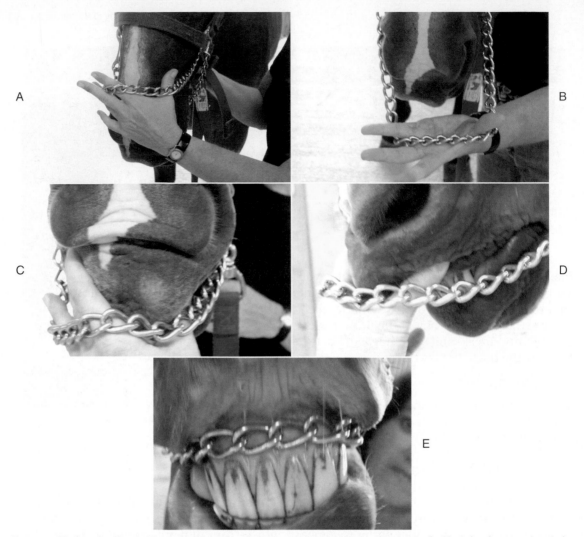

Fig. 3-6. Placing the lip shank. **A,** Holding the chain for placement of the lip shank. **B,** Slack is given to the chain. **C,** Elevating the upper lip to position the chain. **D,** Elevating the upper lip to position the chain. **E,** Proper position of the chain against the upper gum. Note that the chain lays flat against the gums.

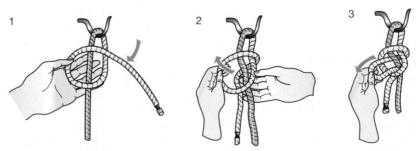

Fig. 3-7. How to make a halter tie (quick release knot).

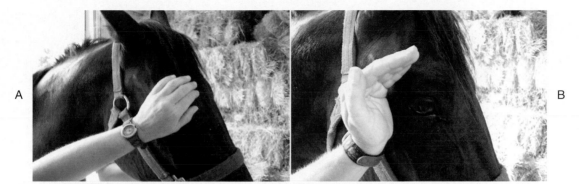

Fig. 3-8. **A,** Improper method for blocking vision. **B,** Proper method for blocking vision.

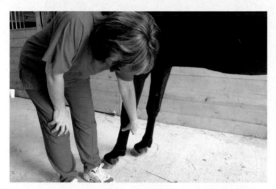

Fig. 3-9. To lift a forelimb, the hand is run down the back of the leg and the tendons or suspensory ligament gently squeezed.

As with other horse-handling procedures, contact with the horse is helpful in communicating intentions. To elevate a forelimb, one hand is placed on the withers or shoulder area and the other hand is run slowly down the back side of the leg to be lifted. When the sliding hand gets to the digital tendons, a gentle squeeze of the tendons usually results in lifting of the leg (Fig. 3-9). If squeezing alone doesn't work, try pressing your shoulder into the horse's shoulder to shift its weight onto the opposite forelimb; once the weight has shifted, the horse will be more inclined to elevate the leg. If you

are lifting a front leg to discourage a horse from kicking with a hind leg, lift the forelimb on the *same* side as the "threatening" hindlimb.

To elevate a hindlimb, face the rear of the horse, and maintain contact with one hand on the horse's hindquarters. Slide the other hand down the leg to the digital tendons, and squeeze the tendons. As with the forelimb, shoulder pressure into the horse's hindquarters can help shift its weight to the opposite hindlimb and encourage lifting the leg.

Once a leg has been lifted, it can be held with the hands or cradled in the lap/thigh area, depending on the procedure to be performed (Figs. 3-10, *A* to *C* and 3-11, *A* and *B*). Do not support the leg so well that you become a substitute leg for the horse, allowing it to kick or move at your expense, or rest so hard on your legs that muscle fatigue or bruising occurs. Horses tend to resist having their legs pulled away from the median plane (abduction) and will stand better when a leg is held as close to its normal position as possible directly underneath it.

TAIL RESTRAINT

Tail restraint is effective for foals and small ponies but not adults. The tail is grasped near its base, and the tail is elevated straight up

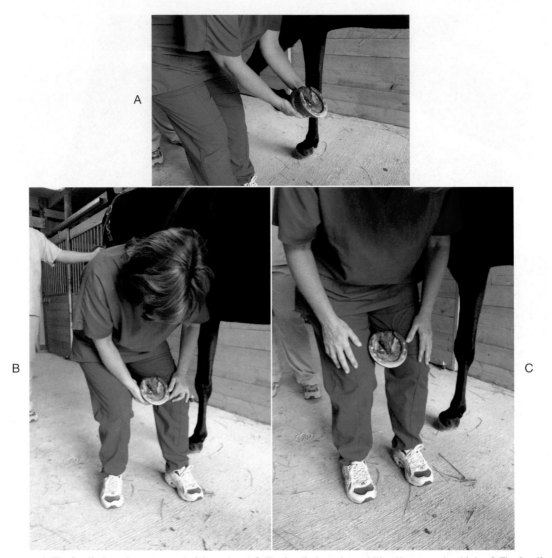

Fig. 3-10. A, The forelimb can be supported with one hand. **B,** The forelimb can be stabilized between the thighs. **C,** The forelimb can be supported between the thighs to free up the hands.

and slightly over the back. At the same time, use the other arm to encircle the shoulders or base of the neck. Be aware that many foals have a tendency to rear when restrained; therefore the restrainer should keep his or her head out of the area immediately above the head and neck to avoid being struck.

TWITCHES

Twitches are among the oldest and most commonly used methods of restraint. Why twitches work has been debated for many years; some people believe that they divert the horse's attention through creating pain that exceeds less painful procedures being

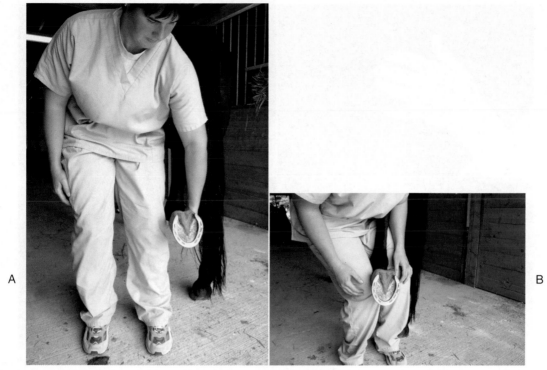

Fig. 3-11. **A,** The hindlimb can be supported with one hand. **B,** The hindlimb can be supported on the thighs to free up the hands.

performed elsewhere on the body, and others believe that acupressure points may be activated, releasing natural endorphins in the brain. Whatever the mechanism, their effectiveness cannot be argued.

There are two classifications of twitches: *natural* and *mechanical*. Natural twitches are applied with the hands directly on the horse; no special equipment is required. Mechanical twitches are manmade devices that are placed directly on the horse. Twitches of any type are *not* appropriate for foals.

Natural twitches are the shoulder (skin) twitch, the ear twitch, and the lip twitch. The shoulder twitch ("shoulder roll" or "skin twitch") is actually applied to the skin over the lateral aspect of the neck. This skin is loose and can be picked up with the fingers

and pinched firmly (Fig. 3-12, *A* and *B*). For added effect, the skin can be picked up with all of the fingers and rolled like a motorcycle accelerator; this can be done with one or both hands (Fig. 3-12, *C* and *D*). This twitch is a mild form of restraint and loses its effectiveness after a few minutes. If applied tightly for long, some horses swell locally after releasing the hold, which produces a welt. Such welts disappear within 24 hours with no special treatment and are not a physical problem but may give the client a bad impression.

The ear twitch is very effective for some horses, but others vehemently resist it. To apply this twitch, do not grab the ear directly; this may startle the horse. Rather, place the hand on the neck and slide it to the

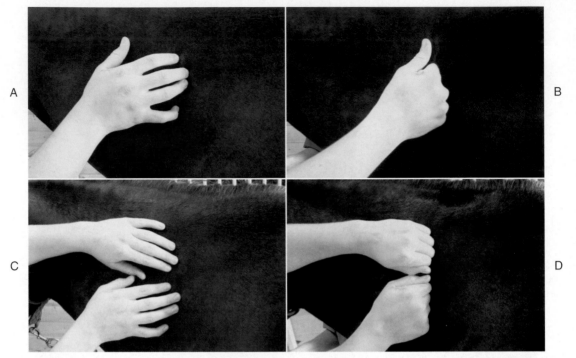

Fig. 3-12. Shoulder twitch. **A,** Placement of the hand. **B,** The skin is grasped and pinched firmly. **C,** Placement of both hands for a two-handed twitch. **D,** The skin is grasped and rolled.

base of the ear. Slowly grasp the base of the ear, squeeze it, and rotate the ear slightly, again like a motorcycle accelerator (Fig. 3-13, *A* to *D*). Like the shoulder twitch, the ear twitch loses its effectiveness in a short period. Grasping at the base of the ear, not in the middle or tip (Fig. 3-14), is important. Realize that the cartilage of the ear pinna can be broken, resulting in permanent deformity, and the nerves to the pinna can be damaged, so if the horse elevates its head or rears, it is best to let go and try another approach.

Biting the horse's ear is still accepted in some parts of the country as a restraint method, but it is not commonly accepted and is not recommended for use by medical professionals.

The upper lip can be twitched with either hand. The lip can simply be grasped and

squeezed and jiggled back and forth if necessary. Grabbing a lip may be enough restraint for many horses. For more force application to the upper lip, mechanical twitches are necessary.

Mechanical twitches can be homemade or commercially bought (Fig. 3-15). They are designed to "pinch" the upper lip. The traditional twitch is constructed from a wooden handle with a rope or chain loop attached to one end. To place the twitch, first control the twitch handle with a hand or tuck it under an armpit while placing the twitch loop; otherwise, the handle is free to swing and hit the handler and/or the horse and cause injury. The upper lip is grasped with the hand, and the loop is transferred from the hand to the lip by sliding the loop over the fingers (Fig. 3-16, *A* to *E*). Once the lip has been

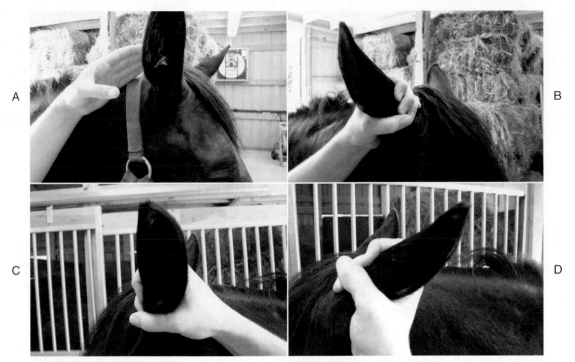

Fig. 3-13. Ear twitch. **A**, The ear is approached by maintaining contact with the horse. **B**, The base of the ear is grasped. **C**, The ear is squeezed. **D**, The ear can be rotated for added effect.

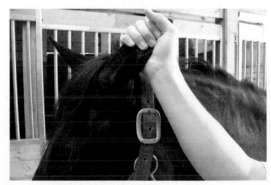

Fig. 3-14. Improper grasping of the ear tip for an ear twitch.

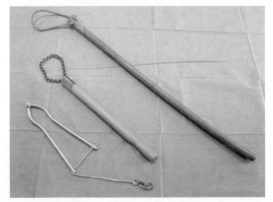

Fig. 3-15. Mechanical twitches. Long wooden handle with rope loop *(top)*. Short wooden handle with chain loop *(middle)*. Aluminum humane twitch *(bottom)*.

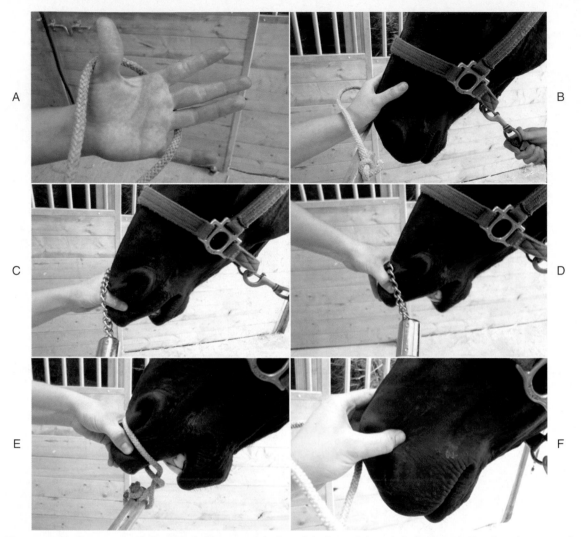

Fig. 3-16. Placing a mechanical twitch. **A,** Proper positioning of the loop of the twitch. **B,** Place the hand on the nose and slide it toward the upper lip. **C,** Grasp the upper lip and elevate it slightly. **D,** Elevate the hand and wrist to help transfer the loop from the hand over the lip. **E,** Transfer the loop onto the upper lip. **F,** Avoid blocking the nostrils while placing the twitch.

placed through the loop, the twitch handle is rotated to twist the loop firmly around the lip. The handle should be rotated as if it were being rolled up the nose toward the ears, not downward toward the lower lip. Avoid occluding the nostrils while placing the twitch; horses cannot mouth breathe and tend to panic when the nostrils are blocked (Fig. 3-16, *F*). By twisting the handle, the loop can be tightened or loosened for varying degrees of control.

The twitch handle comes in various lengths; however, the shorter the handle, the less useful it is if the horse rears, and it places the operator closer to the front feet. Many horsemen prefer a handle 30 to 40 inches long.

The other type of mechanical twitch is called the humane twitch; it consists of two arms that function as a scissors-type "clamp" on the nose. Pressure is controlled by opening or closing the arms of the clamp. This type of twitch is usually made of aluminum and has a string with a clip attached to it so that it can be "self-retaining" by clipping it to the halter. In reality, the humane twitch is limited in usefulness; the arms are short (≈12 inches), and if the horse elevates its head, it is difficult to maintain a grip on the device. When applied as a self-retaining twitch, the string tends to loosen; if the horse then swings its head, the arms become a

potential weapon, injuring the horse or the handler. The humane twitch is useful in some situations but ineffective and potentially harmful in others (Fig. 3-17, *A* to *D*).

After the twitch is in place, one person should hold the twitch handle and the lead rope, being careful not to wrap the lead around the handle or any part of the hand or arm (Fig. 3-18). The twitch does not replace the lead rope. The person on the head still has primary responsibility for control of the horse and the safety of coworkers. The pressure of the twitch is adjusted by twisting the twitch handle to tighten or loosen the chain/rope loop or by squeezing the handles of the humane twitch. Apply only enough pressure with the twitch to accomplish the procedure and only as long as necessary.

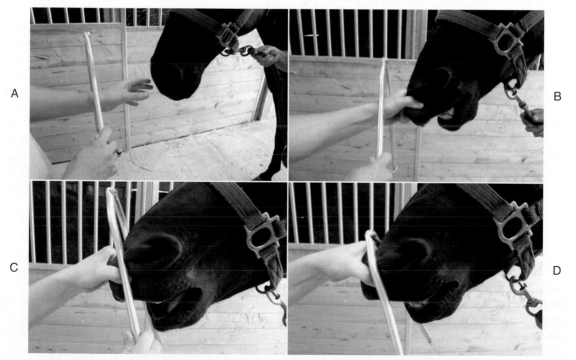

Fig. 3-17. Placing a humane twitch. **A,** Approach to place the humane twitch. **B,** Grasp the upper lip. **C,** Proper placement of the humane twitch, with the lip between the straight portion of the twitch arms. **D,** Improper placement of the humane twitch, with the lip between the rounded portion of the twitch arms.

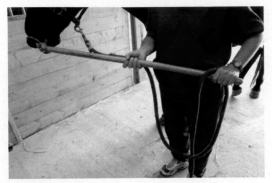

Fig. 3-18. Proper way to hold the twitch. The lead rope is not wrapped around the twitch handle.

Sometimes jiggling the twitch helps to get the horse's attention without having to crank down tightly on the twitch. Also, be aware that the upper lip can become numb after prolonged application. When the lip turns blue and cool to the touch, the twitch has usually lost its effectiveness and should be loosened or removed.

Mechanical twitches should never be applied to foals and should never be applied to the ears. Twitching the lower lip is possible but not advisable, since many horses rear or throw their heads in response.

TAIL TIE

The tail of a horse is considerably more substantial than the tail of a cow; it is strong enough to be used to move, lift, or support the hindquarters. Horses with neurological or musculoskeletal diseases may need assistance to stand and/or remain standing, and horses recovering from anesthesia may need assistance standing. The tail tie can be helpful in these situations; it provides a means of safely securing a rope to the horse's tail, which can then be placed over a supporting beam or through a pulley or block and tackle, where it can be positioned for support.

The tail tie is performed just beyond the end of the last coccygeal vertebrae (Fig. 3-19).

No part of the vertebral column should be included in the tie; only the tail hairs are incorporated into the knot.

A tail rope should *never* be tied to an immovable object. The tail rope is also not a substitute for the hindquarters; if the horse demonstrates that it cannot provide any support of its own rear bodyweight, the horse should not be left dangling by a tail rope.

STOCKS

Stocks are rectangular enclosures made of wood or metal (Fig. 3-20). They are designed to confine the horse to a small area with restricted movement, usually only 1 to 2 feet of lateral movement and 1 to 2 feet of front-to-back movement. Because of the varying sizes of horses, stocks may be adjustable for the width and length of the patient. The side panels or rails of the stocks usually adjust to allow access to the body parts being worked on. Horse stocks typically are open above (i.e., have no ceiling).

Horse stocks and cattle stocks are different in construction. Cattle stocks are purposefully designed to firmly squeeze the cow's neck and sometimes have panels that can be used to firmly squeeze the cow's body. Horses cannot tolerate this type of tight, rigid confinement and typically violently resist it. Therefore horses should never be placed in cattle-type stocks.

Stocks are not necessary for all procedures. They are most often used to protect the clinician from being kicked when working on the hindquarters. Stocks are also useful for standing surgery procedures where the horse must be prevented from wandering. Horses are naturally suspicious of stocks and may need to be tranquilized before leading them into the stocks. Some horses may vehemently resist entering or staying in stocks; therefore they are not suitable or safe for every patient. Good judgment must be used.

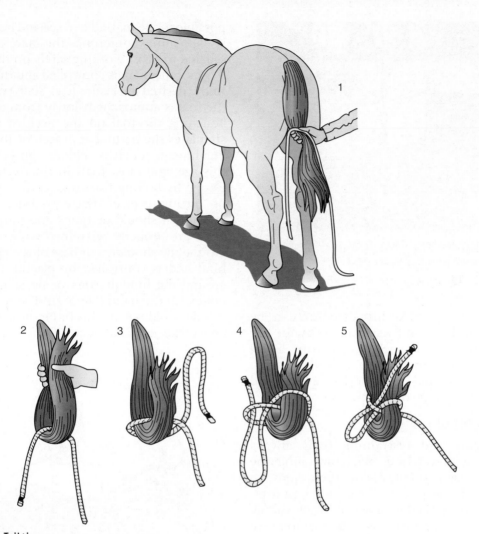

Fig. 3-19. Tail tie.

Stocks usually have two gates, one at each end. Both gates are opened, and the handler leads the horse through the rear gate into the stocks. Once the horse has cleared the rear gate and the handler has cleared the front gate, an assistant quietly closes the rear gate. The handler or assistant closes the front gate. Any adjustments to the side rails can then be made, if necessary, though it is generally best to have adjustments done before the horse enters, since the noise and movement may startle the horse. Occasionally it may be dangerous for the handler to walk through the stocks with the horse. If sedation is not effective or feasible, the handler can remain outside the stocks and carefully try to guide the horse through the gates.

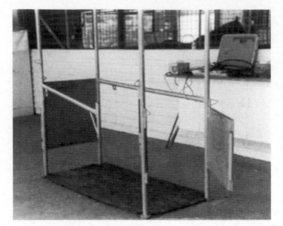

Fig. 3-20. Typical horse stocks. (From Speirs VC: *Clinical examination of horses*, St Louis, 1997, Saunders.)

Temporary makeshift "stocks" can be made on the farm by stacking straw or hay bales to prevent personnel from being kicked or to limit a horse's motion.

Horses should *never* be left unattended while in any type of stocks.

RESTRAINT OF FOALS

Capturing and restraining foals always begins with catching and controlling the mare. Foals naturally follow their dams, so leading the mare essentially results in leading the foal. Having assistants walk calmly behind the pair encourages the foal to move forward and stay close to the mare. Older foals may be accustomed to a halter and lead rope but naturally want to follow and be near the mare.

Controlling the mare is also important for the safety of personnel because some mares may be aggressive in attempting to protect their foals. Therefore someone should always be responsible for restraining the mare. In general, mares become more resistant as the distance between them and the foal increases; best results with the mare usually come when she is allowed to be as close as

possible to the foal, able to see and hear what is happening. Sometimes the mare must be sedated to assist working safely on the foal.

Once the mare is controlled and the foal is in the desired enclosure (e.g., stall, paddock), the foal is approached slowly from the side. Touching the foal on the neck or withers simulates the natural approach of the mare, but human touch is seldom appreciated at this age, and most foals instinctively try to escape by bolting forward, rearing, kicking, or "hitting reverse." Therefore once contact is made, it should be quick and purposeful. Foals are properly restrained with one arm around the shoulders or base of the neck; the hind end is controlled by placing the arm around the hindquarters or by using a tail hold with the hand (Fig. 3-21). The restrainer should avoid putting his or her head directly above the head or neck of the foal, since

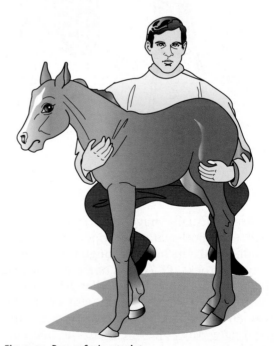

Fig. 3-21. Proper foal restraint.

many foals rear or throw their heads in an effort to resist being held.

Try not to oversupport a foal's bodyweight. Foals have a tendency to sag toward the ground when this is done.

For procedures that need to be performed with the foal in lateral recumbency on the ground, the foal should be sedated first and then gently laid on the ground by lifting the foal's body up and over. Unsedated foals should not be thrown to the ground unless it is medically contraindicated or impossible to sedate them first. Once on the ground, three people can provide ideal restraint. One person keeps pressure on the foal's neck to keep it from struggling to rise; this person may use hand pressure or gentle pressure by kneeling along the crest of the neck (never the ventral aspect of the neck, which could obstruct breathing). Another restrainer is responsible for the front legs and grasps each with the hands just above the carpus;

the hindlimb restrainer grasps both hindlimbs just above the tarsus. Grasping the legs below the carpus or tarsus runs the risk of growth plate fractures of the lower leg if the foal struggles. If the lower legs need to be further controlled, the restrainers may straddle the lower legs and firmly secure them between their own legs, while keeping their hold above the carpus/tarsus.

SUGGESTED READING

Ball MA: Restraint techniques, *The Horse* 34-37, Sept 1998.

French DD, Tully TN: Restraint and handling of animals. In McCurnin DM, Bassert JM, editors: *Clinical textbook for veterinary technicians*, ed 6, St Louis, 2006, Saunders.

Leahy JR, Barrow P: *Restraint of animals*, Ithaca, NY, 1953, Cornell Campus Store, Inc.

Sontsthagen TF: *Restraint of domestic animals*, St Louis, 1991, Mosby.

Equine patients must often receive medications as part of the treatment or management of their medical or surgical conditions. Various substances must also be given to healthy horses as part of their routine health maintenance. The size and anatomy of the horse presents some challenges in delivering these products in an effective manner. The most common routes of medication are oral (per os) and parenteral injection.

ORAL MEDICATION

Many medications are delivered via the oral route. These medications may be supplied in powder, tablet, or liquid form. Different strategies are available to deliver each of these drug forms.

FEED ADDITIVES

Oral medications may be given as feed additives, meaning they are added to the horse's dry feed, usually grain. The advantages of this approach are primarily convenience; powders and liquids can be added to the feed directly. There is no need to catch and restrain the horse with this method.

Placing whole tablets into the feed is seldom successful; therefore crushing the tablets to form a powder is preferred. Tablets can be crushed with a mortar and pestle or by the time-honored method of placing the tablets into a plastic bag and hitting them with a hammer against a hard surface. Large volumes of tablets can be ground with a standard food blender. Many large hospitals grind large volumes of tablets and store them in plastic containers for use over several days.

The disadvantages of this method are many. Medications often have an objectionable taste, leading horses to reject their food. Taste can be disguised with substances such as molasses, syrup, applesauce, pudding, and peanut butter, but some horses still reject the medicated feed. Attempts to hide the medicine in an apple or carrot also have mixed results. Another pitfall of powdered feed additives is a tendency to "fall through" or "sift" through the grain to the bottom of the feed tub as the horse eats. This results in underdosing because much of the dose settles to the bottom of the feed tub and is not consumed. Using sweet feed (which has molasses) or other sticky substances can improve delivery of the powder by preventing it from sifting through the feed. Another problem is that many horses spill grain from their mouths when they eat, leading to medication landing on the ground. Delivering medications by adding them to the feed can be a highly unreliable method of dosing horses and other large animals.

DOSE SYRINGES

Dose syringes can be used to deliver medications directly into the mouth. In order to use this method, the medication must be in a liquid or paste form. Powders can be mixed with liquid mediums such as molasses or applesauce to form a paste but must not be made into thick pastes that will be difficult to push through the opening of the syringe. Contrarily, the liquid medium should not be too watery, which may lead to spillage from the mouth. A thick syrup consistency is ideal (Box 4-1).

Dose syringes that may be bought commercially are usually capable of delivering up to 500 ml of liquid (Fig. 4-1). This large volume

---

BOX 4-1   Suggested Method of Preparing Medications for Delivery by Oral Syringe

The following steps are recommended for preparation of medications in solid or powder form into a mixture suitable for oral delivery directly into the mouth:

1. Convert solid tablets/pills to powder form:
   a. Capsules: Open the capsule to release the contents.
   b. Tablets/pills: Crush them to create a powder. A mortar/pestle is convenient for small numbers of pills. Most clients do not have a mortar and pestle; alternatively, they may put the prescribed number of pills into a sturdy plastic bag, close the bag, and use a hammer to crush the pills against a hard, smooth surface.
   c. In a hospital setting where crushing large numbers of pills for multiple patients by hand is too time consuming, a blender or food processor dedicated to pill grinding is helpful. The volume of powder for each dose of a medication must be determined: If a standard dose of drug X is 10 tablets, put 10 tablets into the blender and grind to powder form. Then retrieve the powder into a measuring spoon or scoop. This volume is recorded so that all staff know that 10 tablets equal a specific (tablespoons, cups, scoops, etc.) volume. This process can be repeated for different doses and for different medications. Large numbers of tablets can then be crushed in the blender, placed in an air-tight plastic container, and used daily for up to several days under proper storage conditions, using the measuring spoon or scoop to retrieve the powder from the container.
2. Place the appropriate dose of medication for the patient (e.g., 2 g phenylbutazone) into a small paper cup. Write the dose (e.g., 2 g PBZ) on a piece of adhesive tape (1 inch wide × 3 inches long); use a waterproof marker to write on the tape. Put the paper cup next to the piece of tape; the tape identifies the contents of the cup. If multiple patients are being treated, use multiple cups and tape markers for the contents of each cup.
   a. Some medications may be safely mixed together. If medications are compatible, place the appropriate doses of each into the cup and write all contents on the corresponding adhesive tape for proper identification.
3. Pour a thick liquid such as syrup or applesauce into each cup; molasses works especially well. Stir with a tongue depressor to mix the powder and liquid. Use only enough liquid to form a thick liquid consistency, like a thick cake batter. Too much liquid produces a runny medication, which tends to run out of the horse's mouth.
4. Choose an appropriate-sized syringe for the volume in the cup. Usually this is a 20-, 35-, or 60-ml syringe. The Luer tip must be removed to enlarge the opening; otherwise, the liquid mixture does not exit the syringe (even 60-ml catheter-tip syringes have difficulty delivering pasty medications; they should be reserved for pure liquids only). After snipping off the Luer tip, a small knife or file is used to enlarge the opening to approximately the size of a dime. Syringes can be premade and, after use, cleaned well with hot water and a brush, disinfected (if needed), rinsed, dried, and reused.
5. Remove the plunger from the syringe. Place the adhesive tape strip firmly across the opening of the syringe to identify the contents and keep them from leaking.
6. Tilt the paper cup and empty the contents into the barrel of the syringe. Use the tongue depressor to help scrape all of the medication into the syringe.
7. Replace the plunger into the syringe barrel. Set the assembled syringe on a slant for several minutes so that the medication settles backward against the plunger and away from the syringe opening. Once settled, depress the plunger to expel the air pocket through the syringe opening. The syringe is now ready for use.
8. Remove the adhesive tape just before administering the contents.

is seldom necessary to deliver most common medications, and a 60-ml catheter tip syringe is useful for smaller volumes. The opening of Luer-tip syringes is too small to make delivery of medication into the mouth feasible; this can be corrected by carefully cutting the Luer tip off of any syringe and enlarging the opening to dime size or slightly smaller. Twenty-, 35-, and 60-ml Luer-tip syringes that have been modified in this way are ideal for delivery of most oral medications.

When using any type of dose syringe, the fingers should be used to open the horse's lips before introducing the syringe (Fig. 4-2, *A*). Jamming the syringe into the mouth without warning may alarm and possibly injure the horse. The syringe should be introduced near the commissure of the lips. The lips should be slightly parted with the fingers or thumb, and the tip of the syringe carefully introduced toward the interdental space (Fig. 4-2, *B*). Once in the mouth, the syringe should be directed caudally between the cheek and the cheek teeth (Fig. 4-2, *C*).

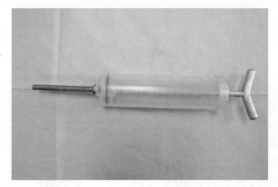

Fig. 4-1. Large dose syringe.

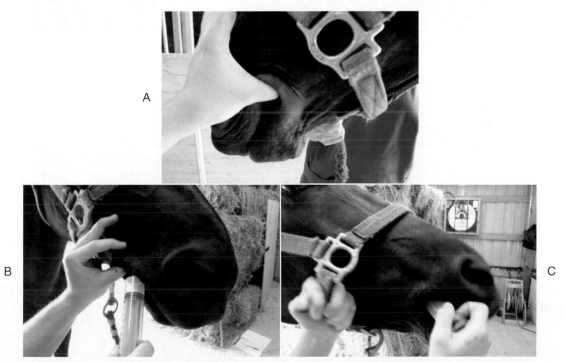

Fig. 4-2. A, Opening the lips before placing the oral syringe in the mouth. **B,** Placement of the dose syringe near the commissure of the lips. **C,** Proper positioning of the oral syringe.

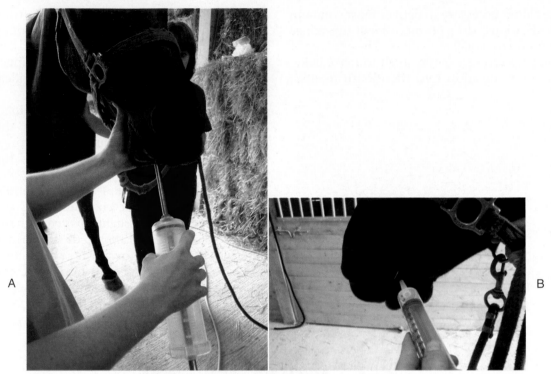

Fig. 4-3. Improper use of the dose syringe. **A,** Avoid placing the syringe over the incisors. **B,** Avoid delivering medication across the interdental space.

Avoid introducing the syringe over the incisors because the horse can bite and break the syringe (Fig. 4-3, *A*). Also avoid aiming the syringe over the base of the tongue, which increases the ability of the horse to spit out the medication and also increases the possibility of squirting the liquid into the trachea (Fig. 4-3, *B*). Most horses try to spit medication out of the mouth; this can be discouraged by elevating the chin after dispensing the medication and waiting for the horse to swallow. "Jiggling" the throat while the chin is elevated is an old trick to encourage swallowing. Regardless of the method used, the technician should *always* observe the horse after delivering oral medication to be sure the dose is consumed, not spit out on the ground.

The balling gun is an instrument designed to administer large tablets to large animals (Fig. 4-4). It is a poor choice for medicating horses. The balling gun must be placed deep into the mouth, over the base of the tongue, and horses typically resist by throwing their heads. Unfortunately, this may lead to lacerations and puncture wounds of the larynx and pharynx.

NASOGASTRIC INTUBATION

Nasogastric intubation is a variation of oral dosing. It involves placing a long, plastic "hose" from the nostril to the pharynx, where it enters the esophagus and is advanced into the stomach. The advantages of nasogastric intubation include reliable delivery of the entire dose to the patient and the ability to

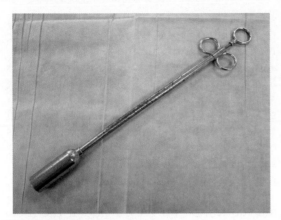

Fig. 4-4. Balling gun.

use the nasogastric tube as a diagnostic tool in addition to a medication tool. Disadvantages include trauma to the horse's turbinates, larynx, and pharynx, which can result in nosebleeds, abscesses, and inflammation and swelling. The turbinates are fragile, and nosebleeds occasionally happen to even the most skilled technician. Nosebleeds are especially likely if the horse throws its head during the procedure. If a nosebleed (epistaxis) occurs, the volume of the resulting hemorrhage may be impressive to the layman, but remember that the quantity is usually small in terms of the total blood volume of a horse. Elevating the head and possibly applying cold water or cold compresses over the nose may help. Unless the horse has a bleeding disorder, the hemorrhage is rarely life threatening and stops on its own. Horses with nosebleeds typically snort frequently, spraying blood droplets in every direction. Be prepared for this response.

Another disadvantage of nasogastric intubation is the possibility of "tubing the lungs," which occurs when the tube enters the trachea rather than the esophagus. Placing the tube in the trachea usually elicits coughing but is *not* a problem if the tube is withdrawn promptly. Problems occur when the tube is left in the trachea and liquids are delivered through the tube; the liquids run down the trachea and bronchi into the lungs, resulting in life-threatening pneumonia. Every precaution must be taken to prevent delivering medications into the trachea.

Another difficulty with nasogastric intubation is the fact that horses resent this procedure. Restraint is necessary with almost all horses, unless they are moribund. Physical restraint may be insufficient, and chemical restraint is often necessary. Since the tube is being placed through a nostril, the personnel involved in the procedure should stand to the side of the head and forequarters, out of reach of a possible strike with the front hooves.

Once a nasogastric tube is placed into the stomach, it should not be allowed to slide in and out, which could lead to accidental entry into the trachea. The person handling the head of the horse is often responsible for stabilizing the tube's position. The tube should be held firmly, and resting the hand against the horse's muzzle or halter helps keep the tube in the desired position if the horse moves its head.

Delivery of medication through the tube may be accomplished in several ways. A funnel may be placed into the opening of the tube, held above the level of the stomach, and the fluid poured into the funnel. This method is slow and somewhat cumbersome. Alternatively, a dose syringe containing the medication can be attached to the tube opening, and the plunger pushed to deliver the medication. The most common method is to place the medication or liquids to be delivered into a bucket or plastic jug and use a stomach pump to deliver the contents (Fig. 4-5). Whatever the method of delivery, liquids should never be forced against back pressure. The capacity of an average (1000 lb) horse's stomach is 4 to 5 gallons, and it is risky to approach or exceed this volume.

Typically, 1 gallon of fluid is the maximum given at one dosing, though this may be repeated at 30-minute or 1-hour intervals in urgent situations.

Most commercial nasogastric tubes are made of clear plastic materials. Nasogastric tubes come in several diameters, from foal size through large horse size (Fig. 4-6, *A*). Nasogastric tubes can be purchased with two options of openings at the stomach end of the tube (Fig. 4-6, *B*). A single opening at the stomach end is available; however, this type of tube tends to plug with debris (undigested material) once it enters the stomach. Tubes are also available with side ports, which are

small holes in the sidewall of the tube, near the end of the tube, in addition to the large main opening at the end of the tube. The addition of side ports makes blockage less likely. Side ports can be added to tubes using a piece of heated metal like a nail to melt several penetrating holes into the tube. All nasogastric tubes should have smooth edges on the main end hole and all side ports; sharp edges tend to grab and tear nasal tissue, resulting in nosebleeds.

Nasogastric tubes are never placed without lubrication on the outside of the tube. Water is the most common lubricant, but petroleum jellies such as obstetrical lubricants (OB lubes) can also be used. The lubricants do not need to be sterile. Mineral oil is a readily available alternative but is irritating to mucous membranes of the nose, and droplets may be inhaled into the lungs; its use for this purpose is discouraged.

An idiosyncrasy of the tubes is their sensitivity to temperature; they stiffen in cold temperatures. Excessively stiff tubes tend to cause nosebleeds. Soaking tubes in warm water before use softens them.

One advantage of using a nasogastric tube is that it can be left in place for 24 to 48 hours, allowing staff to medicate the horse

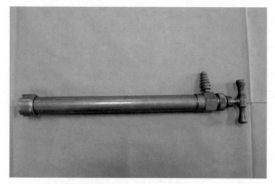

Fig. 4-5. Stomach pump.

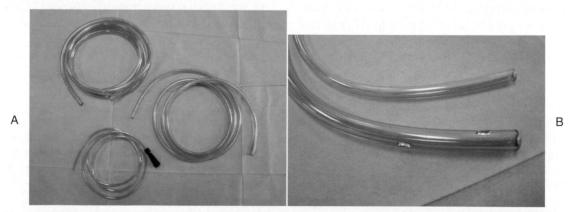

Fig. 4-6. **A,** Nasogastric tubes are available in different diameters. **B,** Single opening *(top)* and multiple side ports *(bottom).*

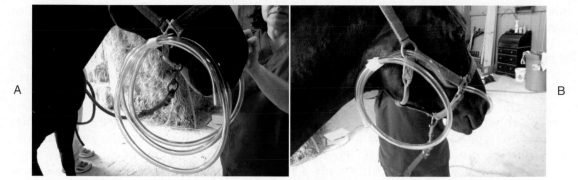

Fig. 4-7. **A,** One way of securing the nasogastric tube to the halter. **B,** Another way.

and/or monitor stomach contents without having to replace a tube every few hours. If the tube is to be left in place, it should be secured to the halter (Fig. 4-7). Adhesive tape is usually used to tape the tube to the halter, though clinicians have preferences as to how and where the tube is secured. Regardless of the method, the tube should not be secured with large loops through which a horse could place a hoof; this is important because horses with indwelling tubes are often being treated for abdominal pain (colic), which is often accompanied by lowering the head and pawing with the front feet. If the feet are put through the tube loops, the tube can be ripped from its position in the stomach. It is helpful to mark the position of an indwelling tube with a simple ring of adhesive tape at the level of the nostril so that the staff can easily see if the horse has dislodged the tube from its original position (Fig. 4-8).

Some clinicians feel that the nasogastric tube provides a possible route for air to enter the stomach, leading to bloat. These clinicians usually cap the external opening of the tube with a syringe plunger or syringe case to prevent aspiration of air. Other clinicians do not feel that aspiration of air is a problem and leave the tube open. This is based on clinician preference, since data

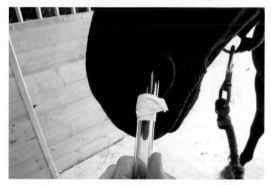

Fig. 4-8. Proper position of the tube is marked with adhesive tape at the level of the nostril.

have not proven that either approach is problematic.

Removal of the nasogastric tube requires some skill to prevent nosebleeds. Removal should not become a "taffy pull," where the operator grabs the tube in one place and pulls it completely out of the nose. The tendency of most horses is to throw their head upward, especially when the last 12 to 24 inches of the tube are removed, effectively turning the tube into an "intranasal whip" and causing a nosebleed. The operator should keep the hands close to the nostril, retrieving a 12-inch section with one hand, then regrasping with the other hand and withdrawing another 12 inches, and so on to remove the tube in short segments and therefore maintain control of the tube at all times.

When a tube is removed, there is often liquid material *inside* the tube. If this material is not controlled, it can dribble out of the tube as it is withdrawn and be inhaled into the lungs as the tube is withdrawn. Covering the external opening of the tube during its removal is important; this prevents liquids from flowing out of the tube. To do this, either cover the external opening with a thumb or finger or crimp the tube by folding it over double during removal.

PARENTERAL INJECTION TECHNIQUES

Syringes and needles can be used to deliver injections by many routes. The route selected depends on many factors, including Food and Drug Administration (FDA)–approved routes of injection (listed on the label of all medications), tractability of the patient, capability of the person performing the injection, toxicities of the medication, and temperament of the patient. The most common routes of injection are intramuscular (IM), intravenous (IV), subcutaneous (SC or SQ), and intradermal (ID).

Before any parenteral injection, the skin should be cleaned appropriately. Some procedures require sterile preparation of the skin, such as IV catheterization and joint injections. However, for most routine injections, cleaning of the skin and hair with isopropyl alcohol is sufficient. The alcohol can be placed on a cotton swab or gauze 4 × 4 and should be used to vigorously wipe the intended injection site. Wipe repeatedly until the cotton or gauze is essentially clean. A common mistake is to just wipe over the hair; the alcohol should *thoroughly* soak the skin. Even if the skin over the site appears to be clean, alcohol should be used, even though it does not thoroughly disinfect the skin. Scrubbing with alcohol removes some

debris and makes a positive impression on the client.

If the horse is being medicated with injectable drugs, multiple injections are often required over a several-day period. This tends to make the horse sore, especially if large volumes of drug are given at each injection. It is helpful to have a rotation plan for the injections, where the location of the shot is rotated to prevent overuse of a single site. For instance, the jugular veins can be alternated at each injection for IV injections. For IM injections, the left neck can be used first, then the left hindquarter, then the right neck, then the right hindquarter, etc.

INTRAMUSCULAR INJECTIONS

Strictly speaking, any skeletal muscle that can be accessed safely can be used for an IM injection. However, several muscles are more readily accessible than others: the brachiocephalicus, pectoral, gluteal, semitendinosus, and triceps brachii.

Muscles do not have unlimited capacity for injection. It is recommended that the maximum volume of injection be limited to 15 ml in any single location; in smaller muscle bellies like the pectoral and semitendinosus, 5 to 10 ml is a maximum volume. In large draft horses, these volumes may be increased by an additional 5 ml. Some common medications such as procaine penicillin G require volumes of approximately 30 ml at each treatment in an average horse; obviously, this dose must be split into two sites of 15 ml each. Two separate injection sites can be used or the needle can be placed for administration of half the dose, then the bevel partially withdrawn to the level of the subcutaneous tissue, redirected at a 45-degree angle to the first injection angle, and reinserted along this new line. The second half of the dose can then be administered.

Some drugs are toxic or injurious if accidentally injected intravenously. Therefore *all* IM injections should be "screened" *before* delivering the drug to ensure that the bevel of the needle is *not* in the lumen of a blood vessel. This is accomplished by stabilizing and aspirating the syringe—pulling *gently* backward on the plunger—before injecting. If blood is seen in the needle hub or syringe, the needle should be withdrawn and discarded, and a new needle inserted and aspirated again, before injecting.

Selecting a diameter and length of syringe needle depends on the size of the muscle to be injected, the volume to be delivered, and the consistency of the medication. Thicker medications require larger diameters. In general, most IM injections are done with a range of 18- to 22-gauge (ga) needles; the length is usually 1 to 1½ inches. Foals and ponies require the shorter length, and smaller muscles like the pectoral also need the 1-inch length. Thin horses with little muscle mass are also candidates for shorter needles.

Following IM injections, bleeding from the injection site is common. This blood is usually from skin vessels that were punctured during insertion of the needle and does *not* imply that the needle bevel was in a blood vessel at the time of injection. The bleeding can be controlled with hand pressure over the site. Bleeding leaves red stains on the haircoat, which is unsightly in light-colored horses. It leaves a better impression to clean this blood from the horse, using peroxide or alcohol, than to leave a large blood stain.

Injection abscesses are a potential complication of IM injections. They are more likely to occur when injections are given through dirty skin and seem to occur more often following biological products such as vaccines than other products. As with any abscess, part of the treatment is providing drainage. Drainage occurs best when it is ventral, allowing gravity to constantly assist the process.

Of the commonly used injection sites, the pectorals and semitendinosus muscles provide the best access for ventral drainage. Conversely, the brachiocephalicus and gluteals provide poor drainage access.

INTRAMUSCULAR INJECTION SITES

Lateral Cervical

The most common site for IM injection is the lateral aspect of the neck, in the brachiocephalicus or serratus ventralis muscle. This area is easy to access, and personnel can stand to the side of the forequarters, where a strike or kick is less likely. The landmarks for safe injection are (1) a hand's width ventral to the crest of the neck (Fig. 4-9, *A*), (2) a hand's width dorsal to the jugular groove (Fig. 4-9, *B*), and (3) a hand's width cranial to the cranial border of the scapula (Fig. 4-9, *C*). These landmarks outline a large triangle (Fig. 4-9, *D*), and the injection can be safely administered anywhere in this area. Following cleansing of the skin, the needle is inserted at an angle perpendicular to the skin and inserted to its full depth. The needle should be stabilized while its position is checked by gentle aspiration, and then the medication is delivered. The skin over the neck is somewhat loose, and the author prefers a technique where the skin is first pinched with one hand before the injection (Fig. 4-10, *A*). While maintaining this skin pinch, the needle is inserted about 1 to 2 inches directly caudal to the skin pinch (Fig. 4-10, *B*). Pinching the skin accomplishes two things: (1) It distracts from the pain of the needle, and (2) when the skin is released, it slides caudally to cover the IM needle track, providing a physiological "bandage."

The lateral cervical area is contraindicated in nursing foals for IM injection. Soreness usually follows IM injection, and foals with sore necks tend to avoid nursing. Other sites such as the semitendinosus are better choices in nursing foals.

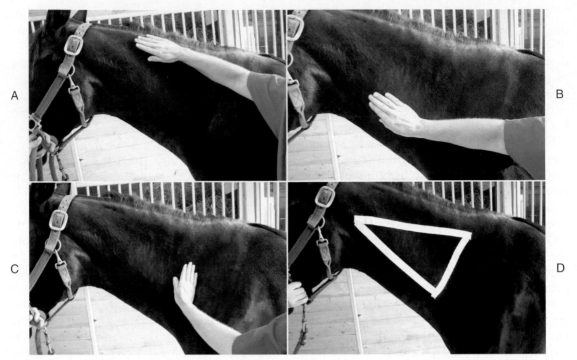

Fig. 4-9. Landmarks for lateral cervical injections. **A,** Landmark ventral to the crest of the neck. **B,** Landmark dorsal to the jugular groove. **C,** Landmark cranial to the scapula. **D,** Borders for intramuscular injections into the lateral cervical area.

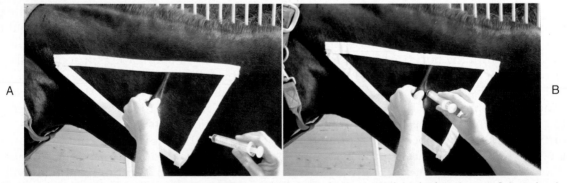

Fig. 4-10. Lateral cervical injection technique. **A,** Pinching the skin before intramuscular injection into the neck. **B,** Inserting the needle caudal to the skin pinch.

Pectoral Muscle

The pectorals are suitable for smaller volumes of injection, less than 5 ml in most cases, though larger horses can receive up to 10 ml per injection. In general, a 1-inch needle is used. This muscle is somewhat movable in the standing horse, and one hand should be used to stabilize the muscle belly while the other hand inserts the needle at a 90-degree angle to the skin (Fig. 4-11). Be sure to stand to the side of the forequarters, out of range of a potential forelimb strike.

The pectorals have good ventral drainage compared with other IM sites, which is an advantage if an injection abscess develops.

Triceps Muscle

The triceps is generally used when all other common sites have been exhausted. It is not suitable for large injection volumes and should be avoided in any performance animal unless absolutely necessary; this is due to fear of soring and/or scarring the triceps, which is the main muscle that propels the forelimb. Soreness and scarring could produce lameness and poor performance.

Gluteal Muscles

The gluteal muscle actually consists of several muscle bellies in the rump area. The skin overlying this area is thick and fairly tight, and more force is required to penetrate it with a needle than in other locations. For this reason, small-diameter needles should be used cautiously, and 18- to 20-ga syringe needles are recommended for most medications.

The landmarks for safe injection are (1) a hand's width lateral to the spine (dorsal midline) (Fig. 4-12, *A*), (2) a hand's width caudal to the tuber coxae (Fig. 4-12, *B*), and (3) a hand's width dorsal to the greater trochanter of the femur (Fig. 4-12, *C*). These landmarks define a circular area, and injections can be safely given within these boundaries (Fig. 4-12, *D*).

The technician should stand beside the flank or area of the point of the hip, facing caudally during the injection. In general, the farther cranial that the technician stands, the more likely he or she is to avoid a kick from a hindleg.

Horses do not like to be surprised with needles, and if the needle is thrust into the animal with no warning, a kick is a common response. One helpful technique is to use the base of the hand to firmly thump the skin three or four times just before inserting the needle; this serves as notice that something is about to happen (alternatively, if the horse's attitude makes thumping unwise, at least try to firmly rub the area). The area is

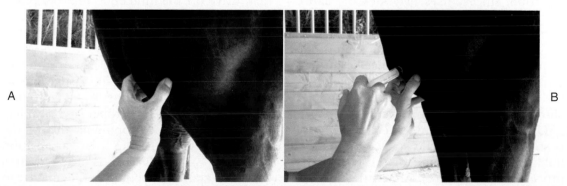

Fig. 4-11. Pectoral muscle intramuscular (IM) injection technique. **A,** Stabilizing a pectoral muscle for IM injection. **B,** Inserting the needle at a 90-degree angle to the skin.

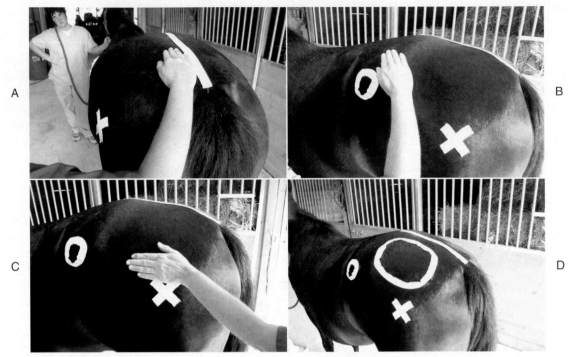

Fig. 4-12. Landmarks for gluteal injections. **A,** Landmark lateral to the spine. **B,** Landmark caudal to the tuber coxae (point of the hip). **C,** Landmark dorsal to the greater trochanter of the femur. **D,** Boundaries for safe intramuscular injection into the gluteal muscle.

thumped, and then the needle is immediately inserted perpendicular to the skin, to its full depth. It is recommended *not* to leave the syringe attached to the needle during insertion, since horses may kick or "dance around" after the needle is inserted. If a horse moves around and the technician cannot hold on to the syringe, the weight of the syringe essentially turns the needle into an intramuscular blade, lacerating muscle fibers and blood vessels as the syringe wobbles above the skin (Fig. 4-13, *A* and *B*).

Once the needle is inserted, and the horse is still, one hand should stay committed to holding the needle hub for the rest of the procedure (Fig. 4-13, *C*). Attach the syringe, aspirate to check position, and then deliver the medication. The syringe and needle are

withdrawn as a unit when the injection is complete.

The gluteal muscles should be avoided in racehorses and other performance horses that "drive off the hind end," to avoid possible muscle soreness or scarring.

Semitendinosus Muscle

The semitendinosus muscle is well suited to smaller injection volumes, less than 10 ml. As with the gluteals, care must be taken to prevent being kicked. The proper site for injection is at the most prominent area of the buttocks as viewed from a lateral position (Fig. 4-14, *A*). The needle is inserted in a caudal-to-cranial direction, perpendicular to the skin (Fig. 4-14, *B* and *C*). The needle must avoid the sciatic nerve, which lies in the

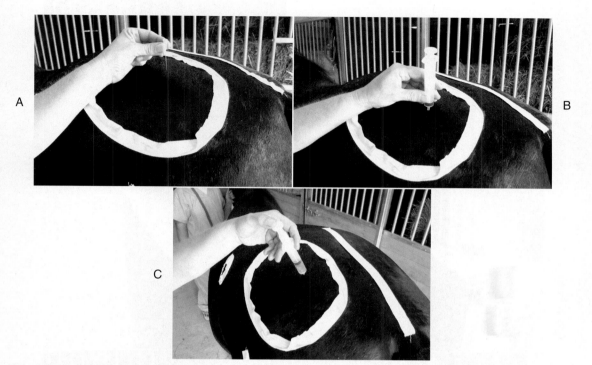

Fig. 4-13. A, Insertion of the needle into the gluteal muscle. **B,** Attachment of the syringe after insertion of the needle. **C,** Avoid giving the injection without stabilizing the syringe hub.

easily visible groove on the caudolateral aspect of the thigh (Fig. 4-14, *D*). The needle should be inserted before attaching the syringe, in case the horse moves or kicks. An alternative approach that provides additional safety from kicks is to stand on the opposite side of the horse (i.e., stand beside the left hindquarters and insert the needle into the right semitendinosus muscle) and reach across the buttocks to insert the needle.

INTRAVENOUS INJECTIONS

Injections can be given into any vein that is visible or palpable and safely accessed. By far, most IV medications are given into the jugular vein.

Needles for IV injections may range from 14- to 22-ga in diameter and be 1- or 1½-inch in length, depending on the viscosity of medication to be injected and size of the vein. The 14-ga needle is used for rapid fluid infusions and administration of euthanasia solutions, which must be injected rapidly. The author prefers a 19-ga × 1½-inch length for most equine IV injections and 20-ga × 1-inch length for foals. It is highly recommended to place the needle first, confirm its position, then stabilize the needle hub while attaching the syringe *and* while injecting.

Some controversy exists as to the direction of IV injections. Some prefer to inject with the flow of blood in the vein, while others inject against the blood flow. Injecting against the direction of blood flow creates turbulence, which some fear may cause clotting of the blood. While there is some intuitive sense to this argument, to the author's

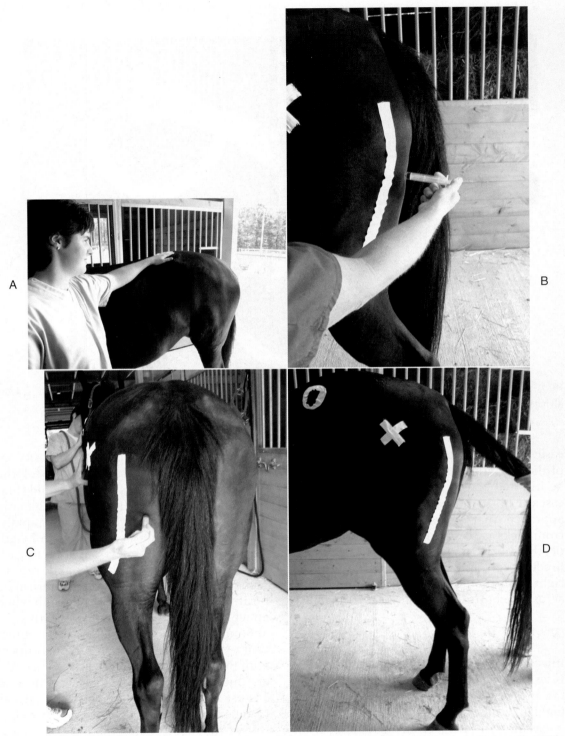

Fig. 4-14. Semitendinosus injection technique. **A**, Location of the most prominent area of the buttocks. **B**, Insertion of the needle from cranial to caudal into the semitendinosus muscle. **C**, Proper technique for intramuscular semitendinosus injection. **D**, Location of the sciatic groove *(curved white line)*.

knowledge it has never been proved that either method is superior to the other. Personal preference dictates the technique used.

Some horses and foals resent IV injections. It may be helpful to firmly pinch the skin over the site of the injection just before inserting the needle; this has a numbing effect on the skin. If using this method, it is unnecessary to pull the skin far—just a simple fingertip pinch is sufficient. Be sure not to contaminate the insertion site with a dirty hand.

IV injections should always begin by distending the vein, then visualizing and/or palpating the vein to identify its course. Best results are obtained when the needle mimics (parallels) the course of the vein; trying to hit a vein from an angled or skewed approach is more difficult to accomplish. Once the needle is aligned over the distended vein, the needle is tilted to a 45-degree angle to the skin and advanced through the skin in a single smooth motion and into the vein. Unlike IM injections, the needle should not enter perpendicularly to the skin.

The speed of injection depends on the intent of the drug and possible side effects. Euthanasia solutions and some anesthetics are intentionally bolused. Other medications have serious complications if given too rapidly intravenously. Most substances are best delivered by a slow injection technique, allowing them to mix and dilute with the blood.

INTRAVENOUS INJECTION SITES

Jugular Vein

The jugular vein is used for most IV procedures in large animals. It is readily accessible, and personnel can position themselves away from strikes and kicks from the hooves. It is also the largest-diameter peripheral vein, which makes identification and puncture easier than other veins.

The jugular vein lies just below the skin in the jugular groove (Fig. 4-15). The anatomy of this area is important; the carotid artery and vagosympathetic nerve trunk lie deep to the jugular vein and parallel to it. It is possible to insert a syringe needle such that it goes completely through or around the jugular, penetrating the carotid artery and, rarely, the vagosympathetic trunk.

There are several consequences of a "carotid stick." Large hematomas can result, and while they are seldom life threatening, they can take days to weeks to resolve and are at risk for infection. The blemish they produce can keep a horse from the sale ring, show ring, or race, causing unhappy clients. Another consequence can occur if medication is injected into the carotid artery; blood in the artery is traveling rapidly to the brain, and when the brain receives boluses of certain drugs, horses may collapse, have seizures, display dementia, and even die from cardiac or respiratory arrest. Horses may recover from these effects but be left with permanent neurological defects. Injecting any compound into the carotid artery must be avoided.

The risk of accidental carotid injection can be minimized in several ways. Whenever possible, the cranial half of the jugular groove should be used for vein access (Fig. 4-16). In the cranial half of the jugular groove, the omohyoideus muscle is interposed between the jugular vein and the carotid artery, affording some protection to the artery (Fig. 4-17). However, this muscle is not thick enough to totally prevent a carotid stick, and other precautions should still be observed.

It is recommended to insert the needle first, without the syringe, so that the needle's position can be confirmed. When the needle is placed in the jugular vein and the vein is distended by manual pressure, blood should flow freely from the hub of the needle. This blood, however, is not under high pressure as it exits the hub, and because it is venous blood, there is no pulse effect of the blood as

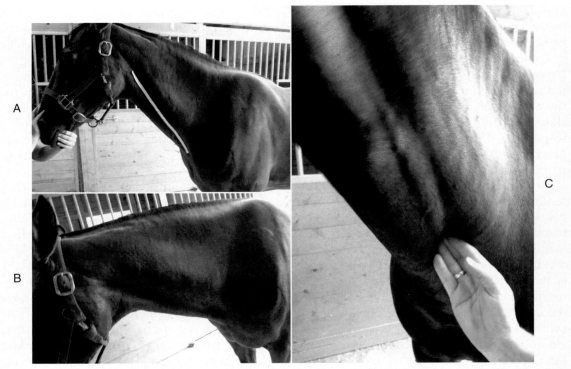

Fig. 4-15. Anatomy of the jugular vein area. **A,** Location of the jugular groove. **B,** The jugular groove. **C,** Distension of the jugular vein.

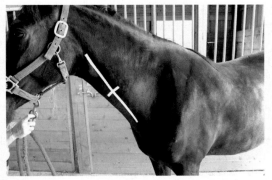

Fig. 4-16. Demarcation of cranial and caudal portions of the jugular groove.

it exits. In contrast, carotid arterial blood is under high pressure and may squirt up to several feet out of the needle hub; additionally, the blood often displays a pulsing effect.

The color of the blood exiting the hub has been used as a criterion for needle location, with dark blood assumed to be jugular venous blood and bright red blood assumed to be arterial. However, this method is highly unreliable and is not recommended.

Once the needle has been inserted and its position in the jugular vein confirmed, one hand should be committed to stabilizing the needle hub while the syringe is attached and the medication delivered. Maintaining the position of the needle prevents accidental advancement into the carotid artery, as well as accidental injection into the perivascular tissues. Some medications are highly irritating when injected outside the vein and can lead to large areas of inflammation, skin slough, and permanent scarring. The technician should be certain that the needle bevel

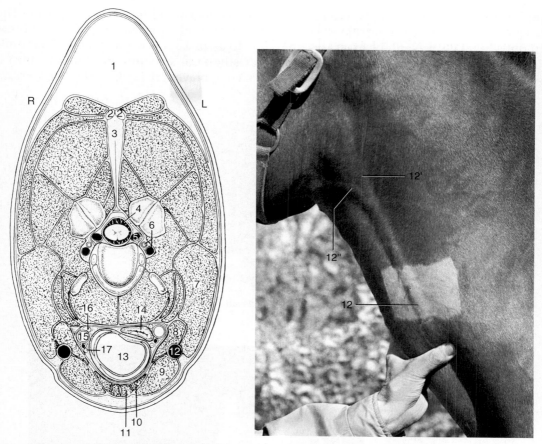

Fig. 4-17. Cross-section of the cranial portion of the neck. *12*, Jugular vein. *12'*, Maxillary vein. *12"*, Linguofacial vein. (From Dyce KM, Sack WO, Wensing CJG: *Textbook of veterinary anatomy*, ed 3, St Louis, 2002, Saunders.)

rests inside the lumen of the jugular vein to avoid these complications.

After the injection, the needle is removed and finger pressure is applied to the venipuncture site to prevent bleeding. Sedated horses or horses that hold the head lower than the heart can experience blood loss into the subcutaneous tissues around the venipuncture site, leading to hematomas. Elevating the head and applying manual pressure can prevent hematoma formation. Similar precautions should be taken with accidental puncture of the carotid artery; elevate the head and apply firm pressure to the area for at least 5 minutes.

Lateral Thoracic Vein, Cephalic Vein, Saphenous Vein, Coccygeal Vein

These veins can be accessed when the jugular vein is not an alternative for IV injection. They are considerably smaller than the jugular vein, and injections of large volumes are slower and technically more difficult. For most purposes, a 1-inch long syringe needle is adequate.

The lateral thoracic vein runs along the ventrolateral aspect of the thorax (Fig. 4-18).

Clipping the hair can facilitate visualizing this vein if the haircoat is long. Blood in the vein flows cranially toward the brachial vein.

The cephalic vein (forelimb) and saphenous vein (hindlimb) are leg veins that are difficult to access in standing horses (Fig. 4-19). They are more useful for sedated patients or horses or foals in lateral recumbency while under anesthesia or sedation. Precautions must be taken to prevent being kicked while accessing

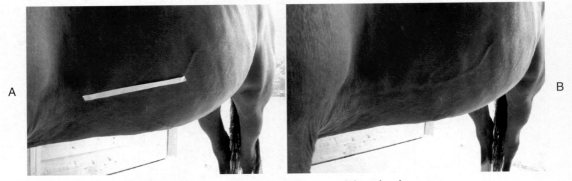

Fig. 4-18. **A,** Location of the lateral thoracic vein. **B,** Closer view of the lateral thoracic vein.

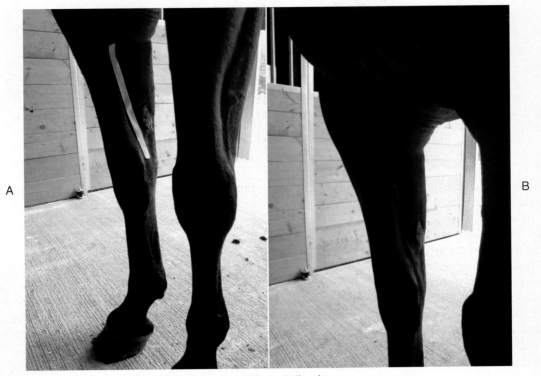

Fig. 4-19. **A,** Location of the cephalic vein. **B,** Closer view of the cephalic vein.

these veins. Motion of the legs can easily dislodge the needle during injection.

The coccygeal vein lies on the ventral midline of the tail, adjacent to the coccygeal artery. It is best accessed near the base of the tail (Fig. 4-20). Use of this vein should be restricted to only small volumes of nonirritating substances; any swelling or perivascular scarring in this area may occlude the coccygeal artery, which is the main (and only) arterial supply to the tail. The entire tail may slough if this occurs.

SUBCUTANEOUS INJECTION

Subcutaneous injections are easiest to perform in fleshy areas where the skin is loose and elastic, allowing the technician to lift the skin and slide the needle between the tented skin and the underlying muscle tissue. The most common place for SC injections in large animals is under the skin of the lateral aspect of the neck.

The skin is tented (Fig. 4-21, *A*), and the needle is advanced into the "tent" at an angle nearly paralleling the surface of the neck (Fig. 4-21, *B*). Once the needle bevel is completely in the subcutaneous space, the skin is released and the injection made; releasing the skin allows the technician to observe the "skin bleb," which usually confirms correct delivery of the injection. When the needle is properly placed, there is little resistance to injection.

SC injections are not suitable for large volumes of fluid in large animals, and therefore the SC route is not used for fluid therapy as it is in small animals. Syringe needles from 20- to 25-ga × 1-inch length are used.

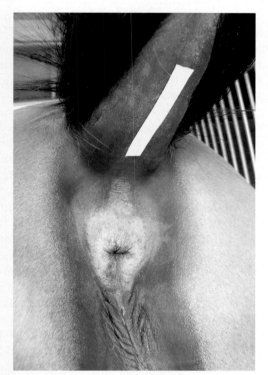

Fig. 4-20. Location of the coccygeal vein.

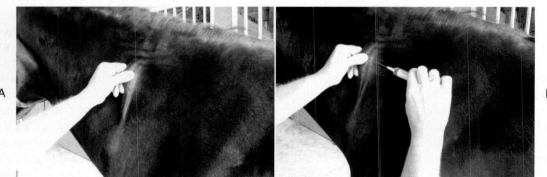

Fig. 4-21. **A,** Elevating the skin for subcutaneous injection. **B,** Injection technique for subcutaneous injection.

INTRADERMAL INJECTION

ID injection is rarely used to administer medications but is used mainly for diagnostic testing in large animals for tuberculosis (cattle) and skin testing for allergies.

Only volumes less than 1 ml can be injected into the skin at a single site. A 25-ga needle is the largest size used for ID injections. After cleaning the skin, the needle is laid nearly parallel to the skin, bevel up, and advanced into the skin. This is a shallow injection, and care must be taken not to enter the subcutaneous tissue. The syringe plunger is gently withdrawn to be sure that the bevel is not within a blood vessel; if no blood is aspirated, the injection is completed. A visible bleb should appear in the skin.

ADVERSE REACTIONS

Adverse reactions may occur following any medication. Some reactions are allergic (hypersensitivity or immune mediated), and the manifestations may be local or generalized (anaphylaxis). Anaphylactic shock may be life threatening, leading to respiratory distress, collapse, and death. Most local allergic reactions (skin wheals, hives, facial edema, etc.) are not life threatening, but they can be uncomfortable for the horse (pruritus). If facial edema is severe, breathing may be compromised. A veterinarian should be consulted when any allergic reaction is suspected.

Adverse vaccine reactions are uncommon. They may produce anaphylactic reactions, but this is very rare. Most vaccine reactions are mild and localized, consisting of muscle soreness at the injection site (especially stiff neck), swelling at the injection site, mildly elevated temperature (<101.5° F), and 24 to 48 hours of depression and loss of appetite. Abscesses may develop. Cold compresses at the injection site and administration of a nonsteroidal antiinflammatory drug such as phenylbutazone may be helpful in the acute

phase of a local reaction. If a firm swelling develops over the next several days, an abscess may be organizing; hot packs may be warranted. If body temperature is greater than 101.5° F at any time or if depression and loss of appetite continue for more than 48 hours, the veterinarian should be consulted.

Reactions may relate to the rate of administration; this is usually a problem with IV medications. Bolus administration of some drugs, especially those with potassium or calcium, may have adverse effects on the cardiovascular system.

Reactions may occur with inadvertent IV injection of drugs that are not intended for IV use or accidental injection into the carotid artery of drugs that are intended for other routes. Effects may include dementia, collapse, and death.

Chemical damage to tissue may occur with improper injection techniques. This is most common with perivascular injection of drugs intended for IV use. Phenylbutazone and barbiturates are the most common examples of this complication; if injected outside a vein, severe tissue inflammation and necrosis may occur.

Procaine penicillin G, a commonly used antibiotic in horses, is approved only for IM injection. Two types of adverse reactions are associated with use of this drug. True penicillin allergy occurs rarely and usually manifests as skin wheals/hives. Horses with true penicillin allergy should not receive penicillin drugs after the allergic reaction is observed. More common than allergy, however, is poor injection technique, which results in accidental injection into the bloodstream, and when the drug reaches the brain, dementia, hyperesthesia, and collapse may occur. This type of reaction is related to the procaine portion of the drug and is not an allergic reaction. Most horses will recover from a procaine reaction. These animals may safely receive future doses of the drug, provided that it is not again injected directly into the bloodstream. These two types of reactions are often confused by clients, who report that their horse had an allergic reaction to penicillin, when in fact it was most likely a reaction to a bloodstream injection. Careful questioning of the client usually distinguishes which type of reaction the horse actually experienced.

Adverse systemic reactions warrant immediate treatment. If the medication is still being administered, it should be stopped immediately and the patient should be evaluated. Treatment may range from simply keeping the animal warm, to treatment with corticosteroids, epinephrine, or IV fluids, to emergency establishment of a patent airway with nasotracheal intubation or even tracheostomy. The clinician should be alerted whenever an adverse reaction is suspected. An emergency "crash kit" containing emergency drugs and tracheostomy equipment is essential in any practice (Box 4-2) and should be readily available.

INTRAVENOUS CATHETERIZATION

Intravenous catheterization has become a readily available, commonplace procedure in equine medicine. Catheters may be placed for short-term use, as for induction/maintenance of anesthesia, emergency fluid administration, and euthanasia. Long-term use is also possible for patients requiring long-term fluid therapy or IV medication. If properly placed and maintained, catheters are safe to use and save the pain and discomfort of multiple IV perforations.

CATHETER SELECTION

Catheters are available in different lengths, diameters, and materials. Selection of catheters should not be a "one-size-fits-all" proposition but should be adaptable to the patient and the patient's needs. To minimize

---

BOX 4-2 Equine Emergency Crash Kit

Drugs
Atropine 1% injection (inj.)
Calcium gluconate 23%
Diazepam 5 mg/ml inj.
Dopamine 200 mg/20 ml inj.
Doxapram 20 mg/ml inj.
Epinephrine 1:1000 inj.
Glycopyrrolate inj.
Lidocaine 2% inj.
Prednisolone sodium succinate inj.
Sodium chloride 0.9%
Xylazine 100 mg/ml inj.
Note: Be sure to have an emergency drug dose/dilution chart readily available.

Syringes / **Needles**
60 ml × 1 — 20-ga × 1 inch (5)
30 ml × 2 — 20-ga × 1½ inch (10)
20 ml × 3 — 18-ga × 1½ inch (10)
12 ml × 5 — 18-ga × 3½ inch (2)
6 ml × 5 — 18-ga × 6 inch (2)
3 ml × 5 — 14-ga × 3 inch (2)

Catheters
10- to 12-ga × 5½ inch (5)
16-ga × 5½ inch (3)
Extension set (2)
Administration set (2)

Airway Supplies
Endotracheal tube 14 mm (1)
Endotracheal tube 9 mm (1)
Oral speculum/bite block (1)
Air syringe 60 ml (1)
KY (sterile lubricating) Jelly (1)
Tracheostomy tube, self-retaining
Disposable scalpel handle (1)
Disposable No. 10 blade (3)
Forceps, Kelly (2)

Miscellaneous
Adhesive tape, 1-inch diameter
Heparin flush
Surgical skin stapler

the risk of thrombophlebitis, the shortest-length, smallest-diameter, least-reactive catheter that will accomplish the treatment goals should be chosen.

The length of the catheter must be carefully considered. Catheters are either long (5 to 6 inches) or short (2 to 3 inches). Short catheters can be used successfully in foals and small ponies but must be used carefully in larger patients. This is because the short lengths are stiff, and if the horse turns its head to the side, there is a possibility of the catheter tip perforating the vein when the horse returns the head to a forward-facing position. Short catheters are not suitable for long-term use. It should be noted, however, that the risk for thrombophlebitis increases with increasing catheter length.

Catheter diameter is another factor that must be considered. The primary factor in choosing diameter is the "need for speed" (i.e., how rapidly the medication or fluid must be delivered). The most commonly used diameters are 10-, 14-, and 16-ga. Ten-gauge catheters are recommended for emergency administration of large fluid volumes. Sixteen-gauge catheters are useful for repeated IV medication, with or without small IV fluid volumes. For most general purposes, a 14-ga diameter is the most commonly used, especially where administration of large volumes of maintenance fluids are necessary. Because the risk of thrombophlebitis rises as catheter diameter increases, the smallest diameter that can accomplish the treatment goals should be chosen.

Catheters may be constructed from different materials. These materials vary in tissue reactivity—the tendency to cause inflammation and/or initiate the clotting cascade. The materials also affect mechanical properties such as the tendency to kink and ease of insertion. Tissue reactivity also affects the tendency to cause thrombophlebitis, and this tendency is related primarily to the softness of the material. Stiff materials are associated with a higher risk of thrombophlebitis. Some of the more commonly available catheter materials are polypropylene, Teflon, polyurethane, and silicone. Polypropylene is the stiffest and most reactive of the materials; polypropylene catheters are usually large in diameter, which makes them desirable for emergency IV fluid administration. However, because of their reactivity, they should not be used beyond 24 hours and should be replaced if IV therapy is still necessary after that time. Teflon and polyurethane have moderate stiffness/reactivity and can be used safely for 7 days on average if properly maintained; these are the most popular IV catheters currently in use. Silicone is the most pliable and least reactive material; with sterile placement and careful maintenance, silicone catheters have been safely left in place for 4 weeks. However, silicone catheters are available only in smaller diameters, restricting their use for fluid therapy to small volumes only. Their low reactivity makes silicone a popular choice for neonates.

CATHETER SITES

Almost all IV catheters in large animals are placed in the jugular vein. Although the esophagus usually lies on the left side of the trachea, penetration of the esophagus by the catheter is unlikely, and either jugular vein may be used with safety. If the jugular veins are not usable, the next choice is usually the lateral thoracic vein (Fig. 4-22). The median, cephalic, and saphenous veins of the legs are available but are difficult to enter because of the tendency of the veins to collapse once the catheter is introduced, making advancing the catheter to its proper depth difficult. Also, even if successfully placed, motion of the legs makes it difficult to prevent kinking and dislodgement. Leg veins are easier to access with the patient in lateral recumbency versus standing.

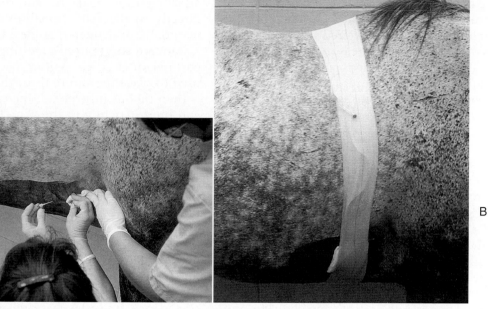

Fig. 4-22. Insertion of a catheter into the lateral thoracic vein. **A,** Note that the direction of insertion is caudal to cranial, which follows the flow of blood through the vein. **B,** The catheter and extension set are secured with elastic adhesive tape. (From Colahan P et al: *Equine medicine and surgery,* ed 5, St Louis, 1999, Mosby.)

INTRAVENOUS CATHETER PLACEMENT TECHNIQUE

In general, the location for perforation of the vein should be as far "upstream" (with regard to the direction of blood flow) as possible. If the first attempt at insertion is unsuccessful, further attempts can be made "downstream." This minimizes irritation to endothelium that is trying to heal from unsuccessful punctures.

Aseptic technique should be followed. The hair is clipped, and shaving is recommended if long-term placement of the catheter (more than 4 to 5 days) is anticipated. Occasionally, owners request that the hair not be clipped; catheters can be inserted safely if aseptic technique is followed, but owners should be warned that there may be an increased risk of infection.

After clipping, the skin should be surgically prepared with an appropriate scrub solution followed with isopropyl alcohol wipes. A minimum of three scrub/alcohol applications should be performed. Examination gloves should be worn for prepping the skin.

Local anesthesia of the skin over the vein is almost never necessary. However, it should always be performed in foals and in individuals that are "needle shy." If local anesthesia is used, no more than 1 ml of anesthetic should be used. Placing large blebs of anesthetic makes visualization and palpation of the vein difficult and is no more effective than the smaller volume. Local anesthetic is delivered with a 25-ga needle into the SC tissue.

Cutdowns are sometimes performed in other species to facilitate IV access. This procedure involves local anesthesia of the skin followed by a small skin incision; the catheter is then introduced directly into the vein. Cutdowns are almost never necessary in horses, unless the desired site of insertion is obscured for some reason.

Insertion technique is similar to the technique for venipuncture. The insertion angle should mimic the course of the vein, and the catheter should enter at a 45-degree angle to the skin (Fig. 4-23, *A* and *B*). Once the tip of the catheter is in the vein, blood should flow freely from the hub. At this point, the catheter stylet should be withdrawn only 1 to 2 inches; this gives the catheter some rigidity as it is advanced fully into the vein (Fig. 4-23, *C*). Full removal of the stylet before advancing the catheter invites kinking of the catheter. With the stylet slightly withdrawn, the catheter/stylet is carefully advanced, as a unit, fully into the vein (Fig. 4-23, *D*). Once the catheter hub is touching the skin and blood flows freely from the catheter, the stylet can be withdrawn and discarded.

One of the most common errors in catheter insertion is to allow the vein to collapse during advancement of the catheter. Distension of the vein greatly enhances the chances for success. The technician should develop a technique that allows advancement of the catheter with one hand while the other hand maintains occlusion of the vein.

Immediately after insertion and confirmation of proper location in the vein, the catheter should be capped with an injection cap, three-way stopcock (Fig. 4-24), or extension set. The type of cap depends on the medications and/or fluids to be delivered. After capping, flushing with heparin flush solution should be done promptly to prevent clotting of the catheter.

The next step is to secure the catheter hub to the skin. Catheter stabilization is extremely important; in humans, catheter motion is the number one factor leading to the development of phlebitis. There are several methods for securing catheters. The most secure attachment is made by suturing the hub directly to the skin. Nonabsorbable suture material (2-0 diameter) is ideal for this use. A standard suture needle (cutting or reverse-cutting) or a 20-ga syringe needle can be used to place the suture through the skin; it is then tied to incorporate the catheter hub and bind it tightly to the skin. One or two skin sutures are usually sufficient. Another stabilization method is the traditional "butterfly" made from adhesive tape and placed around the hub; the butterfly is secured to the skin with sutures or skin staples. Butterflies tend to allow more motion of the catheter than direct suturing and are therefore not suitable for long-term catheters. Using superglue to bond the hub directly to the skin is another method; this should not be the only method of stabilization, since it is the least reliable method available. Superglue is, however, a useful addition to the other methods.

Once the catheter is placed and secured, the skin around the insertion site should be lightly coated with an antibacterial or povidone-iodine ointment. Further dressing of the catheter site depends on the patient's circumstances. All long-term catheters and catheters in foals should be covered with sterile 4 × 4s and secured with an elastic adhesive tape around the neck, being careful not to constrict blood flow in the vein (Fig. 4-25). Recumbent patients should also have their catheters protected to prevent contamination from the bedding and ground. Short-term catheters (<24 hours) do not necessarily require a protective dressing.

CATHETER MAINTENANCE

The principles of IV catheter maintenance are similar in all species. Maintaining cleanliness, minimizing motion, regular flushing to prevent clotting, and close observation for evidence of problems are essential.

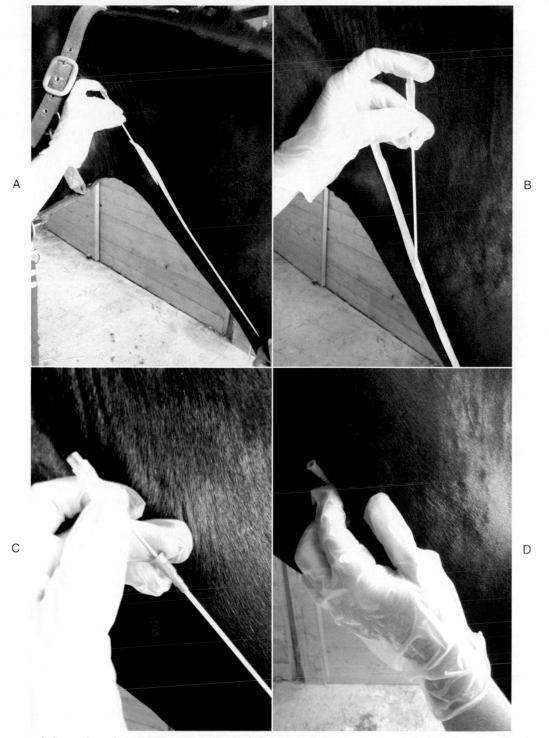

Fig. 4-23. **A,** Proper insertion angle for an intravenous (IV) catheter. **B,** Improper approach for insertion of an IV catheter. **C,** Partial withdrawal of the stylet. **D,** The catheter is advanced until the hub reaches the skin.

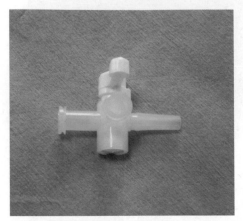

Fig. 4-24. Three-way stopcock.

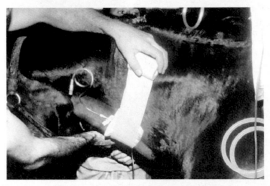

Fig. 4-25. Placement of elastic adhesive tape and gauze 4 × 4s to protect the catheter. (From Jaffe TJ: Diagnostic sampling and therapeutic techniques. In McCurnin DM, Bassert JM, editors: *Clinical textbook for veterinary technicians*, ed 5, St Louis, 2002, Saunders.)

The area around the catheter must be kept clean. If protective dressings are used, they should be changed as needed. Injection caps and three-way stopcocks should be replaced every 24 to 48 hours. If alcohol is used to clean injection caps, it should be allowed to air dry before injecting into the cap. Hands should be clean or covered with gloves whenever the catheter is handled. Whenever the catheter must be manipulated, it should be stabilized to prevent motion, which increases the risk of complications.

Heparin flush can be made by diluting heparin in normal saline (10 international units [IU] heparin per ml of normal saline). Approximately 10 ml of heparin flush are used to thoroughly clear the catheter. The catheter should be flushed after every medication; medications should never be allowed to mix in the catheter, since they may react chemically to form crystals and precipitates that can be harmful to the patient and/or clog the catheter. Catheters should be flushed a minimum of four times daily, even if not being used for medication. Flushing should be easy to perform, with a minimum of resistance. Resistance usually indicates clotting inside the catheter or kinking of the catheter; in either case, it usually will have to be replaced.

Catheters must be closely watched for problems. The catheter itself should be checked for mechanical failure; most catheters fail at the junction of the hub and the barrel. Liquid may be seen to drip from this area while it is being injected; if the patient is on IV fluids, the skin and hair near the insertion site may be wet from leakage. Mechanical failure is an indication for removal of the catheter.

The insertion site should be watched closely for thickening and swelling, pain, and purulent exudate. The vein should be gently palpated beyond the length of the catheter for cordlike swelling, which could indicate thrombus formation (Fig. 4-26). These routine "catheter checks" should be performed several times a day, and the clinician alerted if problems are detected. Most commonly, skin swelling around the insertion site is caused by local subcutaneous infection/inflammation, and less commonly indicates true thrombophlebitis. However, it can be difficult to distinguish subcutaneous inflammation from intravenous inflammation. The catheter should not be removed without *first* consulting the clinician.

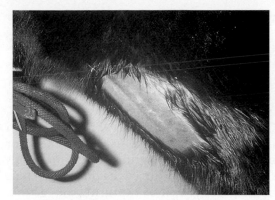

Fig. 4-26. Thrombosed left jugular vein in a horse. Note the ropelike or cordlike swelling of the vein; this area has a solid feel when palpated. (From Colahan P et al: *Equine medicine and surgery*, ed 5, St Louis, 1999, Mosby.)

Use of IV catheters to obtain blood samples is strongly discouraged. This practice increases the risk of clotting in the catheter, and blood samples may be tainted with drug residues inside the catheter.

CATHETER REMOVAL

After removal of a catheter, care must be taken not to allow hematoma formation at the insertion site. Firm pressure directly over the insertion site should be applied for at least a minute or more. Do not occlude the vein downstream from the insertion site, which can cause blood to back up and exit through the puncture site. Elevating the head after removing a jugular catheter minimizes the risk of hematoma formation.

Once bleeding has stopped, the insertion site should be cleaned and an antibacterial ointment placed directly into and around the location. Bandaging the area is optional in most cases.

THROMBOPHLEBITIS

Thrombophlebitis is inflammation of a vein with concurrent thrombus formation. Thrombus formation may begin on the catheter itself or on damaged areas of the vein walls created by insertion or use of the catheter. Once thrombus formation begins, it may grow to a size large enough to completely obstruct blood flow. The thrombus may be complicated by bacterial colonization (septic thrombophlebitis); bacteria may come from the patient's own bloodstream (septicemia) or may travel down the catheter from the catheter hub or insertion site (ascending infection). Poor insertion technique, lack of cleanliness, and excessive motion of the catheter are all associated with increased risk of thrombophlebitis.

If one jugular vein thromboses, the other jugular vein can usually provide adequate drainage of the head. However, if both jugular veins thrombose, severe swelling of the head typically results. There are other veins that drain the head, but they are smaller in diameter and cannot provide enough drainage to prevent the edema formation. Swelling of the head may be life threatening if breathing is compromised. Forced elevation of the head by tying it above the level of the heart will discourage further fluid accumulation, and feed should be offered well above ground level.

If thrombophlebitis is confirmed, the catheter must be removed. The tip of the catheter should be cultured for bacteria by cutting the tip off with sterile scissors and placing it into a sterile container for submission to the lab. The inflamed area should be hotpacked several times a day; once the skin has dried, topical dimethyl sulfoxide (DMSO) gel or liquid can be applied to help reduce swelling. DMSO should not be applied to broken or wet skin. The insertion site should be kept free of exudates and covered with an antibacterial ointment.

Once a vein is affected with any degree of thrombophlebitis, all use of the vein *must* stop. All staff should be alerted to the location of the affected vein, and other veins used instead.

Thrombosis is not always permanent; the body has mechanisms to break down clots and may partially or completely resolve them. However, the lining of the vein is usually left with irregularities that can initiate more thrombi, and other veins should be preferentially used if catheterization is ever necessary in the future.

ENEMAS

This once-popular route is rarely used today for medication of large animals. It is still used for its ability to stimulate bowel movements in some cases of gastrointestinal disease, though its usefulness is debated. Enemas are commonly given to newborn foals to encourage passage of meconium (fetal feces); human pediatric enema solutions may be used for equine neonates and require no special equipment.

Older animals require delivery of larger volumes of fluid. Fluids should be warm and nonirritating. Delivery is accomplished through a tube or hose that has been adapted for this purpose. Enema tubes can be made from any flexible rubber or plastic tubing with smooth siding; side ports should be removed to prevent accidental catching of the rectal mucosa in the ports. A single opening at the end of the tube should be made and the edges smoothed and rounded. Old nasogastric tubes are commonly used for enema tubing.

Insertion begins with restraint of the patient; this procedure is not painful, but it does produce some discomfort. The operator should stand to the side of the horse during the entire procedure. The tip of the hose is lubricated and gently inserted several inches into the rectum; the hose should not be inserted farther than 12 inches and should never be forced if resistance is encountered. Once inserted, the desired enema solution is administered by gravity flow (safest) or use of a large dose syringe or pump; fluids should never be forced against resistance because of the risk of rupturing the rectum. Generally 1 to 3 gallons of liquid can be given to an average (1000 lb) adult horse; when fluids begin to flow out of the anus or when resistance is encountered, the administration is stopped.

The horse's urge to void the rectum is usually rapid, and the enema fluids are expelled in projectile fashion; the operator is encouraged to stand well to the side of the horse's rear end and be prepared for rapid voiding of most of the enema volume.

SUGGESTED READING

Jaffe TJ: Diagnostic sampling and therapeutic techniques. In McCurnin DM, Bassert JM, editors: *Clinical textbook for veterinary technicians,* ed 6, St Louis, 2006, Saunders.

Kemper T, Hayes C: Nursing care of horses. In Pratt PW, editor: *Principles and practice of veterinary technology,* St Louis, 1998, Mosby.

Teeple TN: Nursing care of horses. In Sirois M, editor: *Principles and practice of veterinary technology,* ed 2, St Louis, 2004, Mosby.

Diagnostic sampling refers to obtaining samples of body fluids or tissues for the purpose of analysis. The results of the analysis are then used to aid the clinician in making a diagnosis and planning and monitoring treatment.

Body fluids that can be collected include venous and arterial blood, abdominal fluid, pleural fluid, airway fluid, joint fluid, cerebrospinal fluid, and urine. The technician should be familiar with where the procedure is performed, proper preparation (prep) for the procedure, what tests will be performed on the fluid, and the rationale behind the procedure. Details on processing and performing laboratory tests are beyond the scope of this text and have been covered in detail in many excellent references.

Normal numerical values for fluid analysis are not presented here because of laboratory variation and the fact that "normal" values are commonly debated by clinicians. In general, however, "normal" body fluids (other than blood) have the following characteristics:

- Their clarity is transparent (not cloudy).
- They are nonodorous.
- They have low white blood cell counts.
- They have no or few red blood cells (the procedure itself, i.e., obtaining the sample, can cause some bleeding into the fluid).
- They have no bacteria (if obtained from closed body cavities).
- They have low protein levels.

Tissue samples include skin and mucosal scrapings/swabs, fine needle aspirates, and biopsy tissue sections. These procedures are performed similarly in all species, and the reader is referred to other sources for in-depth coverage of these topics.

BLOOD SAMPLING

Blood samples may be collected from arteries or veins. Preference for arterial or venous blood is dictated by the type of analysis to be performed. Almost all blood samples are venous; veins are more accessible (located more superficially) and less prone to hematoma formation than arteries.

Sites for venous blood sampling have been discussed and include the jugular vein, cephalic vein, lateral thoracic vein, saphenous vein, and coccygeal vein. Any vein that can be identified, occluded, and accessed safely may be used.

Sites for arterial blood sampling are more difficult to access, especially in unsedated patients. The transverse facial artery and the dorsal metatarsal artery are most commonly used, especially in anesthetized patients. Arteries are prone to developing hematomas after withdrawal of the needle, and firm pressure should be applied directly to the puncture site (1 to 2 minutes minimum) to minimize this risk.

Blood can be collected by aspiration into a syringe or Vacutainer tube. If dealing with a foal or needle-shy adult, Vacutainers can be challenging to use because of patient motion, and the author prefers to use a 20-gauge (ga) needle and Luer syringe to aspirate the blood, then transfer it to a vacuum tube. For direct blood draws into Vacutainer tubes, Vacutainer needles 1½ inches long are available for large animal use.

Processing and analysis of blood samples are discussed in detail in other texts.

BLOOD GAS SAMPLES

Blood gas analysis is used most often in assessing patients with respiratory disease and monitoring patients under general anesthesia. The analysis determines the oxygen content, carbon dioxide content, and pH of the blood sample. Arterial blood is usually preferred to venous blood for blood gas analysis, since it more accurately reflects the ventilation status of the animal. Blood gas analysis as an anesthetic monitoring tool is more common in large than small animals.

Samples for blood gas analysis must not clot and must not be contaminated by atmospheric air. Typically, a 25-ga needle and 3-ml syringe are used to obtain the sample. To prevent coagulation of blood, just enough heparin is aspirated to fill the needle and appear in the needle hub. No air or air bubbles should be in the syringe. At least 1 ml of blood is drawn from an artery or vein, and the needle is immediately capped with a rubber stopper to keep air from contacting the sample (the rubber stoppers from blood tubes work well). The syringe/needle/cap combination is placed on ice and promptly analyzed. The sample should be run within 10 minutes, although if maintained on ice and kept airtight, it may yield accurate results for about 1½ hours. The patient's temperature should be taken at the time of collection; the analysis must be corrected for body temperature.

ABDOMINOCENTESIS (ABDOMINAL TAP)

Purpose

Obtain a sample of abdominal (peritoneal) fluid for analysis. The fluid is produced by the cells of the peritoneum, which line the abdominal wall and the outer surfaces of the abdominal organs. Abnormalities of abdominal organs may change the character of the abdominal fluid, providing clues for diagnosis of abdominal disease.

The procedure can be readily performed in the clinic or in the field.

Indications

Abdominal disease, gastrointestinal (GI) or
   non-GI origin
Chronic weight loss

Equipment

Sterile gloves
Ethylenediamine tetraacetic acid (EDTA) and serum
   (plain) blood tubes
Needle: 18- or 19-ga × 1½ inch for most adults
18-ga × 3-inch spinal needle for large or obese horses
20-ga × 1-inch for foals
Blunt trocar or cannula for severely bloated patients
No. 15 scalpel blade if using a trocar or cannula
Local anesthetic/syringe/25-ga × ⅝-inch needle for
   anesthesia of the skin (for foals or if using a trocar
   or cannula)
Sterile 4 × 4 gauze if using a trocar or cannula
Clean ground cloth/towel for foals

Location of Procedure

Usually performed at the most dependent (lowest) point of the abdomen, on ventral midline or slightly to the right of ventral midline (Fig. 5-1).

Patient Position

Adults in standing position
Foals usually restrained in lateral recumbency

Patient Preparation

The hair should be clipped and sterile skin prep performed. Performing the procedure without clipping the hair is possible, but special care must be taken to properly prepare the area and the client should be warned about the slightly increased risk of introducing infection.

Local anesthesia is seldom necessary in most patients when hypodermic or spinal needles are used.

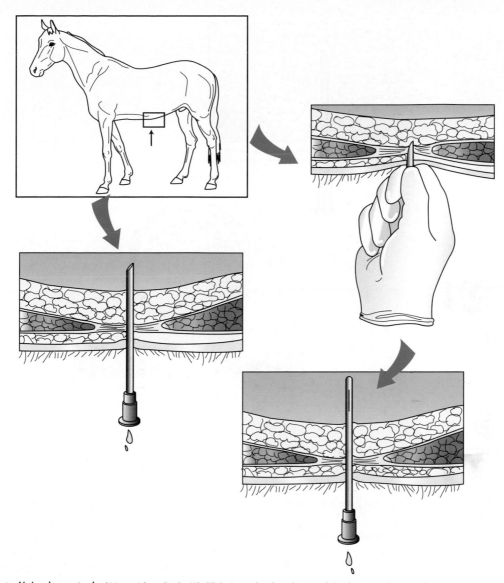

Fig. 5-1. Abdominocentesis. (Adapted from Speirs VC: *Clinical examination of horses,* St Louis, 1997, Saunders.)

Continued.

However, local anesthesia of the skin is routinely performed for foals or whenever a trocar or cannula is used. A final skin prep is performed after the anesthetic is injected subcutaneously.

Patient restraint is sometimes necessary, though the procedure is well tolerated and many horses require minimal, if any, restraint. The patient should be prevented from walking during the procedure.

Procedure Technique

Personnel should stand as far cranially as possible to avoid being kicked during the procedure.

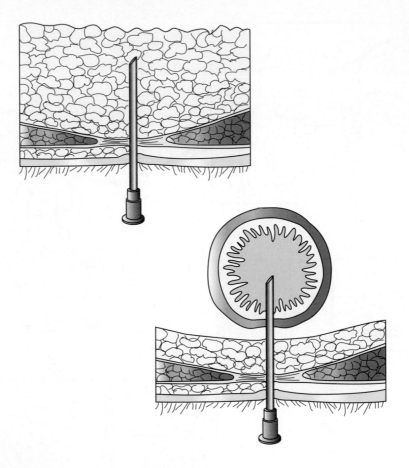

Fig. 5-1. cont'd

Patients typically flinch when the needle is passed through the skin but rarely kick.

A small stab incision through the skin is performed if using the trocar or cannula method; syringe needles do not require a skin incision. The clinician advances the needle/trocar/cannula until fluid is obtained. Fluid is collected by gravity flow into the sample collection tubes. The EDTA tube sample should be collected first, since most of the laboratory analysis will use this sample. At least 1 ml of fluid should be obtained to prevent false laboratory results, which can occur if the ratio of EDTA to abdominal fluid is too high. The serum (plain) tube is used to collect samples for culture if bacterial disease is suspected; as little as one drop of fluid is sufficient for this use.

Abdominal fluid may be difficult to obtain, requiring several attempts before fluid is obtained.

Aftercare

Bleeding is common after removal of the needle. This bleeding is due to incidental perforation of skin vessels, which are difficult to avoid because they can rarely be seen. Manual pressure over the site stops the bleeding. If a stab incision was made, the clinician may elect to place a simple skin suture or skin staple to close the incision.

The area should be cleaned gently, and antibiotic ointment applied daily for 2 to 3 days. Complications such as infection or abscessation of the site are uncommon.

Laboratory Evaluation

Common procedures include the following evaluations and measurements:

- Gross visual examination: Normal abdominal fluid is pale yellow, clear, and odorless. Its consistency is similar to water.
- Total protein level
- Red blood cell (RBC) and white blood cell (WBC) count
- Packed cell volume (PCV)
- Microscopic evaluation:
  Cytology: direct smear, air-dried, stained
  Gram stain: if bacteria are observed
- Microbial culture and sensitivity: if infection is suspected or confirmed
- Ancillary tests: may include pH, enzyme, and other chemistries; seldom necessary

ARTHROCENTESIS (JOINT TAP)

Purpose

Obtain synovial fluid from a synovial joint for analysis. All synovial joints contain synovial fluid, which is produced by the cells of the synovial membrane. Disease of the joint often changes the characteristics of the fluid, and the sample can be used to aid diagnosis of various joint diseases.

Tendon sheaths and bursae are also synovial structures, lined by a synovial membrane that produces synovial fluid. Many tendon sheaths and bursae can be accessed for fluid collection in the same manner as the joints. Analysis of these samples is similar to that of joint fluid.

Arthrocentesis and centesis of other synovial structures can be performed in the clinic or in the field. It is common practice to use the procedure to also medicate the synovial structure; after the fluid sample has been obtained, the selected medication is injected into the structure before removing the needle.

Indications

Joint disease, suspected or confirmed
Tendon sheath/bursal disease, suspected or confirmed

Equipment

Sterile gloves
EDTA and serum (plain) blood tubes
Needle: depends on many factors, especially location and depth of the joint, size of the patient, temperament of the patient, and clinician preference
Sterile 6- or 12-ml syringe
Local anesthetic/syringe/needle if skin block is necessary (foals, deep synovial structures, patients that resist the procedure)
± Medication to be injected

Location of Procedure

Depends on the anatomical location of the structure and clinician preference. Some synovial structures are accessible from more than one location.

Patient Position

Depends on the anatomical location of the synovial structure, restraint methods, and clinician preference. Most arthrocentesis is performed with the horse standing and weight-bearing, though some structures are accessed with the leg elevated.

Patient Preparation

The hair should be clipped and skin sterilely prepped. It is possible to perform the procedure without clipping the hair, but special care must be taken to properly prepare the area and the client should be warned about the slightly increased risk of introducing infection. In either case, following the final alcohol scrub, the author recommends that povidone-iodine solution be applied to the area and allowed to air dry. The solution remains on the patient until the procedure is completed.

Local anesthesia is usually necessary for the skin and subcutaneous tissue if a large needle is to be used, such as for the hip and shoulder joints. Local anesthesia is sometimes required for horses that resist the procedure, and this can be provided as a small anesthetic bleb at the skin puncture site or by regional anesthesia of peripheral nerves on the limbs. Most horses do not require local anesthesia for lower leg arthrocentesis.

Restraint is required for most cases. Restraint depends on many factors and may range from minimal restraint to more severe physical restraint. In some cases chemical sedation or even general anesthesia is necessary. The patient *must* be motionless while the needle is in the joint; motion can bend or break the needle, and the cartilage and synovial membrane surfaces of the joint can be severely lacerated or punctured.

Procedure Technique

Once the needle enters the synovial structure, fluid may flow freely or not at all. Occasionally the clinician may use a sterile syringe to aspirate the synovial fluid. The EDTA tube sample should be collected first, since most of the laboratory analysis will use this sample. At least 1 ml of fluid should be obtained to prevent false laboratory results, which can occur if the ratio of EDTA to fluid is too high. The serum (plain) tube is used to collect samples for culture if bacterial disease is suspected; as little as one drop of fluid is sufficient for this use.

After collecting the fluid samples, medication can be injected through the needle into the synovial space.

Aftercare

Bleeding from the skin is not unusual after withdrawing the needle and is controlled with direct pressure. If bleeding occurs, blood is cleaned from the skin and antibiotic ointment is placed over the injection site.

Bandaging depends on several factors. Often the joint disease itself requires some form of bandaging. Otherwise, many clinicians prefer to cover the injection site for 24 hours to minimize the risk of infection; this becomes more essential with structures closer to the ground (i.e., the distal limbs).

Exercise is also dictated by the nature of the joint disease, the horse's occupation, and the type of medication injected into the joint (if this was performed).

Laboratory Evaluation

Common procedures include the following evaluations and measurements:
- Gross visual examination: Normal synovial fluid is yellow, clear, and odorless. The fluid should have

viscosity (i.e., be "stringy"); watery consistency is abnormal.
- Total protein level
- RBC and WBC count
- PCV
- Microscopic evaluation:
  Cytology: direct smear, air-dried, stained
  Gram stain: if bacteria are observed
- Microbial culture and sensitivity: if infection is suspected or confirmed
- Ancillary tests: may include pH, enzymes, chemical mediators of inflammation, and other chemistries; cartilage fragment analysis and mucin clot tests are no longer routinely performed

CEREBROSPINAL FLUID COLLECTION

Purpose

Obtain cerebrospinal fluid (CSF) from the subarachnoid space for analysis. CSF is produced by ependymal cells in the ventricles of the brain and flows in the subarachnoid space around the brain and spinal cord. CSF also flows through the ventricles of the brain and the central canal of the spinal cord but cannot be safely accessed in these locations.

Diseases of the central nervous system (CNS) may produce changes in the character and composition of CSF; therefore it is used as a diagnostic aid in neurological disease.

CSF in the subarachnoid space may be readily accessed for sampling at two locations: the atlantooccipital space (also referred to as the *cisterna magna*) and the lumbosacral space. These procedures are significantly different in technique, but the CSF obtained from either location is essentially the same and there is no difference in laboratory analysis procedures.

The atlantooccipital space can only be safely accessed with the patient under general anesthesia. Although the procedure carries the risks of general anesthesia, it is a brief procedure and injectable anesthesia can be used. CSF is technically easy to obtain at this location. If the patient is ataxic, as many neurological patients are, the risk of self injury during the anesthetic recovery period is increased and may be unacceptable.

The lumbosacral space is usually accessed in the awake, standing patient; this avoids the risk of recovery from general anesthesia. However, the lumbosacral space is technically more difficult to enter, and patients may display violent reactions to pain from the procedure.

Indications

Diagnosis of CNS (brain and spinal cord) disease
Differentiation of peripheral nervous system disease

Equipment

Sterile gloves
Sterile 12- or 20-ml syringe

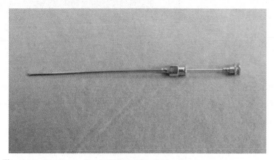

Fig. 5-2. 18-gauge × 3-inch spinal needle.

EDTA and serum (plain) tubes
Needle:
- 18-ga × 3-inch spinal needle for atlantooccipital tap (Fig. 5-2)
- 8-inch spinal needle for lumbosacral tap

Local anesthetic /12-ml syringe/20-ga × 1½-inch needle for lumbosacral tap
General anesthesia (injectable or inhalation) for atlantooccipital tap

Location of Procedure

Atlantooccipital space: Just caudal to the poll, on dorsal midline, at the level of the wings of the atlas (Fig. 5-3)

   Lumbosacral space: On dorsal midline, at the level of the wings of the ilium (Fig. 5-4)

Patient Preparation and Positioning

Atlantooccipital space: This procedure must be performed under general anesthesia; therefore proper preparation for anesthesia is required. The patient is placed in lateral recumbency; a rope is usually placed around the nose and pulled caudally to ventroflex the head and neck; this opens up the atlantooccipital space and facilitates needle placement. The patient is clipped and sterilely prepped for the procedure.

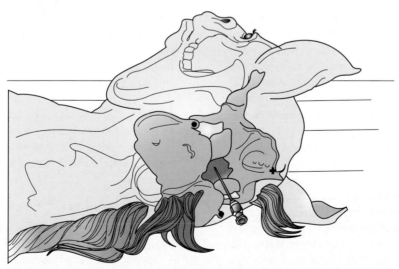

Fig. 5-3. Cerebrospinal fluid collection from the atlantooccipital space.

A

B

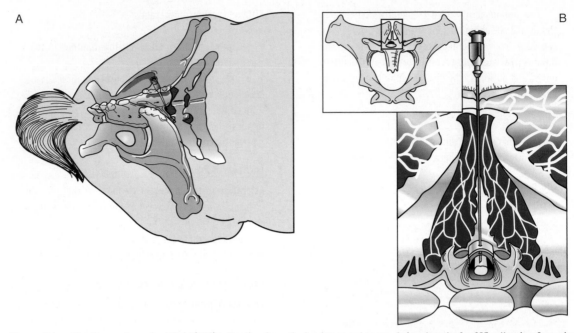

Fig. 5-4. Location for cerebrospinal fluid (CSF) collection from the lumbrosacral space. **A,** Landmarks for CSF collection from the lumbosacral space. **B,** Collection of CSF from the lumbosacral space. (From Speirs VC: *Clinical examination of horses*, St Louis, 1997, Saunders.)

Lumbosacral space: The procedure is performed in the standing patient, usually with sedation. Care must be taken not to overly sedate the horse, which may cause excessive body swaying. The patient *must* stand still during the procedure; therefore stocks are highly desirable to restrict movement. The horse must also stand squarely with weight distributed evenly on all legs; leaning makes the procedure difficult to perform. The patient is clipped and sterilely prepped for the procedure, and local anesthesia of the skin, subcutaneous tissues, and deeper tissues is performed. A final prep is performed after the local anesthetic is injected.

Procedure Technique

The needle is advanced by the clinician, with careful attention to anatomical landmarks, until the bevel is confirmed to be in the subarachnoid space. With atlantooccipital taps, fluid usually flows freely from the needle and may be collected from the needle hub.

Fluid may flow freely from the lumbosacral space but usually needs to be collected by gentle aspiration with a sterile syringe because it cannot be easily collected by gravity flow with the needle in its vertical position. Fluid is usually collected into both EDTA and serum tubes; greater than 1 ml should be placed in the EDTA tube.

Aftercare

Blood is cleaned from the site and antibiotic ointment is placed over the area. Minimal local swelling is expected. Infection and abscessation at the site are uncommon.

Laboratory Evaluation

CSF fluid should be analyzed as soon as possible because of rapid deterioration of cells.

Common procedures include the following evaluations and measurements:

- Gross visual examination: Normal CSF is clear, colorless, and odorless. It has the consistency of water.
- Total protein level
- RBC/WBC count: A hemocytometer is often required for accurate counts.
- Microscopic evaluation:
  Cytology: direct smear, air-dried and stained
  Gram stain: if bacteria are suspected or confirmed
- Microbial culture/sensitivity is performed if infectious etiology is suspected or confirmed.
- Serology: Antibody titers for some neurological diseases are commonly performed on CSF.
- Ancillary procedures: Glucose, pH, electrolyte, and enzyme levels are occasionally measured.

THORACOCENTESIS (CHEST TAP)

Purpose

Obtain a sample of pleural fluid for analysis. Pleural fluid is produced by the cells of the pleura, which line the pleural cavities and surface of the lungs. This fluid surrounds the lungs and is entirely different from samples of fluid and cells collected from the airways of the lungs (transtracheal wash/aspirate, bronchoalveolar lavage). The pleural cavities are normally closed body cavities, whereas the respiratory airways openly communicate with the outside world.

Normally there is little accumulation of pleural fluid in the pleural cavities, and access to the fluid is often difficult in normal horses. However, diseases of the pleural cavity and external surfaces of the lungs may change the character and quantity of the pleural fluid, increasing volume and thereby making access easier.

The right and left pleural cavities communicate in most horses through a small "hole" in the caudal mediastinum. Disease of a pleural cavity may "plug" this communication with fibrin and other exudates. Therefore it is possible to have pleural effusion and/or abnormal pleural fluid in only one pleural cavity, while the other cavity is essentially normal.

Diagnostic ultrasound is extremely valuable in detecting pleural fluid. Ultrasound can identify accumulation of pleural fluid and guide the clinician in selecting the specific location for performing thoracocentesis. The procedure is sometimes performed on both right and left pleural cavities.

Indications

Any disease that produces pleural effusion, including the following:
Diseases of the pleural cavity (pleuritis, pleuropneumonia)
Diseases of the lungs (pneumonia, pleuropneumonia)
Some cardiac diseases
Some neoplastic diseases

Equipment

Sterile gloves
EDTA and serum (plain) tubes
Needle—clinician's preference for:
  Large-gauge syringe needle
  Intravenous (IV) catheter (14- or 16-ga)
  Sharp trocar or cannula
Note: All of the above must be at least 3 inches long to penetrate the chest wall.
Local anesthetic/6-ml syringe/20- or 22-ga × 1 or 1½-inch needle
No. 15 scalpel blade
Sterile 35- or 60-ml Luer tip syringe
Three-way stopcock

Location of Procedure

Right or left lateral thoracic wall, through an intercostal space. The specific location is usually determined following ultrasound examination. The location is usually toward the ventral aspect of the lateral thoracic wall (Fig. 5-5).

Patient Positioning

Standing

Patient Preparation

The procedure is usually performed under sedation, although physical restraint alone may be sufficient for some horses. The patient must stand still for the procedure.

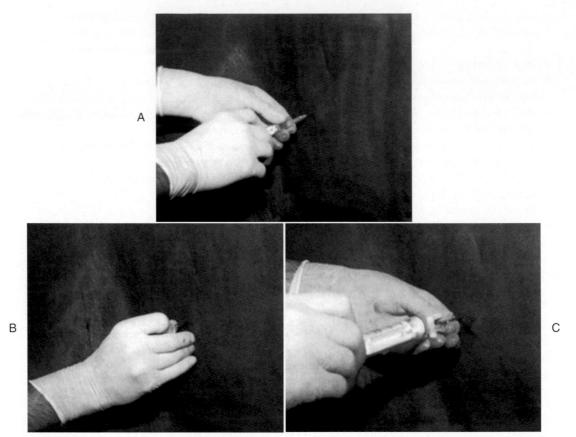

Fig. 5-5. Thoracocentesis. **A,** Injection of local anesthetic. **B,** Making a stab incision with a small scalpel blade. **C,** Insertion of needle/cannula attached to a syringe and 3-way stopcock. (From Speirs VC: *Clinical examination of horses*, St Louis, 1997, Saunders.)

The patient is clipped and sterilely prepped. The prep is performed after the intercostal site is determined by ultrasound and/or physical examination. Local anesthesia of the skin, subcutaneous tissue, and deeper tissues is performed, and a final scrub of the area is performed after the local anesthetic is deposited.

Procedure Technique

The needle is advanced through the intercostal space into the pleural cavity. Care is taken to avoid iatrogenic pneumothorax, which occurs if the needle allows free passage of air from the atmosphere into an open space in the pleural cavity. For this reason, it is common to control the entrance of the needle hub with a three-way stopcock or other valve.

Once the needle bevel enters an area of fluid accumulation, the fluid often flows freely from the needle and can be collected directly into the sample tubes. Sometimes the pleural fluid contains fibrin or other exudates that can occlude the bevel, limiting fluid flow through the needle. Gentle aspiration with a sterile syringe may facilitate sample collection. Samples are collected into both EDTA and serum (plain) tubes.

After diagnostic samples are collected, the needle in often left in place and as much pleural fluid as possible is drained from the pleural cavity. Sometimes drainage must be assisted by manual or machine aspiration.

Aftercare

Bleeding is controlled with manual pressure over the puncture site. The area should be cleaned, and topical antibiotic ointment applied. The patient should be observed for signs of pneumothorax, which include elevated respiratory rate, dyspnea, cyanosis, and possibly collapse.

Laboratory Evaluation

Common procedures include the following evaluations and measurements:

- Gross visual examination: Normal pleural fluid is transparent, clear to light yellow in color, and odorless. It has the consistency of water.
- Total protein level
- RBC/WBC count
- Microscopic evaluation:
  Cytology: direct smear, air-dried, stained
  Gram stain: if bacteria are suspected or confirmed
- Microbial culture/sensitivity: if infectious etiology is suspected or confirmed
- Ancillary procedures: Other chemistries are occasionally performed.

TRANSTRACHEAL ASPIRATION (TRANSTRACHEAL WASH)

Purpose

Obtain a representative sample of material from the lower respiratory tract airways by "washing" the material from the tracheal lumen. It is assumed that the material in the trachea accurately reflects the condition of the lower airways—bronchi, bronchioles, and alveoli.

The respiratory airways are internal epithelial surfaces that communicate with the environment through the nose and mouth. Since this is not a closed body cavity, microorganisms are normally present on the airway surfaces and are commonly recovered in the diagnostic samples; this may make diagnosis of infectious disease and interpretation of culture results difficult.

Two methods can be used to obtain samples:

- **Endoscopic:** A fiberoptic endoscope is placed through the nasal cavity to enter the tracheal lumen. Special tubing is placed through the biopsy channel of the endoscope to perform the wash. The advantages of this method are that it is noninvasive and allows visual examination of the upper airways and trachea. The disadvantages are patient resistance to the presence of the endoscope and questionable accuracy of microbial samples recovered with this technique. Because the endoscope must travel through the nasal cavity, pharynx, and larynx before entering the trachea, the tip of the endoscope may acquire contaminants.
- **Percutaneous:** The tracheal lumen is entered directly through the skin. This method is perceived as a sterile procedure that yields more accurate microbial samples than the endoscopic method. The disadvantage is that it is an invasive procedure with possible complications; however, complications are uncommon.

Indications

Lower respiratory tract disease

Equipment

Endoscopic:
  Fiberoptic endoscope
  Long, narrow-gauge polyethylene tubing (sterile)
  Sterile saline, 100 to 200 ml
  Two to three sterile 60-ml syringes
  EDTA and serum (plain) tubes
Percutaneous:
  Sterile gloves
  Local anesthetic/3-ml syringe/25-ga needle
  No. 15 scalpel blade
  14-ga teat cannula or IV catheter or syringe needle
  Polyethylene or red rubber catheter (small enough to pass through the needle), sterile, at least 12 inches long
  Sterile saline, 100 to 200 ml
  Two to three sterile 60-ml syringes
  Sterile 4×4 gauze squares
  Elastic, adhesive tape
  EDTA and serum (plain) tubes

Location of Procedure

Endoscopic: Endoscope enters through a nostril (Fig. 5-6)

Percutaneous: Ventral midline of the neck, over the middle third of the cervical trachea. The tracheal rings are easily palpated on ventral midline; the needle is placed between tracheal rings (Fig. 5-7).

Patient Positioning

Standing

Patient Preparation

Endoscopic: Most horses resist placement of the endoscope; restraint of the head is essential and usually accomplished with a nose twitch.

Percutaneous: The skin over the ventral trachea is clipped and sterilely prepped. Local anesthetic is deposited subcutaneously, and a final prep is performed.

The patient should be discouraged from elevating the head during the actual wash procedure; holding the head and neck level with the ground is ideal.

Note that chemical sedation may be necessary for some patients, but some sedatives may interfere with the cough reflex. The cough reflex is desired during this procedure to help bring up material from the lower airways.

Personnel should not stand directly in front of the horse to avoid being struck with the forelimbs.

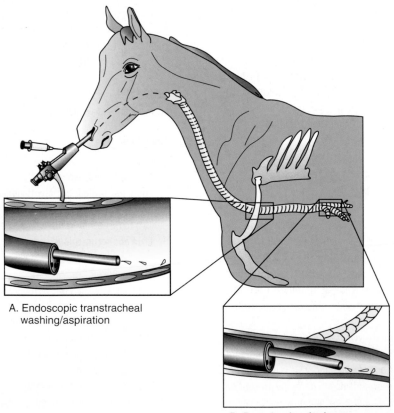

A. Endoscopic transtracheal washing/aspiration

B. Bronchoalveolar lavage

Fig. 5-6. Endoscopic technique for transtracheal wash and bronchoalveolar lavage. (Adapted from Speirs VC: *Clinical examination of horses*, St Louis, 1997, Saunders.)

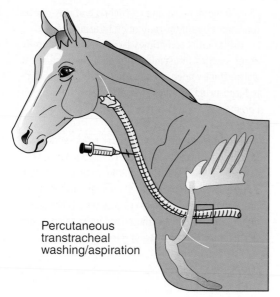

Fig. 5-7. Percutaneous technique for transtracheal wash and bronchoalveolar lavage.

Percutaneous transtracheal washing/aspiration

Procedure Technique

Endoscopic: The endoscope is passed through the nasal cavity into the trachea. The tubing is passed through the biopsy channel of the endoscope until it enters the trachea. Sterile saline in a 60-ml syringe is rapidly injected through the tubing, and then the syringe is used to aspirate as much fluid as possible back into the tubing and syringe. It is common to recover only a few milliliters of the injected saline. Up to 300 ml of saline may safely be used to perform the wash; if saline reaches the alveoli, it will be absorbed by the body. The majority of saline will not be recovered into the syringes.

Percutaneous: A stab incision is made through the skin only. The needle of choice is passed through the incision and enters the trachea between tracheal rings. Once confirmed to be in the trachea, the sterile tubing is placed through the needle to enter the trachea. The wash procedure is identical to the endoscopic technique.

Once fluid has been collected into the syringes, it is injected into the EDTA and serum tubes and other diagnostic media as desired.

Aftercare

Endoscopic: No special aftercare is necessary.

Percutaneous: Bleeding is controlled with manual pressure. The incision site should be cleaned and covered with antibiotic ointment. A light pressure wrap is applied; sterile gauze 4 × 4s are placed over the site and secured by encircling the neck several times with 4-inch diameter elastic adhesive tape, being careful not to occlude blood flow or breathing. The wrap is removed in 24 hours.

Complications may include infection/abscessation of the puncture site and subcutaneous emphysema. Subcutaneous emphysema is common but seldom causes any clinical problem; the air is eventually reabsorbed. Covering the incision with a pressure wrap reduces the amount of air accumulation.

Laboratory Evaluation

Common procedures include the following evaluations and measurements:

- Gross visual examination: Normal samples are odorless and slightly cloudy due to the presence of mucus, cells, microorganisms, and debris.
- Microscopic evaluation:

  Cytology: direct smear, air-dried, stained. Note that mucus is normally seen. Note also that bacteria are normally seen and may represent normal bacterial flora. In herbivores, plant material, pollen, and fungal hyphae may be seen and are not necessarily associated with disease; their presence should be noted, however.

  Gram stain: if bacterial disease is suspected or confirmed

- Microbial culture/sensitivity: if infectious etiology is suspected or confirmed

BRONCHOALVEOLAR LAVAGE

This procedure is another method for collecting lower airway fluid samples and is similar to the transtracheal wash procedures. Usually, an endoscope is passed as far as possible into the trachea or bronchi, and sterile tubing is passed through the endoscope as far as possible into the lower airways, presumably coming to rest in a bronchus or bronchiole (see Fig. 5-6). It is possible to pass tubing directly from the nares through the trachea without using an endoscope. The lavage is performed similarly to transtracheal aspiration, injecting large aliquots of sterile saline and attempting to recover as much of the fluid as possible by aspirating with a syringe after each saline injection. Catheters for bronchoalveolar lavage (BAL) procedures are commercially available. Local anesthetic is often infused into the bronchi to decrease the cough reflex; coughing does not enhance this procedure and is not desirable.

BAL samples are believed to more accurately reflect the condition of the lower airways than transtracheal samples because they are obtained farther down the respiratory tract. The potential disadvantage is that the region of lung sampled with BAL may or may not be abnormal; there is no way to ensure that the tubing lodges in a diseased area of the lung.

Evaluation of the fluid is similar to transtracheal wash samples.

URINE COLLECTION

Purpose

Obtain a sample of urine for laboratory analysis.

Cystocentesis is not feasible in large animals; therefore sampling is limited to voided urine collection and bladder catheterization. Cystocentesis is not used in adults because of the inability to stabilize the bladder and the possibility of the intestines being perforated during the procedure. Cystocentesis has been successfully performed in foals and small ponies/miniature horses, but it is a risky procedure and not often attempted.

Voided urine is not sterile and therefore not suitable for culture and sensitivity testing. Urine is collected into a clean container when the horse urinates. When catching a sample of voided urine, it is best to avoid the initial urine stream and collect a "midstream" sample. The initial urine stream tends to contain more mucus and cell debris and may not be representative of the content of the urine.

Urination is sometimes facilitated with diuretic drugs such as furosemide to reduce the time spent waiting for a voided sample. When analyzing diuretic-induced urine samples, the effects of the drug on parameters such as urine-specific gravity must be considered.

Catheterization of the bladder risks contamination of the urine with bacteria that accumulate on the catheter as it passes through the urethra. Therefore culture results of catheterized samples must be interpreted with caution. Since cystocentesis is not feasible in large animals, catheterized urine samples are the accepted compromise for microbial testing.

Indications

Urinary tract disease
Various systemic diseases
Toxicological/pharmacological analysis

Equipment

Catheterization:
- Urinary catheter: Stallion catheter for males. Mare catheter or metal Chambers catheter for females (Fig. 5-8)
- Sterile gloves
- Sterile 60-ml syringe, catheter or Luer tip, depending on the catheter used
- Sterile lubricating jelly
- Sterile collecting container (plastic or glass)

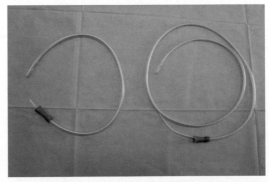

Fig. 5-8. Flexible female urinary catheter and stylet *(left)*. Flexible male urinary catheter and stylet *(right)*.

Voided:
- Clean container
- Examination gloves
- ± Diuretic drugs

Location of Procedure

Catheterization of the bladder is performed through the urethra. In males, the urethral entrance is on the end of the glans penis; in females, the urethral entrance is in the floor of the vestibule/vagina junction.

Patient Positioning

Standing (preferred) or recumbent

Patient Preparation

Voided: possible administration of diuretic drug
  Catheterization:
  Males: Tranquilization is usually required to cause relaxation and extension of the penis. This procedure induces discomfort; therefore personnel should position themselves cranially to avoid being kicked with the hind legs. Additional physical restraint may be necessary.

  Following extension of the penis, the tip of the glans penis is prepared with at least three applications of antimicrobial soap/water rinses. The tip of the catheter should be well lubricated with a sterile lubricant.

  Females: The tail is tied or held to the side, and the perineum prepared with at least three applications of antimicrobial soap/water rinses. The clinician's gloves should be well lubricated with a sterile lubricant. Physical restraint may be necessary; sedation is occasionally necessary.

Procedure Technique

- Voided: Allow the initial portion of the urine stream to pass, then catch the midstream urine in a clean container. Cap the container.
- Catheterization: The urethral opening is identified and the lubricated catheter is passed into the urethra and slowly advanced into the bladder. If the catheter has a stylet, it must be withdrawn to allow urine flow through the catheter. Urine sometimes flows freely from the catheter and may be

collected in a sterile container. If urine does not flow freely, a sterile 60-ml syringe is used to aspirate urine from the bladder.

Aftercare

All soap residues should be removed to prevent scalding of the skin and mucosal surfaces. Catheterization may cause temporary irritation of the urethra, leading to increased frequency of urination for 1 to 2 days.

Laboratory Evaluation (Urinalysis)

Common procedures include the following evaluations and measurements:
- Gross evaluation: Normal horse urine is clear to cloudy and yellow. The cloudiness is due to a relatively large amount of mucus, which is normal in the horse.
- Urine specific gravity
- Chemical analysis: reagent test strips ("dipsticks") and/or machine analysis
- Urine sediment evaluation: Calcium carbonate crystals are normal and common in horses.
- Microbial culture and sensitivity: if infectious disease is suspected or confirmed

FECAL COLLECTION

Purpose

Collection of feces for parasitic and/or microbial culture.

Indications

Suspected intestinal parasite infestation
Suspected intestinal bacterial/viral/protozoal infection

Procedure

Feces can be collected from the ground with a glove or clean container, or from the rectum with a glove or rectal sleeve. A hand is inserted into the glove/sleeve and used to grasp the feces. Then, while maintaining a grasp on the feces with the hand, the glove/sleeve is simply turned inside out. This maneuver keeps the feces inside the glove/sleeve, and physical contact with the fecal material is avoided. The glove/sleeve is tied in a knot above the feces and transported to the laboratory.

Sample sizes for large and small animals are similar; large animals do not require voluminous fecal samples.

Laboratory Evaluation

- Gross evaluation: Normal equine feces are mostly solid, in formed fecal balls. Color is light to dark green. Mucus coating may indicate that the feces have been retained longer than normal.
- Parasitic evaluation: fecal flotation, ± quantitative techniques, ± larval culture
- Fecal culture/sensitivity: This is especially important when Salmonella is suspected. Salmonella testing usually requires daily samples for 3 to 5 days; at least 10 g of feces should be submitted for each sample.

SUGGESTED READING

Colahan PT et al: *Equine medicine and surgery,* ed 5, St Louis, 1999, Mosby.

McCurnin DM, Bassert JM: *Clinical textbook for veterinary technicians,* ed 6, St Louis, 2006, Saunders.

Pratt PW: *Principles and practice of veterinary technology,* St Louis, 1998, Mosby.

Sirois M: *Principles and practice of veterinary technology,* ed 2, St Louis, 2004, Mosby.

Speirs VC: *Clinical examination of horses,* St Louis, 1997, Saunders.

6

External Coaptation in Horses

External coaptation refers to the use of bandages, splints, and casts. It should not be confused with external fixation, which is a method of fracture fixation using metal pins that are placed through bone, exit the skin, and are secured to an external frame.

Indications for external coaptation include the following:

- Reduce (compress) dead space: to prevent formation of hematomas/seromas during treatment of surgical or traumatic wounds
- Reduce skin motion around a surgical or traumatic wound
- Minimize wound contamination by protecting it from environmental exposure and/or absorbing drainage and discharge
- Hold medications against a surgical or traumatic wound
- Prevent further injury to tissues after an initial injury
- Compress open wounds to retard development of exuberant granulation tissue ("proud flesh")
- Prevent self-mutilation of a wound
- Immobilize a limb or joint
- Provide supplemental support to a joint or limb
- Protect limbs during transportation
- Protect limbs during work/performance
- Apply pressure to control hemorrhage

The basis of a good bandage is padding. This becomes especially important on the lower legs (distal to the carpus/tarsus), where there is no muscle tissue to provide protection for the tendons, ligaments, and neurovascular structures. Failure to apply adequate padding can have disastrous consequences, including pressure sores, pressure necrosis, and inflammation of tendons and ligaments, all due to compromise or complete strangulation of blood supply. Tendinitis of the superficial and/or deep digital flexor tendons may result from lack of padding ("bandage bow"). Pressure sores and necrosis of the skin and subcutaneous tissues ("cording") may also occur, with permanent scarring and/or regrowth of white hairs in the damaged area. Complete strangulation of the blood supply to the area may cause gangrene and sloughing of a part; if this occurs in a lower leg area, where there is little collateral circulation, the results may threaten a horse's career or even be life threatening. Usually it is better to use too much padding rather than too little; however, too much padding can prevent a good fit and result in slipping and bunching up of the bandage, which may also lead to compromise of blood flow. Proper bandage fit is as much an art as it is a science; the goal should be a snug, firm fit—not too tight or too loose—and padding is the most important key to achieving proper fit.

Bandages should be applied evenly to prevent problems; this means that the pressure applied by a bandage should be even throughout the length of the bandage. A bandage should not be applied tightly in one region and loosely in another. All layers of a bandage should be applied in the same direction, and each layer of the bandage should be applied under a constant tension that is appropriate for that layer. Each layer of a bandage has a different function and is therefore applied under a different tension from the other layers.

Bandages can cause pressure sores, especially over bony prominences of the legs. The accessory carpal bone, calcaneus (point of the hock), proximal sesamoid bones, and heel bulbs are prone to developing pressure sores and should be well padded in an effort to prevent this complication. Another approach to prevention is to provide relief incisions—small incisions through constrictive layers of the bandage made directly over the pressure point—to effectively remove constriction and rubbing by the bandage at that spot.

Bandages should be monitored at least once daily. Depending on the type of bandage and temperament of the patient, bandage checks may need to be performed several times a day. Bandage checks should include examination for dislodgement, tightness (too tight or too loose), soiling, strike-through (absorbed wound exudate appearing on the surface of the bandage), swelling around the margins of the bandage, and unraveling of material. If any of these problems are seen during the bandage check, the clinician should be alerted. One of the most important parameters to check in patients with leg bandages is *increased* lameness, not only in the bandaged leg but in the other legs, too. Bandages should not increase lameness in any leg, and when observed, the clinician should closely evaluate the bandage. A bandage change is usually required in this circumstance.

Bandages should also be watched for "patient tampering." This is not common in large animals, but it does occur. Patients' chewing on their bandages is the most

common form of tampering and can be difficult to control. One approach is to try to physically limit access to the bandage by tying or cross-tying the patient. Neck cradles are also available; these are the large animal version of the Elizabethan collar used in small animals. Neck cradles are usually constructed from smooth wooden slats, bound together with leather or string (Fig. 6-1). Another strategy is to place bad-tasting liquids or pastes on the outer surface of the bandage; many of these substances are irritating to skin, so care must be taken not to apply them to the skin adjacent to the bandage. Caustic chemicals should not be used to discourage bandage chewing because of possible damage to the tissues of the mouth and eyes if the horse rubs its head or chews on the bandage.

Even if complications are not seen, bandages still need to be routinely changed for sanitation and to inspect the healing of the injured area. The purpose of the bandage and the patient's demeanor dictate how frequently routine bandage changes need to be performed.

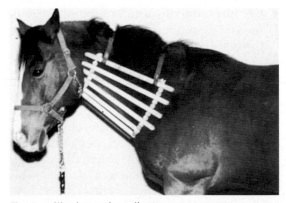

Fig. 6-1. Wooden neck cradle. (From Auer JA, Stick JA: *Equine surgery,* St Louis, 1992, Saunders.)

TYPES OF BANDAGES

Bandages are of many types. Choosing the type of bandage for a patient depends on several factors:

- Anatomical location of the bandage
- Available materials
- Patient factors: confinement, temperament, training, etc.
- Experience of the personnel applying the bandage
- Purpose of the bandage

Always ask, "What am I trying to accomplish with this bandage?", and then select the most appropriate bandage for the situation. The best bandage may not be the same for every patient or every situation.

LEG BANDAGES AND SPLINTS

There are many types of leg bandages and splints. This discussion emphasizes bandages and splints with primarily medical uses.

EXERCISE BANDAGES/WRAPS

These bandages are designed to provide additional support and/or protection for the legs during exercise. The need for exercise bandages is determined by the horse's "profession" and also by its tendency to accidentally strike its own legs (interfering). The bandages are usually worn only during exercise or turnout and are removed afterward. Indications include the following:

- Protection of lower legs during turnout or exercise: this may be accomplished by wrapping only the metacarpus/metatarsus (cannon area) or the entire distal limb down to the coronary band. For protection of a specific anatomical part, commercial "boots" are available to protect specific areas such as the splint bones or the fetlocks; these boots usually have padding incorporated into them and are secured with Velcro or buckle straps. They are constructed of leather or neoprene rubber (Fig. 6-2).
- Protection of the hoof/heel bulbs: If a horse has a tendency to step on the heels of its front feet with its back feet, commercial rubber "bell boots" can be placed around the pasterns of the forelimbs to cover the heels. Bell boots can be combined with lower limb wraps to provide complete coverage of the lower leg, heels, and coronary band (Fig. 6-3).
- Support of lower legs during turnout or exercise: It is commonly believed that bandages can provide significant support to the tendons and ligaments of the lower legs. However, when the bodyweight and biomechanical force of a horse moving at speed are compared to the strength of bandaging materials, it is probably not possible to provide more than 5% to 10% additional support to the lower leg with a support wrap. Nevertheless, support wraps are commonly used.

SHIPPING BANDAGES

When horses are transported, they are subject to sudden vehicle stops, starts, and turns. If thrown off balance, the horse may slip, fall, or step on itself, causing serious injury. Some horses kick while in the transportation stall, which can also produce injury. Some individuals strongly resist loading into the trailer/van and can injure themselves in the struggle. Protecting the legs of the horse for transportation is essential.

Proper protection includes, at the minimum, complete lower leg coverage from below the carpus/tarsus to the hoof, including the coronary band. This can be provided by bandaging the cannon and pastern, plus covering the coronary band with the bandage or a bell boot.

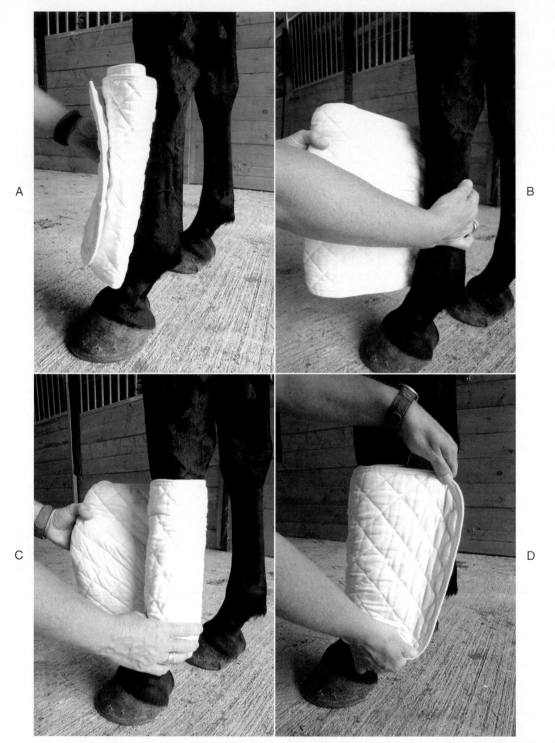

Fig. 6-2. Protection of lower legs. **A,** Proper sizing of quilted cotton to cover the metacarpus/metatarsus. **B,** The bandage is started by placing the edge of the roll on the medial aspect of the limb and unrolling it in a cranial direction. **C,** The padding is unrolled evenly, avoiding wrinkles. **D,** Completed padding layer.

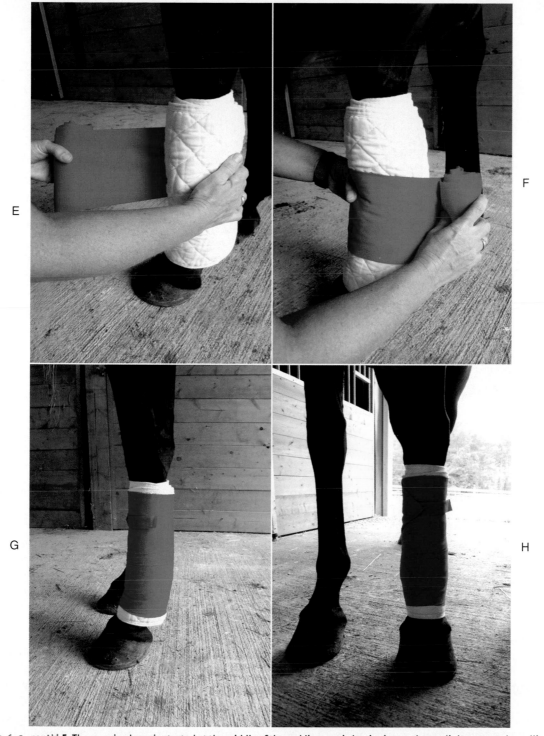

Fig. 6-2. cont'd **E**, The securing layer is started at the middle of the padding, again beginning on the medial aspect and unrolling in a cranial direction. **F**, Note use of the free hand to stabilize the bandage to prevent "spin-out." **G**, Side view of finished bandage. Note that 1 inch of padding is exposed at the top and bottom of the bandage. **H**, Front view of finished bandage.

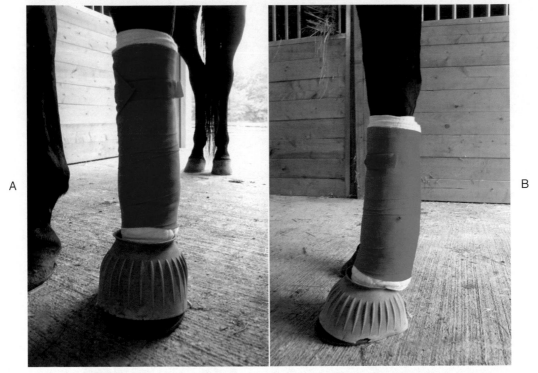

Fig. 6-3. **A,** Addition of a bell boot to protect the heels and coronary band. **B,** Side view of bell boot.

Commercially available shipping wraps that cover the entire lower leg, including the coronary band, are available. They offer some padding for protection and are washable. Shipping boots come in lower leg and full leg lengths (Fig. 6-4).

HOOF BANDAGES

This family of bandages is generally used to cover open surgical or traumatic hoof wounds. Hoof bandages may also be used to protect the hoof from external damage, such as preventing chipping of the hoof wall after removal of horseshoes (especially useful for lameness examinations on hard surfaces). Hoof bandages, wraps, and covers may be made from standard bandaging materials,

applied as prescription horseshoes by farriers, or purchased commercially.

Before placing a hoof bandage, any open wounds should be cleaned and appropriate topical medications applied. The rest of the hoof should be clean and dry. Performing the treatments and bandaging on a clean surface is a good idea; this can be provided by spreading paper or cloth towels under the horse; if the horse accidentally sets the foot down during treatment, the clean towel will prevent contamination of open wounds. Once open wounds have been treated, a bandage or other covering must be placed for protection.

One way to cover the entire hoof is with a commercial hoof boot. Commercial hoof boots (e.g., EZ Boots) are made of rubber and

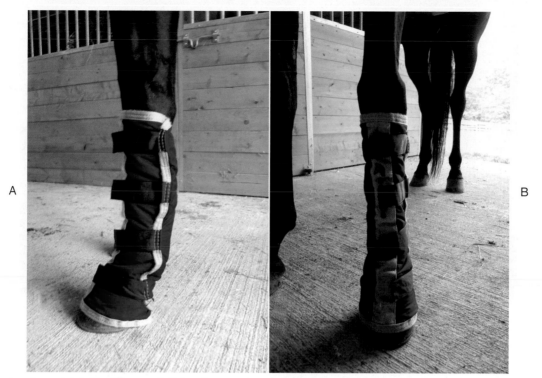

Fig. 6-4. Commercial shipping wrap. **A,** Velcro fasteners are positioned on the lateral aspect of the leg to prevent catching. **B,** Note coverage of heels and coronary band.

are available to fit all sizes of hooves. These boots have metal bindings that secure them in position. Boots must fit snugly or they are easily dislodged, especially in wet or muddy conditions; this can have disastrous consequences if an open wound is exposed by loss of a boot.

Hooves can also be protected by bandaging. In general, the material for hoof bandages should be waterproof and durable. Elastic and nonelastic bandaging tape can be used for wrapping the foot, but duct tape is more durable, more waterproof, and less expensive.

Several rules apply to using tape "booties." Because of the risk of constricting blood flow to the hoof, nonelastic tapes should not be applied on or above the coronary band and

elastic tapes should be used cautiously above the coronary band. As long as tape is confined to the hoof wall only, it can be applied tightly to produce a snug fit. Too much tape on the *sole* can cause discomfort; therefore use only enough to provide a reasonably thick covering that will stay in place.

Horseshoes can be designed to protect and cover healing hoof wounds. Hoof pads can be applied to cover an injured area and are appropriate when the injury does not require direct topical care. Treatment plates (i.e., "boiler plates") are metal plates that are fixed to a horseshoe with three to four screws; the metal plate completely covers the sole but can be removed with a screwdriver to allow full access to the sole (Fig. 6-5). Treatment plate shoes are useful for protecting

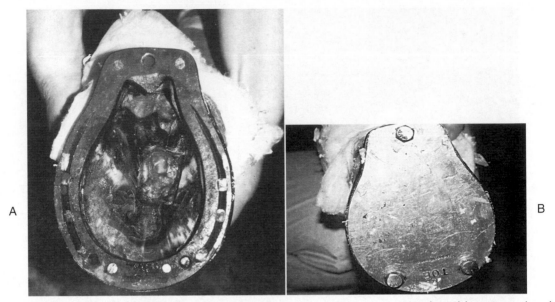

Fig. 6-5. A, Screw holes have been added to this treatment plate shoe. **B,** The treatment plate in position to cover the sole.
(From Wildenstein MJ: Horseshoeing. In Colahan PT et al: *Equine medicine and surgery,* vol 2, ed 5, St Louis, 1999, Mosby.)

open sole wounds between topical treatments such as soaking and application of topical medications. Owners can be easily instructed in maintaining and removing treatment plates and frequently find them more convenient and less expensive than the alternative of daily bandage changes. Depending on the construction of the shoe, the horse may or may not be able to have limited turnout exercise; this depends on whether the screw heads are exposed or recessed into the shoe.

DISTAL LIMB BANDAGES

This is the most common bandage used for medical purposes. It is used almost exclusively for inflammatory conditions of the lower leg but can also be used for protection and support.

Inflammatory conditions are accompanied by swelling, and one of the main purposes of this type of bandage is to limit or reduce swelling by applying firm compression. The distal limb bandage is applied from the top of the metacarpus/metatarsus to just below the coronary band. It should not be placed to cover only the cannon area; because it is designed to apply compression, lymphatic and venous drainage of parts of the leg distal to the compression may be compromised (this is true of any bandage). Swelling of the pastern often results if compression is applied only to the cannon area; therefore the entire pastern down to and including the coronary band should be included in the bandage. Compression is not an issue below the coronary band.

Before applying the bandage, topical medications are applied if indicated. If wounds are present, they are cleaned and an appropriate topical wound medication is applied (if indicated; some wounds may be left dry). If no wound is present, topical medications are seldom necessary, though occasionally topical treatments such as sweats[1] or poultices[2] are applied.

Restraint of the patient is *critical* to the successful application of the bandage; it is not possible to properly bandage a moving target. If the horse moves the leg during application, the layers already applied often have to be removed and the whole bandaging process started again from the beginning. Most horses are easily bandaged with no restraint, but some may require mild or moderate restraint such as elevating one leg or using a twitch. Ideally the horse should bear weight on the leg during application, though sometimes pain from an inflammatory condition makes weight-bearing difficult or impossible.

Having all bandaging materials assembled beforehand, unwrapped and ready for use, and within easy reach of the person applying the bandage is important.

The five standard layers of the distal limb bandage can be modified slightly to accommodate the underlying condition of the leg. Layers 1 and 2 are necessary only if wounds are present; otherwise, they may be omitted. The standard layers are, from innermost to outermost:

Wound Dressing

If an open or sutured wound is present, a wound covering is usually placed directly against the wound (Fig. 6-6). The nature of the wound determines the type of covering. The thickness of the covering is dictated by the amount of compression to be applied to the wound by the bandage and the anticipated amount of exudate absorption needed. Common choices include the following:

- Dry 4 × 4 gauze squares are useful if wound exudation or bleeding is expected,

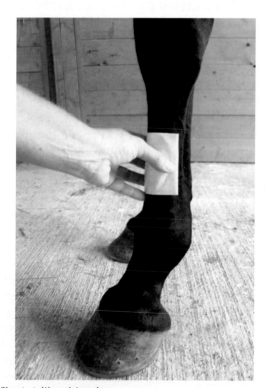

Fig. 6-6. Wound dressing.

---

[1]Sweats are mild chemical counterirritants, in liquid or gel form, applied to unbroken skin with the purpose of increasing local blood flow and therefore creating warmth. They are often used to *reduce* swelling in an area but can *create* swelling if the horse's skin is sensitive to the chemicals in the sweat. After applying the sweat, the area is sometimes loosely covered with a single layer of plastic wrap to enhance the effects of the chemicals by preventing their evaporation and absorption into the bandage. Because of irritation to the skin, sweats are removed by thorough washing 12 to 24 hours after application; a decision may then be made as to whether another application is warranted.

---

[2]Poultices are topical kaolin-based pastes, usually with additives designed to reduce swelling. They can be purchased in ready-to-use paste form or as a powder to be mixed with water to form a paste. They are applied by hand to the affected area and often covered with a layer of paper (brown paper bag or similar paper) before the bandage is applied. Poultices have a cooling effect on the skin and local tissues; however, as with sweats, some horses may be sensitive to the chemical contents and respond with local inflammation.

to absorb fluid. The gauze may be sterile or nonsterile, according to the needs of the wound.

- Nonstick pads (e.g., Telfa) are useful during the epithelialization phase of wound healing, to minimize trauma to the new epithelial cells.
- Wet saline-soaked gauze is sometimes useful to encourage wound granulation.
- Petrolatum-impregnated wound coverings are useful to cover clean, sutured incisions and lacerations; the petrolatum prevents the pad from sticking to the sutures and incision line.
- Gauze rolls can lay passively over suture lines to increase the amount of pressure applied by the securing layer of the bandage.

Layer to Hold Wound Dressing

If a wound dressing is used, it must be held in place against the wound. This layer must NOT be used to apply compression; the goal is to passively keep the wound dressing in position over the wound. Elastic materials are generally preferred to minimize the risk of strangulation. Common choices for this layer include the following:

- Roll gauze, brown or white. For large animals, the gauze rolls should not be less than 3 inches wide; 4 or 6 inches is preferable. The gauze may need to be sterile, depending on the nature of the wound. Roll gauze is rather inelastic and can cause constriction of blood flow if applied too tightly. Kling roll gauze has more elasticity than standard roll gauze.
- Elastic foam rubber (Foam-air): This material is self adherent and very flexible. It tears easily under tension, which makes the possibility of strangulation extremely low. It is easy to apply without any special instruments and readily conforms to the leg (Fig. 6-7).
- Elastic adhesive tape

Padding

Whenever compression is applied, adequate padding must be used to prevent strangulation of the blood supply. In general, the more compression to be applied, the thicker the padding required. The padding layer is applied passively, without pressure. Quilted cloth pads, towels, and even disposable diapers can be used for the padding layer. However, sheet cotton is the preferred material.

Sheet cotton is available by the dozen or in large quantities by the bale (200+ sheets). If indicated, sheet cotton may be wrapped and sterilized in an autoclave. The sheets are rectangular in shape and must be folded over to reduce their size in order to fit the lower leg. The length of the horse's lower leg dictates the pattern used to fold the sheets. Regardless of the folding pattern, the cardinal rule for adequate padding is to use a *minimum of three* sheets in a distal limb bandage (when folded over, this produces six layers of cotton). Occasionally, the sheets may be so thin that four sheets are required to produce sufficient padding.

When sheet cottons are used, the securing layer may have difficulty "biting" into it, since the material has a fairly smooth surface. Nonsterile, 6-inch wide, brown roll gauze can be applied circumferentially over the sheet cottons to provide a better "bite" for the securing layer. The gauze also helps to conform the padding more closely to the leg (Fig. 6-8).

Roll cotton can be used for padding, but it is difficult to work with and often leads to uneven thickness and bunching of the layer. Roll cotton is, however, useful for adding bulk *over* a distal limb bandage, as is done in the application of splints.

Securing Layer

This is the *only* layer that is used to apply compression. Compression is applied from distal to proximal, as evenly as possible over the entire length of the wrap. The layer is

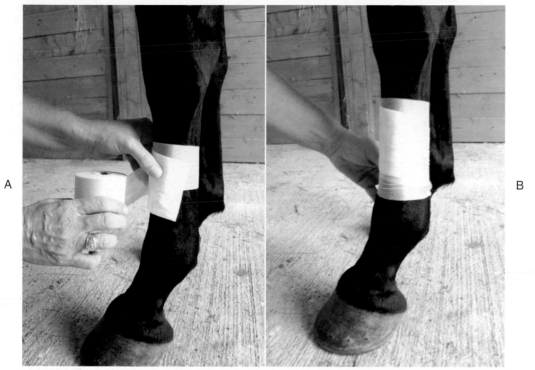

Fig. 6-7. A, Use of Foam-air over wound dressing. **B,** Completed layer to hold wound dressing in position.

applied by spiraling the bandage material around the leg; compression is applied by placing the layer under tension as it is unrolled. The amount of tension controls the amount of compression; for more compression, pull the layer into more tension as it is applied. Common securing materials are the following:

- Cloth bandages: These are usually supplied as rolls of cloth material referred to as *derby wraps* or *flannel wraps.* Ace bandages can also be used. Cloth bandages are washable but tend to lose their elasticity over time. Because they stretch markedly and unevenly, they are difficult to use to apply evenly distributed compression. They are usually secured with Velcro straps, tape, or large safety pins, making reliable compression difficult to maintain. Also, cloth

bandages are typically too short in length to adequately cover the full length of the bandage.

- Elastic self-adhesive tape (Table 6-1): For large animals, the minimum width is 3 inches, but 4- to 6-inch tape is preferable. The self-adhesive properties of the tape help to provide consistent compression throughout the length of the bandage. This is the most popular choice for the securing layer.

- Elastic adhesive tape: The minimum width for large animal use is 3 inches, but 4 inches is preferable. The expense of these types of tapes often precludes their use for this layer. They are most often used for the finishing layer.

- Nonelastic adhesive tape: The lack of elasticity increases the chance of strangulation; therefore these tapes are not often

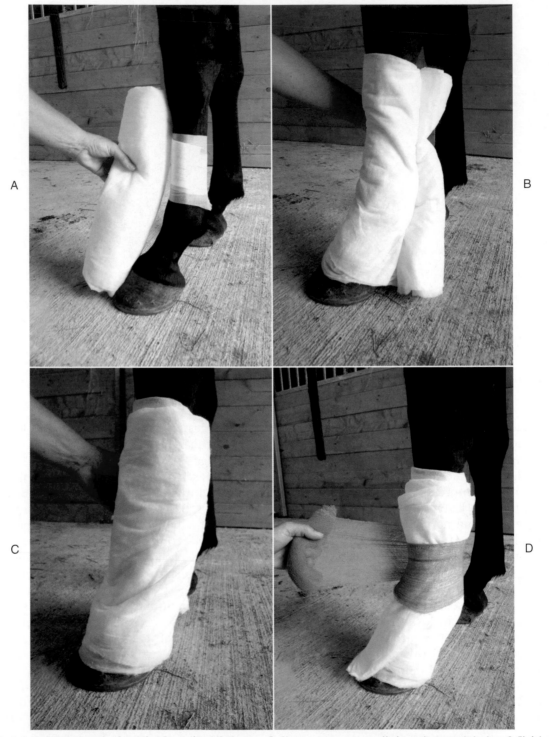

Fig. 6-8. A, Proper length of padding for a distal limb wrap. **B,** Sheet cottons are unrolled evenly around the leg. **C,** Finished padding layer. Note the smoothness of the material. **D,** Brown gauze is used to further conform the padding, beginning at the middle of the bandage.

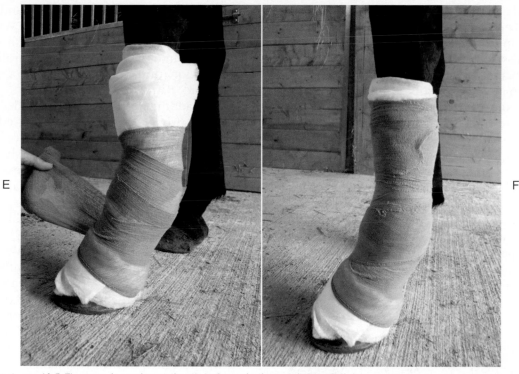

Fig. 6-8. cont'd **E,** The gauze is continued distally before spiraling proximally. **F,** Finished gauze layer.

<table>
</table>

TABLE
6-1   BANDAGING TAPES

Type	Properties	Trade and Common Names
Elastic, self adhesive	Adheres to itself but not other surfaces	Vetwrap, Coflex
Elastic, adhesive	Has adhesive coating that allows it to adhere to itself and other surfaces	Elastikon, Conform
Nonelastic, adhesive	Has adhesive coating that allows it to adhere to itself and other surfaces	Adhesive tape Duct tape

used for the securing layer. However, this material is suitable for holding splints in place over a padded distal limb wrap.

Finishing Layer

This layer is optional, depending on the underlying condition and clinician preference. Finishing is provided by covering the top and/or bottom of the bandage with elastic adhesive tape. The purpose is to prevent bedding and other debris from entering the bandage; it can also help prevent slipping of the bandage, though it should not be relied upon as 100% effective for this purpose.

Typically the tape is wrapped two to three times around the top and/or bottom of the bandage, overlapping the bandage and the adjacent skin or hoof wall. The tape should not apply compression; it should be applied to passively stick to the skin or hoof (Fig. 6-9).

To apply the bandage, first gather bandaging materials, scissors, topical medications, etc., and have them ready to use. If necessary, restrain the patient and try to keep the leg in a fully weight-bearing position. The principles to be followed include:

1. Apply any topical medications or treatments, and clean and dress wounds. Clean and dry the leg before applying the padding.
2. When unrolling bandage materials, it is standard practice to begin on the medial aspect of the leg and unroll cranially to establish the direction of the "bandage spiral" (Fig. 6-10, *A*). Once a direction has been established, all layers of the bandage should follow the same direction. When unrolling materials, the material should unroll around the leg like a carpet unrolling on a floor (think of the leg as the floor) (Fig. 6-10, *B* and *C*).
3. If the padding material has been folded (to achieve proper length), open (free) edges of the material should be placed distally.
4. The length of the padding layer should cover the coronary band distally and extend proximally to the top of the metacarpus/metatarsus. Always leave at least 1 inch of padding exposed at the proximal and distal ends of the bandage.
5. The securing layer must usually be "seated" before it can be pulled tautly to apply compression. Seating the material involves circling the padding layer several times, starting near the middle of the bandage and proceeding distally with minimal tension. When the securing material is within 1 inch of the distal margin of the padding layer, the seating is complete, and compression can now be applied in a proximal direction. Once seated, it is easier to apply compression, and the padding is less likely to "spin out" (spin around the leg while the bandage is being applied) (Fig. 6-11).
6. After seating, the securing layer is applied tautly to apply compression. The layer is applied by spiraling around the leg from distal to proximal, overlapping each previous spiral by half the width of the material. The tension on the tape should be even with every pass, over the entire length of the bandage (Fig. 6-12, *A*). The purpose of the bandage determines the amount of tension; some conditions require more compression than others.

Most elastic tapes have a waffle or ribbed appearance on the roll; pulling the tape tautly until the waffle/rib pattern disappears is the *minimum* amount of tension

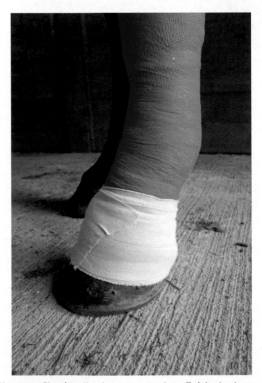

Fig. 6-9. Elastic adhesive tape used to finish the bottom of a distal limb bandage.

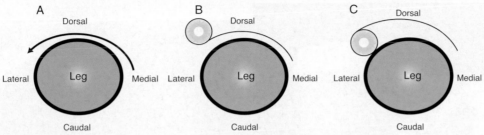

Fig. 6-10. **A,** Proper direction to unroll bandage material. **B,** Proper way to unroll bandage materials. **C,** Improper way to unroll bandage material.

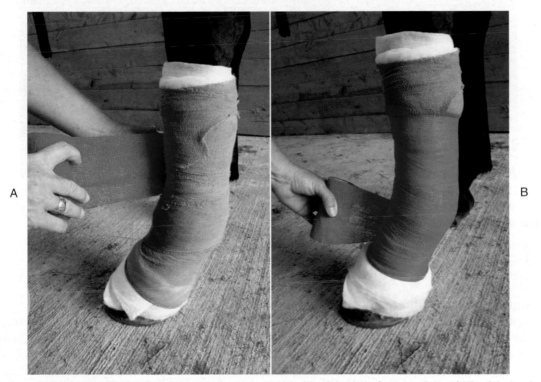

Fig. 6-11. **A,** The securing layer is seated by applying the material with minimal tension around the middle of the bandage. **B,** The tape is then applied distally.

to apply (Fig. 6-12, *B* and *C*). The bandage should be stabilized with the free hand (the hand not holding the tape roll) to prevent spin out during application of the tape.
7. Be sure that the padding layer does not bunch up as the securing layer is placed;

bunched up areas tend to rub and cause pressure sores. This tends to occur at the pastern-fetlock area, where the change in angulation and diameter of the leg makes it difficult to get a good form fit. Using 6-inch brown roll gauze over the padding helps

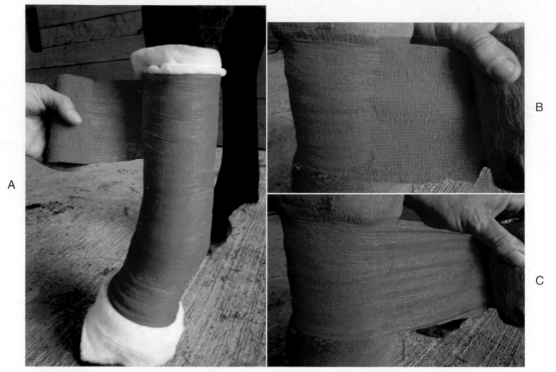

Fig. 6-12. A, Compression is applied from distal to proximal direction by pulling the tape to the desired tension as it is unrolled. **B,** The waffle pattern of the tape is visible when the tape is under insufficient tension. **C,** The waffle pattern disappears when the proper tension is applied to the tape.

conform the padding to the leg, making application of the securing tape easier.

8. Check the bandage for proper fit: this should be done before finishing the bandage. One finger should be able to fit snugly between the bandage and the skin at the proximal and distal ends of the bandage; if two or more fingers can be inserted, the bandage may be too loose. The midsection of the bandage can be checked by thumping the wrap with a finger; proper compression usually results in a "watermelon thump" sound. Be sure that 1 inch of padding is exposed at the top and bottom of the wrap (Fig. 6-13).

FULL LIMB BANDAGES

For conditions of the carpus and/or upper limb (antebrachium) of the forelimb and tarsus and/or upper limb (gaskin) of the hindlimb, a full limb bandage should be used. A common error is trying to bandage these areas with a wrap that encircles only the upper leg. This practice should be avoided for two reasons. First, applying compression to only the upper leg can lead to edema of the lower leg. Second, even with use of adhesive tapes, these bandages are usually doomed to slip down the leg. Therefore they must be "buttressed" against a supporting structure to prevent slipping.

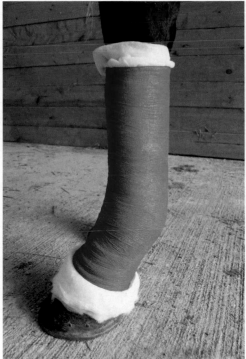

Fig. 6-13. Finished distal limb bandage, lateral view. Note that padding is exposed at both ends of the bandage, that there are no bunches or wrinkles, and that there is no "waffling" pattern to the tape.

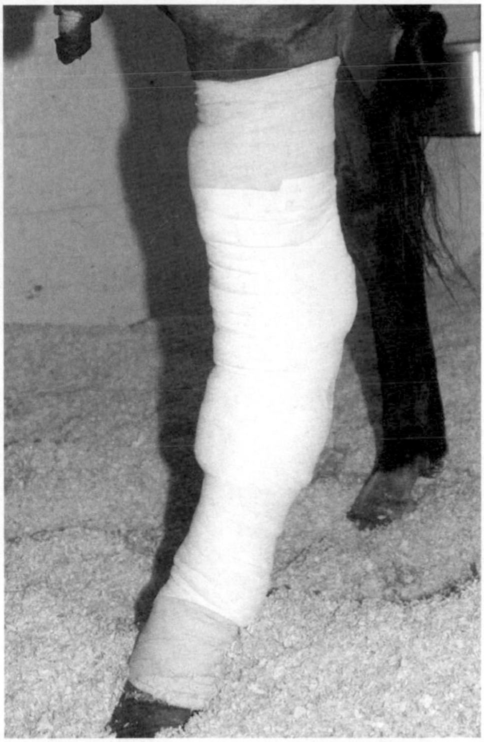

Fig. 6-14. A full limb bandage of the hindlimb. Note the "double-decker" bandaging and finishing tape across the top and bottom of the bandage. (From Auer JA, Stick JA: *Equine surgery*, ed 2, St Louis, 1999, Saunders.)

For these reasons, the full limb bandage is applied in two parts (commonly referred to as a *double-decker bandage*) (Fig. 6-14).

A standard distal limb bandage (padding and securing layer) is applied to the lower leg *first;* this bandage acts to support the upper leg bandage and also applies compression to the lower leg. The upper bandage is applied next and is essentially a repeat of the distal limb bandage, using wound dressings as necessary; it is applied to overlap the lower bandage by 2 to 3 inches (Fig. 6-15).

Pressure sores are likely to form over the point of the accessory carpal bone and the point of the calcaneus (point of the hock).

Use of extra padding over these bony prominences may decrease this complication, but relief incisions may achieve the same result. A relief incision is a small, vertical incision made through the securing and padding layers, directly over the bony prominence. The incision provides spot relief of compression and rubbing. Relief incisions must be made carefully to prevent accidental laceration of the skin (Fig. 6-16).

Additional concerns exist for strangulation and pressure sores over the gastrocnemius tendon (Achilles tendon) in the hindlimb. This area should be liberally padded if any compression is to be applied. The bandage should be monitored closely for complications.

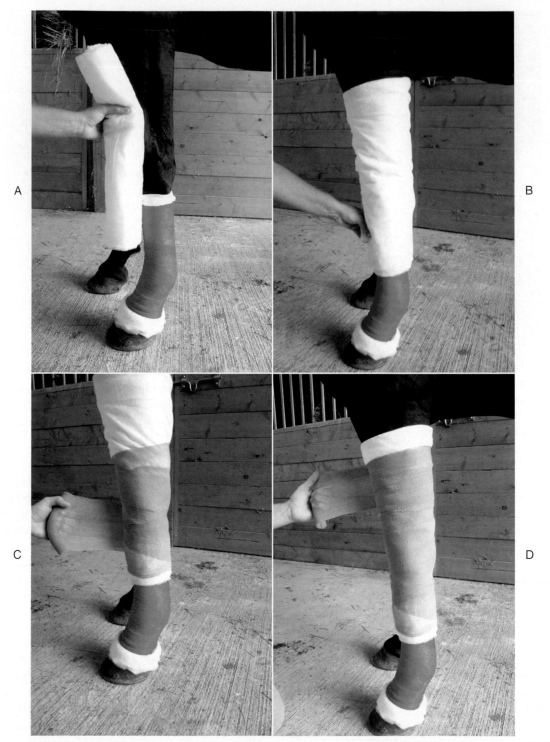

Fig. 6-15. Applying a double-decker bandage. **A,** A standard distal limb bandage is applied first, then the "double-deck" is positioned. **B,** Completed padding layer. **C,** The gauze is seated similarly to a distal limb bandage. **D,** Completed gauze layer.

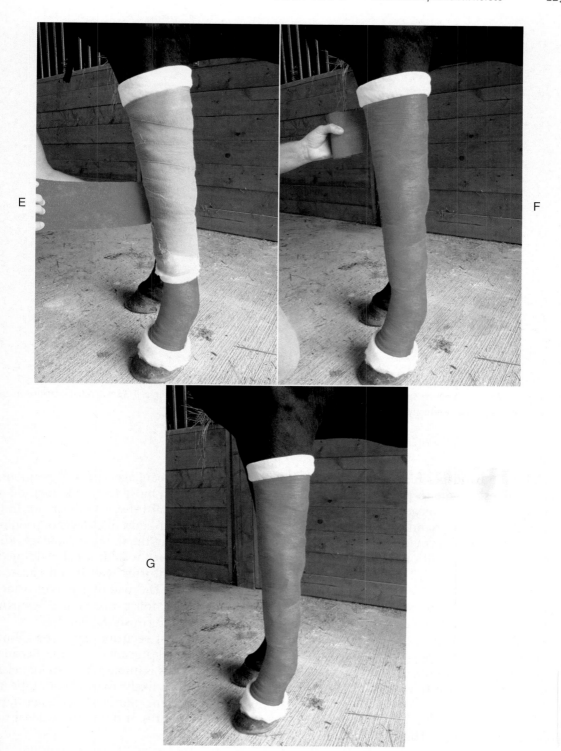

Fig. 6-15. cont'd E, The securing layer is seated at the middle of the padding layer, similarly to a distal limb bandage. **F,** Compression is applied from distal to proximal direction. **G,** Finished securing layer.

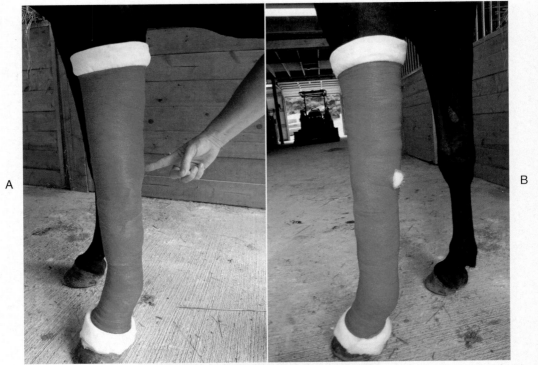

Fig. 6-16. A, Bony prominences such as the accessory carpal bone are prone to pressure sores. **B,** A small relief incision through the securing layer is made directly over the bony prominence to prevent a pressure sore.

Full limb bandages may be finished with elastic adhesive tape to prevent debris from getting under the bandage. The double-decker method can allow bandage changes of the upper wrap only, provided that the lower wrap is in good condition.

LIMB SPLINTS

Splints are applied to try to immobilize a joint, bone, or soft tissues following severe, destabilizing injuries. They may be used temporarily to transport an injured patient or used long term to support healing of tissues during conservative treatment or following surgery.

The simplest type of splint is the Robert-Jones splint bandage. This is basically a distal limb or full limb bandage with a large amount of padding. The most common method is to apply a standard distal limb or full limb bandage first, then add a thick layer of padding over the outside of the standard bandage. Roll cotton is ideal for the additional padding; it is bulky but conforms well if roll gauze is used to seat it. The padding is conformed and seated with roll gauze, and a securing layer is applied to finish the bandage.

The outermost securing layer for splints should be a nonelastic adhesive tape. Because the goal of splints is immobilization, nonelastic tape is more likely than elastic tape to restrict movement. Standard adhesive tape (3- to 4-inch width) or duct tape is ideal for this use.

Splints are usually made with supporting struts incorporated into them for additional support and immobilization. Struts can be made from wooden poles, broomsticks, metal rods, and casting tape (molded to the patient's leg). Polyvinyl chloride pipe is extremely strong and can be cut to fit the patient using a hacksaw and metal file (Fig. 6-17). Struts should be cut to fit the entire length of the splint bandage, being careful to remove, contour, or pad any sharp edges that could injure the patient.

A standard distal limb or full limb wrap is applied to the leg first. Then additional padding may be added over the standard wrap to increase the bulk of the padding layer; enough padding should be added to reduce mobility of the leg and protect the leg from rubbing by the struts. One or more struts are then positioned and secured firmly with nonelastic adhesive tape or duct tape (Fig. 6-18).

The anatomy of the leg dictates the proper location of struts. All joints of the forelimb (below the shoulder) and hindlimb (below the hip) can normally move only in a cranial-caudal direction. Therefore to prevent cranial-caudal motion, struts should be placed on the cranial and/or caudal aspects of the limb. If placed medially and/or laterally, there will be nothing solid to prevent motion in the cranial-caudal plane. The patient's injury dictates whether one or two struts are necessary.

Immobilization of a joint usually requires immobilization of the joint above and the joint below the injured joint. Therefore the shoulder and hip are located too proximally to be supported by a bandage or splint. Similarly, the elbow and stifle cannot be completely immobilized by splints because of the inability to immobilize the joints above (i.e., the shoulder and hip joints). Modified Thomas splints have been adapted for large animal patients; they restrict, but do not completely immobilize, the elbow and stifle joints.

Commercially prepared metal splints have been developed (e.g., Kimsey splint) and can be purchased in different lengths and sizes (Fig. 6-19). These splints are used mostly for emergency immobilization of a part, usually for transportation and protection until the wound can be evaluated at a hospital/clinic. The splint is secured with Velcro straps; a standard distal limb bandage or full limb bandage can be applied under the splint for additional protection of soft tissues.

Splints can provide good immobilization if properly applied, but because they use bandaging materials that are not rigid, complete immobilization is not possible. If complete immobilization is required from external coaptation, a cast must be used.

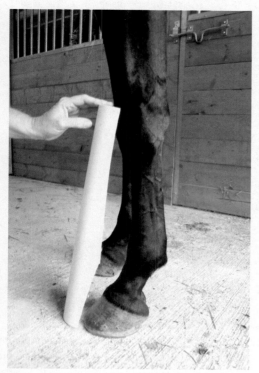

Fig. 6-17. Sizing a polyvinyl chloride strut to the desired length. This strut is suitable for a distal limb splint.

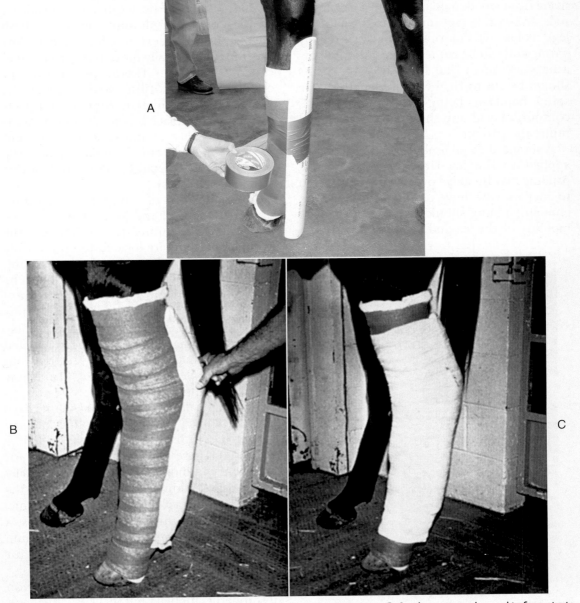

Fig. 6-18. **A,** Applying a distal limb splint with a polyvinyl chloride supporting strut. **B,** Casting tape can be used to form struts for splints. A distal limb bandage is applied first, then the tape is molded to fit the bandage. **C,** The strut is secured with a nonelastic adhesive tape. (**A** from McCurnin DM, Bassert JM: *Clinical textbook for veterinary technicians,* ed 6, St Louis, 2006, Saunders; **B** and **C** from Stashak TS: *Equine wound management,* Philadelphia, 1991, Lea & Febiger.)

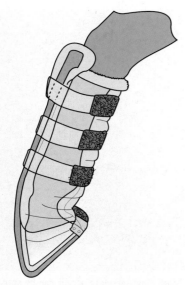

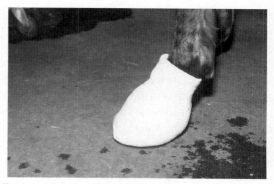

Fig. 6-20. Foot cast. The top of the cast should be finished with elastic adhesive tape. (From Auer JA, Stick JA: *Equine surgery,* ed 2, St Louis, 1999, Saunders.)

Fig. 6-19. Emergency metal splint applied over a distal limb bandage. (Adapted from White NA, Moore JN: *Current practice of equine surgery,* Philadelphia, 1990, Lippincott.)

LIMB CASTS

Casts are superior to splints for providing immobilization of the limbs. However, they are subject to the same mechanical limitations as splints for treating the upper joints of the forelimbs and hindlimbs.

Casting material is usually a combination of fiberglass with resins. For large animal use, 3- to 4-inch width is preferred. Fiberglass is lighter and stronger than older plaster materials and cures faster. Fiberglass is difficult to conform to the leg, but this is easily overcome with experience. Fiberglass is also relatively radiolucent, which allows some ability to monitor healing of bone with radiographs without having to remove the cast.

Large animal casts are of several types:

1. Foot cast: incorporates the entire hoof and extends proximally to a level between the coronary band and the fetlock, depending on the underlying condition. This cast is used for conditions of the hoof and some pastern conditions (Fig. 6-20).

2. Lower limb cast: incorporates the entire hoof and extends proximally to the top of the metacarpus or metatarsus.

3. Full limb cast: incorporates the entire hoof and extends to just below the level of the elbow on the forelimb or just below the stifle on the hindlimb.

4. Tube cast (sleeve cast): the only type of cast that does not enclose the hoof. The cast extends from the fetlock to just below the elbow or stifle. This cast is used mostly for foals with angular limb deformities or flexural deformities of the lower leg. Use of the foot and pastern are maintained with this type of cast.

Cast application is almost always done under general anesthesia; this is necessary because the patient must be motionless during application and initial curing of the cast material. Also, awake patients may be in too much pain to allow manipulation of the leg into the proper position for a cast. The risks of general anesthesia and especially recovery from anesthesia must be weighed against the risks of an improperly applied cast. The consequences of a poorly fitting cast are potentially disastrous. Strangulation, ulceration, fractures, dislocations, and refusal to bear weight on the cast are real concerns with *any* cast, and poor fit *greatly* increases the likelihood of these complications. The exception is the foot cast, which can be placed on awake, standing, cooperative patients under ideal circumstances. In some emergency situations where anesthesia is impossible or impractical, temporary limb casts have been placed without general anesthesia, allowing transportation of the patient to a treatment facility.

Clinicians have individual preferences for how to clean the leg and prepare it for the cast, whether or not to use orthopedic felt padding, and what type of additional padding/covering to use underneath the cast. Talcum powder, powdered boric acid, or corn starch are sometimes rubbed into the skin to help absorb moisture. The underlying condition of the leg determines the need for topical medications and additional wound dressings. Bulkiness of materials should be minimized. In general, the less bulk beneath the cast, the better the fit that can be obtained.

The bottom (weight-bearing) surface of the cast in large animals requires an additional protective layer to prevent wearing away of the cast; clinicians may prefer to add a metal walking bar, a piece of rubber tread, a piece of plywood, or an acrylic such as methylmethacrylate that can be spread over the bottom of the cast (Fig. 6-21). All casting materials to be used should be identified and assembled before inducing anesthesia.

Because the hoof is included in almost all casts, it should be cleaned as thoroughly as possible. It is not wise to enclose a dirty hoof in a high moisture, poorly aerated environment such as a cast; fungal/bacterial infections ("thrush") of the hoof can easily result. Trimming/paring of the frog, sole, and hoof wall helps remove the outer layer of debris and contaminants; any infected areas should

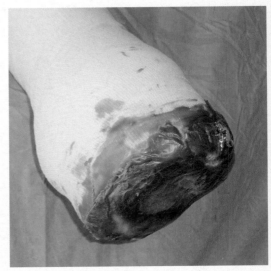

Fig. 6-21. Methylmethacrylate acrylic can be spread across the bottom of the cast for protection. (From McCurnin DM, Bassert JM: *Clinical textbook for veterinary technicians*, ed 6, St Louis, 2006, Saunders.)

also be removed by trimming. A scrub brush is used to completely scrub all surfaces of the hoof, using a povidone-iodine scrub or solution. The hoof should then be rinsed and dried. The sulci of the sole and frog can be packed with cotton or gauze soaked in povidone-iodine solution if thrush is a concern.

Casting tape is available in rolls; 3- to 4-inch width is appropriate for large animals. The rolls are activated by immersing them in warm water. The application of the casting tapes on the patient typically requires at least three people (in addition to the anesthetist)— one person to unwrap and moisten the tape rolls, one to two people to hold the leg in proper position, and one to two people to actually apply and mold the casting material. The step-by-step casting process is similar to casting in small animals. When molding the material to the limb, it is important not to make indentations in the casting tape; keeping the hands open and holding the fingers

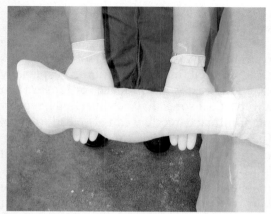

Fig. 6-22. Preventing indentations. When assisting in cast application, keep the hands open to avoid leaving indentations. (From McCurnin JM, Bassert JM: *Clinical textbook for veterinary technicians*, ed 6, St Louis, 2006, Saunders.)

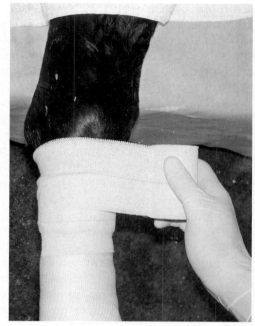

Fig. 6-23. Placing elastic adhesive tape on top of the cast to form a seal, thus preventing debris from getting down inside the cast. (From McCurnin DM, Bassert JM: *Clinical textbook for veterinary technicians*, ed 6, St Louis, 2006, Saunders.)

together helps prevent making indentations, which can lead to pressure sores (Fig. 6-22).

Some anesthetic time must be devoted to the curing process; the cast should be hard before allowing the patient to recover. Finishing the proximal end of a cast with an elastic adhesive tape is common to prevent bedding, feces, and other debris from getting inside the cast and causing pressure sores and irritation (Fig. 6-23).

Strict stall rest is mandatory for casted patients. The most common cause of cast complications is excessive motion of the leg in the cast. Horses should not be forced to move unless *absolutely* necessary. Contrary to popular belief, excessively deep stall bedding can cause the patient to stumble and should be avoided.

Patients with casts are high priority with regard to monitoring and case care. Many things can go wrong in a hurry with a cast, with grave consequences. A clinic or hospital setting is highly preferred for these cases so that trained personnel can monitor the patient. Complete patient and cast monitoring

should be done at least twice a day. The "cast check" should include evaluation of the following:

1. Temperature, pulse, and respiration (TPR): Elevation in temperature, pulse, or respiration may indicate inflammation or infection. Even mild increases in pulse or respiration may be early indicators of pain associated with inflammation; close evaluation of the casted limb and the contralateral limb (especially the hoof for laminitis) should be performed.
2. Feel the cast for hot spots (areas of heat), which often indicate underlying inflammation such as a pressure sore. Some heat directly over wounds is expected. Pressure sores also generate heat and commonly develop over the heel bulbs, proximal

sesamoid bones, accessory carpal bone, and calcaneus. Distal limb casts also tend to form sores at the top of the cast, over the dorsal aspect of the cannon bone. This area should be watched carefully for cast pressure sores.

3. Odor
4. Exudate: The porous nature of fiberglass may allow exudates to appear on the surface of the cast. Depending on the nature of the underlying condition, exudation may or may not be expected. The clinician should be alerted if exudate is seen.
5. Check the areas around the margins of the cast for swelling.
6. The bottom of the cast over the sole of the foot must be closely examined for excessive wear. If the leg shifts distally in the cast due to excessive wear, pressure sores and even strangulation of the leg may occur.
7. Check the integrity of the cast (cracks, separation of layers).
8. Check the opposite limb for inflammation, especially over the digital tendons and the hoof. All hooves should be closely monitored for laminitis (heat, increased rate and strength of pulse, constantly shifting weight, reluctance to bear weight).
9. The *most important* assessment is how the horse uses the cast, including willingness to bear weight. This should be observed several times a day. Any change in use, such as going from willingness to bear weight to refusal to bear weight on the cast, frequently indicates an underlying problem that must be carefully and immediately investigated.

Suspected complications warrant immediate evaluation; life-threatening consequences are possible, and a "let's look at it in the morning" attitude is not prudent. When casts are confirmed or suspected of causing a problem, a cast change is often necessary. A decision will be made as to whether or not to recast the leg; general anesthesia is necessary if another cast is contemplated.

Client education for casts should include warnings about cast (pressure) sores. Cast sores are expected in most patients, especially when the cast is left in place for longer than a week. Cast sores may be superficial, requiring minimal care; they can also lead to deep, full-thickness wounds that may require significant care, including the possibility of skin grafts, to heal. These sores may lead to permanent scarring, including regrowth of white hair. The consequences of skin damage must be weighed against the consequences of trying to heal the leg's injury without a cast.

Clients should always be warned about complications developing in the other legs, especially laminitis. One of the most common complications of casts is laminitis in the other legs, especially in the contralateral limb; this is related to pain in the casted leg (from the cast or the underlying condition, or both), which forces the horse to spend increased time supporting its weight on the opposite, uncasted leg. The increase in weight-bearing may also cause significant inflammation of tendons and ligaments in the opposite leg. When laminitis develops in uncasted legs, the prognosis for survival is significantly worsened. Laminitis is less likely to occur when the casted leg is comfortable, because the patient will bear more weight on the casted leg, providing some relief to the other legs. Still, laminitis may occur at any time, even in patients who appear comfortable on their casts. A firm distal limb wrap should always be placed on the contralateral limb to provide additional support to tendons and ligaments, and it should be reset daily to maintain firm compression. Some clinicians may also use frog supports to increase support and comfort of the opposite hoof.

Sedation may be required to calm active or anxious horses, since motion and activity tend to increase the complication rate. Most horses tolerate casts extremely well; others may require sedation/tranquilization to facilitate acceptance of the cast. Usually a horse does not completely reject a cast, but it does occur, and the client should be prepared for this possibility.

Cast removal at the end of treatment is preferably done with the patient standing, to avoid reinjury of the leg during recovery from anesthesia. Restraint, and often sedation, are necessary, since horses tend to move in response to the noise and vibration of the cast saw. The cast saw is used to bivalve (score) the cast along its medial and lateral aspects; medial and lateral scoring is preferred to prevent accidental lacerations of the superficial digital flexor tendon. The score lines are then connected by scoring across the bottom of the cast. Cast spreaders are used to open the cast in preparation for removal (Fig. 6-24). Bandage scissors are used to cut through the underlying stockinette and wound dressings, and the cast is removed. Once the cast is removed, the leg should be cleansed, and a splint or heavy bandage wrap applied. Radiographs may be necessary following cast removal; materials and radiographic equipment should be assembled beforehand.

HEAD/FACE BANDAGES

Because of the anatomy of the head, it is not possible to apply firm compression bandages without compromising circulation, breathing, or vision. It is possible, however, to protect wounds from environmental contamination by covering them, and sometimes light compression can be applied.

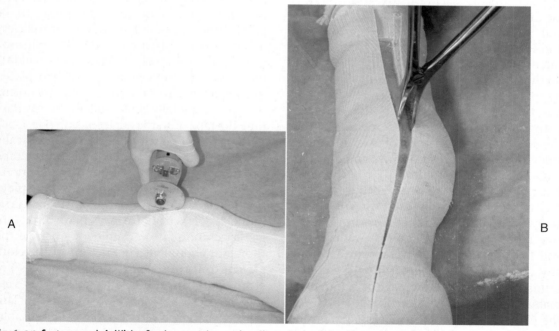

Fig. 6-24. Cast removal. **A,** With a Stryker saw, the cast is split on the medial and lateral surfaces, and the cut is continued under the foot. **B,** Once the cast is completely cut, the two halves are separated with cast spreaders. (From McCurnin D, Bassert JM: *Clinical textbook for veterinary technicians,* ed 6, St Louis, 2006, Saunders.)

In some situations, elastic adhesive tape can be used to circle the head and secure underlying wound dressings. The tape can be applied with moderate tension, being careful not to compromise breathing.

More commonly, orthopedic stockinette is used to create a "head sleeve" bandage. Foals and small equids can use 4-inch stockinette, but most equine patients require 6-inch width. The length of the stockinette should be approximately twice as long as the length of coverage desired on the head. The stockinette is rolled up into a donut shape, placed around the nose, and unrolled toward the ears. Eye and ear holes need to be cut out of the stockinette for the horse's comfort. This is best accomplished by marking the location of these structures on the stockinette with a marking pen; the stockinette is then removed from the horse, and circular 1- to 2-inch openings are created with bandage scissors at each of the four marked locations. The stockinette is rolled up again, and the injured area is cleaned, medicated, and covered with a wound dressing if indicated. The stockinette is then placed back on the horse. Each of the openings can easily be enlarged for a custom fit, usually by using the fingers to carefully rip the material. Using scissors to enlarge the openings while the stockinette is on the horse is not advisable; if the horse moves, injury could result.

Once positioned, the stockinette wrap must be secured in order to keep it in place. The rostral aspect is secured directly to the skin with two to three circles of elastic adhesive tape, placed to contact the stockinette and the adjacent skin but carefully avoiding any compromise to the nasal passages. The caudal aspect of the bandage is secured by making a small slit in the stockinette between the ears; the forelock or mane hairs can be passed through this hole and secured with adhesive tape to form a securing loop of hair, which keeps the bandage from sliding down the face. If hair is not available, tape or string can be passed through the slit and around the top of the halter. Elastic adhesive tape can also be used, with caution not to obstruct breathing or blood flow around the throatlatch (Fig. 6-25).

ABDOMINAL ("BELLY BAND") WRAPS/ THORACIC ("CHEST") WRAPS

These bandages are similar in materials and placement. They are used to cover wounds, incisions, and drains placed in the pleural or abdominal cavity. They may be placed to passively cover the affected area or placed with moderate tension to provide some compression or support to an area.

The basic material is 3- to 4-inch wide, elastic adhesive tape. Multiple rolls of tape are usually necessary. The bandage is started cranially and spiraled caudally around the patient's body to cover the desired area. Because removal of the tape tends to be painful (the tape pulls hairs out of the follicles), it is common to first cover the skin with roll gauze (or a minimal thickness of a padding material). The bandaging tape is then placed to completely cover the gauze, plus anchoring the gauze cranially and caudally by overlapping the tape onto the adjacent skin (Fig. 6-26).

Removal of elastic adhesive tape typically pulls out hair. Short, quick pulls on the tape can help to minimize patient discomfort.

An alternative to the above is the spider bandage. A large, heavy cloth material (nonelastic) is cut to form a square or rectangle large enough to completely encircle the thorax or abdomen. The borders of the cloth are cut to form several extensions ("legs") of cloth that are long enough to be tied together across the back of the patient. This type of bandage is washable and reusable, which is cost saving to the client. However, it is difficult to achieve uniform, firm compression with this type of wrap.

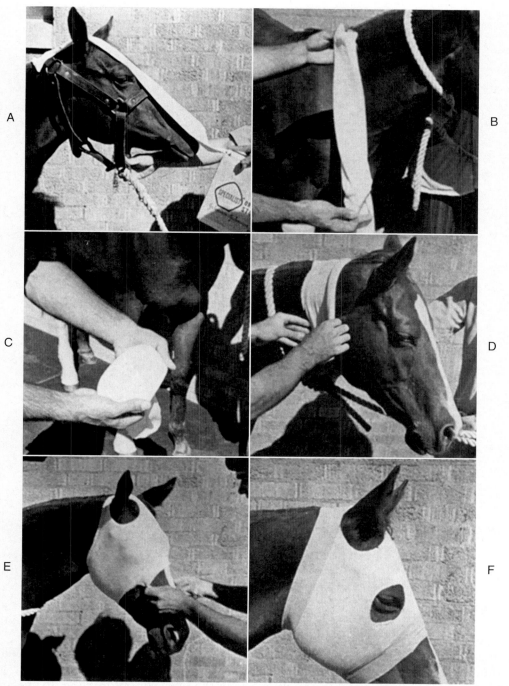

Fig. 6-25. Application of a stockinette head bandage. **A,** Six-inch orthopedic stockinette is measured. The measured length is doubled. **B,** Stockinette is doubled. **C,** Stockinette is rolled. **D,** Stockinette is placed over the horse's head and rolled rostrad. **E,** Ear and eye holes are created and the stockinette is held in place with elastic tape. **F,** Head bandage is complete. (From Stashak TS: *Equine wound management,* Philadelphia, 1991, Lea & Febiger.)

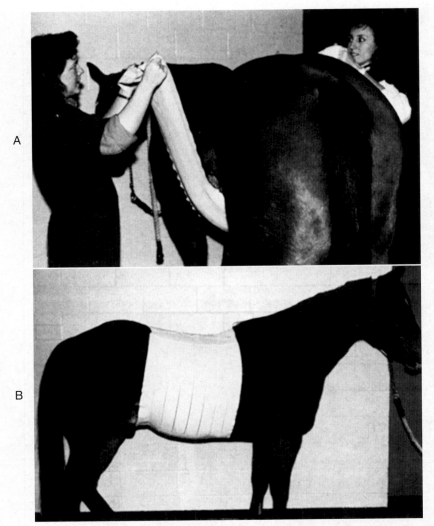

Fig. 6-26. A, Application of an abdominal bandage requires two people. **B,** Completed abdominal bandage. (From Lindsay WA: *Vet Clin North Am Equine Pract* 5:513-538, 1989.)

TAIL BANDAGES/WRAPS

Tails are bandaged for protection during shipping; for protection from feces, urine, or fetal fluids; and to prevent contamination of the vulva/perineum during medical and surgical reproductive procedures. Tail bandages are used when it is impractical or impossible to have an assistant simply hold the tail out of the way.

The arterial supply to the tail is via a single major artery, the coccygeal artery, located on the tail's ventral midline. If this artery is strangulated, the entire tail can be sloughed. For this reason, it is best to avoid circling the living portion of the tail with nonelastic materials (these materials can, however, be used safely on the tail hairs alone). If an elastic material is used to circle the tail, it should not be applied tightly. Tail wraps should be changed daily, and the tail checked closely for signs of strangulation (swelling, cool temperature, discoloration of the skin, loss of sensation).

Commercial tail wraps are available; they are made of neoprene rubber and secured with Velcro. Moisture tends to form under the rubber; therefore the wrap should be removed and cleaned, and the tail dried daily (Fig. 6-27).

The tail can also be wrapped with roll gauze; 6-inch nonsterile gauze is ideal because it can be used to contain the tail

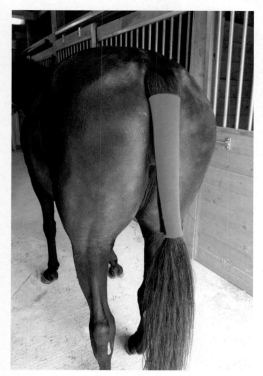

Fig. 6-27. Commercial neoprene tail wrap with Velcro fastener.

hairs and still have enough length left to be passed around the neck and tied. This maneuver avoids having an assistant hold the tail out of the way while the clinician performs reproductive procedures and surgery. The gauze is spiraled around the tail to a level below the vulva, being careful not to strangulate the coccygeal artery. The gauze is seated at the base of the tail by circling it two to three times; then, the gauze is spiraled distally to the desired level. As each spiral passes over the dorsal aspect of the tail, a small loop of tail hair is grasped and pulled proximally over the gauze; this forms a series of "locking loops" of tail hairs that keep the gauze from sliding off the tail (Fig. 6-28, *A* to *C*).

Once the desired level below the vulva is reached, a simple knot is tied for security (distal to the coccygeal vertebrae), and the gauze is then passed cranially and circled around the neck once from ventral to dorsal and back, where it is tied with a quick-release knot (Fig. 6-28, *D* to *H*).

The neck loop will partially obstruct blood flow through the jugular veins, and distension will be seen cranially to the loop; this will not present a problem if the loop is only used for a few minutes. However, if longer use is necessary, the person attending the horse's head should be instructed to "burp" (relieve) the jugular veins every 1 to 2 minutes by simply pulling the gauze loop away from the neck and allowing the jugular distension to subside (Fig. 6-29). If this is not done, horses can develop dyspnea from nasal swelling and can even lose consciousness (pass out) in rare instances.

To remove the tail wrap, the encircling neck loop is released by pulling the quick-release knot. The tail portion of the wrap is removed by grasping the wrap at the proximal end and pulling it distally in one smooth motion (Fig. 6-30).

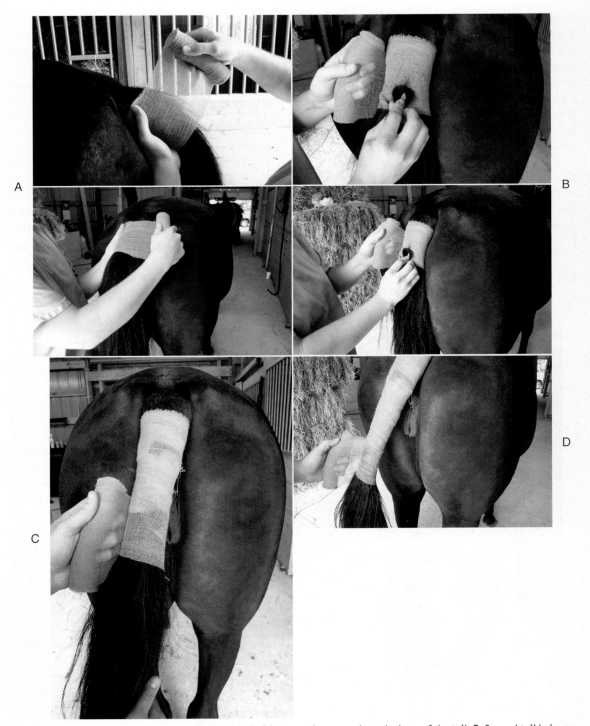

Fig. 6-28. **A,** To wrap a tail, the gauze wrap is started with two to three rounds at the base of the tail. **B,** Several tail hairs are pulled proximally to form a locking loop between each pass of the gauze. **C,** For female reproductive procedures, the wrap should extend at least to the ventralmost aspect of the vulva. **D,** The wrap is commonly continued several inches below the vulva.

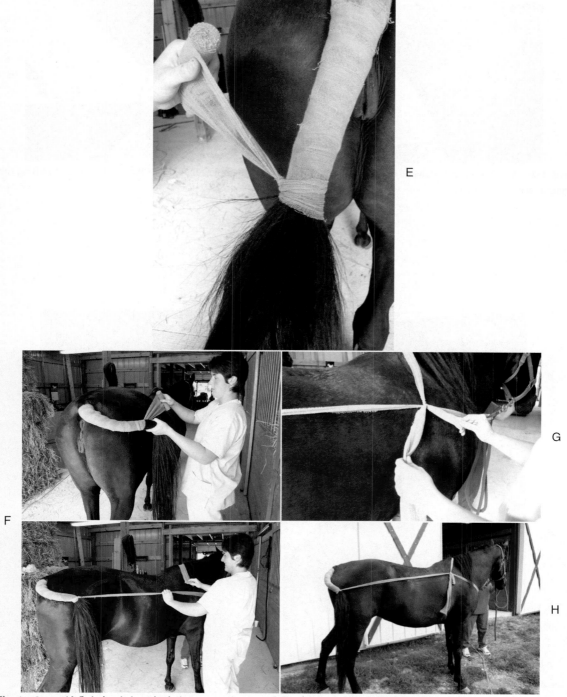

Fig. 6-28. cont'd E, A simple knot is tied to secure the wrap. **F,** The tail is supported while the gauze is passed cranially around the neck. **G,** A quick-release knot secures the wrap around the neck. **H,** Completed tail wrap.

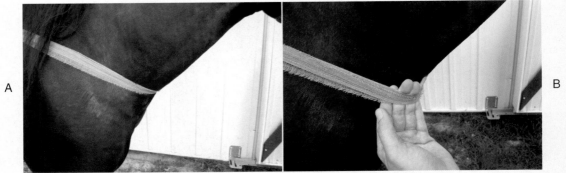

Fig. 6-29. A, Jugular vein distension results from partial occlusion by the tail wrap. **B,** Relieving the distension by lifting the gauze away from the neck.

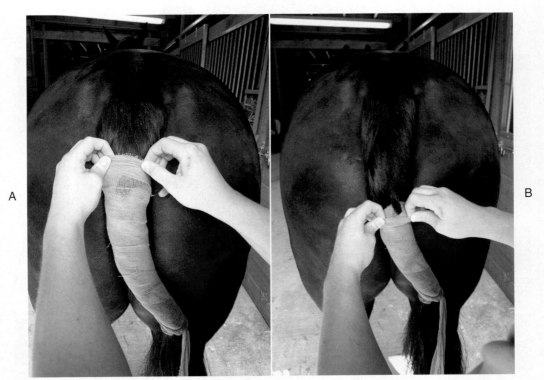

Fig. 6-30. A, To remove the tail wrap, grasp the gauze at the base of the tail. **B,** Pull the gauze distally to remove it.

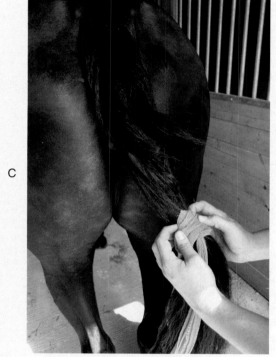

C

Fig. 6-30. cont'd C, Remove the wrap easily by sliding it off the tail.

TAIL BAGS

Horses with conditions such as diarrhea, impending foaling, or paralysis of the tail tend to soil the tail. Soiling then requires a tail bath, which is time consuming and, in the case of infectious diarrhea such as *Salmonella,* places the technician at risk of exposure to the infectious organisms. A plastic tail bag can be useful in these cases; it prevents soiling of the tail and can be changed daily or as needed. A rectal sleeve with the hand portion removed makes an ideal plastic tail "sleeve." Removal of the hand portion is necessary to allow good airflow under the sleeve; otherwise, moisture tends to build and can cause skin irritation.

The tail hairs are braided or taped (distal to the coccygeal vertebrae) so that they will be contained within the length of the plastic sleeve. The sleeve is then slid over the tail and secured near the base of the tail with two to three circles of an elastic adhesive tape, placing the tape to contact the skin adjacent to the proximal extent of the plastic sleeve. The anchoring tape should be placed passively (without applying compression) to avoid strangulation of the arterial supply (Fig. 6-31).

SUGGESTED READING

Hosgood G, Burba DJ: Wound healing, wound management, and bandaging. In McCurnin DM, Bassert JM: *Clinical textbook for veterinary technicians,* ed 6, St Louis, 2006, Saunders.

Sirois M: *Principles and practice of veterinary technology,* ed 2, St Louis, 2004, Mosby.

Stashak TS: *Equine wound management,* Philadelphia, 1991, Lea & Febiger.

Stone WC: Drains, dressings and external coaptation. In Auer JA, Stick JA: *Equine surgery,* St Louis, 1999, Saunders.

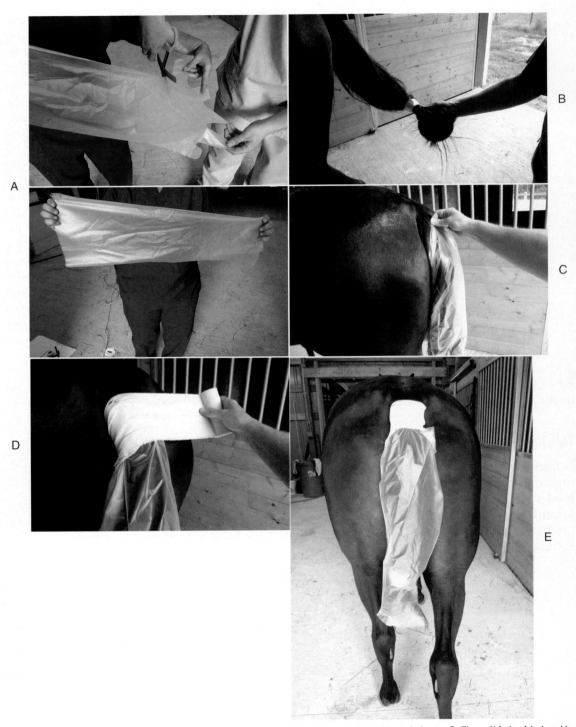

Fig. 6-31. A, The tail bag is created by removing the hand portion from a standard rectal sleeve. **B,** The tail is braided and/or taped to a length that will be totally covered by the tail bag. **C,** The tail is placed inside the sleeve. **D,** Elastic adhesive tape is placed around the base of the tail to hold the sleeve in place. **E,** Completed tail bag.

7

Diagnostic Imaging of Horses

Diagnostic imaging of large animals is similar to imaging of small animals. All of the imaging modalities used for small animals are also possible in large animals, though they may be limited in usefulness and availability because of the larger size of the animal. The limitations are usually related to an inability of the equipment to accommodate the size of the large animal patient or to penetrate into the patient to a sufficient depth. Another restriction is that large animal imaging often takes place on the farm, requiring use of portable equipment; portable equipment frequently lacks the output power of stationary equipment, thus limiting the ability to obtain diagnostic quality images of thick body parts.

Many excellent texts are available to the technician that detail the principles of diagnostic imaging. The actual principles of imaging are basically the same for small and large animals; they need only be adapted for the patient's location, size, and available equipment. This chapter emphasizes practical concerns and adaptations for large animals. The reader is encouraged to refer to other texts for in-depth discussion of imaging physics, specific techniques, and patient positioning.

DIAGNOSTIC RADIOLOGY

The principles of taking a quality, diagnostic radiograph are the same for large and small animals. However, large animal radiology is unique due to the conformation of the patient and the fact that most radiographs are performed on a standing, awake patient. The temperament of the animal often further limits the ability to position the patient for ideal film studies.

SAFETY

The physical safety of the people handling the horse and the safety of the horse must always be the first concern. Horses tend to be apprehensive about radiographs. Most radiograph machines make strange noises, generate a bright light for collimation, and generally must be positioned within 30 to 40 inches of the patient. Ideally the film cassette should be placed to contact the patient's skin, which may alarm the horse, causing it to move away or perhaps kick. The patient is often in pain from the injury or condition for which the radiograph is being taken, adding to the "fear factor." Personnel and equipment are therefore in vulnerable positions, with a patient that is often suspicious of the situation. Physical and/or chemical restraints must be selected carefully, and personnel should not be placed in dangerous, compromising positions. Common sense handling—moving slowly and speaking calmly—are necessary. It also helps to let the horse know what is coming (i.e., rather than slapping a cassette against the leg with no warning, it helps to gently rub the area a few times to accustom the horse to touch at that location, and then place the cassette against the skin). If the machine produces noise, the rotor can be activated once or twice to reproduce the noise before positioning the patient for the actual film.

Radiation safety is the next concern, once physical safety has been addressed. Small, portable radiograph machines present no less danger than the larger, fixed machines in hospitals and clinics; radiation is dangerous, regardless of the source. Personal protective equipment, such as lead aprons and thyroid collars, are recommended for everyone involved in the procedure. The person holding the cassette should always wear lead gloves, even if a mechanical cassette holder with an extension arm is used (Fig. 7-1).

In general, taking a radiograph requires three people: one to tend the horse's head, one to operate the radiograph machine, and one to position the film cassette. Whenever possible, these people should distance themselves from the primary x-ray beam. Cassette holders can be purchased or homemade to provide distance from the primary beam. Hay bales and buckets can also serve to prop up film cassettes for cooperative patients.

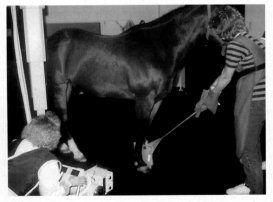

Fig. 7-1. Extension arm cassette holder for large animal radiography. Note that the technician is wearing lead gloves, even though the cassette holder is in use. (From Partington BP: Diagnostic imaging. In McCurnin DM, Bassert JM: *Clinical textbook for veterinary technicians*, ed 6, St Louis, 2006, Saunders.)

These devices should be used whenever the situation allows (Fig. 7-2).

The safety of the equipment must also enter the safety equation; radiograph machines and film cassettes are expensive, and they can also injure the patient. Because of the close distance of these items to the patient, the equipment is vulnerable and must be protected while the radiograph is taken. After the film is taken, the equipment should be removed from the immediate vicinity of the patient. Exposed and unexposed cassettes should be kept out of the area of the procedure for protection; they should also be kept in distinctly separate stacks to prevent accidental double exposure. Having a marking system to identify exposed cassettes provides an additional safeguard against double exposure.

EQUIPMENT

Radiograph machines are either mobile, fixed, or portable.

Mobile machines are the least frequently used; these are large machines designed for human hospitals to be rolled from room to room. In large animal practice, they are found only in hospital settings and are somewhat cumbersome to move and position. However, they are powerful and useful for thick body parts that smaller machines cannot penetrate (Fig. 7-3).

Fixed machines are mounted to either floor or ceiling tracks, which allow limited mobility within the radiograph procedure room. These machines have the highest output capabilities of any of the radiograph machine types; even so, they may not be able to penetrate thick body parts such as the pelvis on large individuals. Collimation and illumination tend to be superior; however, the noise generated by the rotors tends to be louder than the other machines (Fig. 7-4).

Most large animal radiographs are made with portable machines; these "farm call"

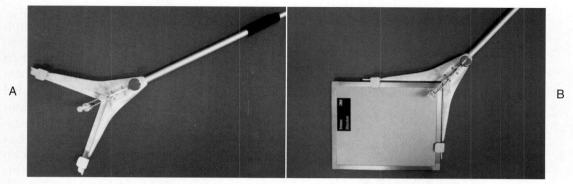

Fig. 7-2. **A**, Radiograph cassette holder. **B**, Film cassette inserted in the cassette holder.

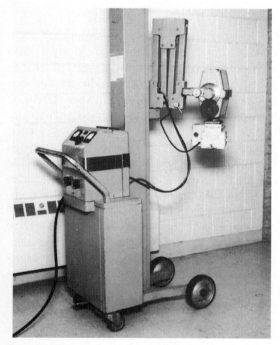

Fig. 7-3. **Mobile radiograph unit.** (From Lavin LM: *Radiography in veterinary technology,* ed 3, St Louis, 2003, Saunders.)

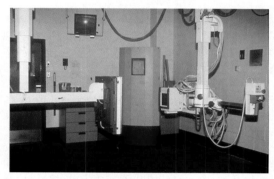

Fig. 7-4. **Fixed radiograph machine for large animals, with ceiling-mounted x-ray tube and film cassette holder.** (From Partington BP: Diagnostic imaging. In McCurnin DM, Bassert JM: *Clinical textbook for veterinary technicians,* ed 6, St Louis, 2006, Saunders.)

units are small enough to be taken almost anywhere there is an electrical power source (Fig. 7-5). They have limited output capability in terms of kVp (average 90 kVp maximum) and mA (average 20 mA maximum); therefore longer exposure times (S) must be used to compensate. The collimators on some portables may not be lighted, creating an inability to reliably aim the primary beam and control the exposure field.

Portable machines are usually used on the farm, in barns or paddocks where the quality of electricity—the "line voltage"—may be low or erratic. Portable machines have a minimum line voltage required to produce quality radiographs; there is a line voltage indicator on the machine that measures the strength of the incoming electricity. If the line voltage

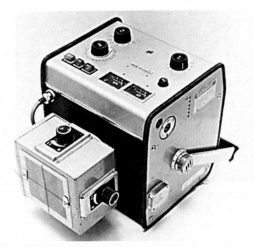

Fig. 7-5. Portable radiograph machine with a light collimator. (From Partington BP: Diagnostic imaging. In McCurnin DM, Bassert JM: *Clinical textbook for veterinary technicians*, ed 5, St Louis, 2002, Saunders.)

is low, turning off radios, electrical fences, barn lights, heaters, etc. often increases the voltage to an acceptable range.

Because of the limited power of portable machines, their ability to penetrate thick body parts is restricted. Assuming an average 1000-lb horse, the quality of radiographs of the following areas is usually compromised when a portable machine is used:
- Caudal areas of the skull
- Caudal cervical vertebrae
- Shoulder joint
- Craniocaudal view of the elbow joint
- Cranioventral thorax
- Pelvis
- Caudocranial view of the stifle joint
- Abdomen

When studies of these areas are necessary, the patient usually needs to be referred to a facility with a more powerful radiograph machine.

OTHER TYPES OF RADIOGRAPHY

Most radiographs are made using standard radiograph machines and radiographic film and cassettes. Xeroradiographs ("blue pictures") are also made with standard radiograph machines but use electrostatically charged plates to form latent images, which are then exposed to a charged powder (toner) to form a heat-transferred image to plastic-coated paper. Xeroradiographs provide excellent bone detail and better soft tissue visualization than conventional radiographs but require much higher exposures to form an image (as much as seven times higher); this creates additional safety risks to personnel. Also, the equipment is expensive and not economical for most practices. "Xeros" are useful when routine radiographs do not provide sufficient detail for a diagnosis.

Digital radiography is an emerging technology that is becoming more popular and affordable. Standard radiograph machines are used to generate the radiographs, but instead of conventional film cassettes, a phosphor-imaging plate is used to capture the radiographic image. The plate is then placed in a laser reader, where it is scanned with a laser beam and digitized for viewing on a computer monitor. The images can be enhanced and manipulated by the computer and printed out as hardcopy. Storage of images as computer files saves office space, and images can be transferred electronically to other veterinarians and veterinary radiologists.

COMMON PROBLEMS

Motion

The most common error in large animal radiography that prevents diagnostic quality radiographs is motion, which produces a blurred image ("moving picture") (Fig. 7-6). Long exposure times are frequently necessary in large animal radiography, especially with portable machines. Longer exposure times mean that there is more time for motion to occur as the image is being made.

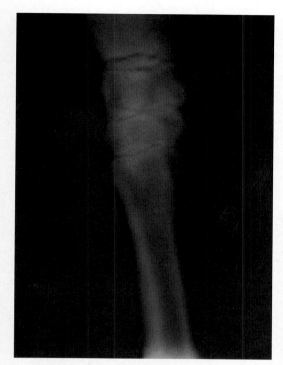

Fig. 7-6. Motion produces a blurred radiographic image.

There are three possible sources of motion:
1. Radiograph machine: This problem is associated with portable machines, which are often handheld during film taking. This motion source can be alleviated by using tripods or other stands that can be purchased for the machines or by improvising support with hay bales, buckets, or boxes when possible.
2. Patient: This is difficult to control with an awake patient. Even swaying from leg to leg can be enough to ruin the quality of an image. Effective restraint is essential. Chemical restraint must be used judiciously; oversedation can make a patient wobbly and unable to stand still.
3. Film cassette: Because cassettes are usually handheld directly or with a mechanical extension arm, the person holding the cassette must hold it as still as possible.

This is a difficult task, given the weight of the cassette and lead-lined gloves. Whenever possible, resting the cassette on the ground or a solid object may help to steady the cassette. Also, only high speed film/screen combinations should be used for general large animal radiography.

Movement of any one of the above during an exposure will be captured on the radiograph film. Before each radiograph is taken, all three sources should be evaluated as part of a mental checklist, with the goal of making each one as stationary as possible.

Height of Primary Beam

The object of most large animal radiographs is the distal limb, especially the foot. Radiographic principles require that the anatomical part of interest be positioned in the center of the x-ray beam; this minimizes distortion. When the hoof is on the ground, the center of the hoof will be 1 to 2 inches above the ground. Unfortunately, no radiograph machine can center a beam at that level. Even small portable machines generate a beam that is centered at a minimum of 3 to 4 inches above ground. Therefore, for foot films, since the beam cannot be lowered to foot level, the foot must be raised to the level of the center of the beam (Fig. 7-7, *A*). This can be accomplished by using positioning blocks or foot stands (Fig. 7-7, *B*). These can be commercially obtained or made from wood (wood blocks that are 4 × 4 inches and 2 × 4 inches are popular), Plexiglas, or other sturdy material that can support the horse's weight (Fig. 7-8). The device should be wide enough to prevent it from tipping over while the horse is standing on it; this will be at least the width of the horse's hoof. The horse's foot is placed on the positioning device only while the film is taken. Once the film is made, the device should be removed and set safely aside; the horse should not be allowed to stand on the support unattended.

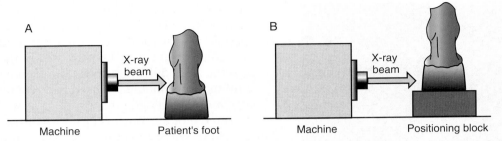

Fig. 7-7. A, Even with the machine resting on the ground, the x-ray beam is too high for structures in the foot. **B,** Elevation of the foot to the level of the x-ray beam, using a positioning block.

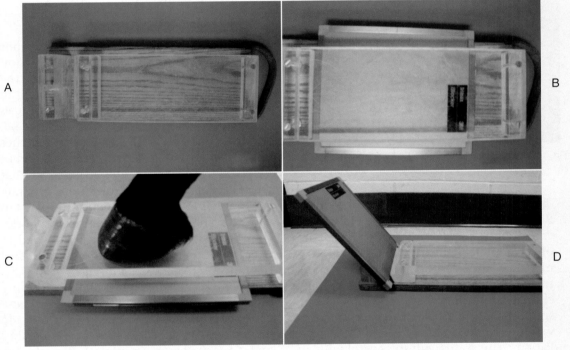

Fig. 7-8. A, Wood and Plexiglas positioning block for the equine foot. This design also has a cassette tunnel that protects the cassette for stand-on views. **B,** Position of the cassette for stand-on radiographic views. **C,** Position of foot and cassette for stand-on views of the foot. **D,** Slots provide additional support for film cassettes.

Marking System for Distal Limb Radiographs

Understanding that the distal limb of one leg is *indistinguishable* radiographically from the distal limb of any other leg is essential. This is because of the similar bone structure of *all* limbs distal to the carpus/tarsus. Without proper identification the clinician cannot tell a right distal limb from a left one or a front distal limb from a rear limb. Horses have had surgical procedures performed on the wrong leg because of errors in film identification. Lower leg films must always be accurately identified with some type of marker as either "right" or "left," *and* either "front" or "hind."

Radiographic views are named by the direction of the x-ray beam, from the radiograph machine to the film cassette. The first word (or initial) of the view identifies the location of the radiograph machine, and the second word (or initial) indicates the location of the film cassette. For example, if the machine is on the lateral aspect of the limb, and the film cassette is placed on the medial aspect of the leg, a lateromedial (LM) radiograph is produced. If the positions of the machine and cassette are reversed, a mediolateral (ML) view results.

The standard radiographic views used for the lower legs are, as in small animals, the LM view and the dorsal-palmar/plantar view.

To obtain additional information to the two standard 90-degree views, it is common in large animals to also obtain oblique (angled) views of the lower legs. There are four common oblique radiographic views, named by the direction of the radiograph beam (from radiograph machine to film cassette). The oblique views are made at 45-degree angles to the standard 90-degree views (Fig. 7-9). Oblique views of the distal limbs must be accurately marked, since they are also indistinguishable from one another below the carpus/tarsus.

Patient Preparation

The surface of the patient should be cleaned before taking radiographs. Shavings, dried mud, and other debris can create subtle images that interfere with interpretation of the film. Some topical medications contain iodine, and because iodine is radiopaque, it should be washed thoroughly from the area.

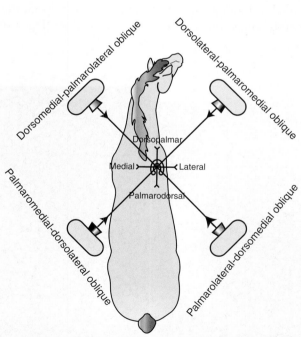

Fig. 7-9. Proper terminology for the standard and oblique views of the right forelimb of a horse, according to the position of the radiograph machine. (Adapted from Lavin LM: *Radiography in veterinary technology,* ed 3, St Louis, 2003, Saunders.)

Bandages should be removed if possible. Although radiographs can penetrate bandages and even casts, these materials may obscure subtle anatomical lesions. If it is not safe or feasible to remove a bandage or cast, slightly longer exposure time or higher kVp can be used to help compensate for the added thickness.

Foot Radiographs

Preparation of the foot is important for good quality films. The hoof should always be cleaned to remove dirt, gravel, and bedding. If necessary, a brush and water with mild soap can be used to clean the hoof wall, sole, and recesses of the frog.

Horseshoes should be removed whenever possible. Metallic horseshoes and nails obscure clear vision of the anatomical structures within the hoof (Fig. 7-10). However, owners are understandably reluctant to have the shoes removed; there is additional expense and time involved in having the farrier replace the shoe. Rarely, the veterinarian

may be able to see hoof lesions without removing shoes, but in most cases, the owner should be advised that the shoes should be removed to have the best chance of obtaining diagnostic-quality radiographs. Client consent should always be obtained *before* pulling the horse's shoes. Because many horses tend to chip and crack their hooves if left unprotected, a temporary duct tape "hoof bootie" or commercial rubber boot can be used to protect the hoof until the farrier can return to replace the horseshoe.

The deep grooves of the sole (central sulcus of the frog and lateral sulci of the frog) are naturally occupied by air. The air creates artifacts—dark gas lines—on dorsopalmar/plantar (straight and oblique) hoof radiographs. These gas lines mimic fracture lines and may obscure true lesions. The gas lines can be eliminated by filling the grooves with something other than gas; semisolid radiolucent materials such as Play-Doh or putty are commonly used to pack the grooves and eliminate the air pockets (Fig. 7-11). The packing material

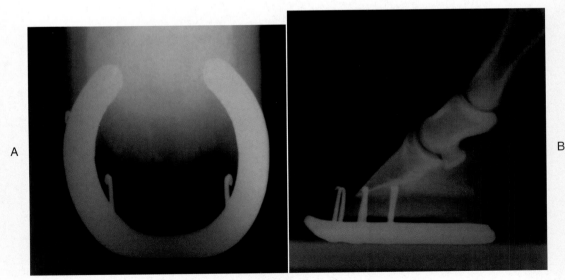

A   B

Fig. 7-10. A and **B,** Horseshoes interfere with interpretation of radiographs.

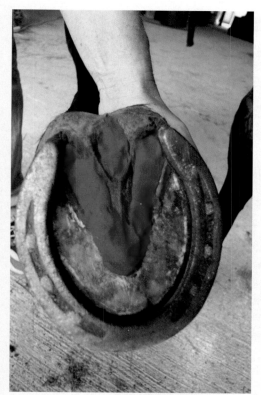

Fig. 7-11. Packing of the grooves of the sole for radiographs.

should be pressed firmly into the grooves to fill them deeply and completely; however, overfilling should be avoided. Filling beyond the margins of the grooves is unnecessary, and overfilling may actually create more artifacts that obscure accurate interpretation of the film.

After packing the hoof grooves, the packing material should be covered before the horse is allowed to set the foot down on the ground. Covering the material is necessary to prevent gravel, bedding, and other debris from sticking to the material and causing artifacts. A paper towel or piece of brown paper pressed over the packing is all that is necessary to cover and protect the area (Fig. 7-12).

Head/Throat Radiographs

Metallic buckles and billets are radiopaque. Halters with metal should be removed and replaced with halters without metal.

Because of the machine lights and noise, as well as pressing film cassettes against the head, most horses do not stand quietly for radiographs of the head area. Sedation is almost always required to obtain diagnostic films of this highly detailed region.

Pelvic Radiographs

Because of the extreme thickness and anatomical structure of the pelvic region, lateral views of the pelvis are only possible on small equids. The ventrodorsal view is available for larger animals but requires a frog-leg position in dorsal recumbency, obtainable only with the patient under general anesthesia. Patient preparation for general anesthesia is therefore required for this procedure.

STANDARD RADIOGRAPHIC VIEWS

Although the number of radiographic views of an anatomical part is limited only by the imagination, standardized views for each part have emerged to provide consistency in interpretation of radiographic films. Table 7-1 lists the standard radiographic views for the limbs, plus common supplemental views.

NUCLEAR SCINTIGRAPHY

Scintigraphy is a method of imaging that emphasizes physiology rather than anatomy. Whereas a radiograph or ultrasound takes an image of a patient's anatomy, scintigraphy takes an image of a patient's physiological processes. This is accomplished by administering a radioactive compound, allowing the compound to accumulate within the patient, and then measuring the amount of radioactivity emitted from the patient. A gamma camera is used to measure the radioactivity.

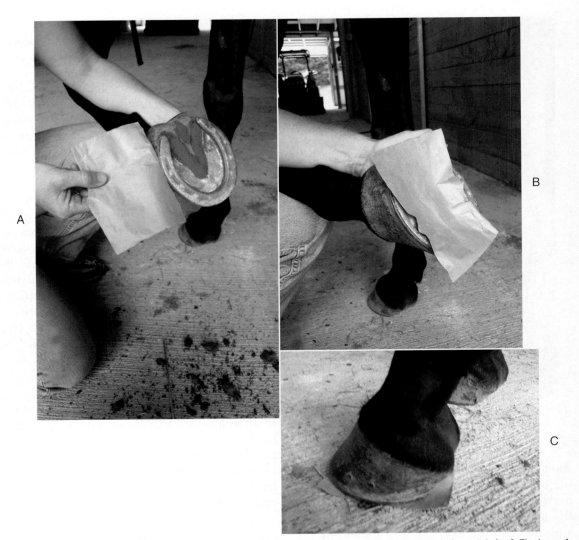

Fig. 7-12. A and **B,** A small piece of brown paper is pressed over the packing material to protect it from debris. **C,** The horse is allowed to set the hoof down once the packing material has been covered.

The properties of the radioactive compound determine where in the body the compound is likely to accumulate, according to the body organs that process the compound; this is the physiological part of the image process. The radioactive compound, or radiopharmaceutical, is made by attaching a radioisotope to another compound that has an affinity for certain body organs, such as iodine for the thyroid or phosphonates for bone. Technetium-99m is the most common radioisotope used for the radiolabel.

Most large animal scintigraphy is performed to evaluate the musculoskeletal system; skeletal scintigraphy is also known as a "bone scan." The patient is sedated for

TABLE

7-1 RADIOGRAPHIC VIEWS OF THE EQUINE LIMBS

Anatomical Part	Standard Radiographic Views	Supplemental Views
P3/Hoof	Straight DP 60 degrees DP (stand-on) Lateromedial	60 degrees DP obliques (stand-on)
Navicular bone	Lateromedial 60 degrees DP(stand-on) 45 degrees flexor tangential (stand-on)	30 degrees DP (stand-on) 45 degrees DP (stand-on) 60 degrees DP obliques (stand-on)
Pastern	Lateromedial Straight DP Obliques (MLO, LMO)	30 degrees DP
Fetlock	Lateromedial Flexed lateromedial Straight DP Obliques (MLO, LMO)	Hanging DP Flexor skyline Proximal-distal obliques (MLO, LMO)
Metacarpus /metatarsus	Lateromedial DP Obliques (MLO, LMO)	
Carpus	Lateromedial Flexed lateromedial DP Obliques (MLO, LMO)	Flexed skyline (distal radius) Flexed skyline (proximal row carpal bones) Flexed skyline (distal row carpal bones)
Radius	Lateromedial Craniocaudal (AP)	Obliques (MLO, LMO)
Elbow	Mediolateral Craniocaudal (AP)	
Shoulder	Mediolateral	
Tarsus	Lateromedial DP Obliques (MLO, LMO)	Flexed skyline Flexed lateromedial
Tibia	Lateromedial Craniocaudal (AP)	Obliques (MLO, LMO)
Stifle	Lateromedial Caudocranial (PA)	Flexed lateromedial Flexed skyline Obliques (MLO, LMO)
Pelvis	Ventrodorsal	Ventrodorsal obliques

DP, *Dorsopalmar/dorsoplantar;* MLO, *mediolateral oblique;* LMO, *lateromedial oblique;* AP, *anteroposterior;* PA, *posteroanterior.*

the procedure. Technetium-labeled diphosphonate is given intravenously to the patient, and the diphosphonates are incorporated into the patient's bone, taking the radioactive technetium "tags" with them. The radioactivity over the bone is then measured, and high emission of radiation is assumed to reflect areas of increased blood flow in the bone and/or uptake by osteoblasts—an indication of inflammation and/or new bone formation. These areas of increased radioactivity are commonly called "hot spots."

Scintigraphy is helpful in detecting lesions when radiography and ultrasonography have not confirmed a diagnosis or cannot penetrate deeply enough, especially in the regions of the upper limbs, shoulders, and pelvis. Scintigraphy can also screen large areas of the patient (Fig. 7-13).

Only clinics or hospitals that are licensed to handle and dispose of radioactive materials and waste can perform this procedure. The patient must usually be isolated for several days until the radioactive material is cleared from the body; excrement requires special handling requirements. Each state has regulations for licensing and operating these facilities.

COMPUTED TOMOGRAPHY

Computed tomography (CT), or "CAT scan," was unavailable to large animal patients until recent years. Technical modifications have been necessary to adapt CT for large animal patients, and its use is still restricted to examination of the head, cranial cervical spine, and distal limbs in the adult horse. The spinal cord, thorax, and abdomen can be imaged in miniature horses and small foals, depending on the diameter of the equipment. CT equipment is expensive; therefore it is only found in specialized facilities. Another consideration is that the patient must be under general anesthesia to prevent motion during the scan. The cost of a CT scan, therefore, is expensive—reflecting the cost of the equipment and the cost of general anesthesia. CT is used only when other diagnostic methods have failed to provide a diagnosis (Fig. 7-14).

CT is essentially a series of thin, cross-sectional radiographs. The part to be imaged

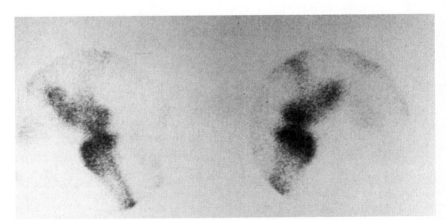

Fig. 7-13. Nuclear scintigraphic scan of both stifle joints in a lame horse. Note the increased radioactivity *(blackness)* of the right stifle as compared to the left stifle joint. The horse had degenerative joint disease (chronic arthritis) in the right stifle.
(From Lavin LM: *Radiography in veterinary technology,* ed 3, St Louis, 2003, Saunders.)

is placed inside a donut-shaped ring called a gantry. The gantry contains a small x-ray tube and multiple radiation detectors to receive the radiograph beam from different angles. The gantry rotates around the patient, taking multiple radiographic images. The images are collected and assimilated by a computer, resulting in a gray-scale cross-sectional image of the part. The computer can be used to digitally enhance different types of tissue.

As technology progresses, larger gantries may allow CT scans of larger body parts in adult horses. CT is generally superior to

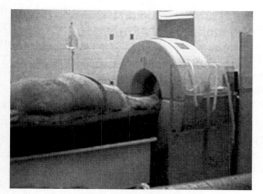

Fig. 7-14. Computed tomography scan of the equine head. (From Kraft SL, Gavin P: *Vet Clin North Am Equine Pract* 17:115-130, 2001.)

magnetic resonance imaging (MRI) for bone lesions.

MAGNETIC RESONANCE IMAGING

MRI is now possible for large animals. The physics of MRI are complex but basically involve placing the body part to be studied in a powerful magnetic field. The magnetic field causes alignment of all of the hydrogen nuclei (protons) in the body part; then, radiofrequency pulses are sent through the part. This temporarily excites the magnetized protons, which emit radiofrequency signals when they return to the original magnetized state. These signals are detected and transformed into images by computer. Ionizing radiation is not used in the procedure (Fig. 7-15).

The usefulness of MRI in large animals is currently restricted by the physical capacity of the equipment. The head, cervical spinal cord, and lower legs can be imaged in an adult horse. The cost of the equipment is quite high, and therefore MRI is not widely available at this time. Similar to CT, general anesthesia is required, and the cost of the procedure is high due to the expensive equipment and cost of general anesthesia. MRI tends to be superior to CT for soft tissue imaging.

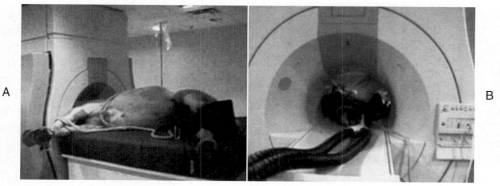

Fig. 7-15. Magnetic resonance imaging scan of the equine head. **A,** Patient position in the magnetic resonance gantry. **B,** View of horse's head within the gantry, with anesthetic tubing. (From Kraft SL, Gavin P: *Vet Clin North Am Equine Pract* 17:115-130, 2001.)

THERMOGRAPHY

Diagnostic thermography uses a "heat camera" to scan the body surface temperature of the patient. This technique is popular because it is noninvasive, and the equipment has become more affordable and portable. Thermography can be used to examine specific body parts or used for whole body screens as part of regular "wellness" examinations of the legs. The primary use of thermography is to locate "hot spots," which may indicate inflammation (Fig. 7-16). Heat is one of the cardinal signs of inflammation. Thermography is best used to locate inflammation near the body surface. Areas of inflammation deep within the thorax or abdomen cannot be seen with thermography.

False-positive (increased heat) readings are likely with thermography unless the conditions of the examination are closely controlled. The patient should be shielded from environmental heat sources such as the sun. Bandages, tack, and blankets can all cause a local increase in heat; patients should have these removed 2 hours before the examination. Topical medications should also be removed. The area of the examination should be less than 86° F to prevent sweating; 70° F is ideal. The area should be free of drafts.

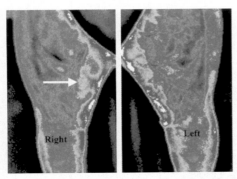

Fig. 7-16. Thermogram of both stifles. The right stifle shows a "hot spot" over the medial femorotibial joint. (From Turner TA: *Vet Clin North Am Equine Pract* 17:95-113, 2001.)

The patient should be placed in the examination area and allowed approximately 20 to 30 minutes to acclimate to the room's temperature.

Artifacts are easily produced on a thermogram, and any hot spots should be closely inspected for possible insignificant sources of heat or cold. Insects and insect bites can produce artifact hot spots on a thermogram. Injection procedures such as diagnostic nerve and joint blocks produce inflammation and cause artifact hot spots on the scan; it may be necessary to wait up to a week before performing thermography on patients that have had injections in the area of interest. Also, areas where the hair has been clipped alter the surface temperature of the skin and may create artifacts. Generally, if possible, the thermogram should be performed before the horse is clipped or injected.

Thermography is useful to locate the general area of an injury but lacks the detail necessary for a specific diagnosis in most cases. Typically, once a hot spot is identified with thermography, radiography or ultrasound must be used to accurately define the problem.

DIAGNOSTIC ULTRASOUND

Ultrasound employs high-frequency sound waves that are beyond the range of human hearing. Depending on the frequency, ultrasound waves can be used for either diagnostic imaging (diagnostic ultrasound or "sonogram") or for therapeutic treatment of soft tissue injuries (therapeutic ultrasound). Because diagnostic ultrasound and therapeutic ultrasound serve different purposes, they require different equipment, and the equipment is not interchangeable (Fig. 7-17).

Ultrasound is generally superior to standard radiographs for visualizing soft tissues. Radiographs are generally superior for imaging bony structures (Fig. 7-18).

Diagnostic ultrasound commonly uses sound waves in the frequency range of 2 to 10 megahertz (MHz). The waves are generated by a transducer, which is a handheld attachment to the ultrasound machine. The sound waves penetrate the patient's tissues and are reflected by tissue interfaces (i.e., the junctions between different tissue types and tissue contents) (Fig. 7-19). The transducer receives these reflected waves or "echoes" and relays them to the ultrasound machine. The ultrasound machine processes the waves into a visual image that displays on a video screen. The image is generated as a series of dots; the brightness of each dot corresponds to the amplitude of the reflected sound wave. Very bright areas are called *hyperechoic* and generally indicate a more solid tissue; black areas are called *anechoic* and generally indicate liquid. If an area generates less brightness than expected, the area is called *hypoechoic.*

The frequency of the ultrasound waves greatly influences the quality of the ultrasound examination. The higher the frequency, the shorter the wavelength; this leads to better resolution (definition) of the image, but the trade-off is low penetration (depth) of the scan. Conversely, low frequency waves penetrate more deeply into the patient but with less resolution. Transducers are usually limited

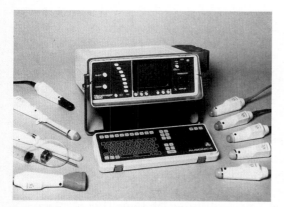

Fig. 7-17. Portable ultrasound machine (Ausonics Microimager) and compatible ultrasound probes. (From Lavin LM: *Radiography in veterinary technology,* ed 3, St Louis, 2003, Saunders.)

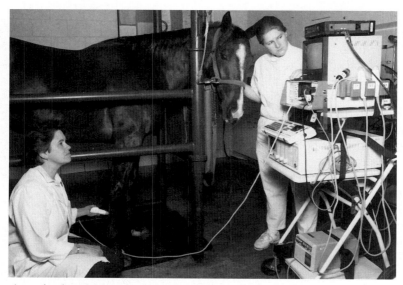

Fig. 7-18. Ultrasound examination of the metacarpal region of the horse. (From Lavin LM: *Radiography in veterinary technology,* ed 3, St Louis, 2003, Saunders.)

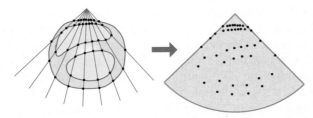

Fig. 7-19. Ultrasound waves are reflected by tissue interfaces *(left)*. The images are converted into a series of dots to form a B-mode sonogram. (Adapted from Powis RL: *Vet Clin North Am Equine Pract* 2:3-27, 1986.)

TABLE 7-2 **ULTRASOUND TRANSDUCER PROBES AND COMMON APPLICATIONS**

Frequency (MHz)	Common Applications
10.0	Superficial tendons, ligaments, bone surfaces, eyes, jugular vein, umbilicus
7.5	Superficial tendons, ligaments, bone surfaces, eyes, jugular vein, umbilicus, male reproductive organs
5.0	Female reproductive system (per rectum), abdominal viscera (per rectum), muscles
2.5-3.0	Heart, pleural cavity, superficial aspects of lungs, kidneys, liver, spleen, abdomen (outer 10-18 inches), cranial mediastinum, deep muscle, and bone surfaces

to the production of a single frequency; therefore several transducers must be purchased to give the practitioner the ability to scan a variety of anatomical structures (Table 7-2).

There are two basic types of transducers. Linear array transducers have ultrasound crystals, which emit the ultrasound waves, arranged in a row (Fig. 7-20). This emits ultrasound from multiple points along the transducer, producing a rectangular image (Fig. 7-21). Sector scanner transducers have one or more ultrasound crystals that rotate or oscillate to produce a pie-shaped image (Fig. 7-22). Variations of sector scanners, such as the annular array and phased array, are also available for some machines; these are more expensive machines used mostly for cardiac studies such as color-flow Doppler echocardiography.

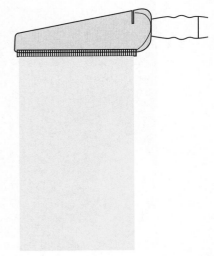

Fig. 7-20. A standard linear array transducer. (Adapted from Reef VB: *Equine diagnostic ultrasound*, St Louis, 1998, Saunders.)

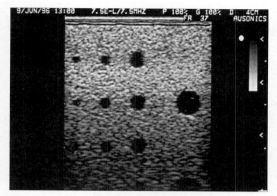

Fig. 7-21. Sonogram produced by a linear array transducer.
(From Reef VB: *Equine diagnostic ultrasound*, St Louis, 1998, Saunders.)

There are two common types of display modes used for ultrasound examinations. B (brightness) mode is the most commonly used; the brightness of the dots corresponds to the strength of the returning echoes. The examination is conducted in real time, but the real-time image can be frozen at any time on the screen for closer study or for recording onto camera or video film. The other type of display is M (motion) mode, which is used primarily for echocardiography (Fig. 7-23). M mode is essentially "B mode in motion" across the viewing screen. The image is a "trace" over time of the movements of the heart structures, allowing measurement of wall thickness, valve motions, and chamber capacities.

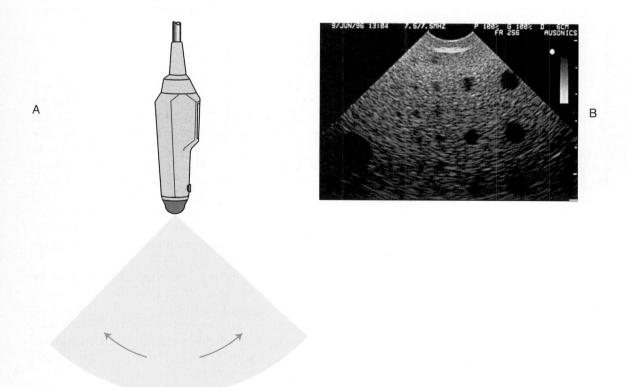

Fig. 7-22. A, Sector-scanner transducer. **B,** Sonogram produced by a sector scanner transducer. (Adapted from Reef VB: *Equine diagnostic ultrasound*, St Louis, 1998, Saunders.)

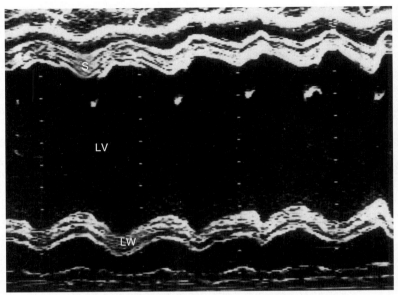

Fig. 7-23. Echocardiogram. *S*, Interventricular septum; *LV*, left ventricle; *LW*, left ventricular wall. (From Lavin LM: *Radiography in veterinary technology*, ed 3, St Louis, 2003, Saunders.)

The maximum depth of penetration for most ultrasound machines is 30 to 40 cm. This depth does *not* allow complete examination of the entire thoracic or abdominal cavity from the exterior of the patient. The abdomen has the additional option of internal ultrasound via the rectum; however, rectal examinations are limited by the length of the examiner's arm, and there are regions of the abdomen that cannot be completely evaluated. Despite these limitations, ultrasound is an invaluable tool in the examination of these body cavities.

PATIENT PREPARATION

Air reflects sound waves, which produces an essentially meaningless image. For this reason, there must be no air between the patient and the transducer during the examination.

The patient's haircoat traps air and creates numerous little air pockets. The best quality images are obtained if the hair is clipped; if the hair is coarse, shaving may also be necessary (Fig. 7-24). The owner's permission should be obtained before clipping the patient; occasionally an owner may object to this procedure. The owner must understand that failure to remove hair can compromise the scan, especially when trying to find subtle lesions. In these cases, thoroughly soaking the area with water for several minutes before the examination may improve the results.

After clipping, the clipped hairs must be thoroughly wiped from the surface to avoid creating artifact reflections. Also, skin scurf creates artifacts; softening the scurf with warm water helps to remove it. Dirt, topical medications, and any other debris should also be removed.

A coupling medium is used to provide a continuous path for the ultrasound waves between the transducer and the patient,

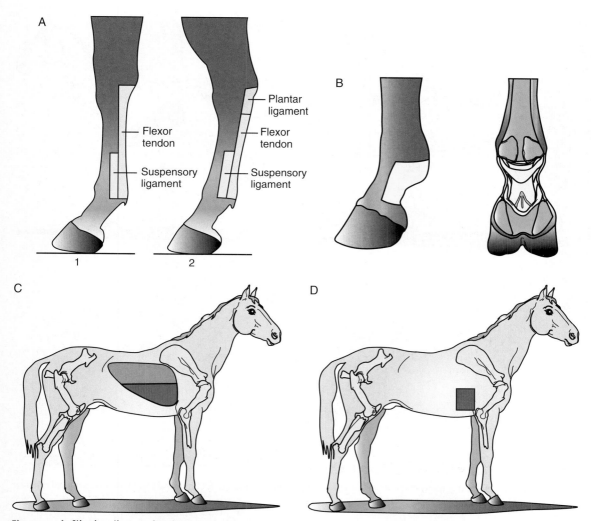

Fig. 7-24. A, Clipping diagram for ultrasound examination of the tendons and ligaments of the metacarpus *(1)* and metatarsus *(2)*. The areas marked "Suspensory ligament" are clipped if the suspensory branches are to be evaluated. **B,** Clipping diagram for ultrasound examination of the tendons and ligaments of the pastern. **C,** Clipping diagram for noncardiac ultrasound examination of the right thorax *(dark gray).* The *lighter gray area* is added if abnormal lung sounds are ausculted in the dorsal lung field. **D,** Clipping diagram for cardiac ultrasound from the right side. The window is centered over the right fourth intercostal space and covers the area from the point of the elbow to the point of the shoulder. For examination from the left, the window is centered over the third to fifth intercostal spaces. Note that the forelimb is positioned cranially to open up the window.

Continued.

E

F

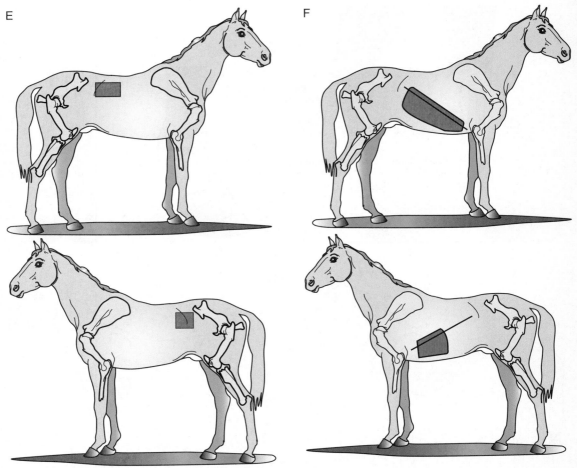

Fig. 7-24. cont'd E, Clipping diagram for ultrasound of the right and left kidneys. **F,** Clipping diagram for ultrasound of the liver from both sides of the horse.

free of air. Usually, commercial ultrasound coupling gel is used. Coupling gel can be bought in bulk and portioned into individual containers for more convenient use. Other gels such as OB lubricant and KY Jelly can be used. The use of mineral oil is discouraged for use on the skin; it causes many horses to scurf, is difficult to remove, and can damage the transducer head. Coupling gels should be thoroughly removed from the skin after the examination, since they may be irritating to the skin if allowed to dry.

The ultrasound waves emitted from the transducer have a focal zone, similar to a camera or radiograph machine (Fig. 7-25). Objects that are closer to the transducer than the focal zone, or beyond the focal zone, will not be in focus. This commonly occurs when trying to examine structures that are superficial (near the skin) and is referred

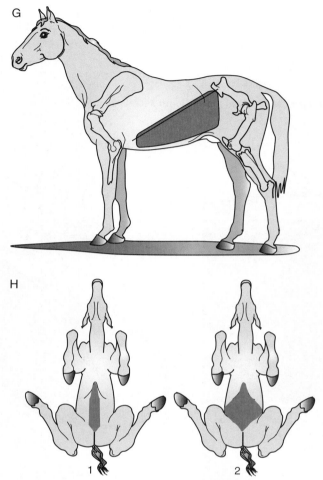

Fig. 7-24. cont'd G, Clipping diagram for ultrasound examination of the spleen. **H,** Clipping diagram for umbilical or bladder examination *(1)* and general abdominal examination *(2)* in the foal. (Adapted from Reef VB: *Equine diagnostic ultrasound*, St Louis, 1998, Saunders.)

to as a near-field artifact. To compensate, "standoffs"—jellylike synthetic pads—are used to back the transducer away from the skin, allowing the skin and structures just beneath the skin to fall within the transducer's focal zone. Standoffs may be built into some transducer heads, while others are handheld. Standoffs are easily damaged by excessive pressure and sharp objects, and they should be handled carefully. The handheld pads are usually stored in a refrigerator and should be allowed to warm to room temperature for best results.

REPRODUCTIVE ULTRASOUND

Reproductive ultrasound examinations are commonly used in large animal practice to image the ovaries and uterus. These examinations are performed to diagnose pregnancy (as early as 10 days), detect twin pregnancies,

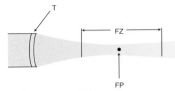

Fig. 7-25. The transducer *(T)* operates in a focal zone *(FZ)* with a focal point *(FP).* (From Powis RL: *Vet Clin North Am Equine Pract* 2:3-27, 1986.)

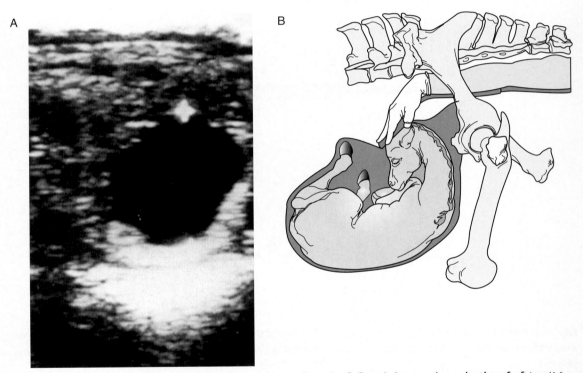

A

B

Fig. 7-26. A, A 16-day pregnancy, visualized rectally with a 5-mHz probe. **B,** Rectal ultrasound examination of a fetus. (**A** from Torbeck RL: *Vet Clin North Am Equine Pract* 2:227-252, 1986; **B** adapted from Reef VB: *Equine diagnostic ultrasound,* St Louis, 1998, Saunders.)

determine the sex of a fetus, identify pathology of the uterus and ovaries, and confirm the stage of the female's estrous cycle (Fig. 7-26). These examinations are performed via the rectum, except in the case of late gestation, when the fetus is best imaged from the exterior (Fig. 7-27). Some individuals resent rectal examination; care must be taken to protect

the operator and the equipment from kicks and patient movement. Stocks, hay bales, stall doors, and doorways can be used as barriers against kicking and excessive movement.

Fetal sex determination ("sexing") is best performed between days 60 and 75 of gestation. Sexing requires locating the genital tubercle. In males the genital tubercle is located near

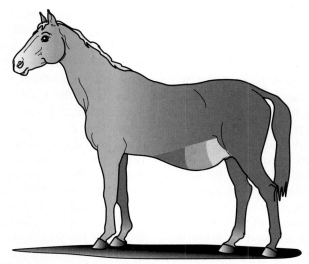

Fig. 7-27. Clipping diagram for a mare for late gestation external ultrasound. (Adapted from Reef VB: *Equine diagnostic ultrasound,* St Louis, 1998, Saunders.)

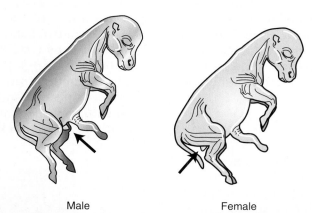

Male   Female

Fig. 7-28. The genital tubercle is located closer to the umbilicus in the male and closer to the tail in the female. (Adapted from Reef VB: *Equine diagnostic ultrasound,* St Louis, 1998, Saunders.)

the umbilicus, and in females the genital tubercle is closer to the tail (Fig. 7-28). Before day 60, the genital tubercle is located between the hindlimbs and has not yet migrated sufficiently to easily predict sex. After day 75, the fetus has grown to a size and location that often prevents visualization of the genital tubercle.

CARE OF ULTRASOUND EQUIPMENT

Transducers are expensive and are the most easily damaged part of an ultrasound machine. Hard impacts can damage the ultrasound crystals. The surface is susceptible to scratching from abrasive materials. Built-in stand-offs are susceptible to punctures and cuts. The transducer cable should never be folded;

rather, it should be loosely coiled to prevent breaking the cable wires.

The manufacturer specifies which cleaning agents are safe to use on the transducer. These instructions should be followed to prevent damage to the surface of the transducer. Abrasive cleaning agents and pads should never be used to clean transducer heads.

Cold weather can affect ultrasound examinations by altering the properties of coupling gels and standoff pads. If possible, examinations should not be performed in extreme cold. When performing examinations in a cold environment, the coupling gel should be applied and allowed to warm to the patient's skin temperature before conducting the examination. Standoff pads also benefit from warming before use; placing the pad against the body for several minutes can warm the pad in a cold environment if another heat source is not available.

Ultrasound machines should be kept covered when not in use. If the machine is to be used for ambulatory work, a hard case is desirable to protect the unit while it is being transported.

ENDOSCOPY

Endoscopes come in two basic varieties: rigid and flexible. Rigid endoscopes are used for arthroscopy, laparoscopy, thoracoscopy, and rhinoscopy (especially evaluation of the sinuses). An external light source provides illumination for the procedure. The insertion tube is made of metal and should not be bent or flexed. The operator can observe directly through the eyepiece, but more commonly a video camera and screen are used for viewing. Rigid endoscopes are relatively short in length (most are <18 inches) compared to flexible endoscopes, which are up to 3 m (9 feet) long.

The flexible fiberoptic endoscope is basically a flexible, nonmetallic tube that houses two bundles of fibers; one bundle carries light from an external, stationary light source to the tip of the endoscope, and the other bundle returns a visual image from the tip back to the operator's eyepiece. The tube also contains a system of wires and interlocking rings that allow the tip to be moved or deflected in different planes; this allows the endoscope to be directed around curves and corners and provide views in multiple directions. Most endoscopes have additional internal channels for passing instruments (such as biopsy or grasping forceps) and channels for air, water, and/or suction systems (Fig. 7-29).

The flexible endoscope consists of three main parts: The *control handpiece* contains the eyepiece, deflection knobs, air, suction and water controls, and entrances to instrument channels. The *insertion tubing* is the long tube that is inserted into the patient; it is usually marked with gradations for length at 10 cm intervals. The *light guide cable* connects the control handpiece to the external light source and transmits light to the light fiber bundle (Fig. 7-30).

The operator controls the endoscope with the control handpiece by observing through the eyepiece and manipulating the tip with the deflection knobs. An assistant is

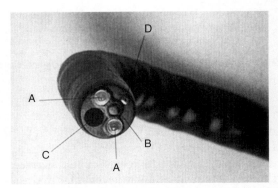

Fig. 7-29. Distal tip of the endoscope insertion tube. A, Illumination lenses; B, viewing lens; C, instrument channel; D, air/water channel. (From Traub-Dargatz JL, Brown CM: *Equine endoscopy*, ed 2, St Louis, 1997, Mosby.)

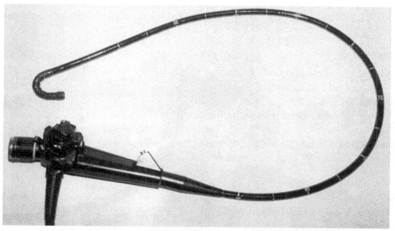

Fig. 7-30. Control handpiece and insertion tube of the flexible endoscope. The light guide cable exits the bottom of the photo.
(From Traub-Dargatz JL, Brown CM: *Equine endoscopy*, ed 2, St Louis, 1997, Mosby.)

usually necessary to support and advance the insertion tubing into the patient, under the guidance of the operator. Since endoscopy is usually performed on standing, awake horses, additional staff may be required to restrain the patient.

Only the operator can view the conveyed images through the eyepiece. Video endoscope systems that project images onto a larger video viewing screen are available; this is made possible by attaching an external video camera to the endoscope eyepiece. The video screen allows bystanders to view the examination. Video image endoscopes that use a microchip and electric charges instead of a fiberoptic bundles to carry images back to a viewing screen are also available. Permanent records of an endoscopic examination can be made with still photographs and video recordings, either by using a video recording system or attaching still cameras to the eyepiece with an adapter ring.

The most common use of endoscopy in equine practice is for examination of the upper respiratory tract. These examinations are usually performed with the horse at rest,

but with the advent of the treadmill, a dynamic examination can now be performed to visualize problems that may not be apparent at rest (Fig. 7-31). Upper respiratory examinations are conducted by introducing the endoscope through a nostril and passing it through the nasal cavity; most horses resent this procedure and must be physically and/or chemically restrained. The procedure is similar to nasogastric intubation, and the same safety precautions used for nasogastric intubation should be followed whenever the endoscope is introduced through the nares.

Gastroscopy, the next most common use of endoscopy, was developed primarily to assess gastric ulceration in horses. Standard endoscopes (<110 cm) are not long enough to reach the stomach except perhaps in miniature horses and young foals; for adults, a scope 3 meters long is recommended. Endoscopes for gastroscopy are therefore more expensive than standard scopes. The endoscope is passed through a nostril to the pharynx and then down the esophagus to the stomach, similar to the path used for nasogastric intubation. Once the endoscope tip is in the

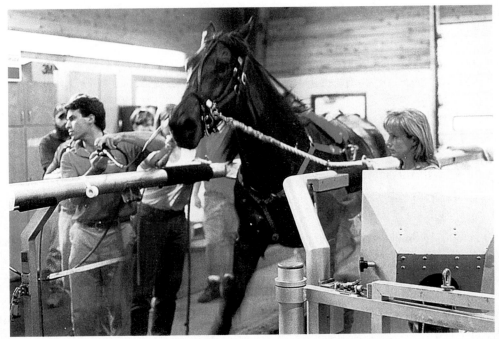

Fig. 7-31. Endoscope examination of a Standardbred exercising on a treadmill. The endoscopist is observing the examination on a video monitor (not included in the photograph). The equipment to the horse's left is the treadmill control panel. (From Traub-Dargatz JL, Brown CM: *Equine endoscopy*, ed 2, St Louis, 1997, Mosby.)

stomach, the stomach is inflated with air to facilitate visualization; this may produce some patient discomfort. Gastroscopy requires patient fasting before the examination and sedation during the examination for best results.

Urinary tract endoscopy is also possible in both sexes. By passing the endoscope through the urethral orifice, the urethra and bladder of both males and females can be visualized. Sedation of the male is necessary to relax and extend the penis for passage of the endoscope through the urethra; females have wider and shorter urethras and may be more tolerant of the procedure (Fig. 7-32). To reduce the risk of introducing bacteria into the urinary bladder, the endoscope should be cold sterilized and the patient properly cleansed, similar to preparation for passing a urinary catheter. (Clean the glans penis in the male and vulva in the female.)

In the female, the endoscope can be used to evaluate the vagina, cervix, and uterus. The tail should be wrapped and held or tied to keep it away from the perineum during prepping and examination. The perineal area is thoroughly cleansed with water and mild soap, centering on the vulvar lips and progressing outwardly 4 to 6 inches, similar to preparation for vaginal and uterine reproductive procedures. The person passing the endoscope should wear sterile gloves. Sterile lubricating jelly is applied to the outer surface of the endoscope *except* over the optic surface of the tip. Depositing lubricant over the endoscope tip should be avoided because the lubricant can obscure the lenses and instrument channels. Alternatively, sterile

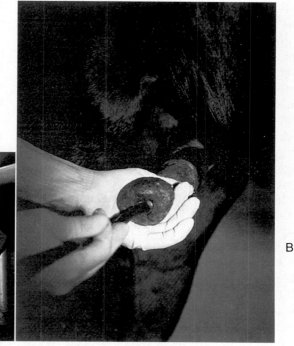

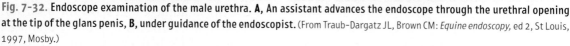

Fig. 7-32. Endoscope examination of the male urethra. **A,** An assistant advances the endoscope through the urethral opening at the tip of the glans penis, **B,** under guidance of the endoscopist. (From Traub-Dargatz JL, Brown CM: *Equine endoscopy,* ed 2, St Louis, 1997, Mosby.)

water can be used to lubricate the tip and does not obscure vision through the lenses. The uterus must be inflated with air to balloon the walls of the uterus; this is necessary for visualization within the organ. Sedation in usually required, since the procedure produces some discomfort when the uterus is inflated with air.

Surgical procedures can be performed through the endoscope. Most of the procedures are performed on the upper respiratory tract in standing, sedated horses and are well tolerated. Electrosurgery can be performed by passing coagulation electrodes or snares through the instrument channel of the endoscope and applying extreme heat to a lesion. More recently, laser surgery has been performed in horses using the endoscope for visualization and guidance of the laser. Laser light energy can be carried through special flexible fiber bundles, which are small enough to pass through the instrument channel of the endoscope. The surgeon can visualize lesions through the endoscope and advance the laser fiber tip to deliver the laser energy to the affected area.

CARE OF THE ENDOSCOPE

The endoscope should be inspected before each use for cracks in the external surface of the insertion tubing and debris on the tip. Damage to the fiber bundles is assessed by looking through the eyepiece; if the image is blurred or dim, and cleaning the lenses and adjusting the eyepiece focus do not improve the image, it is likely that fiber damage has occurred. The endoscope should not be used if it is damaged; repairs are necessary.

Mobility of the tip should be checked by turning the deflection knobs and watching the response of the tip; do not manually bend the tip to check its mobility. Deflection cables can stretch or even break; if the scope does not bend appropriately, the deflection cables may need to be replaced.

All connections of the endoscope to the light source, including air, water, and suction systems, should be checked before use. The water source should be filled before the examination; distilled water is preferred to tap water. In some cases, sterile fluids may be indicated.

Perhaps the most important rules for handling an endoscope are *never* to bend any part of the tubing at an acute angle and *never* twist or crush the insertion tubing. Sharp bending and/or twisting can break fibers. Likewise, compression can break fibers. Broken fibers cause small black dots (pixels) to appear on the image, and if the image is compromised by the black dots, expensive repairs will be necessary to replace the fiber bundles. An important note to remember is that cold conditions increase the likelihood of fiber breakage.

Immediately after an endoscopic examination, the equipment should be cleaned thoroughly. Secretions, lubricants, and medications can dry and crust on the outer surface and tip of the insertion tube and clog the tube's internal channels. The manufacturer's specific cleaning instructions should be followed. The external surface of the endoscope tubing can be cleaned with water and mild surgical soap, using a soft cloth or soft brush. Cotton swabs can be used to clean the tip of the scope, especially the lenses and channel openings.

The internal channels of the scope are cleaned by immersing the tip of the endoscope in a solution of water and mild soap or mild surgical soap and then applying suction.

If suction cannot be applied, cleaning solutions can be flushed through the channels with large syringes. A channel cleaning brush (provided with the scope) is used to further clean the instrument channels of debris. All soap should be thoroughly rinsed before storing the scope or using it on another patient. Clean water or distilled water is then used for a final rinse of the channels. Residual water should be flushed from the channels with an air flush or air suction.

Endoscope control handpieces are either fully immersible or nonimmersible. Immersible scopes can be placed in disinfecting solutions or water after protective caps are placed on the handpiece. The control handpiece on nonimmersible scopes should not get wet and must be cleaned with a damp cloth.

The outside of the instrument should be dried with a soft towel, and the endoscope hung to dry. The drying rack should support the control handpiece and allow the insertion tubing to hang vertically for gravity drainage.

If disinfection is necessary, the manufacturer's recommendations for acceptable disinfectant solutions should be followed. A tray, plastic basin, or clean sink can serve as a reservoir for the disinfectant solution, allowing the endoscope tubing to be loosely coiled and immersed in the disinfectant for the appropriate contact time. Disinfecting solutions cannot substitute for proper physical cleaning of the instrument.

Sterilization may be required, especially after use on suspected infectious cases. Cold sterilization by immersing the control handpiece and insertion tube in liquid sterilizing solutions is the most common way to sterilize an endoscope. Special sterilizing basins are available for immersion of the scope. Gas sterilization with ethylene oxide may sometimes be used to sterilize an endoscope. Steam autoclaving is not a sterilizing option for the endoscope but may be possible for some of the endoscope accessories. The manufacturer's recommendations for sterilization procedures should be consulted.

SUGGESTED READING

Han C, Hurd C: *Practical diagnostic imaging,* ed 3, St Louis, 2005, Mosby.

Han C, Hurd C, Bretz C: Diagnostic imaging. In Sirois M: *Principles and practice of veterinary technology,* ed 2, St Louis, 2004, Mosby.

Kraft SL, Roberts GD: Modern diagnostic imaging, *Vet Clin North Am Equine Pract* 17:1-189, 2001.

Lavin LM: *Radiography in veterinary technology,* ed 3, St Louis, 2003, Saunders.

McCurnin DM, Bassert JM: *Clinical textbook for veterinary technicians,* ed 6, St Louis, 2006, Saunders.

Rantanen NW: Diagnostic ultrasound, *Vet Clin North Am Equine Pract* 2:1-261, 1986.

Reef VB: *Equine diagnostic ultrasound,* St Louis, 1998, Saunders.

Traub-Dargatz JL, Brown CM: *Equine endoscopy,* ed 2, St Louis, 1997, Mosby.

8

Equine Surgery and Anesthesia

Remarkable advances in large animal anesthesia and surgical techniques have occurred in the past 30 years, leading to a vast array of surgical procedures currently available to the equine patient. Surgical procedures range from simple laceration repair to laser surgery and laparoscopy. Most of the instrumentation and surgical techniques have been borrowed from human surgery and adapted for veterinary use. The variety of procedures and expertise in techniques continue to grow.

The availability of surgical procedures depends on the following considerations:

- Availability of surgical facilities
- Expertise of available surgeons
- Patient health status
- Ability to provide aftercare and follow-up
- Prognosis
- Economic constraints

Surgical procedures can be divided into two major categories:

1. Standing surgery procedures
2. General anesthesia (recumbent) procedures

STANDING SURGERY

Most large animal surgical procedures are performed on standing, awake patients. Most of these procedures are performed for treatment and repair of traumatic injuries such as lacerations and punctures. Other common procedures are castration, female reproductive surgery, laser and endoscopic surgery of the upper respiratory tract, and minor hoof and lower leg procedures. Less common are abdominal and thoracic procedures, ophthalmic surgery, and sinus and dental procedures. Many of these procedures can be performed on the farm, saving the expense and risks associated with transportation.

Generally, the primary benefit of standing surgery is avoiding the risks associated with general anesthesia, especially recovery from general anesthesia. Recovery from general anesthesia is the single largest risk for surgical patients, even the healthy elective surgery patient. Also, some surgical procedures are technically easier to perform on a standing patient for anatomical or physiological reasons. It is in the patient's best interest to use a standing procedure whenever possible.

Criteria and indications for standing surgery include the following:

- The surgical technique must be one that is safe to perform on a standing horse. This implies safety for the horse, the surgeon and other personnel, and the equipment.
- Because the risks of general anesthesia are avoided, standing surgery may be beneficial for sick, debilitated, or elderly patients.
- The risks associated with recumbency under anesthesia (such as compartment syndrome) are avoided; therefore large or heavily muscled horses such as draft

breeds should have standing procedures whenever possible.

- If the patient has undergone extreme stress or trauma, avoiding general anesthesia may be better for the patient.
- If the patient has a history of problems under general anesthesia or has had a difficult recovery, standing surgery may be preferable.
- Usually standing procedures are less expensive than comparable general anesthetic procedures. Fewer drugs, less patient monitoring, and fewer staff members are generally required, all of which reduces costs.

Standing surgery has drawbacks, however. Surgeon comfort is often compromised, especially if operating on the lower legs. The surgeon's visualization of the surgical field is often compromised because of the inability to use retractors and often poor lighting. It is very difficult to drape and maintain a sterile surgical field, and control contamination of instruments, especially under farm conditions. Finally, because the patient is awake, *the patient can move,* presenting a danger to itself, personnel, and equipment. Even with heavy sedation and physical restraint, the possibility of motion must *always* be considered and precautions taken.

PREPARATION FOR STANDING SURGERY

Patient preparation depends totally on the procedure and whether it is being performed on an emergency or elective basis. If the procedure is scheduled in advance, it is preferable to restrict the patient's food intake. Most procedures use some form of chemical restraint; all of the drugs used to produce sedation and tranquilization cause some degree of depression of gastrointestinal (GI) motility. Food restriction can reduce bulk in the intestines and reduce intake of highly fermentable foodstuffs. Clinicians have individual preferences for how to restrict food intake, but generally, grain is withheld for 12 hours, and only small amounts of hay are allowed until 2 to 6 hours before the procedure. Water is not withheld. If the procedure is being performed on an emergency basis, the client should be instructed to remove all hay and grain immediately until the veterinarian arrives and evaluates the situation.

Optimally the procedure should be performed in a clean, dry, dust-free area. Drafts should be prevented, as they can blow dust and debris into the surgical field. Noise and motion must be minimized to prevent arousing the horse.

Surgical instruments must be available to the surgeon, yet out of the way of the horse if it moves. Every attempt should be made to elevate the instruments above ground level, where contamination by dust and debris is most likely. A hay bale, stool, or overturned bucket covered with a towel are simple ways to get instrument packs off the ground. The instrument pack can then be opened and used by surgical team members.

Restraint of the patient depends on the location of the procedure, duration of the procedure, "pain factor" of the procedure, temperament of the horse, facilities, and skill and number of available personnel. Physical restraint may vary from a halter and lead shank to mechanical devices such as twitches and ropes. Chemical restraint (sedation or tranquilization) is often used; sometimes heavy sedation must be employed (Fig. 8-1). Every procedure and patient is different; therefore restraint must be tailored for the situation.

The pharmacology and effects of drugs used for restraint and analgesia are thoroughly discussed in numerous excellent references on anesthesia and pharmacology. The clinical effects of the most commonly used chemical restraining agents are shown in Box 8-1.

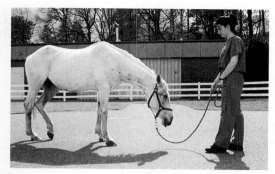

Fig. 8-1. Characteristic stance of a horse sedated with xylazine. (From Trim CM: Principles of chemical restraint and general anesthesia. In Colahan PT et al, editors: *Equine medicine & surgery,* ed 5, St Louis, 1999, Mosby.)

CONTROL OF PAIN

Most surgical procedures either create pain or address a painful condition, or both. Analgesia must be provided to minimize patient discomfort. Many of the drugs used for chemical restraint have analgesic properties but are insufficient to control moderately or markedly painful procedures. Therefore local anesthesia is usually employed for pain control.

Local anesthesia may be applied in several ways.

Nerve Blocks

If a nerve can be reached with a hypodermic needle, then local anesthetic drugs can be deposited over the nerve. The anesthetic diffuses into the nerve and interferes with impulse transmission for variable periods of time. The effects of blocking a nerve must be known in advance, in order to select the proper nerves to desensitize the surgical area and also to prevent unwanted anesthesia of important structures. Anatomical and sensation "maps" for the major nerves are available and help guide the clinician in selecting which nerves to anesthetize. Local anesthetic drugs are primarily chosen according to their duration of action, matched with the anticipated length of surgery.

Field Blocks

These blocks are usually performed to desensitize the skin and subcutaneous tissue around a surgical area, without blocking specific nerves. Rather, a line of anesthetic is deposited subcutaneously around the perimeter of the surgical area ("line block") to produce an area of desensitization. If deeper anesthesia is required, the depth of the line can be extended into underlying muscle tissue (if available). This type of block may produce small or large areas of anesthesia, depending on where the anesthetic is placed. The line block is very useful for suturing lacerations. Large field blocks are commonly used for abdominal surgery through the flank.

Epidural Anesthesia

Caudal epidural anesthesia is routinely used for analgesia of the tail, perineum, anus/rectum, vulva, and vagina. Caudal epidurals are also used to decrease straining associated with obstetrical procedures for dystocias and other reproductive procedures.

Three classes of drugs can be used for caudal epidurals:
- *Local anesthetics* block not only sensory fibers but also motor fibers and sympathetic fibers. Loss of motor control can cause ataxia and even collapse of the hindlimbs; this is a rare occurrence but can be disastrous if it does occur.
- *Alpha-2 agonists* selectively block sensory fibers, with minimal effects on hindlimb function.
- *Opioids* selectively block sensory fibers, with minimal effects on hindlimb function.

Caudal epidural anesthesia is easily performed on large animals. The site of injection is between the first and second coccygeal vertebrae, on the dorsal midline (Fig. 8-2). An estimate of this location is made by moving

BOX

BOX 8-1   Clinical Effects of Commonly Used Chemical Restraining Agents

Acepromazine (tranquilizer)
- Peripheral vasodilation
  - Tendency for hypotension, especially if dehydrated or debilitated
  - Tendency for mild hypothermia
- Delayed onset of action (20-30 minutes after IV injection)
- Long duration of action (3-4 hours)
  - May result in prolonged period of ataxia
  - Penis may remain extended for prolonged time; subject to trauma
- Lowers seizure threshold of the brain
- Tranquilization is not profound; can still respond vigorously to stimuli
- No analgesic properties
- Respiratory rate decreases, but tidal volume increases; net effect maintains relatively normal ventilation

Xylazine (sedative-hypnotic)
- IM route is irritating to foals; warn owner of irritation and swelling at injection site. Avoid neck if foal is nursing.
- Rapid onset of action ($\approx$1-2 minutes after IV injection)
- Good muscle relaxation; shifts weight to forelimbs, lowers head/neck
  - Can still respond to stimuli by kicking with hind limbs; use caution
- Good analgesia (for 20-30 minutes)
- Bradycardia, often with second-degree A-V block
  - Second-degree A-V block is usually transient (5-8 minutes)
  - Reduce dosage if patient has low resting HR or preexisting second-degree A-V block
- Peripheral vasoconstriction
  - Helps maintain blood pressure
- Decreases respiratory rate
- Increases urine output (up to 10×) for 2-4 hours
- Causes sweating
- Decreases GI motility
- Increases blood glucose up to 40%

Detomidine (sedative-hypnotic)
Similar to xylazine, except:
- Longer duration of action ($\approx$60 minutes)
- More potent analgesia
- More profound sedation
- Bradycardia may be more severe

Butorphanol (opiate)
- Opiates cannot be used alone in equids; must first give a tranquilizer or sedative-hypnotic and allow it to take effect before giving the opiate
- Profound sedation and excellent analgesia when used in combination with sedative hypnotics; xylazine/butorphanol is most often used
- Minimal cardiovascular effects
- Minimal or no adverse respiratory effects
- CONTROLLED substance

IV, *Intravenous;* IM, *intramuscular;* A-V, *atrioventricular;* HR, *heart rate;* GI, *gastrointestinal.*

Anticholinergics are, however, very useful for treating bradycardia and second- and third-degree atrioventricular (A-V) block; they should be available for emergency use. Anticholinergics are sometimes used during ophthalmic surgery, when manipulation of the eyeball may create excessive vagal tone.

Because the Risks of General Anesthesia Increase with Time, Every Effort to Decrease Anesthetic Time Should Be Made

This includes the following:

- Surgical clip/prep: Perform as much of the surgical clipping and prepping as possible *before* induction of anesthesia. The disposition of some patients may make this impossible; clippers should be available after induction for these patients. Note that razors are often used for final removal of hair; use of razors on awake patients is difficult and often results in cuts and abrasions of the patient's skin. Therefore if razors are necessary, they should be made available for use after induction of anesthesia.
- Intravenous (IV) catheterization: If IV catheters are to be used, they are placed before induction.
- Preparation of equipment and supplies: All surgical instruments and supplies should be assembled and brought to the surgical area. Equipment should be checked for proper function. Anesthetic supplies and equipment, including IV fluids, must also be anticipated. If gas anesthesia is to be used, the anesthetic machine should be checked for leaks and properly prepared.
- Patient positioning: Positioning should be discussed with the surgeon, so that the operating table and patient padding and support can be set up before the induction.

The Mouth of the Patient May Harbor Feed Material and Other Debris

Feed material tends to accumulate between the cheek teeth and cheek tissue. This material may be pushed into the trachea during endotracheal intubation. The patient's mouth is always flushed with a dose syringe or water hose if endotracheal intubation is anticipated.

The Patient Should Be Thoroughly Cleaned to Prevent Contamination of the Surgical Room

Thorough grooming should always be performed; the patient is brushed and bathed as needed. The tail is often braided or taped to keep tail hairs out of the surgical field and to minimize contamination if the horse defecates while under anesthesia. The hooves should be cleaned and scrubbed with soapy water. If the patient is wearing horseshoes, they are usually removed at this time. The feet should be covered either before entering the surgery room, or immediately upon entering the surgery room. Latex examination gloves, rectal sleeves, plastic bags, and bandaging tape are commonly used for this purpose.

Occasionally it may be desirable to leave horseshoes on, especially if they are being used to correct or treat a medical condition. In such cases the hooves should still be cleaned, and some type of protective boot or hoof bandage placed over the shod hoof for anesthetic induction.

The Lower Legs Should Be Protected during Induction and Recovery

Leg wraps or bandages should be placed on the horse to protect the tendons and ligaments of the lower legs. If it is necessary to remove the leg protection for the surgical procedure, the wraps should be replaced for recovery from anesthesia.

The Eyes Should Be Protected

The wide-set anatomical location of the equine eyes makes them susceptible to trauma. Halters with metal buckles/billets should be removed and replaced with a halter without metal attachments. Padded walls or helmets may be placed to further protect the eyes. The head should be controlled during induction to prevent it from striking the floor or walls as the horse falls to the ground. Sharp objects and corners should be removed from the induction/recovery area or covered with padding if possible. In field settings, the lower (down) eye should be protected from the ground surface with a towel.

Preoperative Patient Examination and Laboratory Evaluation Should Be Performed

The depth and extent of the physical examination and laboratory testing depend on the patient's condition and the nature of the surgical procedure. The clinician prescribes the necessary laboratory tests to be performed. At a *minimum*, a physical examination should include temperature, pulse, and respiration; heart/lung auscultation; and body weight assessment before any general anesthetic episode. It is important to also assess the patient's temperament and manageability; these individual characteristics may influence the choice of induction and recovery techniques.

Fluid, Electrolyte, and Acid-Base Imbalances Should Be Corrected If Possible before Induction of General Anesthesia

Fluid therapy before induction is important to correct dehydration and other imbalances. Sometimes, the emergency nature of a case may preclude complete correction of imbalances; in these cases, provide as much therapy as possible before induction and continue therapy once the patient has been successfully induced.

INDUCTION AND MAINTENANCE OF GENERAL ANESTHESIA

General considerations for induction and maintenance of general anesthesia include the following:

Large Animals Are Prone to Develop Compartment Syndrome

Compartment syndrome is not uncommon in recumbent large animals, regardless of the cause of recumbency. All recumbent animals are susceptible to compartment syndrome, but the heavy bodyweight of large animals exacerbates the problem. Draft horse breeds and heavily muscled individuals are predisposed to developing the condition. Muscle "compartments" refer to muscles and muscle groups in the body that are encased in a dense connective tissue called *fascia*, which has little elasticity. Muscles that are enclosed in these nonelastic envelopes cannot swell outwardly because the fascia prevents it.

There are four clinically significant muscle compartments:
- Gluteals
- Triceps
- Masseters
- Quadriceps

Normally, arteries pump blood into a muscle compartment to nourish the muscle, and veins and lymphatic vessels drain blood and tissue fluid (lymph) out of the compartment. In recumbent animals, however, the vessels may be sandwiched between the animal's own bodyweight pressing down from above and the ground surface below. Compartment syndrome begins with the collapse (partial or complete) of the veins and lymphatics draining the compartment; these vessels have very low pressure inside their walls, and external pressure (such as bodyweight) pressing on them easily collapses them. Arteries, on the other hand, have much higher internal pressures and can therefore resist higher compressive forces. Therefore arteries remain open longer than veins and lymphatics.

As the arterial supply continues to pump blood into the compartment, the pressure inside the compartment starts to rise because the blood and tissue fluid cannot drain adequately through the collapsed veins and lymphatics. A vicious cycle of increasing pressure and increasing collapse of vessels inside the compartment develops. Eventually, the muscle and nerve cells in the compartment begin to suffer because they cannot receive proper nutrition or eliminate their cell waste. Various degrees of muscle and nerve dysfunction result, and the cells may even die if the condition is not successfully treated. The severity of compartment syndrome often correlates with the length of time that the conditions persist.

Compartment syndrome is the primary cause of postanesthetic myopathy (muscle dysfunction) and neuropathy (nerve dysfunction). Postanesthetic myopathy/neuropathy is the leading cause of injury and death in healthy horses undergoing elective surgery; incidence rates as high as 5% of general anesthesia cases have been reported. General anesthesia increases the risk of compartment syndrome because the drugs used to induce and maintain anesthesia usually depress the cardiovascular system and lower blood pressure. Blood pressure is the only pressure inside a vessel that resists external compression; good blood pressure is therefore the primary protection against developing the condition.

Compartment syndrome may affect only one compartment or multiple compartments and may be mild, moderate, or severe in its effects. Clinical signs may include difficulty or inability to stand following general anesthesia, palpable hardening of the affected compartment, paresis/paralysis, and lameness. Acute renal failure or even complete renal shutdown may occasionally result from damage to kidney tubules from myoglobin, which is released from the damaged skeletal muscle cells. Myoglobin may cause dark urine; however, dark urine is not seen in every case. The condition is quite painful, and increased heart rate, respiratory rate, sweating, and anxiety may be observed.

Although the syndrome is usually observed on the patient's "down" side, it may also affect the "up" side if the limbs are not positioned properly or if prolonged hypotension is allowed to occur.

Severely affected animals may have irreversible damage to muscles, nerves, or kidneys and may cause severe damage to themselves by trying to stand on legs that cannot support their weight because of muscle and/or nerve damage. Euthanasia is not an uncommon ending for many affected animals; complications result in euthanasia in up to 25% of cases.

Compartment syndrome is a serious and realistic concern and is frustrating for clinicians and anesthetists—there is no reliable method for predicting or detecting the problem while the patient is under general anesthesia, and it is usually not until the patient tries to stand in the recovery area that the problem is apparent. Even when all precautions to prevent it are strictly followed, some individuals nonetheless develop the condition. Still, the incidence of compartment syndrome *can* be significantly reduced by following certain precautions:

- Minimize anesthetic time: The incidence of compartment syndrome increases with anesthesia time, especially in procedures lasting longer than about 1 hour. As much prepping of the patient and setup of the surgical area as possible should be done before induction.
- Maintain anesthesia only as deeply as necessary: Blood pressure drops as the depth of anesthesia increases, increasing the risk to the patient.
- Use adequate padding: Facilities vary on the type of padding used, but thick foam mattresses (15 to 20 cm thick), conventional mattresses, air mattresses, and waterbed mattresses may be used successfully.

- Position the patient properly:

  Lateral recumbency: Place the forelimbs in a "staggered" position by pulling the lower forelimb forward (cranially) to rotate the shoulder girdle. This decreases the bodyweight pressing down on the triceps muscle. The hindlimbs are not staggered. Elevate the upper limbs (both forelimb and hindlimb) to a horizontal position, parallel to the ground. Do not elevate the upper limbs above this level (Fig. 8-4).

  Protect the masseter muscle by removing or loosening the halter after induction and padding the area supporting the head.

  Dorsal recumbency: Keep the forelimbs folded naturally at the carpus. The hindlimbs are allowed to frogleg naturally at most hospitals, but some clinicians prefer to suspend the hindlimbs in an extended position.

- Reduce carbohydrate intake: Because of the suspected relationship between high carbohydrate diets and postanesthetic myositis, horses on a high grain diet should undergo a "taper down" period of grain reduction for 1 to 2 weeks before general anesthesia.

- Maintain good systemic blood pressure during anesthesia: Correct dehydration before induction, if possible. Consider IV fluids for any procedure lasting longer than 1 hour. Research has shown that mean arterial blood pressure should be kept above 70 mm Hg to minimize the risk of postanesthetic myopathy/neuropathy. Blood pressure monitoring should be considered for any procedure lasting longer than 1 hour, and when hypotension is identified, it should be treated promptly and aggressively.

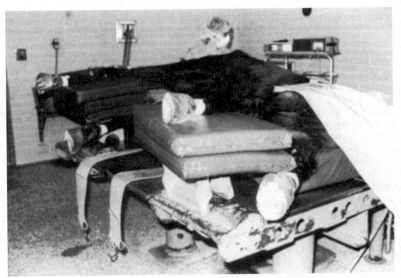

Fig. 8-4. Proper positioning of an anesthetized horse in lateral recumbency. The "down" forelimb has been pulled cranially to "stagger" the shoulder girdle. Both upper limbs have been elevated to a horizontal position, but no higher. (From Auer JA: *Equine surgery,* St Louis, 1992, Saunders.)

Three Methods of Induction and Maintenance of General Anesthesia Are Available

1. Induction with injectable drugs/maintenance with injectable drugs: This is the most common method for procedures in the field and for short procedures (<1 hour). Induction must be rapid; it is desirable for the patient to lose consciousness and fall directly to the ground. If the induction drugs are not given rapidly, the patient may resist the effects of the drugs by wandering or going over backwards.

2. Induction with injectable drugs/maintenance with gas anesthesia: This is the preferred method for procedures lasting longer than 1 hour. Because large animals are prone to ventilation difficulties under general anesthesia and because these difficulties worsen with time, the ability to provide oxygen and assist ventilation with a gas anesthesia machine is valuable for longer procedures.

3. Induction with gas anesthesia/maintenance with gas anesthesia: This method is generally suitable only for foals; gas induction cannot be delivered rapidly enough to adults, leading to prolonged induction with patient resistance to the effects of the anesthetic gas. Gas induction in foals is usually done by facemask, followed by intubation through the nasotracheal or orotracheal route for maintenance.

Foals Are Usually Induced in the Company of the Mare

Unless they are extremely ill, foals panic when separated from their dam, leading to difficult induction of anesthesia. Typically, the foal is induced with the mare at its side, then the mare is sedated and returned to her stall or holding area. When the foal has recovered from anesthesia, the two are reunited. The mare should be observed closely during the separation, since removal of the foal typically causes the mare to become frantic. Heavy sedation of the mare may be necessary.

There Are Three Routes of Tracheal Intubation in Horses

As with other species, great trauma can be done to the patient if intubation is performed aggressively. Just because the animal is bigger does not mean that the larynx, pharynx, and trachea are tougher. Care must be taken during insertion of the tracheal tube and inflation of the cuff (if present).

Three routes are possible for intubation; the route selected depends on patient age, size, and the surgical procedure to be performed:

- *Orotracheal intubation:* the most common method. An oral speculum must be used to maintain separation of the teeth. Oral speculums may be purchased commercially or easily made using 3- to 4-inch diameter polyvinyl chloride (PVC) pipe cut to a 2- to 3-inch length; the slick outer surface of the PVC is covered with duct tape or an adhesive tape to facilitate seating of the PVC between the incisors. The endotracheal tube is inserted through the center of the PVC speculum (Fig. 8-5).

Intubation may be performed in either lateral recumbency or sternal recumbency.

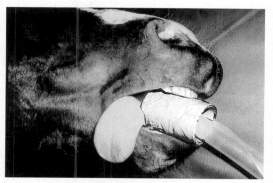

Fig. 8-5. Orotracheal intubation through a polyvinyl chloride speculum placed between the incisors. (From Muir WW et al: *Veterinary anesthesia*, ed 3, St Louis, 2000, Mosby.)

Orotracheal intubation is performed blindly and is usually readily accomplished by following two recommendations. First, position the head and neck in the same plane and extend the head to form a *straight line* from the mouth to the trachea; it is difficult to intubate along a crooked line. Second, grasp the tongue and pull it from the mouth to reduce the bulk of the base of the tongue, which may block the entrance to the trachea. The tube should be lubricated with sterile, water-soluble lubricating jelly.

- *Nasotracheal intubation:* This method is used primarily for foals and small individuals (<100 kg). Because of the small diameter of nasotracheal tubes, it may be difficult or impossible to provide adequate movement of anesthetic gases and oxygen to adult horses. Foals are usually induced with a facemask or injectable drugs, then intubated via the nasotracheal route. Although it is possible to induce foals via the nasotracheal tube, they may resist intubation while conscious; local anesthetic may be added to the lubricating jelly to decrease patient sensitivity of the nasal cavity. As with orotracheal intubation, the head and neck should be aligned and the head extended to straighten the course of intubation. The tube should be well lubricated with sterile, water-soluble lubricating jelly.

- *Direct tracheal intubation:* Tracheal intubation is uncommonly performed. It is reserved for procedures where orotracheal or nasotracheal tubes would interfere with the surgical procedure; this occurs primarily with procedures of the larynx and pharynx. The intubation procedure is accomplished by first performing a tracheostomy, then inserting a standard, cuffed endotracheal tube directly through the tracheostomy into the trachea (Fig. 8-6). Care should be taken not to advance the tube so far that it enters a primary bronchus; this would lead to gas delivery to only one lung, with negative consequences. Care must also be taken not to

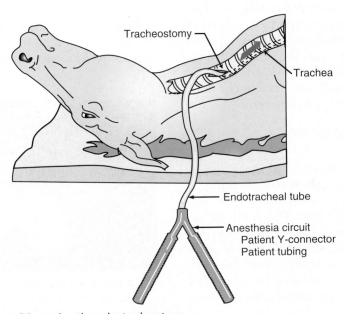

Fig. 8-6. Direct intubation of the trachea through a tracheostomy.

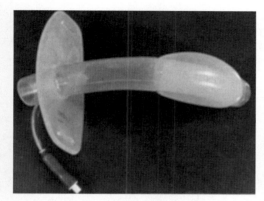

Fig. 8-7. Cuffed silicone tracheostomy tube. (From Riebold TW: *Vet Clin North Am Equine Pract* 6:485-741, 1990.)

bend the endotracheal tube at a sharp angle, which would decrease the diameter of the tube and compromise ventilation. The endotracheal tube should be the same diameter as would be used for orotracheal intubation. In place of standard endotracheal tubes, a cuffed tracheostomy tube can be used (Fig. 8-7).

Following the surgical procedure, the endotracheal tube is withdrawn and replaced with a standard tracheostomy tube; this allows the patient to breathe while laryngeal/pharyngeal swelling from the surgical procedure subsides (usually over several days). When the patient can breathe adequately through the normal route, the tracheostomy tube is removed and the site is managed as a healing tracheostomy (see Chapter 11).

Large Animal Anesthesia Machines Contain the Same Basic Components as Small Animal Anesthesia Machines

However, many of the components of large animal anesthesia machines are larger than those of small animal anesthesia machines (Fig. 8-8). Large animals require larger volumes of carbon dioxide absorber, larger reservoir

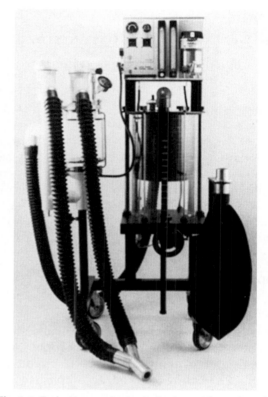

Fig. 8-8. Typical large animal anesthesia machine and ventilator. (From Shawley RV, Mandsager RE: Clinical use of positive-pressure ventilation in the horse. In Riebold TW, editor: *Vet Clin North Am Equine Pract* 6:485-741, 1990.)

bags, and larger-diameter patient tubing (Table 8-1). The large amount of rubber surfaces in large animal anesthesia circuits tend to absorb fairly large quantities of anesthetic gas; absorption of gas by rubber makes the concentration of gas in the circuit lower than the desired concentration on the anesthetic vaporizer. This effect continues until the rubber becomes saturated with anesthetic gas, typically requiring at least 10 to 15 minutes. It may be difficult to achieve surgical anesthesia depth during this time because the rubber competes with absorption of gas by the patient. Therefore the circuit should be "preloaded" with anesthetic

TABLE 8-1   LARGE ANIMAL GAS ANESTHESIA MACHINE AND CIRCUIT COMPONENTS

Carbon dioxide absorber (soda lime)	2 lb	Foal
	5 lb	Pony, small adult
	10 lb	Adult
Reservoir bag	5 L	Foal
	15 L	Pony, small adult
	30 L	Adult
Patient Y-tubing	2 cm	Foal
	5 cm	Adult
Endotracheal tubes (mm ID)	10-16 mm	35-135 kg bodyweight
	16-20 mm	135-250 kg
	20-25 mm	250-350 kg
	25-30 mm	350-450 kg
	30 mm	≥450 kg

ID, *Internal diameter.*

gas before attaching the patient. Preloading allows time for the rubber to become saturated, and it denitrogenates the circuit as well. Preloading can be accomplished by plugging or covering the patient connector of the Y-tubing with duct tape, then turning on the anesthetic gas to moderate levels for at least 10 to 15 minutes before attaching the patient. Preloading is part of routine preparation of the anesthesia machine and circuit.

Patient Monitoring Is Essential

Patient monitoring is essential, especially for procedures lasting longer than 1 hour and for compromised patients. Anesthetic records should always be kept, regardless of the length of the procedure. Large animal anesthetic records are similar to small animal records (Fig. 8-9). The primary concerns for equine patients under anesthesia are hypothermia, hypoventilation, hypotension, and bradycardia (Table 8-2). Basic parameters such as temperature, pulse rate and rhythm, respiratory rate and depth, capillary refill time, and mucous membrane color should always be monitored. Additional monitoring may include the following:

• *Body temperature* is measured rectally. Hypothermia may develop during long procedures, especially in cold environments or air-conditioned surgery rooms. A rectal temperature below 35.6° C (96° F) has been associated with increased ataxia during the recovery period. Efforts to warm the patient should be instituted before the temperature reaches this level; fluid bags warmed in a microwave oven can be packed adjacent to the patient's body, and exposed skin outside the operating field may be covered with clean blankets.

Hyperthermia is rare under anesthesia, but malignant hyperthermia syndrome has been reported in horses under gas anesthetic. Treatment must be aggressive when this condition is identified, cooling the patient and terminating anesthesia as soon as possible.

• *Electrocardiogram monitoring* of cardiac activity is highly desirable for all general anesthesia procedures. Aside from using

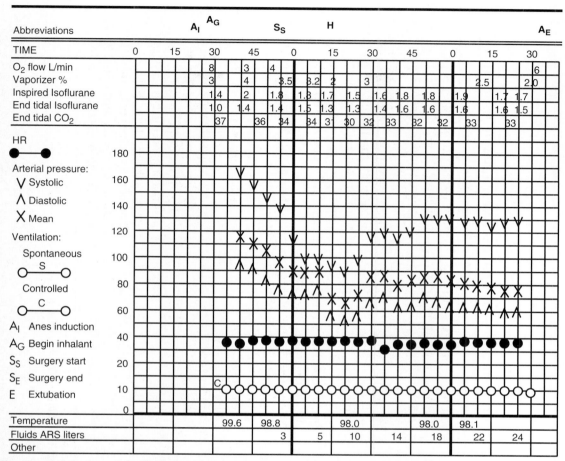

Fig. 8-9. Anesthetic record of a Thoroughbred anesthetized for molar extraction. The *H* abbreviation denotes onset of a period of significant hemorrhage. (From Trim CM: Principles of chemical restraint and general anesthesia. In Colahan PT et al, editors: *Equine medicine & surgery,* ed 5, St Louis, 1999, Mosby.)

longer lead wires, no special equipment is required for monitoring large animal patients.

- *Blood pressure monitoring* is recommended for any procedure lasting longer than 1 hour. Palpating the strength of arterial pulses is misleading when relied on for indicating blood pressure and is discouraged; mechanical measurements are preferred. Blood pressure can be measured directly or indirectly:

- Direct measurement is performed with an intraarterial catheter and a pressure transducer; the most common arteries used are the transverse facial artery (located caudal to the lateral canthus of the eye, below the zygomatic arch) and the dorsal metatarsal artery (located on the lateral aspect of each hindlimb, between metatarsals 3 and 4). Direct measurement is technically more difficult to perform but yields more

TABLE 8-2   GUIDELINES FOR TREATING COMMON COMPLICATIONS OF GENERAL ANESTHESIA IN ADULT HORSES

Complication	Recognition	Comments	Treatment Considerations
Hypothermia	Rectal temp < 35.6° C (96° F)	Best to begin treatment before temperature reaches this level	1. Warm with warm water bags, blankets. 2. Increase temperature in room
Hypotension	Mean arterial pressure < 70 mm Hg* Mean arterial pressure < 63 mm Hg	Begin treatment Emergency	1. Decrease vaporizer setting 2. Increase IV fluid rate 3. Cardiovascular stimulants (especially sympathomimetics)
Hypoventilation	Respiratory rate < 6/min Decreased tidal volume < 10 mL/kg	Best assessed by arterial blood gas (especially CO_2) measurement; respiratory rate, mucous membrane color, and depth of breathing can be misleading	1. Decrease vaporizer setting 2. Institute assisted or controlled ventilation
Bradycardia	HR < 30/min HR < 25/min	Consider treatment Emergency	1. Decrease vaporizer setting 2. Administer anticholinergic or sympathomimetic drugs 3. If surgical procedure is causing increased vagal tone, stop procedure temporarily until HR responds to treatment (most likely with GI and ocular sx)

HR, Heart rate; GI, gastrointestinal; IV, intravenous; sx, surgery.
*Mean arterial pressure = 0.33 (systolic pressure − diastolic pressure) + diastolic pressure.

accurate results than indirect measurement (Fig. 8-10).

- Indirect measurement is usually performed using a Doppler ultrasound unit and an inflatable tail cuff (sphygmomanometer) over the coccygeal artery

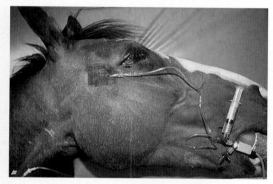

Fig. 8-10. Direct measurement of blood pressure in the transverse facial artery. The intraarterial catheter is connected to a pressure transducer with heparinized saline-filled plastic tubing. (From Trim CM: Principles of chemical restraint and general anesthesia. In Colahan PT et al, editors: *Equine medicine & surgery,* ed 5, St Louis, 1999, Mosby.)

(Fig. 8-11). Alternatively, a rear leg artery may be used. Ideally the level of the cuff should be at the same level as the heart for accurate readings.

Alternative instruments that use oscillometry with an inflatable tail cuff to take pulse and blood pressure readings, as well as calculate mean arterial pressure, are available. These instruments are convenient but expensive and sensitive to vibrations and motion (Fig. 8-12). They are less reliable when the heart rate is low (especially when second-degree A-V block is present).

Blood pressures from 100 to 120 mm Hg systolic/70 to 80 mm Hg (70 to 60 for foals) diastolic, or mean arterial pressure greater than 70 mm Hg, are desirable for adults. Treatment for hypotension may be necessary if pressures fall below these levels.

Because of the tendency for hypotension under general anesthesia, the use of IV fluids is recommended to support

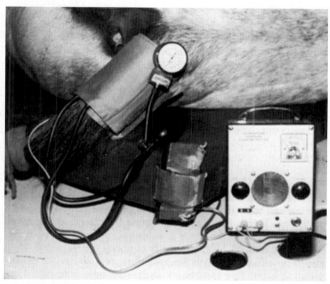

Fig. 8-11. Use of a tail cuff and Doppler ultrasound unit for indirect measurement of blood pressure. (From Riebold TW: *Vet Clin North Am Equine Pract* 6:485-741, 1990.)

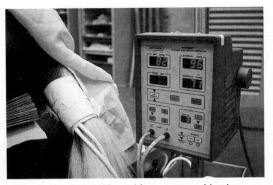

Fig. 8-12. The DINAMAP machine measures blood pressure via a tail cuff over the coccygeal artery. (From Trim CM: Principles of chemical restraint and general anesthesia. In Colahan PT et al, editors: *Equine medicine & surgery,* ed 5, St Louis, 1999, Mosby.)

compromised patients or whenever the procedure is anticipated to last more than 1 hour. Lactated Ringer solution (LRS) is typically given at 10 ml/kg/hr for the first hour, then the rate is reduced to 5 ml/kg/hr for the remainder of the procedure. The rate can be increased if necessary to treat hypotension or hypovolemia from blood loss.

Hypertension (mean arterial pressure > 90 mm Hg) is usually related to light anesthesia and often corresponds to the amount of pain produced by the surgical procedure. Increasing delivery of anesthetic to return the patient to an appropriate level of anesthesia is required.

- *Oxygenation/ventilation* is best assessed by arterial blood gas sampling. Arterial blood can be rapidly analyzed for oxygen and carbon dioxide levels, as well as blood pH. This information is invaluable to the anesthetist for assessing adequacy of ventilation and acid-base imbalances. The equipment for analysis is usually found only at larger hospitals and clinics and is currently not practical in field situations.

An alternative for measuring oxygen levels in the blood is the pulse oximeter; in large animals, the transducer is placed on the tongue. The thickness of the tongue and motion may interfere with the accuracy of this instrument. Hemoglobin oxygen saturation levels above 90% are critical for proper oxygenation of the blood. Note, however, that the oxygen must still be delivered to the tissues; low blood pressure and/or bradycardia can lead to decreased cardiac output and may interfere with oxygen delivery, even when the blood is well saturated.

Ideally, adults should maintain a respiratory rate between 8 and 12/min (>20 for foals). A respiratory rate below 6 warrants immediate assistance. It is very important to note that respiratory rate is *not* the only factor needed for adequate ventilation; each breath must also *exchange* a sufficient tidal volume of air (a tidal volume of 10 mL/kg is ideal for spontaneous breathing under general anesthesia). In other words, an adult breathing at the desired rate of 12 breaths/min may be severely hypoventilating if the breaths are shallow and not exchanging enough air. Another factor that adds to hypoventilation is ventilation/perfusion mismatch; this occurs when the parts of the lungs that are well oxygenated do not correspond to the parts of the lungs that are well perfused with blood (Fig. 8-13). Ventilation/perfusion mismatch is accentuated in large animals because of the size and weight of the lungs; atelectasis (collapse) of the lower (dependent) portions of the lungs begins quickly once the animal becomes recumbent. This results in poor ventilation in the lower portions of the lung as the alveoli collapse under the weight. However, the effects of gravity also tend to "pull" more blood into the lower regions of the lung. The net effect is more blood and less oxygen and anesthetic gases in the lower lung areas. The ultimate result is poor

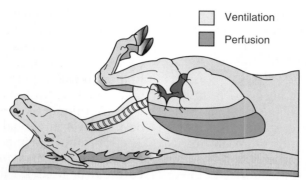

☐ Ventilation
■ Perfusion

Fig. 8-13. Ventilation-perfusion differences in the lung of the anesthetized horse in dorsal recumbency. Similar effects are seen in lateral recumbency. (Adapted from Greene SA, Keegan RD: Special considerations in the management of equine anesthesia. In Auer JA, editor: *Equine surgery*, St Louis, 1992, Saunders.)

exchange between gases and the blood, regardless of the patient's rate or depth of breathing. For these reasons, respiratory rate alone cannot be relied on to indicate the patient's respiratory status.

It is standard practice to "sigh" the animal by squeezing the reservoir bag once every 1 to 2 minutes to visibly expand the chest; this is thought to reopen collapsed airways and alveoli, helping to maintain ventilation. "Sighing" is not the same as intermittent positive pressure ventilation (IPPV), or "bagging," which is a treatment for hypoventilation. Sighing is intended to help maintain normal ventilation, not treat hypoventilation, and should not be used for that purpose.

- *Pulse rate* can be assessed by palpation, without any special equipment. Ideally, adults should maintain a pulse rate of at least 30 to 50 per minute (minimum 80 to 100 in foals). If the pulse rate falls below these ranges, treatment for bradycardia should be instituted.

- *Depth of anesthesia* is best assessed through eye position and reflexes. A slow palpebral reflex is desirable, and a prompt, strong corneal reflex should always be present. With inhalant (gas) maintenance, the eye rotates from a central to rostral position as the horse progresses from light to moderate anesthesia; the eye returns to a central position when anesthesia is excessively deep. Note that Ketamine, a common agent for inducing and/or maintaining anesthesia, tends to keep the eye in a central position as long as its effects persist (≈20 to 30 minutes).

Light anesthesia will be signaled in several ways. Nystagmus usually indicates that anesthesia is too light. Respiratory rate, heart rate, and blood pressure also increase. Patients may begin to move the limbs, sometimes violently, when anesthesia becomes too light. The anesthetist should be alert to the signs of light anesthesia and treat it promptly by increasing the vaporizer gas concentration, improving delivery of gas anesthetic with assisted ventilation (if hypoventilation is contributing to the problem), and possibly adding supplemental injectable anesthetics until the proper anesthetic depth is achieved. If surgery has begun, the anesthetist might also request that the surgeon temporarily halt the procedure to minimize stimulation of the patient until the proper depth of anesthesia can be restored.

Patient motion presents a real danger to personnel and equipment.

Rolling Patients under General Anesthesia Presents Unique Ventilation Concerns

Uncommonly a patient needs to be rolled from one recumbency to another in a single surgery, but there are some procedures that the surgeon can only approach in this fashion. As mentioned earlier, when a patient is in lateral recumbency, the "down" or lower lung tends to partially collapse from the weight of the upper lung and intestinal contents. This lung does not exchange air as well as the "top" or upper lung. If the patient is rolled rapidly to the opposite lateral recumbency, the partially collapsed and congested lower lung quickly becomes the upper lung, not immediately capable of normal gas exchange. Also, the former upper lung has now become the down lung, and immediately begins to collapse. The patient may suffer extreme hypoventilation during this time. Still, rolling can be performed safely by allowing some time for the lungs to adjust to their new positions. The patient is first slowly rolled from lateral to dorsal recumbency and held there for several minutes to allow the congestion/collapse of the previously lower lung to improve. Then, the roll is slowly completed. The patient should also be monitored for hypotension during any rolling procedure.

ADDITIONAL CONSIDERATIONS

Control of bleeding during surgery is obviously necessary for patient health but is also necessary for the surgeon's visualization of the surgical field. One popular method of maintaining a "bloodless" surgical field for procedures on the distal limbs is to temporarily occlude the blood flow to the area with a tourniquet. Properly applied tourniquets prevent inflow of arterial blood but also prevent venous drainage; this venous blood can exit through a surgical incision and block the surgeon's vision. Therefore before activating a tourniquet, it is common to first try to "push" as much blood out of the distal limb as possible with an Esmarch bandage (also known as an Esmarch tourniquet).

A tourniquet is first positioned at the desired level, proximal to the surgical area. The tourniquet may be made from surgical rubber tubing, or a pneumatic tourniquet cuff may be used. If tubing is used, minimal foam or cloth padding should be placed beneath the tubing to protect tendons and other underlying structures. If a pneumatic cuff is used, gauze rolls are placed over the major vessels to maximize occlusion when the cuff is inflated. The tourniquet is positioned but not yet "activated" at this time.

The Esmarch bandage is then applied. The Esmarch is a long strip of latex or other rubber material that is wrapped around the leg with as much tension as possible, beginning just below the coronary band. The wrapping proceeds proximally, overlapping each preceding layer by half, until the level of the tourniquet is reached. The Esmarch essentially forces blood proximally, out of the distal limb. Once the level of the tourniquet is reached, the tourniquet is activated (tied or inflated). The Esmarch is then removed, and the surgical area is prepared for surgery (Fig. 8-14, *A* and *B*).

Tourniquets are painful. If the patient has not reached a surgical plane of anesthesia, or had local anesthesia in the area, lightening of anesthesia may occur. An increase in heart rate and blood pressure may also result. Tourniquets are generally safe to use for up to 2 hours, although tissue damage may begin to occur as early as 30 minutes after activation. The anesthetist should make note on the anesthetic record of the time of activation and periodically notify the surgeon of the time that the tourniquet has been in place. The tourniquet should be removed

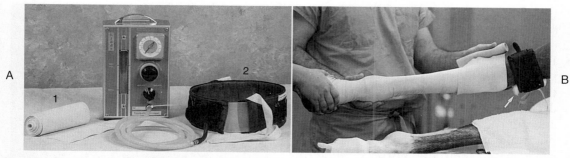

Fig. 8-14. A, An Esmarch *(1)* and a pneumatic tourniquet *(2)* are used for occluding blood flow in a limb. **B,** Application of an Esmarch around the limb to the level of the pneumatic tourniquet. Gauze rolls are placed over vascular pressure points under the tourniquet *(arrow).* (From Auer JA, Stick JA: *Equine surgery,* ed 2, St Louis, 1999, Saunders.)

as soon as possible, and the time of removal also noted in the record.

RECOVERY

In small animal species, recovery is usually the time when most anesthetic danger has passed and the anesthetist can relax somewhat; most small animals recover from general anesthesia with minimal assistance and monitoring. In contrast, recovery from general anesthesia in large animals is perhaps the most nerve-racking part of the whole procedure. Recovery poses more risk to the equine patient than induction or maintenance. The "nature of the beast" is primarily responsible for the risk; horses are a species of prey, therefore they resist being recumbent unless by their own choice. Their natural instinct upon awakening from anesthesia is to get up, NOW. Unfortunately, horses almost always regain consciousness faster than the anesthetic drugs are metabolized, leaving a brain that says "stand" to legs that are not yet capable. In some patients, compartment syndrome may also contribute to the inability to stand. Some individuals will struggle violently in their attempts to rise and can even damage themselves to the extent of creating lacerations, fractures, and

other trauma, which may be severe enough to require euthanasia.

One anesthetic combination that is an exception is xylazine/ketamine. This is the most commonly used drug combination to induce and maintain general anesthesia in horses, used primarily for short procedures (20 to 35 minutes). Horses tend to have uneventful recoveries from this drug combination, especially when allowed sufficient time to remain recumbent, and most stand on the first attempt with a minimum of difficulty.

Even when standard recommendations for recovering horses from general anesthesia are followed, some patients nonetheless have a rough recovery. Therefore emergency drugs and equipment should be readily available. More than one staff member should be available in case an assisted recovery is necessary. In order to provide the best conditions for a successful recovery, these recommendations should be followed:

- Recover horses in lateral recumbency. If the surgical procedure was performed in lateral recumbency, recover the patient in the *same* recumbency, unless an underlying orthopedic or neurological condition makes it unwise to do so. If necessary to roll the patient for recovery, follow the same precautions for rolling (discussed earlier).

- Do *not* encourage the patient to try to stand before the drugs have had sufficient time to wear off. The time necessary depends on the type of drugs used, the amount used, and the patient's underlying physical condition. Recovery usually proceeds best when the horse is allowed to rest quietly until it decides to rise on its own. Therefore during the recovery period, avoid external stimuli such as bright lights, loud noise, and excessive physical manipulation, especially when consciousness begins to return. If recovering under field conditions, cover the eyes to prevent stimulation from sunlight.

  Some individuals try to stand well before they are able. Low doses of a sedative such as xylazine may encourage the horse to lie quietly, allowing more time for metabolism of the primary anesthetic drugs. Conversely, some horses will remain recumbent long after the effects of anesthesia have worn off. Prolonged recumbency can contribute to compartment syndrome and should be discouraged. It is a judgment call as to when sufficient time has passed and when the horse should actually be *encouraged* to stand.

- Supplemental oxygen is desirable during recovery, especially if the procedure lasted longer than 1 hour. Humidified oxygen should be used if possible. Oxygen lines can be placed in the endotracheal tube, and inserted into a nostril or nasotracheal tube (if used), and oxygen administered at a rate of approximately 15 L/min. This can boost blood oxygen levels by as much as 30%. Oxygen demand valves, hand activated intermittently by the anesthetist for 1 to 2 seconds, can be useful for intubated patients who fail to breathe spontaneously at an adequate rate or depth (Fig. 8-15).

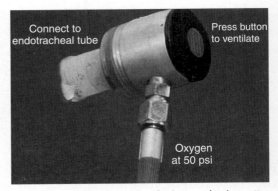

Fig. 8-15. Oxygen demand valve for large animal use. (From Trim CM: Principles of chemical restraint and general anesthesia. In Colahan PT et al, editors: *Equine medicine & surgery*, ed 5, St Louis, 1999, Mosby.)

- If the horse was intubated for the procedure, a staff member should remain with the patient until attempts to swallow are observed. At that time, the tracheal tube can be withdrawn. Swallowing also signals that return to consciousness is not far away—at this time it becomes dangerous to stay in the immediate area where the horse is recovering.

- Do not leave the patient unobserved during any phase of recovery. The patient is attended closely until swallowing occurs. At that time, if the patient is in a recovery stall or other enclosure, leave the enclosure; the risks of being crushed or pinned during the horse's attempts to stand are too great. No one should stay inside an enclosed area with an actively recovering horse. In an open field recovery, all unnecessary personnel should be instructed to clear the area; typically only one person will remain with the horse to control the head during recovery, and this should be a person with training in equine anesthesia techniques.

  Even after leaving the recovery room, continue to observe the patient, either from outside the stall or via video cameras.

The patient may experience trauma or become cast (pinned and unable to rise) against a wall, in a corner, or under mattresses and pads. Compartment syndrome and other painful conditions may make it difficult for the horse to stand. These problems must be identified and addressed promptly; frequently they require assistance. If unusual difficulty in rising is observed, an assisted recovery using head, leg, and/or tail ropes may be necessary (Fig. 8-16).

- Foals are always closely attended during all phases of recovery; they are never left alone. Two people typically stay with the foal; one person attends the head, and one person holds the tail to assist the foal in standing. The risk to personnel is minimal during recovery of a foal, but they should position themselves safely out of reach of the hooves.

- Occasionally, after extubation, the patient may make a loud rattling or snorting noise, especially during inspiration. This is usually caused by edema of the nasal turbinates (less commonly laryngeal spasm or edema), which develops during anesthesia; however, it is not possible to recognize this condition until extubation returns the horse to being an obligate nose breather. Nasal turbinate edema may severely compromise breathing and warrants immediate treatment when identified. Elevate the head, with the nose tilted slightly higher than the rest of the head. A nasotracheal tube (15 to 25 mm inner diameter endotracheal tube) should be placed in one nostril so that it enters the trachea; this will assure a patent airway (Fig. 8-17). *Firmly secure nasotracheal tubes with tape or straps to the halter*

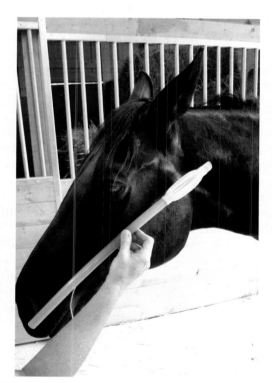

Fig. 8-17. A large canine endotracheal tube of sufficient length to reach the trachea can be used for nasotracheal intubation; it is not necessary to inflate the cuff unless assisted ventilation is needed.

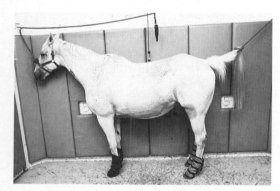

Fig. 8-16. Assisted recovery using head and tail ropes passed to personnel outside the recovery stall. The horse must still provide the effort to stand, but the ropes can provide some lift and help to steady the horse. (From Trim CM: Principles of chemical restraint and general anesthesia. In Colahan PT et al, editors: *Equine medicine & surgery*, ed 5, St Louis, 1999, Mosby.)

or muzzle of the horse to prevent aspiration of the tube into the trachea. Intranasal 1% phenylephrine (Neo-Synephrine) (3 to 5 ml in each nostril) may also help reduce the nasal swelling but is not a substitute for establishing a patent airway when it is needed. Once the patient is standing, the nasotracheal tube can be removed. Resolution of the edema usually proceeds without complication.

To minimize the incidence of nasal turbinate edema, the head ideally should not be positioned lower than the heart during the anesthetic period.

Once the horse is standing, staff may quietly reenter the area. The horse should be checked closely for trauma, and IV catheters should be checked and flushed. The horse should be allowed to stand quietly as long as necessary until its legs are stable enough to walk safely. The horse can then be moved to its stall or paddock, with caution; many horses at this stage are still slightly ataxic and do not negotiate corners well, especially with the hindquarters. The horse should be led in a wide arc around corners and carefully through doorways. A sharp blow to the point of the hip (tuber coxae), even at a walk, can produce a fracture, but is easily avoided if precautions are followed. Often a second person is useful to help guide the hindquarters around these obstacles.

Horses should not be allowed to eat or drink immediately following general anesthesia. Some horses will be so hungry that they will eat their stall bedding; these patients should be placed in a stall without bedding or muzzled. Some horses are talented at eating through or around muzzles; therefore muzzled horses should be watched closely.

The clinician will determine whether oral intake is allowed, based on the patient's underlying condition. Water is returned first, allowing only a few sips to ensure that the patient can swallow without coughing or refluxing from the nostrils. Larger volumes of water are returned gradually over several hours and then a handful of grass or grass hay can be offered (usually after 2 hours). If the swallowing reflex appears coordinated, small amounts of hay or grass can be given. High carbohydrate feedstuffs and larger volumes of solid food are usually not returned until the following day. Intestinal motility and bowel movements should be closely monitored in the initial hours following general anesthesia; the risk of postanesthetic colic is increased by the depressive effects of anesthetic drugs on GI motility. Foals should be muzzled for 1 hour after their return to the mare; this allows time for normal swallowing reflexes to return.

SUGGESTED READING

McKelvey D, Hollingshead KW: *Veterinary anesthesia and analgesia,* ed 3, St Louis, 2003, Mosby.

Muir WW et al: *Handbook of veterinary anesthesia,* ed 3, St Louis, 2000, Mosby.

Pettifer G: Veterinary anesthesia. In McCurnin DM, Bassert JM, editors: *Clinical textbook for veterinary technicians,* ed 6, St Louis, 2006, Saunders.

Riebold TW: Principles and techniques of equine anesthesia, *Vet Clin North Am Equine Pract* 6:485-741, 1990.

Tyner CL, Rundell SW: Anesthesia, analgesia, and anesthetic nursing. In Pratt PW, editor: *Principles and practice of veterinary technology,* St Louis, 1998, Mosby.

Tyner CL, Rundell SW: Anesthesia and perioperative analgesia. In Sirois M, editor: *Principles and practice of veterinary technology,* ed 2, St Louis, 2004, Mosby.

9

Fluid Therapy in Horses

The animal body consists primarily of water. The body's water is divided among three "compartments": intracellular (inside cells), extracellular (plasma water and tissue fluid [lymph]), and transcellular (body cavities such as joints, gastrointestinal [GI] lumen, cerebrospinal fluid, thorax, and abdomen). In a normal animal, the total amount of water in its body is allocated roughly as follows:

Total body water = 60% intracellular fluid +
30% extracellular fluid +
10% transcellular fluid

Animals may experience diseases or conditions that cause imbalances in one or more of the compartments. Severe diarrhea, profuse sweating, and a frozen water bucket are examples of things that can cause problems with water balance. Fortunately, during times of imbalance, water can shift between the compartments to try to maintain health. However, there are limits to the amount of water that can shift without doing harm; when this limit is reached, medical intervention in the form of water supplementation is necessary to prevent complications and possibly death.

Imbalances are not limited to water. Electrolytes, pH, and nutritional substances (protein, carbohydrate, fat) may also become compromised, and medical therapy to replace or balance them may be necessary.

In the natural state, an animal has only one body system for intake of fluids and electrolytes: the GI tract. However, it has four body systems that can lose fluids and electrolytes:

- GI tract: through loss of luminal water and electrolytes
- Respiratory tract: through water vapor in expired air and respiratory exudates
- Urinary tract (kidneys): through the urine
- Integument: through sweat

An additional "route" of loss is via external or internal hemorrhage. The body may recover water and electrolytes from internal hemorrhage by reabsorption, but this reabsorption is a gradual process and may not be rapid enough to prevent death in severe cases. External hemorrhage, of course, is a total loss.

Fluid therapy is basically an alternative to an animal's normal ability to drink and balance its own fluid compartments. Fluid therapy is indicated to:

- Maintain fluid, electrolyte, or nutrient balance when disease prevents the animal from its normal oral intake.
- Maintain fluid, electrolyte, or nutrient balance while under anesthesia.
- Replace fluid or electrolytes when normal oral intake would be too slow.

Calculations for replacement of water are different from calculations to replace substances such as electrolytes and nutrients. The calculations will be considered separately.

FLUID (H$_2$O) CALCULATIONS

An animal exists in one of three states at any given moment:

- Overhydrated: rarely occurs naturally; usually due to iatrogenic overadministration of fluids
- Normally hydrated: the animal does not need fluids (unless necessary to maintain hydration, such as during anesthesia)
- Dehydrated: the animal needs fluid therapy (if unable to replace deficits by mouth)

The dehydrated animal is recognized by laboratory data (packed cell volume/total solids [PCV/TS] measurement) and/or clinical signs. Dehydration is estimated on the basis of PCV/TS and clinical signs. Guidelines are available for estimating percent dehydration on the basis of clinical signs (Table 9-1).

Fluid calculations have been extensively covered in other texts. Fluid calculations in large animals are basically no different from small animal calculations; the same formulas apply. What can be difficult to appreciate is the large volume of fluids necessary in large animals, compared to small animals. Not only do large animals have a large amount of total body water, but herbivores cycle a tremendous volume of water and electrolytes through their GI tracts in a 24-hour day. Literally gallons of saliva, gastric, and intestinal fluids are produced and secreted into the GI tract lumen, and the animal must recover most all of these fluids in order to remain normally hydrated. GI diseases can be especially devastating to a large animal's hydration.

The basic formula for calculating fluid needs in any animal is as follows:

$$\text{Fluids needed} = \text{maintenance fluids} \\ + \text{ongoing losses} \\ + \text{deficit replacement}$$

MAINTENANCE FLUIDS

The term *maintenance fluids* refers to the volume of water necessary to maintain life. This is the volume necessary to supply all of the body's cells and also to remove cell waste. Whether drinking water normally by mouth

TABLE 9-1 **ESTIMATING DEHYDRATION IN THE HORSE**

% Dehydration	Heart Rate (bpm)	Capillary Refill Time (sec)	PCV/TS	Comments
<5	Normal (28-40)	Normal (<2)	Normal	Clinically silent
6-7	40-60	2	40/7	Mild dehydration; mildly delayed skin tent (2-3 sec)
8-9	61-80	3	45/7.5	Moderate dehydration; obviously delayed skin tent (3-5 sec); tacky mucous membranes
10-11	81-100	4	50/8	Approaching severe dehydration/shock; weak peripheral pulse; "sunken" eyes; dry mucous membranes; delayed skin tent >5 sec
12-15	>100	>4	>50/>8	Shock, collapse, death if untreated

bpm, *Beats per minute;* PCV/TS, *packed cell volume/total solids.*

or whether on fluid therapy, an animal must have at least this amount of water: 2 to 4 ml/kg/hr. This amount may need to be slightly increased during late pregnancy and during lactation. Heavily lactating animals need approximately 1 L extra for each liter of milk produced. Fever can also increase maintenance requirements.

To emphasize the amount of fluids required in large animals, using the minimum amount of 2 ml/kg/hr, an average 500-kg horse requires at least 1 L of water/hr (24 L/day) just to sustain its life.

ONGOING LOSSES

Ongoing losses are due to the animal's primary disease or environmental conditions. Diseases may include diarrhea, gastric reflux, GI ileus, kidney disease, profuse and prolonged sweating, severe edema, hemorrhage, and loss of fluids into body cavities. Most ongoing losses cannot be strictly measured; therefore the amount is usually an estimate. However, some losses such as gastric reflux (via nasogastric intubation) and urine output (via indwelling urinary catheter) can be accurately measured.

If the animal is healthy, this factor is zero. If the animal has a disease that causes ongoing fluid losses, medical/surgical therapy is used to try to resolve the primary disease. Once the primary disease is under control, the ongoing losses should end, and this factor will drop to zero and may be eliminated from the equation.

DEFICIT REPLACEMENT

Deficit replacement applies only to a dehydrated animal. Animals that are overhydrated or normally hydrated obviously do not have a deficit to replace. The formula for replacement of water deficit is as follows:

$$\text{Bodyweight (kg)} \times \%\text{ dehydration} = \text{liters to replace}$$

Once the animal's deficit has been replaced, this factor becomes zero and may be eliminated from the equation.

The speed of deficit replacement is determined by the status of the patient. Mild and moderate deficits are replaced over 12 to 24 hours. Severe dehydration, evidenced by cardiovascular shock, is an emergency situation, and replacement is often necessary within 1 to 2 hours if the patient is to have any chance of survival.

Again, once the deficit has been replaced and the ongoing losses have been controlled, the animal needs only maintenance fluids in order to survive. If intravenous (IV) fluids are used for fluid therapy, the animal is weaned off of maintenance fluids as soon as possible and returned slowly to oral intake.

SUBSTANCE CALCULATIONS

The term *substances* refers to all nonwater items that can be measured in the laboratory, including the following:
- Electrolytes: especially sodium, potassium, and chloride
- Minerals: especially calcium and phosphorus
- Nutrients: primarily glucose and protein
- pH buffers: primarily bicarbonate

If normal values are known, the patient's values can be compared with the normal levels. For any given substance, an animal will be in one of three states at any given moment:
- Substance excess: the animal does not need replacement
- Normal value: the animal does not need replacement (but may need maintenance amounts in order to stay normal)
- Substance deficit: the animal may need medical therapy to replace the deficit and return the animal to normal levels (depending on the severity of the deficit and primary disease)

The formula for replacing the deficit of any measurable substance is as follows:

$$(\text{Normal value} - \text{patient's value}) \times \text{extracellular fluid [ECF] factor} \times \text{bodyweight (kg)} = \text{amount to replace}$$

The *ECF factor* refers to the percentage of an animal's total body water that is extracellular fluid. The percentage is age dependent; younger animals have a higher percentage of ECF. The following factors are used:

- 0.3   adults
- 0.4   older foals
- 0.5   neonates

The mathematical units for the amount to replace depend on how the laboratory measures the substance in question; for instance, if the substance is measured in milliequivalents (mEq), the answer (amount to be replaced) will also be in mEq. If the substance is measured in milligrams (mg), the answer will be in milligrams, etc.

Substance replacement must be done cautiously to avoid complications. The patient's blood substance levels should be monitored periodically while the patient is receiving supplementation. Bolus administration is dangerous and should be prevented. The most common substances replaced in horses are potassium, calcium, and bicarbonate.

POTASSIUM

Herbivores are highly dependent on dietary potassium to maintain normal potassium levels in the body. Horses that are off feed longer than 24 hours must typically receive potassium supplements.

If a deficiency has developed, potassium replacement can be accomplished by adding potassium chloride (KCl) solution (commercially available) to the animal's IV fluids. Potassium replacement should not exceed a rate of 1 mEq/kg/hr. Excessively rapid administration can lead to life-threatening hyperkalemia, with subsequent cardiac standstill.

Once deficits have been replaced and the patient is on maintenance fluid levels, maintenance potassium may be given. Maintenance potassium chloride can usually be safely added to IV fluids at 20 mEq KCl/L, for as long as the animal is off feed.

CALCIUM

Animals that are off feed, lactating, or sweating profusely may experience excessive calcium loss. If calcium is deficient, calcium can be given intravenously. This can be accomplished in several ways. Calcium borogluconate (23%) is perhaps the most common IV supplement used. If given too fast, life-threatening cardiac arrhythmias may result; patients should be closely monitored during administration of any calcium supplement. Generally, the maximum rate of calcium borogluconate given intravenously is 250 ml/20 to 30 min. Unless under emergency conditions, calcium should be given as a gradual IV drip, with caution. Calcium-containing solutions should not be allowed to physically mix with bicarbonate solutions.

BICARBONATE

Most pH imbalances in herbivores result in acidosis and accompanying low levels of bicarbonate in the blood (Table 9-2). In order to restore normal bicarbonate levels, sodium bicarbonate solutions are usually given intravenously. Replacement must be gradual. Typically, half of the calculated deficit is

TABLE 9-2	pH OF EQUINE BLOOD
Normal pH	7.32-7.44
Acidemia	7.2-7.31
Life-threatening acidemia	<7.2

replaced over several hours, and the second half over the next 12 to 24 hours. Rapid administration can cause central nervous system dysfunction (severe depression and possible coma).

ROUTES AND METHODS OF ADMINISTRATION

The route of fluid therapy depends on the urgency for correction of the patient's deficits, as well as the patient's underlying health or disease status. If the GI tract is functional and the patient's needs are not critical, then the GI tract may be used for treatment. This may be as simple as adding substances such as electrolytes, glucose, or bicarbonate to a bucket of water. Some additives are not highly palatable or may be added excessively, leading to poor taste. Voluntary consumption is therefore unreliable. Whenever a water source is supplemented with additives, another source of plain, fresh water should still be available at all times to provide the horse with a choice. Patient intake of both plain and supplemented water should be monitored closely.

The GI tract may also be used for replacement of fluids and other substances via nasogastric intubation. Fluids do not have to be sterile, which saves cost. Nasogastric intubation also eliminates "patient choice" in selecting what to consume. However, there is a limit to the capacity of the stomach and the speed that it can empty; if exceeded, colic can result. For an average adult horse with an immediate need for replacement, a maximum volume of 8 L of fluid may be given every 30 to 60 minutes; however, this may be too much for some individuals, and less aggressive volumes given less frequently should be used whenever possible. Note that administering the fluid directly into the stomach does not mean that it will be absorbed rapidly or completely; absorption is

a different process from gastric emptying. Absorption is a slower process and is seldom quick enough to successfully treat shock or severe imbalances.

Subcutaneous (SQ) fluids are not used in large animals in the same fashion as in small animals. The SQ route is not used to replace fluid deficits in large animals; the volumes of fluid that are usually required are so large that subcutaneous tissues would likely be compromised by the pressure and distension. SQ fluids tend to gravitate to dependent areas of the body, where absorption is slow. Also, there are few areas of loose, elastic skin that are suitable for SQ fluids; the lateral cervical regions and the lateral aspect of the triceps muscle mass have enough elasticity to allow small volumes of fluid (<500 ml) to be administered. This is occasionally done (especially in ruminants) for supplementation of calcium or magnesium.

For all other situations, fluids are given intravenously. For short-term administration, a large-diameter hypodermic needle (14- to 18-gauge [ga]) can be inserted directly into a vein and supported manually or taped to hold it in position. Fluids can be given directly through the needle into the vein via sterile rubber tubing. This method is commonly used for small volumes (<1 L) and for emergency situations when an IV catheter is not readily available. If longer-term IV fluid therapy is necessary, an IV catheter should be placed.

The tubing used for administration should be sterile and flexible. Standard IV fluid administration sets, arthroscopy tubing, "bell" IV lines, and many other choices are available (Fig. 9-1). Large-bore tubing should be used when rapid administration is necessary. If the patient is allowed freedom to wander around the stall while fluids are given, the tubing must be long enough to allow the patient to reach the borders of the stall and also to lie down if it chooses. If the

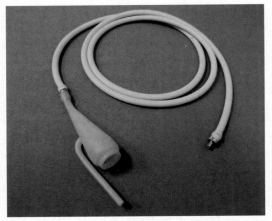

Fig. 9-1. The bell IV line is designed to deliver fluids from bottles, by sliding the "bell" portion over the mouth of the bottle and inserting the Luer tip into a catheter or needle inserted into a vein.

patient's movement is restricted, shorter tubing may be used. Special coil-style tubing for large animals is available; it stretches like a telephone cord to allow the patient to move around the stall or lie down yet takes up slack as the patient moves. This tubing is also rigid enough to provide some resistance to kinking.

One of the greatest challenges in large animal fluid administration is preventing kinking and/or disconnection of the administration tubing, or both. This is most likely to occur when the patient roams around the stall or lays down and tangles the tubing around its neck or legs. Sometimes it is necessary to place a patient in stocks or tie the head to try to prevent wandering or lying down while fluids are being given. Regardless, large animals *must* be closely supervised when they are on IV fluids. Kinking can lead to blood clotting inside the catheter because of stagnation of fluid movement through the catheter; in this case, the catheter will likely have to be replaced. Disconnection of administration tubing from the catheter can result in either aspiration of air through the

catheter into the bloodstream (air embolism) or massive external hemorrhage from the catheter, depending on the level of the catheter in relation to the heart. In either case, death can result.

Fluids can be purchased in 1-, 3-, 5- or 6-L bags. Administration sets (especially arthroscopy tubing) can be obtained with one, two, or four heads; multiple heads allow attachment to multiple fluid bags, for convenience. For most patients, the larger volume fluid bags (5 to 6 L) are more convenient to manage, especially if the patient requires large volumes of fluid.

Fluids can be given by gravity flow or with pressurized flow. For gravity flow, fluid bags may be hung from the ceiling on a rope and pulley system or from any point higher than the patient's catheter or needle. For pressurized administration, pressurized "squeeze" sleeves that wrap around fluid bags can be purchased. Alternatively, the fluids can be pressurized by injecting air into the fluid bag or bottle with a large syringe or hand pump. High-pressure administration is reserved for rapid, emergency administration.

Mechanized IV fluid pumps can be used for large animals but are typically used only for delivery of smaller volumes of fluids, primarily for foals and for low-volume parenteral nutrition in adults. Standard IV fluid pumps cannot exceed 999 ml/hr.

ENTERAL AND PARENTERAL NUTRITION

Various disease conditions may render an animal's GI tract incapable of intake, digestion, or absorption of food and water. For example, a mandibular fracture may prevent chewing; a pharyngeal abscess may prevent normal swallowing; and many conditions of the stomach, intestines, and colon can prevent normal digestion or absorption, or both. Non-GI diseases may also affect an animal's desire to eat and drink, such as during fever, severe pain, or diseases of the central nervous system. Failure to consume adequate carbohydrates, proteins, and lipids forces the body to process its reserves and perhaps its own tissues in order to prevent starvation. Malnutrition has well-known deleterious effects on health and on the ability of a sick or injured animal to heal and return to health.

Patients can be partially or totally nutritionally supported. Formulas are available to calculate an animal's energy, protein, and lipid requirements; vitamins and minerals can also be added if necessary. The formulas attempt to account for patient age, bodyweight, and energy requirements. The patient's underlying disease may affect the calculated nutritional requirements; for instance, sepsis in foals greatly increases energy needs above maintenance levels. Once the requirements have been calculated, the clinician can prescribe substances to precisely meet the nutritional needs of the patient.

Nutritional support can be given by enteral (GI) or parenteral routes.

ENTERAL FEEDING

Enteral feeding is only feasible if the GI tract is capable of digestion and absorption. Liquid diets can be formulated from readily available materials and given by stomach tube. Standard nasogastric tubes can be used; however, many horses resent repeated intubation, and long-term intubation with standard nasogastric tubes is often traumatic to tissues and interferes with swallowing. To minimize the effects of repeated or long-term use of standard tubes, commercially available nasogastric feeding tubes have been developed. The tubes are narrow in diameter and made from soft plastic, resulting in less tissue trauma. The tubes are secured to the muzzle or halter and, if properly maintained, allow long-term fluid and nutritional support (Fig. 9-2). If giving a

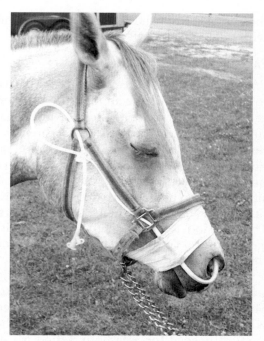

Fig. 9-2. Commercial nasogastric feeding tube for administration of fluids or enteral feeding. (From Hardy J: Critical care. In Reed SM, Bayly WM, Sellon DC, editors: *Equine internal medicine*, ed 2, St Louis, 2004, Saunders.)

slurry-type diet or sticky substances through any feeding tube, the tube should be flushed well after each use to prevent clogging.

Because of the interference with swallowing and possibility of aspiration, patients with indwelling nasogastric tubes, especially large diameter tubes, should not attempt to eat around the tube. Muzzles or stripped stalls may be necessary. If the patient is allowed access to water, it should be watched closely for coughing or reflux from the nostrils, which indicate difficulty swallowing. Removal of the water source may be necessary.

Occasionally a patient may have a condition that prevents passing a nasogastric tube through the nasal cavity or pharynx. Enteral feeding is still possible by placing a feeding tube directly into the esophagus via an esophagostomy. Once the tube is removed, the esophagostomy heals by second-intention with only topical care.

PARENTERAL NUTRITION

Parenteral routes are used as an alternative to the GI tract. In large animals the IV route is the parenteral route of choice. Nutritional support can be either partial (partial parenteral nutrition or PPN) or total (total parenteral nutrition or TPN). Calculations of the patient's nutritional needs are performed, and a decision is made whether to try to meet all (TPN) or part (PPN) of the patient's requirements. The decision is based on the patient's disease, physical condition, and length of time that support will be necessary.

Sterile carbohydrate, lipid, and amino acid solutions are commercially available for IV use. The content of each solution is compared with the calculated patient needs, and the amount needed for a 24-hour period is calculated and delivered through an IV catheter.

BLOOD AND PLASMA ADMINISTRATION

Whole blood is used to treat life-threatening blood loss, red blood cell (RBC) deficit, or platelet loss. Currently, whole blood for large animals is not commercially available because of inability to freeze it or store it under refrigeration for more than several days. Therefore whole blood is collected and used on an "as needed" basis.

Fresh, whole blood is collected from donor horses that are confirmed negative for equine infectious anemia (EIA) and current on their vaccines. With regard to blood types, more than 30 different RBC alloantigens exist in horses, leading to more than 400,000 possible alloantigen combinations! Therefore there is no such thing as a "universal donor." However, two alloantigens, Aa and Qa, are highly immunoreactive and are also very prevalent in horses. The most desirable blood donors would be negative for these alloantigens. Blood typing can be performed to identify the best potential donors (Standardbreds and Belgians have the lowest reported incidence of Qa and Aa, followed by Quarter Horses). While negative Aa and Qa donors should reduce the risk of incompatibility, they do not totally eliminate the risk.

Major and minor cross-matching should always be done to confirm a compatible donor, even when blood types are known (Table 9-3). Unmatched transfusions, though not preferred, may need to be performed in emergency situations. They can be performed with slightly increased risk; most horses can receive one or more transfusions over 3 to 4 days from a single, unmatched donor. Unmatched donors should preferably be geldings; the next choice would be a female that has never been bred. A healthy adult horse can donate 15% to 20% of its total blood

TABLE 9-3 **MAJOR AND MINOR CROSS-MATCHES**

	Components	Perform for Whole Blood Transfusion?	Perform for Plasma Transfusion?
Major cross-match	Donor RBC × recipient serum	Yes	No
Minor cross-match	Donor serum × Recipient RBC	Yes	Yes

RBC, *Red blood cell.*

volume (≈5 to 10 L of blood at one collection, or up to 20 ml/kg every 3 to 4 weeks). Blood volume of the adult horse is estimated as follows:

$$\text{Bodyweight (kg)} \times 8\% \text{ to } 10\% = \text{total blood volume (liters)}$$

Whole blood is collected using strict aseptic technique. The patient is clipped and prepped over a jugular vein. The operator should wear sterile gloves. A large-diameter needle or catheter (preferably 12- to 14-ga) is inserted into the jugular vein (*against* the direction of blood flow to facilitate collection), sterile tubing attached, and blood collected by gravity or vacuum-assisted flow. Gravity collection is preferred because of less damage to RBCs.

Whole blood can be collected into a sterile glass or plastic container; plastic is preferred because glass can potentially activate platelets and coagulation factors. Anticoagulant (usually citrate based) must be added to the collection container. Commercially available acid citrate dextrose (ACD) solution (2.5% to 4%) is used at a ratio of 9 parts blood/1 part ACD. Sodium citrate (3.2%) can also be used, in the same blood-to-citrate ratio. Commercial blood collection kits are available and convenient and provide plastic collection bags or bottles with premeasured anticoagulant and transfer tubing. Periodically during the collection procedure, the collection container should be gently swirled or rotated to assist mixing of the blood with the anticoagulant. The effects of storage on equine blood are not well known; therefore whole blood is preferably collected and transfused promptly. Short-term refrigerated storage for several days has been reported, using citrate phosphate dextrose (CPD) as the anticoagulant, at 4° C (39.2° F).

The volume of blood given to the recipient depends on the underlying disease and the reason for the transfusion. Usually, whole blood is given to replace RBCs. The volume of blood to be given is related to the patient's current RBC count versus the normal RBC count that the patient should have. Several formulas have been reported and used successfully for calculating transfusion volumes. One suggested formula is as follows:

$$\text{Liters required} = \text{bodyweight (kg)} \times \text{blood volume factor (ml/kg)} \times \frac{(PCV\ desired - PCV\ measured)}{PCV\ of\ donor}$$

Blood volume is factored as follows:
151 ml/kg   neonate <4 weeks old
93 ml/kg   neonate 4-12 weeks old
82 ml/kg   foal 12 weeks-6 months old
72 ml/kg   6 months old-adult

This formula provides only an estimate of blood to be replaced. In reality, administration of the entire calculated amount is seldom necessary.

Whole blood is given to the recipient through an IV catheter of at least 14-ga diameter. The administration system should have an in-line filter to remove clots; the filter should be replaced after filtering every 3 to 4 L. Even when cross-matching between donor and recipient indicates compatibility, adverse allergic reactions may still occur. Before beginning the transfusion, heart rate, respiratory rate, and temperature are recorded. The first 50 ml of blood should be given slowly over 15 to 30 minutes, and the recipient closely monitored for changes in heart rate, respiratory rate, and attitude (Box 9-1). If the patient's parameters remain stable over the introduction period, the administration rate may be increased to 15 to 20 ml/kg/hr. The patient should still be closely monitored throughout the entire transfusion. The transfusion should be immediately stopped if any reactions are observed. Because of the possibility of bacterial contamination being responsible for the reaction, the blood being administered should be cultured if adverse

BOX

9-1 Possible Clinical Signs of Adverse Transfusion Reactions

Tachycardia
Tachypnea
Dyspnea
Fever
Trembling
Shivering/piloerection
Weakness/collapse
Abdominal pain
Diarrhea
Hypotension
Hemolysis (with possible anemia, hemoglobinemia, hemoglobinuria)
Disseminated intravascular coagulation (DIC)
Pulmonary edema
Shock
Death

reactions are observed. Delayed reactions to transfusions may occur; therefore close monitoring should continue for at least 24 hours after the procedure.

Transfused equine RBCs live only 2 to 5 days on average. In rare instances when an animal is able to receive its own RBCs (autotransfusion), the life span of the cells may extend to 14 days.

Plasma transfusion is readily accomplished in the horse, due to the availability of commercial plasma. Plasma may be needed to replace plasma proteins, clotting factors, or antibodies (especially in foals with failure of passive transfer). Plasma may be made "hyperimmune" to certain antigens; by exposing the plasma donor to the antigen, antibodies will be produced, with passive transfer of immunity to the recipient.

Plasma may be collected fresh or bought commercially. Fresh plasma can be collected by harvesting whole blood from donor horses and performing plasmapheresis of the whole blood; equipment is expensive and is usually only found at large equine facilities. A less costly method is to collect whole blood and allow the cells to settle by gravity for several hours (at room temperature) or by centrifugation; the plasma may then be aseptically aspirated or siphoned from the settled RBCs and given to the recipient intravenously after passing it through an in-line microfilter. Plasma collected in this fashion is seldom completely free of cells and is prone to bacterial contamination.

Commercial plasma is collected from donors that are free of Aa and Qa alloantigens, and it is cell free. Controlled exposure of donor horses may produce plasma that is rich in antibodies against certain diseases. Compatibility (cross-match) testing is not usually necessary; however, if deemed necessary, only the minor cross-match is applicable. Commercial plasma is usually sold in 1-L plastic bags and is stored frozen. Plasma should never be thawed in a microwave oven, to avoid denaturing the plasma proteins. Rather, thawing should occur slowly in warm water. Plasma should reach at least 37° C (98.6° F) before administration. Frozen plasma generally stores safely for up to 1 year. It will have an expiration date that should not be exceeded. If an accidental partial or complete thaw occurs, refreezing is not recommended.

The amount of plasma given to a patient varies widely, depending on the reason for the transfusion, the rate of protein breakdown and redistribution, and the quality (protein levels) of the plasma being given. There is no single formula to perform universal calculations. The veterinarian will calculate replacement volumes based on patient and plasma variables. Typically, foals require 1 to 2 L to treat failure of passive transfer, and adults being treated for hypoproteinemia require at least 6 L for treatment. Administration of plasma is similar to whole blood, via a 16-ga or larger IV catheter.

An administration set with an in-line filter is appropriate.

Although the incidence is low, allergic reactions to plasma administration do occur. Reactions usually occur during the infusion, manifesting as shivering, difficult or rapid breathing, weakness, colic, or shock. If observed, the infusion should be stopped immediately and a clinician alerted to the situation.

SUGGESTED READING

Colahan PT et al: *Equine medicine and surgery,* ed 5, St Louis, 1999, Mosby.

Pratt PW: *Principles and practice of veterinary technology,* St Louis, 1998, Mosby.

Teeple TN: Nursing care of horses. In Sirois M: *Principles and practice of veterinary technology,* ed 2, St Louis, 1998, Mosby.

The neonatal period is the period following birth, which most clinicians consider the first 4 to 5 days of life. This period is one of susceptibility to many diseases and conditions that can be threatening to the immediate and long-term health of the foal; indeed, many of the diseases are life threatening. An estimated 2% of all foals born alive die before they are 48 hours old. Long-term consequences of neonatal diseases may alter the animal to the point of preventing it from achieving its intended use or athletic potential.

The outward appearance of a foal can be deceiving. Some foal diseases are obvious to the observer through external clinical signs; unfortunately, however, many foal diseases begin with only vague clinical signs that untrained personnel fail to recognize (Table 10-1). Failure to recognize these early signs leads to delays in diagnosis and

treatment and, combined with the tendency of foals to deteriorate rapidly, results in many foals being presented to the clinician in emergency conditions—too late for successful treatment.

Good neonatal care is a combination of sound management practices and recognition of normal and abnormal conditions. This chapter discusses the basics of neonatal care and examination.

PARTURITION

Gestation in the horse averages 330 to 345 days, though it is not uncommonly up to 360 days. Mares commonly have a longer gestation with their first foal, with subsequent pregnancies lasting approximately 5 days less. Statistically, most foalings (80%) occur at night.

The time of parturition is indicated by clinical signs, though they are not reliable enough to predict the exact time with certainty. Edema of the legs and a plaque of edema on the ventral abdomen are commonly seen in late pregnancy but are not helpful in predicting the time of foaling. The udder enlarges about 2 to 4 weeks before foaling, though enlargement may be minimal in maiden mares. The teats may "wax"; this refers to the leakage and subsequent drying of a small quantity of colostrum from each teat, producing a waxlike cap on the end of each teat. Parturition often follows in 24 to 48 hours after waxing is observed; however, this is not always reliable, and some mares

TABLE 10-1 NEONATAL TIMELINE

Time after Birth	Normal Clinical Findings
30-60 sec	Spontaneous breathing begins
5 min	Heart rate ≥60 Respiratory rate ≥60
30-60 min	Foal stands
60-180 min	Foal nurses
<10 hr	First urination
<24 hr	First defecation (meconium)

do not wax. Other possible signs are mild swelling of the vulva, discharge from the vulva, and relaxation of the pelvic ligaments (which is indicated by palpating the muscles around the tailhead for a soft "jiggling like Jell-O" effect).

Rectal temperature may be helpful in some mares. Normally, body temperature is slightly higher at night than in the morning. If the nighttime temperature is not higher than the morning temperature, the mare may foal within 36 hours. This method is not highly accurate.

In order to improve the ability to predict parturition, tests for the calcium level in mammary secretions have been developed. Calcium concentration rises sharply as the time of foaling approaches. The test is actually more accurate for predicting when foaling is *not likely* to occur than for when it *will* occur; calcium levels less than 400 ppm (10 mM/L) usually mean that foaling is unlikely. At levels above 400 ppm, most mares foal within 48 hours, and the remainder within another 48 hours. Samples can be run in a laboratory, or commercially available test kits can be used. Water hardness test kits can also be used. Distilled water should be used for diluting the milk samples, since the calcium in tap water alters the results.

As the mare actually begins stage 1 of labor (preparatory stage), restlessness, pacing, sweating, and disinterest in food are common. Many mares lie down and get up repeatedly and may posture to urinate frequently. Stage 1 may last from 2 to 4 hours on average. The mare should be separated from other horses. The tail should be wrapped, and the perineal area washed with mild soap. If a Caslick's operation has been performed and not yet opened, it should be opened with sharp, disinfected surgical scissors; no anesthetic is necessary, since the scar tissue bridge lacks innervation. The mare should be observed closely for the second stage of labor.

The delivery of the fetus (stage 2 of labor) in horses is rapid, compared with other species. Survival of the species requires that the foal be delivered and quickly stand and be capable of keeping up with the moving herd. Some mares even remain standing during the birth procedure. Supervising or "attending" a foaling is desirable to assure the well-being of both mare and newborn foal. The delivery can be observed and emergency assistance provided if dystocia is identified. It is best not to interfere with the birth process and remain at a distance unless difficulty is suspected or observed.

Once stage 2 of labor begins with the release of several gallons (8 to 20 L) of chorioallantoic fluid ("water breaking"), delivery of the fetus is usually complete within 20 to 30 minutes. The normal presentation is head and front limbs first, in a "head-dive" position; the soles of the hooves should face the ground. The feet rupture the white amnion, which is the membrane immediately surrounding the fetus; a small volume of additional fluid may be expelled. Because the equine placenta separates rapidly from the uterine wall, the foal loses its "oxygen line" and cannot survive being retained in the uterus or pelvic canal for long periods of time (unlike other species where the placenta separates gradually from the uterine wall). If no part of the fetus is seen from the vulva within 20 minutes of the water breaking, the likelihood of dystocia is high. If the foal is not fully delivered and breathing on its own within 30 to 45 minutes, dystocia should be assumed, and emergency assistance should be obtained. Dystocias are *always* true emergencies.

Stage 3 of labor, passage of the placenta and fetal membranes, should occur within 2 to 4 hours. If not passed within 4 to 6 hours, the placenta is considered to be retained, and a veterinarian should be consulted. Equines are susceptible to developing uterine infection, with possible septicemia and endotoxemia, as complications of retained placentas. Clients should never be encouraged to pull on the retained membranes or tie weights to the placenta. Rather, the mare should be confined and the tail wrapped; the exposed membranes may be tied to themselves (with twine) to keep them from dragging on the ground or being kicked at by the mare until the veterinarian arrives.

ROUTINE CARE OF THE NEONATAL FOAL

Once delivery is complete, the following needs of the newborn must be addressed:
1. Oxygenation/Pulse assessment
2. Temperature regulation
3. Care of the umbilical cord and umbilicus
4. Nutrition (nursing)
5. Bonding of mare and foal
6. Passage of meconium
7. Adequacy of passive transfer of antibodies
8. Physical examination of the foal

OXYGENATION/PULSE ASSESSMENT

The first priority immediately after delivery is to assure a clear airway. If amnion (whitish fetal membrane) remains over the nostrils, it should be removed. The force of passing through the birth canal squeezes most of the fluid from the upper airways; even so, the nostrils should be cleared with the fingers and wiped with a clean towel. A large bulb syringe can be used to aspirate fluid from each nostril. The foal is placed in a sternal position with the head and neck extended, and the body rubbed vigorously with dry towels to stimulate breathing. If breathing does not occur within 1 minute, resuscitation should be given. First, the foal's neck should be extended. The mouth and one nostril should be held shut, and the open nostril used to blow air into the lungs (confirmed by observing the chest rising). Both nostrils should be open for exhaling. The process is

repeated several times and, if unsuccessful, continued at a respiratory rate of 20 to 30/min until the foal makes its own efforts to breathe. Alternatively, a nasotracheal tube (8 to 10 mm internal diameter, 45 to 55 cm length) can be inserted through one nostril, the cuff inflated, and the foal manually resuscitated as described earlier or mechanically ventilated with an Ambu-bag or mechanical ventilator at a rate of 20 to 30/min.

The respiratory rate can be quite variable immediately after birth but should be at least 60/min at 5 minutes after birth. This rate will stabilize at 60 to 80/min over the first hour after birth and then decline over the next few hours to 30 to 40/min; this rate will persist for the first few weeks of life.

The pulse should be evaluated for rate and strength. The pulse should be at least 60 at 5 minutes after birth. The pulse rate usually *elevates* above 100 over the first hour, and then declines to 75 to 100 for the first week of life.

The respiratory rate and pulse rate are highly useful indicators of well-being in the newborn foal. If either remains less than 60 at 5 minutes after birth, a veterinarian should be consulted promptly.

TEMPERATURE REGULATION

Neonatal foals are highly sensitive to hypothermia. Drying the foal with towels removes amniotic fluids from the haircoat and is the first step to warming the body. If the environmental temperature is cold, heat lamps may be used. Heat lamps should be kept at least 4 feet away from the foal to prevent overheating and burns, which occur at approximately 103° F (39.4° C). Deep bedding helps to keep foals warm; straw is generally the preferred bedding for foals. Drafts should be prevented.

Rectal temperature of the neonate ranges from 99 to 101.5° F (37.2 to 38.6° C). Efforts to warm a foal should begin at a rectal temperature of 100° F (37.8° C). Heat lamps, warm water pads/bottles, and blankets can be used. Electric heating blankets and heating pads should not be placed directly against the skin due to the possibility of causing thermal burns.

CARE OF THE UMBILICAL CORD/UMBILICUS

The umbilical cord should not be cut unless necessary to prevent strangulation of the foal or entanglement around the mare's legs; these are rare occurrences. If the cord must be cut, hemostats should be placed over the stump to prevent hemorrhage. Once the strangulation or entanglement is relieved, the stump should be shortened to within several inches of the foal's abdomen and hemostats kept in place for 4 to 6 hours to prevent hemorrhage.

Whenever possible, nature should be allowed to take its course. Usually the mare and foal lie quietly for several minutes, and then the cord breaks naturally when the mare stands. The umbilical cord has a natural breakpoint about 1 to 2 inches from the foal's abdomen. The process of natural rupture causes spasm of the blood vessel walls, helping to control hemorrhage. If the cord continues to bleed actively and manual pressure for several minutes fails to stop it, a hemostat can be placed across the stump for several hours. The smallest size hemostat possible that will control the hemorrhage should be used; large hemostats tend to dislodge easily when a foal tries to stand and move around.

Traction should never be put on the umbilical cord such that the tension pulls directly on the foal's abdominal wall. If it is necessary to manually rupture the cord, one hand should press flat against the umbilicus for support of the abdominal wall and the other hand should grasp the cord several inches from the abdomen and apply traction to take advantage of the natural breakpoint.

The umbilical stump should be dipped in an antiseptic solution to cauterize the stump and minimize the bacterial population. Dilute povidone-iodine solution (3%) and dilute chlorhexidine solution (1:4 dilution) have been successfully used; tincture of iodine may cause unnecessary tissue damage. Dipping of the stump is done two to three times daily for the first week of life; a large, clean syringe case (20 or 35 ml size) makes a convenient container for the antiseptic and helps minimize splashing. Fill the container with antiseptic, center the opening over the umbilical stump, and press the container upward against the abdominal wall to effectively "dunk" the umbilical stump several times. Antiseptic should never be forced up or poured into the umbilical stump; the urachus, which is included in the stump, is short and communicates directly with the bladder, providing a potential pathway for the irritating antiseptic to enter the bladder and cause a chemical cystitis. Special care is necessary to avoid this complication if the procedure is done on a recumbent foal; it is less likely to occur if performed on a standing foal.

The umbilicus should be checked at least twice daily for omphalophlebitis and possible abscessation. Moisture, redness, swelling, pain, and exudation indicate the need for veterinary evaluation. Other common complications include persistent patent urachus and umbilical hernia (Boxes 10-1 and 10-2).

NUTRITION/NURSING

The suckling reflex is assessed by placing one or two fingers in the foal's mouth; this should stimulate a vigorous suckling effort in response. The suckling reflex is not present at birth; it develops rapidly after birth, beginning at about 5 minutes, and should be vigorous by 20 minutes.

The foal must stand in order to nurse. On average, a foal should make efforts to stand by 30 to 60 minutes after birth and should be nursing between 60 to 180 minutes

---

BOX **10-1**   **Persistent Patent Urachus**

Common Complaint

The foal appears to dribble or stream urine from the umbilicus. It may urinate from the urethra at the same time, producing two separate streams of urine. The umbilical area is constantly moist.

Etiology

Patent urachus. The urachus is usually patent at birth and closes naturally within 48 hours as the umbilical stump withers and dries.

When It Is a Problem

If urine passes through the umbilicus beyond 48 hours of age, this is referred to as a persistent patent urachus. A veterinarian should be consulted.

Treatment

- Keep the umbilicus clean and dry. Continue application of antiseptics.
- Monitor rectal temperature two to three times daily.
- Prophylactic antibiotics may be prescribed.
- Assist closure of the urachus; usually chemical cautery is tried first, using silver nitrate, tincture of iodine, phenol, or other cauterizing agent.
- If the foal does not respond after several days of treatment or if signs of local or systemic infection are seen, surgical resection of the umbilicus with ligation of the urachus may be recommended.

(2 hours is average). Just observing the foal's head in the vicinity of the mare's udder is not an indication that the foal is actually nursing. The foal should actually be observed taking the teat into the mouth and swallowing. Milk should be seen on and around the lips. A foal may need assistance finding the teat and getting it into the mouth the first few times it tries to nurse.

Some mares resent the foal's attempts to nurse and may even try to kick the foal. These are usually maiden mares or mares with painful udders. The mare may need to be twitched or sedated to allow the foal to nurse. The problem usually gets better over several days; warm compresses may help lessen udder swelling and pain.

Foals are totally dependent on milk for a source of energy because they are not born with large stores of carbohydrate or fat; hypoglycemia develops *rapidly* in foals that

do not nurse or that nurse poorly, and it is potentially life threatening. Foals should naturally nurse every 1 to 2 hours. One possible clue to decreased nursing by the foal may be the mare's development of a distended udder with excess milk. Milk may be observed streaming from the teats. Failure to nurse or infrequent attempts to nurse usually signal a more significant problem, and complete physical examination of the foal is warranted. Hypoglycemia is confirmed by analysis of blood glucose levels; supplementation should begin when blood glucose falls below 90 mg/dl. Blood glucose of 60 mg/dl requires emergency treatment, and death may occur at 40 mg/dl.

Several options are available for feeding orphan or rejected foals. Pan/bucket feeding and bottle feeding are most commonly used (Box 10-3). If bottle feeding, nature should be simulated as best possible. Rubber ewe nipples for lambs are preferred to cow nipples.

BOX 10-2 Umbilical Hernia

Clinical Signs

Soft, fluctuant swelling at the umbilicus. Rarely, the swelling may appear to change size, depending on the contents of the hernia, which may shift in and out of the hernia sac. A hard, firm swelling may indicate strangulation of the hernia contents.

Etiology

The natural opening in the abdominal wall for the umbilical cord should close down after birth as the umbilical cord atrophies. If the opening fails to close completely, a defect up to 3 to 4 inches long may remain. Segments of bowel or omentum may slide through this "hole" and come to rest beneath the skin, but outside the body wall; the presence of these contents outside the body wall is referred to as an *umbilical hernia.* The abnormal contents may slip back into the abdomen, only to reappear later; this cycle may continue for months, perhaps years in some cases. Umbilical hernias are always palpable and usually visible, especially when intestine or omentum is within the hernia sac.

When It Is a Problem

- Occasionally, the contents may become strangulated in the hernia sac (strangulating hernia); this is an emergency situation. Strangulating hernias are recognized by colic and usually an increasing size and firmness of the hernia as the strangulated tissues swell.
- Some owners may find that the visual appearance of a nonstrangulating hernia is an unacceptable cosmetic problem.

Treatment

Treatment depends on the size of the hernia ring, presence or likelihood of strangulation, age of the foal, and ability of the owner to closely monitor the foal.

- Many small hernia rings (<2 inches) close spontaneously, if abnormal contents are kept out of the ring. Hernia rings less than 1 inch in diameter have the best chance for spontaneous closure. Experienced horse owners can be instructed how to reduce the hernia and monitor the foal for signs of bowel entrapment. Closure may continue until 6 to 12 months of age, after which time complete closure is unlikely.
- Historically, hernia clamps have been used to "treat" umbilical hernias. After reducing the contents, the clamp is placed over the hernia sac like a large "chip clip," causing strangulation necrosis of the skin and underlying hernia sac. The clamp falls off in 2 to 3 weeks. However, it is questionable whether this method produces true closure of the abdominal wall defect, and there is risk of infection from the necrosis. Hernia clamps may improve the cosmetic appearance of small hernias. Generally, they are not commonly used.
- Surgical closure (umbilical herniorrhaphy) is intended for cases of confirmed strangulation, cases where strangulation is likely, cases where the owner does not want to risk strangulation, cases with large (>2 inches) hernia rings, or cases where the cosmetic appearance is objectionable to the owner.

Comments

- Umbilical hernias are the second most common congenital defect in horses; some veterinarians believe there is a genetic predisposition to the condition and advise against breeding these animals.
- Predicting whether a hernia will lead to strangulation and if so, when, is impossible. Client education can be challenging!

> | BOX 10-3 | Guidelines for Feeding Orphan and Rejected Foals |

Options for Feeding

- Mare's milk: This is the best choice.
- Cow's milk: Use 2% milkfat. Add 80 g dextrose or glucose/1 gal milk or 4 tsp jelly pectin/1 quart milk (20 g/L). Do not add table sugar (sucrose), corn syrup, or honey. Do not use long term.
- Goat's milk: Feed unaltered. If gastrointestinal (GI) disturbances occur, modify as recommended for cow's milk. Do not use long term.
- Commercial mare's milk replacers: These are sold as powders and are reconstituted with warm water. Foals may find these unpalatable. Soft stools are common and are not of concern. GI problems, especially diarrhea, tend to occur with milk replacers, especially when foals are not gradually introduced to the product or when the product is not changed regularly. Discard any unused, unrefrigerated, reconstituted product at each feeding or at least two to three times daily. Keep feeding containers clean.

Feeding Schedule

0-1 weeks of age: Feed at least every 2-3 hours.
1-2 weeks of age: Feed every 3-6 hours. Sick foals may need more frequent (every 2 hours) feedings.
2-4 weeks of age: 3-6 feedings per day. Begin offering solid food (creep feed or grain) and small quantities of hay or fresh pasture grass. A salt/mineral block should be provided, and fresh water at all times.
4-6 weeks of age: Feed two to three times daily. Increase solid food intake.
>6 weeks of age: Stop feeding milk/milk substitute if solid food intake is adequate.

Amount to Feed

Divide daily total into the number of feedings:
Day 0-2: 10%-15% bodyweight (kg) daily in milk or milk substitute
Day 3-4: Increase to 20%-25% bodyweight daily in milk or milk substitute; continue until 5 weeks of age
>5 weeks: 17%-20% bodyweight daily in milk or milk replacer
Formulas to calculate precise energy needs are available. Healthy foals need a minimum of 100 Kcal/kg/day. Sick foals need a minimum of 180 Kcal/kg/day.
In general, healthy average-sized foals should gain an average 0.5 to 1.5 kg/day bodyweight.

Human infant nipples can be used for neonates, sometimes requiring slight enlargement of the nipple hole. The head and neck should be extended during the feeding but not elevated above the level of the withers; elevating the head and neck increases the chance of aspiration of milk into the lungs. Some veterinarians recommend offering the bottle under the handler's armpit to simulate natural bumping and udder-seeking behavior. Foals should be encouraged to use a pan or bucket as soon as possible, to minimize human imprinting. Buckets and pans should be shallow and wide. There should be enough liquid in the container to prevent the foal from bumping its nose on the bottom of the container; this may startle the foal and make it reluctant to "trust" the container. The foal may need to be introduced to drinking from the container by taking advantage of the suckling reflex; the person doing so should moisten his or her fingers with the milk substance, place the fingers in the foal's mouth, and slowly guide its mouth to the liquid by submerging the fingers.

Nurse (foster) mares provide another alternative but are seldom available in most parts of the country. Nurse mares are mares that have lost their foals or had their foals intentionally removed; the lactating mare is then leased to the client in hopes that she will accept the client's motherless foal and nurse it as her own. Draft horse breeds and draft cross breeds are popular for nurse mares because of their temperament and milk production. However, draft mares may actually produce volumes of milk that are excessive for smaller light horse breed foals, resulting in excessively rapid weight gain and growth and related developmental orthopedic diseases. Lactating goats have occasionally been successfully used as "nurse goats."

BONDING OF MARE AND FOAL

The mare and foal should be interfered with as little as possible so that natural bonding can occur. Rarely a mare rejects her foal; usually the rejection is related to the immediate environment of the mare—too much human interference, loud noises, dogs, or other horses that can be seen or heard by the new mother have all been associated with rejection. If housed indoors, mares and newborns are best kept in fairly isolated stalls in low traffic areas.

Mares tend to be very protective of their foals; some mares may even show aggression toward humans. One person should be responsible for handling the mare when it is necessary to work on or around the foal. The mare should be restrained first before attempting to approach or restrain the foal. The handler should not try to prevent the mare from seeing or being close to the foal; this will upset even "good" mares. Let the mare be as close to the "action" as possible, and keep procedures organized and brief.

PASSAGE OF MECONIUM

Meconium is the term for fetal feces. The fetus naturally swallows amniotic fluid, which is processed by the gastrointestinal (GI) tract to a waste material that accumulates in the colon and rectum. The material is usually hard, dark, and in the form of clumped pellets. Meconium should be defecated after birth; however, it is often difficult and painful to pass. Foals typically strain to pass the material, and it may take several attempts to expel the clumped mass. For this reason, it is routine to give newborn foals an enema. A standard human pediatric sodium phosphate enema (Fleet enema) is commonly used; no more than 1 pint total volume should be instilled at a time. An alternative is a warm mild soap water enema given via soft rubber tubing with gravity flow. The enema must *never* be forced; if resistance is encountered, the enema should be stopped, and a veterinarian consulted.

Enemas may be repeated every 4 to 6 hours until the meconium passes. If not passed in 24 hours or if colic is observed at any time, a veterinarian should be consulted; more aggressive therapy may be necessary. Owners should never be advised to try to remove the meconium themselves. Meconium impactions are the leading cause of colic in neonatal foals and may be severe enough to require surgical correction. Signs of meconium impaction are frequent posturing and straining to defecate without producing feces, frequent swishing of the tail as if agitated, restlessness, decreased nursing, rolling, and possible abdominal distension.

ADEQUACY OF PASSIVE TRANSFER OF ANTIBODIES

Colostrum (first milk) is essential for passive transfer of immunity to foals. Equids are unique in that passive transfer of antibodies across the placenta does not occur; therefore the foal is completely dependent on colostrum for passive antibody transfer until its own immune system matures. The foal's immune system is not fully capable of producing protective antibody levels until close to 8 weeks of age.

TABLE

10-2	**ANTIBODY LEVELS**	
Antibody Level	*Category of Protection*	*Risk for Development of Neonatal Septicemia*
>800 mg/dl	Excellent	Minimal
400-800 mg/dl	Adequate	Low
200-400 mg/dl	Partial failure of passive transfer	Increased
<200 mg/dl	Total failure of passive transfer	High

still have plenty for their own foal. After the mare gives birth, the foal is allowed to nurse. Then, the udder is cleaned with mild soap and water and a soft cloth, and colostrum is milked into a clean glass jar or Ziploc bag, sealed, and marked with the mare's name and date of collection. The colostrum can be used immediately or stored frozen for up to 1 year. Frozen colostrum should not be thawed in a microwave oven to avoid denaturing proteins (antibodies are proteins) and destroying normal bacterial flora (which the foal's intestinal tract needs). Instead, colostrum can be thawed gradually in a warm water bath. The colostrum can then be given to a foal in need via bottle or nasogastric intubation. Administration must occur during the first 18 hours after birth to be effective.

How much colostrum is necessary to protect a foal depends on the amount ingested and the amount of antibody in the colostrum. The amount of antibody in colostrum can be measured by sending a sample to a laboratory for protein analysis, but this may incur needless time delay. For field measurements, a colostrometer is easy and quick to use. Commercial kits for assessing colostrum are also available. The colostrometer measures the specific gravity of colostrum, which correlates to the IgG level. Readings should be made with the colostrum at room temperature (i.e., at the same temperature as the instrument). Good colostrum has more than

3000 mg/dl IgG; this corresponds to a specific gravity greater than 1.060 on the colostrometer. Once the IgG content has been determined, the specific volume of colostrum necessary to provide greater than or equal to 70 g total of IgG can be calculated and given to the foal. As a rule of thumb, 2 pints of colostrum (with adequate antibody level) is the minimum goal for most foals. To prevent overdistending the stomach, up to 1 pint can usually be given per feeding, and at least 1 hour should be allowed between feedings.

If colostrum is not available, commercial plasma can be given by nasogastric tube. This reduces the complications of placing an intravenous (IV) catheter and minimizes the risk of adverse reactions. Recently, nonplasma high-level antibody products have become available for nasogastric intubation. Bovine colostrum is tolerated and absorbed by the foal's GI system but is likely to afford only partial and short-lived protection for the foal. Mild diarrhea has been observed following administration of bovine colostrum to foals.

Foals older than 18 hours of age and those with GI diseases cannot be supplemented via the GI tract. The only option available for these foals is IV plasma or immune serum transfusion. Plasma transfusion in foals is performed similarly to adults, except that it is preferable to sedate the foal and restrain it in lateral recumbency for the IV catheterization and transfusion procedures.

As a rule of thumb, 1 L of "regular" (not hyperimmune) commercial plasma will elevate the IgG level of a normal foal by 200 mg/dl.

Regardless of the route of therapy, the foal should be retested after treatment to ensure that adequate protection has been achieved. Serum IgG levels should be rechecked in 8 to 12 hours after treatment.

PHYSICAL EXAMINATION OF THE FOAL

Basic Evaluation

Basic evaluation of the neonatal foal includes the following:

Temperature	99-101.5° F
	>102° F is febrile
Pulse rate	≥60 at 5 minutes
	75-100 for first week of life
Respiratory rate	≥60 at 5 minutes 60-80 for first 1-2 hours; decreases to 30-40 for first month
Mucous membrane color	Dark pink to pink to pale pink. Mild icterus is not uncommon; it is usually a normal finding but may indicate disease
Capillary refill time	1-2 seconds
Ear pinnae	Examine for icterus and petechiae, which may indicate septicemia

Heart Auscultation

A continuous "machinery murmur" over the left heart base indicates a patent ductus arteriosus (PDA). In horses this is normal and should gradually disappear by 4 days of age.

Lung Auscultation

Lung sounds are moist for the first hours after birth due to the presence of fetal fluids. Even after fetal fluids have cleared, foal lungs continue to sound harsh. Auscultation is NOT a reliable indicator of lung disease in foals; foals can have normal lung sounds yet have severe lung disease. This is due to the prevalence of interstitial pneumonia in foals, which does not affect the alveoli and airways. If alveoli and airways are not affected, the classic signs of cough, nasal discharge, and abnormal lung sounds are not present. Therefore lung disease in foals is best detected by external signs: increased respiratory rate, increased respiratory effort ("pumping"), abdominal breathing, and flared nostrils.

Gastrointestinal Tract

Reflux of milk from the nostrils may indicate a cleft palate. Foals should be watched for abdominal distension. GI motility sounds, which are primarily fluid and gas sounds in the neonate, should occur every 10 to 20 seconds.

After the foal passes meconium, normal "milk feces" should be seen. Milk feces are soft or pasty consistency and yellowish to tan in color.

Mild diarrhea normally occurs around day 5 to 10, corresponding with the mare's first heat cycle after parturition ("foal heat"); this is referred to as "foal heat diarrhea." It is seldom severe, is not normally accompanied by fever, and seldom requires any treatment; it is self-limiting within several days of onset. The cause is unknown.

A veterinarian should be consulted for any diarrhea that is accompanied by fever, dehydration, or loss of appetite or that persists more than 2 to 3 days.

Urination

The first urination should occur by 10 hours of age. Normal urine volume in a foal is 148 ml/kg/day. Urine specific gravity is low compared to adults, with a range of 1.001 to 1.012.

Ocular

Scleral and conjunctival hemorrhage is commonly observed after birth and usually affects both eyes. Increased pressure during passage through the pelvic canal is believed to cause the hemorrhage; it will resolve without treatment over several days.

The corneas and lenses should be clear and transparent; however, congenital cataracts are seen sometimes. The menace reflex, which evaluates cranial nerves 2 (optic) and 7 (facial), is not fully developed until 2 weeks of age; the pupillary light response may also be slow (but present) during this time.

Foals must be watched carefully for entropion of the lower eyelid. Dehydrated foals quickly develop entropion, which results in hairs rubbing on the cornea and subsequent development of corneal ulcers. Corneal ulcers can form rapidly and quickly progress to infection or rupture, or both, of the globe. Treatment of entropion is an urgent situation. Entropion is treated by everting the affected lid with a subcutaneously injected "bleb" of procaine penicillin G (PPG) or by temporary suturing of the lid in the correct position.

Blepharospasm (squinting) and tearing are the hallmarks of corneal ulcers and are the earliest clinical signs. Cloudiness of the cornea and "milk spots" may not be present initially; therefore they cannot be relied upon as the only telltale signs of an ulcer. When any of these signs are observed, a veterinarian should be consulted *immediately*. The eye will need thorough evaluation, and topical and systemic medication may be necessary. Severe cases may require surgical treatment.

Musculoskeletal System

The hooves of the neonate are covered by fetal hoof pads; these appear as irregular, yellowish, soft material covering the sole of each hoof. The hoof pads fall off or wear away quickly as the foal bears weight; no special treatment is required.

Fractured ribs, which are due to the high pressures on the foal as it passes through the pelvic canal of the mare, are not uncommon. When they occur, it is common for multiple adjacent ribs to be involved. Swelling may or may not be seen initially but typically develops and is mild. Palpation may reveal the fractured ends if they are displaced. Auscultation over the fracture may reveal a clicking sound with each inspiration. Ultrasound can be used to identify questionable fractures. Fractured ribs almost always heal without special treatment, but occasionally bleeding into the pleural cavity and punctured heart or lungs may occur. The foal should be restricted to a stall for approximately 3 weeks to allow the fracture to stabilize. Pressure in the area of fractured ribs should be avoided.

Joints should be watched for effusion (swelling), heat, and pain. Any joint swelling, with or without lameness, should be considered suspicious for a septic process (bacterial infection), and a veterinarian should be consulted.

The gait of the neonate can be difficult to assess; exaggerated leg movements are normal, and spinal reflexes may be increased (hyperreflexive). Foals may naturally stand with a base-wide stance.

Legs should be evaluated for limb deformities. There are two primary types of limb deformities:
- **Flexural deformity:** assessed by viewing the legs from the lateral (side) position. Before birth, the musculoskeletal soft tissues (muscles, tendons, and ligaments) of the limbs have not supported weight. When the foal first stands and bears weight, these unused soft tissues are seldom accustomed to the tension and flexural deformities commonly occur. One or more legs may be affected. There are two varieties

of flexural deformity: (1) soft tissues that are too "loose" and (2) soft tissues that are too "tight."

When too loose, the fetlock is hyperextended and appears as a "dropped ankle." As the foal begins to move around, the soft tissues adapt to weightbearing and the condition usually corrects spontaneously within several days. In more advanced cases, the hoof may not sit flat on the ground; the toe is elevated off the ground and the weight is rocked back on the heels (Fig. 10-1). Veterinary evaluation should be sought for these cases. These foals are at risk for damaging the lower leg joints and tendons and severely bruising (often abscessing) the heels; they should be confined to a stall or small pen to prevent running and excessive exercise until the tissues strengthen and the hoof rests normally on the ground. A common practice is to place heel extensions (using special shoes or thin plywood blocks) on the affected hooves; the heel extensions force

the hoof to sit flat on the ground by preventing the ability to rock back on the heels. They are worn until the legs have strengthened.

When the tissues are too tight, commonly referred to as *contracted tendons,* the appearance of the leg depends on which tendons and ligaments are involved. The forelimbs are more commonly affected than the hindlimbs. The normal fetlock angle may diminish, giving an upright, straight, "post-legged" appearance; knuckling over at the fetlock may occur in severe cases. Other cases may have a clubfoot appearance, and the heel may not rest flat on the ground (Fig. 10-2). Veterinary evaluation is necessary to identify which structures are too tight and to select the appropriate therapy; radiographs may be necessary to assess the health of bones and joints. Therapy may include dietary management, IV administration of tetracycline, applying extended toe shoes, use of splints or casts, and even surgery in some cases.

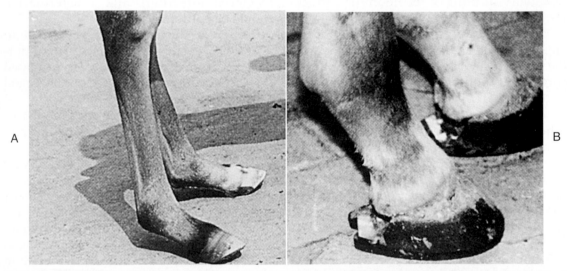

Fig. 10-1. **A,** Severe flexor tendon laxity in a neonatal foal. Note the dropped fetlock appearance and the weight "rocked" back on the heels with the toes elevated off the ground. **B,** Same foal after application of glue-on heel extension shoes. (From Auer JA, Stick JA: *Equine surgery,* ed 2, St Louis, 1999, Saunders. Photo courtesy H. Dallmer, FRG.)

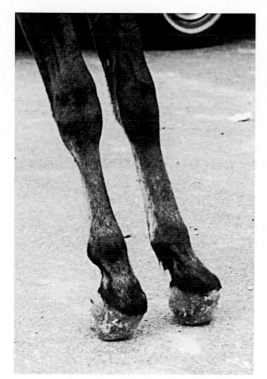

Fig. 10-2. Contractural deformity of a foal resulting in club-foot appearance and upright fetlocks. (From Auer JA, Stick JA: *Equine surgery*, ed 2, St Louis, 1999, Saunders.)

Severe cases may not respond to any combination of medical or surgical therapy.

- **Angular deformity:** assessed by viewing the legs from a cranial-caudal (front-back) position. The leg appears crooked or deviated from the midline, usually in the vicinity of the carpus or tarsus, though less commonly the fetlock area is affected. There are two varieties of angular deformities. When the deviation is away from the body's median plane, the deformity is referred to as *valgus*. When the deviation is toward the median plane, the deformity is referred to as *varus* (Figs. 10-3 and 10-4).

Occasionally a foal is born with a varus deformity of one limb and a matching valgus deformity of the opposite limb. This occurs more commonly in the

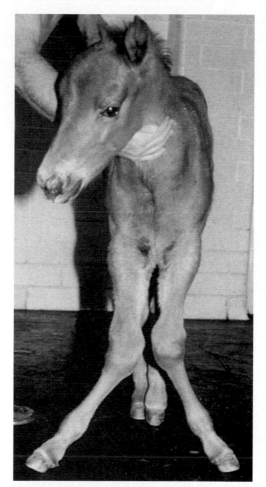

Fig. 10-3. Foal with severe bilateral valgus deformities of the forelimbs, centered around the carpal regions ("carpal valgus"). (From Colahan PT et al: *Equine medicine and surgery*, ed 5, St Louis, 1999, Mosby.)

hindlimbs and is believed to be due to malpositioning in the uterus during late gestation. Foals with this appearance are referred to as *windswept* foals. Depending on the severity, treatment may or may not be required.

Radiographs are recommended to determine the cause of the deformity so that therapy can be prescribed. Mild angulations may respond to corrective trimming

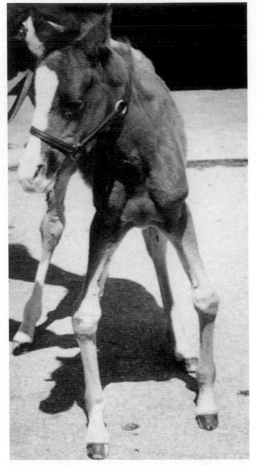

Fig. 10-4. Foal with severe varus carpal deformity. (From Colahan PT et al: *Equine medicine and surgery*, ed 5, St Louis, 1999, Mosby.)

or shoeing. More severe angulations may require splints or even surgery to correct the deformity. If bone damage is involved, it may not be possible to straighten the leg completely, even with surgery.

IDENTIFICATION AND CARE OF THE SICK NEONATAL FOAL

A foal is not simply a miniature version of an adult. The function of organ systems, nutritional needs, and distribution of body water are quite different in neonates. Some neonatal problems are obvious—crooked legs, hernias, and lameness can be readily seen by most observers. However, many serious neonatal diseases begin with vague clinical signs that untrained personnel may fail to detect. One of the most important characteristics of sick neonates is their tendency to "crash and burn," often within a matter of hours. Adopting a "wait and see" attitude frequently leads to disaster, requiring heroic measures to try and save the foal—often without success.

Certain conditions may predispose a foal to developing illness. When any of the following are observed, the foal is considered to be a "high risk" foal:

- Mare with fever, systemic disease, or vaginal discharge during pregnancy
- Abnormal placenta
- Prolonged delivery or dystocia
- Mare with agalactia or colostrum leakage before parturition
- Premature or dysmature foal
- Twin foal
- Orphaned or rejected foal
- Failure to ingest colostrum
- Delivery by caesarean section

High-risk foals should be watched very closely for development of abnormalities. Frequent monitoring of TPR and frequent physical examinations should be performed. Passive transfer status should be determined with a blood test for IgG, and treatment instituted as necessary. Attention to stall sanitation and a warm, dry environment is essential. The umbilicus should be treated three to four times daily and watched closely for signs of infection. If any abnormalities are detected in these foals, early evaluation and treatment offer the best chance of a successful outcome.

Sick foals seldom have only one problem, though often only one problem is readily apparent. Astute clinicians carefully evaluate *all* body systems for problems and provide treatment as necessary. Also, because the immune system does not respond well until several weeks after birth, careful attention must be paid to sanitation and sterile technique when treating and examining foals to avoid creating additional problems from iatrogenic contamination. Injections, diagnostic sampling, and IV catheter and feeding tube maintenance require strict attention to cleanliness. Stall sanitation is a must; urine and feces should be removed frequently. Hand washing before and after contact with the foal is important. Many procedures on foals are performed by restraining the foal on the ground in lateral recumbency; working at ground level requires extra care to prevent contamination of equipment and supplies. The ground under the foal should be covered with a clean sheet, towel, or drape to form a barrier against bedding and excrement.

The level of care required for a sick foal may range from a heat lamp and blanket to complete 24-hour care in a neonatal intensive care unit. Some recumbent foals may struggle frequently, risking tangling fluid and oxygen lines, and require at least one person to literally sit with them at all times (Fig. 10-5). Once a sick foal has been evaluated and its needs determined, client communication is important to determine what treatment options are available and reasonable to pursue. Care for many foal diseases is labor intensive and expensive.

The following patient needs may need to be addressed:
- Nursing care: warmth, cleanliness, complications of recumbency (pressure sores, constipation, urine scalding, etc.)
- Nutritional care: pan/bottle feeding, indwelling nasogastric tube, or intravenous feeding (partial or total parenteral nutrition). Hypoglycemia develops rapidly in neonates that are not nursing normally; blood glucose levels may need to be monitored three to four times daily.

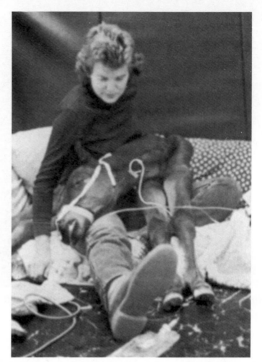

Fig. 10-5. An attendant may be required to monitor a sick neonate and prevent entanglement with fluid and oxygen lines. (From Vaala WE: *Vet Clin North Am Equine Pract* 10:1-271, 1994.)

- Immune status: treatment if antibody levels are low.
- Respiratory support: supplemental nasal oxygen, mechanical ventilator for severe cases (Fig. 10-6).
- Fluid therapy: IV fluids to maintain normal hydration, electrolyte, and acid-base balance.
- GI ulceration: the incidence of gastric (and duodenal) ulceration is *very high* in sick equine neonates; many receive oral or IV anti-ulcer medications for prophylaxis or treatment.
- Disease-specific medication and treatment: antibiotics, antiinflammatories, joint lavage, etc., depending on the foal's specific medical/surgical problems.

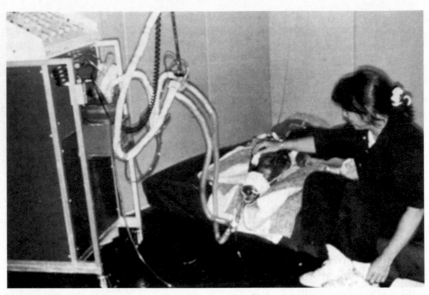

Fig. 10-6. Four-day-old septic foal with respiratory failure, on mechanical ventilation. (From Paradis MR: *Vet Clin North Am Equine Pract* 10:109-135, 1994.)

Neonatal diseases that typically require intensive nursing care include prematurity (Box 10-5), peripartum asphyxia syndrome (Box 10-6), and neonatal bacterial septicemia (see Box 10-4).

Depending on the facilities, severity of the foal's disease, and other factors, the mare may or may not be able to stay with the foal during its medical treatment. This decision is not always an easy one. If the mare is to remain with the foal, she should be allowed as close to the foal as possible. If necessary to use a partition to keep the mare physically apart from the foal, as is often necessary to prevent entanglement in fluid or oxygen lines, the partition should allow the mare to be as close to the foal as possible and maintain visual contact. If the foal is unable to nurse, the mare should be milked every 2 to 4 hours to encourage continued lactation while the foal recovers. Occasionally it is in the best interest of the mare, foal, and staff to remove the mare from the foal, which

is essentially early weaning. Separation must be complete, removing sight, smell, and sound of the foal. Sedation of the mare may be required. To end lactation, hand-milking is stopped and carbohydrates in the mare's diet are reduced.

Restraint of the foal in lateral recumbency is often necessary. One person should be responsible for restraining the head and neck, taking care to protect the down (lower) eye. Care should also be taken to avoid interfering with breathing by accidentally compressing the trachea or throat or occluding the nostrils. If the foal is capable of leg motion, it is usually necessary to have one person restrain the forelimbs and one person restrain the hindlimbs. Limbs should never be restrained by grasping only the distal parts of the limbs, such as the pasterns; the primary restraining force should be applied just proximal to the carpus or tarsus, and lighter force applied to the distal limbs if necessary.

BOX

10-5 Premature Foals

Definition

Gestation averages 330 to 345 days in the equine. Prematurity is usually defined as delivery before gestational age of 320 days; however, the presence of clinical signs may occur at gestational ages older than 320 days. These cases are properly referred to as *dysmature.*

Clinical Signs

Small size and bodyweight
Generalized weakness
Delayed time to stand
Poor suckling reflex
Silky haircoat
Floppy ears
Prominent forehead (normal in Miniature Horses)
Hyperextension of fetlocks (flexural limb deformity)

Clinical Significance

Premature foals are at high risk for respiratory, metabolic, musculoskeletal, and infectious problems.

Treatment

No specific therapy. Provide nursing care as needed for the foal's individual problems. Closely monitor foals (temperature, pulse, and respiration/physical examination) and provide a clean, dry, warm environment. Adequate antibody levels should be confirmed with a blood test and treated if they are deficient.

BOX

10-6 Peripartum Asphyxia Syndrome (Neonatal Maladjustment Syndrome, "Dummy" Foals)

Common Complaint

These foals are usually born without apparent difficulty and act normally for the first hours of life. However, by 24 hours, they appear to lose the suckling reflex and affinity for the mare. They may wander aimlessly, appear blind, become recumbent, and possibly seizure.

Etiology

The cause of peripartum asphyxia syndrome is not yet confirmed but is believed to be a derangement in cerebral blood circulation and blood pressure, combined with low oxygen levels, during birth. Histopathology shows cerebral edema and hemorrhages.

Clinical Signs

Clinical signs are primarily neurological and develop after birth. Because infection is not part of the syndrome, temperature, pulse, and respiration and complete blood count are usually normal. If febrile, a separate infectious process (such as septicemia) should be suspected in addition to peripartum asphyxia syndrome.

Treatment

No specific therapy exists; provide supportive care as needed. A high level of supportive care may be necessary for recumbent foals. If not complicated by infectious processes, at least 50% of foals recover with proper supportive care, and recovery is usually complete.

NEW MARE AND FOAL CHECK

After an uncomplicated delivery, it is common practice for the veterinarian to examine both mare and foal within the first 24 hours after birth. The client should be instructed to save the placenta for examination by placing it in a plastic garbage bag (wear gloves) and refrigerating it (if possible) until the veterinarian arrives. The placenta should be kept out of reach of dogs and cats, since they often try to eat or carry it away.

The veterinarian will give the mare a thorough physical examination, followed by a rectal, vaginal, and perineal examination to check for trauma from parturition. The uterus is commonly lavaged to dilute and expel lochia (postpartum accumulation of fetal fluids and blood in the uterus). The veterinarian will examine the placenta to ensure that it has been completely expelled and also check for thickening and discoloration, which might indicate placentitis or other abnormalities.

The foal will receive a thorough physical examination as described earlier. Blood is drawn for passive transfer (antibody) testing, and often a complete blood count (CBC) is obtained. Further examination and blood work depends on any abnormalities that are detected during the course of the evaluation.

SUGGESTED READING

Beech J: Neonatal equine disease, *Vet Clin North Am Equine Pract* 1:1-263, 1985.

Lewis LD: Feeding and care of the horse, ed 2, Baltimore, 1996, Williams & Wilkins.

McCurnin DM, Bassert JM: *Clinical textbook for veterinary technicians*, ed 6, St Louis, 2006, Saunders.

Pratt PW: *Principles and practice of veterinary technology*, St Louis, 1998, Mosby.

Vaala WE: Perinatology, *Vet Clin North Am Equine Pract* 10:1-271, 1994.

IDENTIFICATION

ELECTRONIC IDENTIFICATION

Implantation of a coded microchip beneath the skin that can be read with an electronic sensor is available for equines. The microchip, about the size of a rice grain, is encoded with the horse's registration or other identification number. Although microchipping is not yet common, it is gaining popularity.

The location for implantation is halfway between the withers and poll, about $1\frac{1}{2}$ inches below the crest of the neck. The chip is injected about 1 to $1\frac{1}{2}$ inches beneath the skin, into the nuchal ligament. Recent studies in horses indicate that migration of the chip away from the implant site is not likely to occur.

PROCEDURE

Clipping is preferred but optional. Local anesthetic is optional. The injection site should be sterilely prepared (prepped). The horse is restrained as necessary. The chip is implanted by injection, using a specially designed syringe and 12-gauge (ga) needle.

AFTERCARE

The injection site should be kept clean. Antibiotic ointment may be applied to the site for several days.

LIP TATTOOING

Horses are tattooed on the mucosal side of the upper lip. Several racing authorities require lip tattoos as a method of identification; tattoos are applied by tattoo technicians employed by the breed or racing governing bodies. The horse must be properly registered with its breed registry in order to receive the official tattoo. However, any horse owner can have his/her horses privately tattooed with any letter/number combination he/she desires. Tattoo equipment is readily available from livestock supply companies.

Most official tattoos begin with a letter that corresponds to the year of birth, followed by a number sequence that matches the registration number. Thoroughbreds use all letters of the alphabet; the letter A was used in 1971, B in 1972, etc., until the letter A was used again in 1997. Standardbreds began a new system in 1982 (=A) but do not use the letters I, O, Q, or U; therefore the letter Z was used for 2003.

Horses should preferably be at least 1 year old so that the lip is large enough for the tattoo gun to be applied. Once applied, the tattoo grows with the horse.

PROCEDURE

Restraint of the head is necessary; a standard lip twitch obviously cannot be applied. The upper lip is retained in a metal lip clamp that exposes and spreads the lip and helps in restraint by mimicking the effect of a twitch. Sedation may be necessary for some individuals.

After applying the lip clamp, the area is cleaned with alcohol. The tattoo gun is checked for accuracy of the tattoo pattern and is dipped into antiseptic solution. Tattoo ink is spread across the tissue, and then the tattoo gun is applied to the lip. The tattoo gun contains metal dies with sharp needles that make tiny punctures in the tissue, carrying the ink into the tissue. The tattoo gun is applied by squeezing the handles and is then promptly removed; the fingers are used to rub the remaining ink into the perforations.

AFTERCARE

The tissue quickly heals over the punctures, capturing the ink. No special aftercare is necessary. Complications are rare.

RESPIRATORY SYSTEM

SINUS TREPHINATION/SINOCENTESIS

Horses have an extensive network of paranasal sinuses, which are subject to a variety of diseases, most of which are infectious. Signs of sinus disease include nasal discharge, facial swelling, and possible malodor. The anatomy of the sinuses and their openings is complex and prevents visual examination with the endoscope and insertion of instruments through the natural internal openings. In order to examine and treat sinus diseases, alternate entrances directly into the sinuses through the skin must be made. Centesis (sinocentesis) refers to making a small-diameter hole (perforation) through bone into a sinus; trephining is the process of making a larger-diameter hole into a sinus by removal of a small, circular piece of bone. Depending on the diameter of the hole, endoscopes, instruments, and tubing for flushing can be inserted for diagnostic and therapeutic purposes. Repulsion of cheek teeth can also be performed through trephine holes.

Sinocentesis and trephination can be performed under general anesthesia or on a standing horse using sedation and local anesthesia.

PATIENT PREPARATION

Standing procedure: appropriate physical and chemical restraint
General anesthesia: follow anesthetic protocol

PROCEDURE

The location depends on which sinus is to be entered (Fig. 11-1). The area is clipped and sterilely prepped. Local anesthesia (3 to 5 ml) is required if the procedure is performed standing. A stab or small incision is made through the skin with a scalpel.

The size of the intended hole determines the instrument used to penetrate the bone. Small holes (centesis) can be made with a

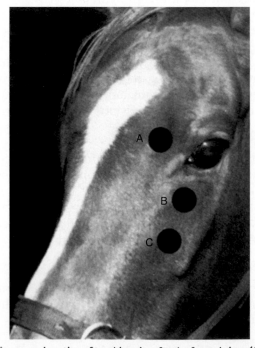

Fig. 11-1. Location of trephine sites for the frontal sinus (A), caudal maxillary sinus (B), and rostral maxillary sinus (C). (From Speirs VC: *Clinical examination of horses*, St Louis, 1997, Saunders.)

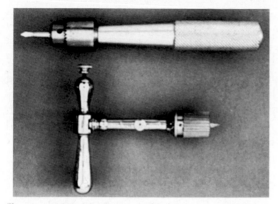

Fig. 11-2. A handchuck and pin *(top)* are used to make small holes in the sinus, and a trephine *(bottom)* is used to remove a circular piece of bone. (From Bertone AL: *Vet Clin North Am Equine Pract* 7:485-735, 1991.)

Jacobs hand chuck and Steinmann pin or a bone drill. Larger holes are made with a stainless steel trephine (Fig. 11-2). A depth of approximately 2 to 3 cm is all that is necessary to penetrate into the sinus.

The diagnostic or therapeutic procedure (endoscopy, sinus lavage, etc.) is then performed. Sometimes a rubber catheter or other tubing may be placed through the hole and secured to the skin for long-term flushing of the sinus (Fig. 11-3). Small stab incisions for sinocentesis may be left to heal by second intention or closed with a simple skin suture. Trephine sites may be left open to heal or closure of the incision may be performed, depending on the size of the trephine hole. In either case, the bone disk is discarded and not replaced. The skin can be closed with sutures or skin staples.

Open trephine holes should be covered to prevent material from entering the sinus; a head bandage using stockinette may be used to cover and protect the site. Otherwise, bandaging is optional. Pressure bandages are difficult to apply in this area, but light pressure may be possible with gauze 4 × 4's and elastic adhesive tape used to carefully encircle the head.

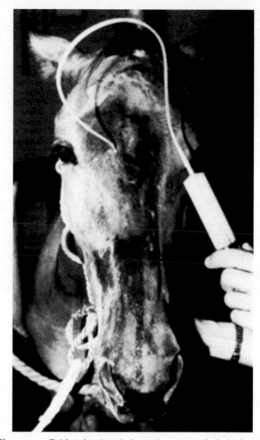

Fig. 11-3. Tubing is placed through a centesis hole in the frontal sinus for diagnostic and treatment purposes. The tubing can be sutured to the skin for use as an indwelling catheter for sinus lavage. (From Bertone AL: *Vet Clin North Am Equine Pract* 7:485-735, 1991.)

AFTERCARE

The incision is kept clean, and antibiotic ointment is applied until the area heals. Sutures/staples are removed in 5 to 10 days. The area should be watched for signs of infection, including excessive swelling and discharge.

TRACHEOTOMY/TRACHEOSTOMY

Tracheostomy may be performed as an emergency or elective procedure (Box 11-1).

11-1   Emergency Tracheostomy Pack

1. Local anesthetic
2. 20- to 25-gauge syringe needles
3. 3 ml or 6 ml syringes
4. Disposable scalpel blade (No. 10) and handle
5. Metzenbaum scissors
6. Mosquito hemostats
7. J-type, self-retaining, or cuffed tracheostomy tube

Obstructions of the upper airway such as swelling due to snakebite, compression or blockage by tumors, and lymph node swelling may create life-threatening compromise to breathing. Elective tracheostomy is performed whenever severe postoperative swelling is anticipated following surgery on the nasal, pharyngeal, or laryngeal regions. Elective tracheotomy/tracheostomy is also performed to administer gas anesthesia when an orotracheal or nasotracheal tube would interfere with surgical access to the mouth, nose, or throat.

Rarely, permanent tracheostomy may be required. Patients with permanent tracheostomy lose the natural defense mechanisms of the upper airways (filtration and humidification) because these defenses are essentially bypassed and are therefore susceptible to lower respiratory tract infections. These patients should be maintained in a dust-free environment and watched closely for signs of disease. Daily cleaning of the site is necessary to remove secretions.

Tracheostomy is usually performed with the horse standing but may be performed under general anesthesia. The usual location is at the junction of the cranial and middle third of the neck.

PATIENT PREPARATION

Appropriate physical and chemical restraint is applied. The neck should be positioned in a straight line, regardless of whether the patient is standing or recumbent.

PROCEDURE

If possible, the area over the trachea should be clipped and sterilely prepped. In an emergency situation, complete sterile preparation may not be possible; the trachea is penetrated with a sharp object, and any tube available is used to provide an airway. Local anesthesia (3 to 5 ml) is required if the procedure is performed on a conscious patient.

A longitudinal 5 to 10 cm incision is made directly on the ventral midline through the skin and subcutaneous tissue. The muscle bellies of the sternothyrohyoideus muscles are divided on ventral midline to expose the trachea. Two tracheal rings are identified, and an incision is made in the tissue between them by rotating the scalpel blade 90 degrees and "stabbing" the blade through the tissue. This horizontal stab incision is then extended about 2 cm to either side. Care is taken not to cut the cartilage rings (Fig. 11-4). When the incision is complete, a tracheostomy tube or endotracheal tube is inserted, depending on the patient's needs (Fig. 11-5).

AFTERCARE

While the tracheostomy tube is in place, it should be inspected frequently for proper positioning and possible obstruction by secretions. It should be removed once or twice daily and replaced or cleaned in an antiseptic solution. The tracheostomy site is cleaned with a sterile dilute antiseptic solution (such as dilute povidone-iodine) before replacing the tracheostomy tube. Discharge from the skin wound often occurs and may scald the skin; petroleum jelly applied to the "run-off" area ventral to the tracheostomy site helps to prevent skin scald.

After removal of the tracheostomy tube, the incision is left to heal by second intention. Healing is usually complete in about 3 weeks.

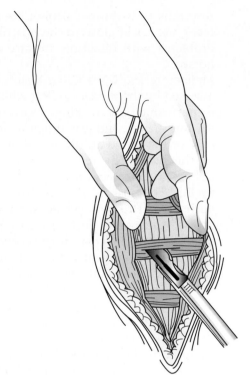

Fig. 11-4. Longitudinal skin incision and horizontal incision between tracheal rings for tracheotomy. (From Orsini JA, Divers TJ: *Manual of equine emergencies*, ed 2, St Louis, 2003, Saunders.)

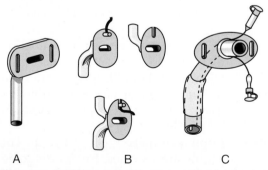

A   B   C

Fig. 11-5. McKillip J-tube **(A)**, Dyson self-retaining tracheotomy tube with male and female parts **(B)**, and cuffed tracheotomy tube **(C)**. (From Colahan PT et al: *Equine medicine and surgery*, ed 5, vol 1, St Louis, 1999, Mosby.)

The site is cleaned once or twice daily with sterile dilute antiseptic solution, and an antibacterial ointment is applied to the healing skin edges, being careful not to place ointment inside the wound where it could accidentally enter the trachea.

Subcutaneous emphysema may develop adjacent to the tracheostomy site. It is recognized by swelling and a crepitant or "bubble wrap" texture on palpation. There is no specific treatment. The body gradually reabsorbs the subcutaneous air.

NERVOUS SYSTEM

NEUROLOGICAL EXAMINATION

The purpose of the "neuro exam" is threefold: (1) confirm that neurological disease is present, (2) localize where in the nervous system the disease is occurring (Box 11-2), and (3) arrive at a diagnosis or formulate a list of possible diagnoses (rule-out list). Further diagnostic tests are usually required to confirm the specific neurological disease from a list of rule-outs.

The technician may assist in the performance of neurological exams. Truly neurologically affected animals must be handled cautiously; certain diseases can produce ataxia and other deficits that predispose the animal

---

BOX 11-2 Basic Localization of Neurological Lesions

Central Nervous System

- Cerebrum
- Cerebellum
- Brainstem (medulla)
- Spinal cord

Peripheral Nervous System

- Peripheral nerves
- Neuromuscular junctions

to stumbling and perhaps falling, injuring the handler. Even recumbent "neuro" cases (unless completely paralyzed) must be respected for the potential damage that can be done by thrashing legs and struggling efforts to stand.

The neurological exam is similar to that performed in small animals, with a few modifications. If the patient is presented in recumbency, additional modifications may be necessary. Minimal equipment is necessary for the basic exam; however, if further diagnostics are necessary, referral to a well-equipped hospital may be necessary.

The basic neurological exam consists of the following steps:

1. History and general physical exam
2. Observation
   a. Behavior
   b. Mental status (level of awareness or consciousness)
   c. Posture and coordination: The head, body, and limbs are observed for abnormalities such as head tilt, weakness, ataxia, and involuntary movements such as tremors, tetany, and myoclonus.
3. Cranial nerve exam (Box 11-3)
   a. Smell: CN 1: Smell is difficult to assess but is usually evaluated by noting

---

BOX 11-3 Cranial Nerves

CN 1 = Olfactory nerve
CN 2 = Optic nerve
CN 3 = Oculomotor nerve
CN 4 = Trochlear nerve
CN 5 = Trigeminal nerve
CN 6 = Abducens nerve
CN 7 = Facial nerve
CN 8 = Vestibulocochlear (auditory) nerve
CN 9 = Glossopharyngeal nerve
CN 10 = Vagus nerve
CN 11 = Spinal accessory nerve
CN 12 = Hypoglossal nerve

---

reactions to isopropyl alcohol, food, feces, etc., held close to the nostrils. Problems with olfaction are rare in horses.

b. Menace reflex: CN 2/CN 7: Vision is assessed by the menace reflex, which is performed by making a gesture toward the eye and watching for closure of the eyelid and/or withdrawal of the head. The test also assesses CN 7, which is necessary to close the eyelid. The test is best performed with several fingers spread apart to avoid creating and pushing a current of air against the cornea. The cornea can feel air currents and initiates closure of the eyelid, even in a blind animal. The menace reflex is not fully developed in neonatal foals until approximately 2 weeks of age.

Vision may also be assessed by walking the horse through an obstacle course. To prevent "cheating," one eye may need to be blindfolded to accurately assess vision in the opposite eye.

c. Pupillary light reflex: CN 2/CN 3: When a light is directed into one eye, the pupils of both eyes should constrict in response. The "direct response" is the constriction of the pupil on the same side as the light, and the "consensual response" is constriction of the opposite eye. Proper function of both CN 2 and CN 3 is necessary for a normal pupillary light reflex but it is *not* a test of vision; blind horses may have normal pupillary light responses.

d. Pupil symmetry: CN 2/CN 3: The pupils are assessed for miosis (constriction), mydriasis (dilation), and anisocoria (pupils of different size).

e. Eye position: CN 3/CN 4/CN 6/CN 8: The position of the eye within the orbit is assessed at rest and also while the head is rotated slowly from side to side. Abnormal position at rest (strabismus) and abnormal eye movement (nystagmus) may occur. When the head of the horse is elevated, the normal response is for the eyes to try to remain horizontal, causing a natural ventral rotation; this is sometimes referred to as the *doll's eye effect*.

f. Facial sensation: CN 5/CN 7: A blunt object is used to touch or lightly pinch the areas of the face, ears, and mouth. The horse should respond with movement of muscles in the area or withdrawal of the head.

g. Facial symmetry: CN 5/CN 7: The muscles of the head are observed for atrophy and loss of muscle tone. Drooping of the ear, lips, and/or eyelids is abnormal. Deviation of the muzzle to one side is also abnormal (Fig. 11-6).

h. Hearing: CN 8: Hearing is difficult to evaluate and is usually done by clapping or producing a loud noise and watching for a response. Deafness in horses is rare.

i. Tongue pull: CN 12: The tongue is pulled out of the mouth to one side, and the horse should retract it back into the mouth within several seconds. The test is repeated to the opposite side (Fig. 11-7). The tongue should also be inspected for atrophy of one or both sides of the tongue, which occasionally occurs.

j. Swallowing: CN 9/CN 10: Abnormal swallowing may result in water, feed, or saliva dribbling from the mouth or nostrils.

4. Gait assessment

a. Observation at the walk and trot: performed on a straight line and in circles.

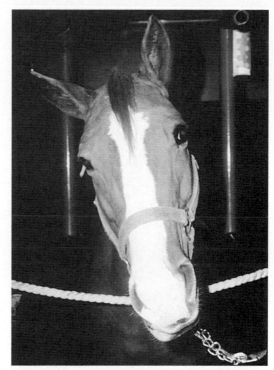

Fig. 11-6. Thoroughbred with head tilt to the right, ptosis (drooping) of the right eyelid, drooping right ear pinna, and deviation of the muzzle to the left. (From Reed SM, Bayly WM, Sellon DC: *Equine internal medicine*, ed 2, St Louis, 2004, Saunders.)

b. Circling: sometimes called "spinning," the horse is turned in very tight circles, and the coordination of the limbs is observed. The handler should turn the head sharply to one side so that the hindquarters respond by moving away from the handler. This is maintained until the horse has turned 360 degrees several times. The procedure is repeated on both sides of the horse. Falling, stepping on itself, failing to lift the legs, or wide circumduction of the outside limb may be abnormal behavior (Fig. 11-8).

c. Backing: limb coordination is observed. Dragging the legs or stepping on itself may be abnormal.

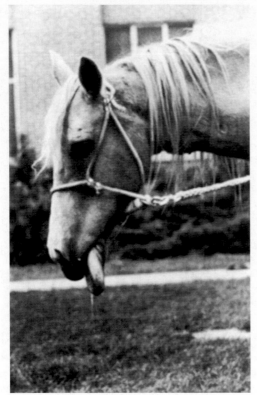

Fig. 11-7. Paralysis of the tongue seen with dysfunction of cranial nerve XII. (From Reed SM: *Vet Clin North Am Equine Pract* 3:255-440, 1987.)

d. Incline walking: the horse is walked up and down an incline while limb coordination is observed.

e. Elevated head walking: the handler holds the lead rope in one hand and uses the other hand to elevate the head (beneath the chin) so that the nostrils are level with the poll. The horse is then walked in a straight line. Elevating the head may accentuate proprioceptive deficits. This test may also be performed on an incline; the handler must be extremely careful not to position himself or herself

directly in front of the horse, in case the horse stumbles and falls.

5. Postural reactions
   a. Sway reaction: This test is performed either by pushing sideways on the horse's forequarters or hindquarters or by pulling the horse sideways by the tail ("tail pull" or "tail sway" test). Normal horses should make an effort to resist the push or pull. The tail pull must be performed cautiously to avoid being kicked; it is safest to grasp the tail near its end in order to create some space between the handler and the horse. The handler should stay laterally even with the hindquarters, not lagging behind the hindquarters where a kick is possible. The test is repeated on both sides and may also be performed while the horse is walked in a straight line.
   b. Placing responses: A leg is lifted and set down in an abnormal position, such as in a base-wide stance or in a cross-legged position (Fig. 11-9). The normal response is for the horse to reposition the leg directly beneath itself within several seconds. This test is variable in individuals and may be difficult to evaluate.
   c. Hopping: This test is difficult to perform in large animals. One person handles the head, and one performs the maneuver. One of the horse's legs is elevated while applying lateral pressure to the shoulder (for a forelimb) or hip (for a hindlimb) area to encourage the horse to hop sideways on three legs (Fig. 11-10).

6. Spinal reflexes
   a. Anal/perineal reflex: The anus and perineal area are gently prodded with a blunt instrument. The anus should contract in response. Care must be taken to stand to the side of the horse

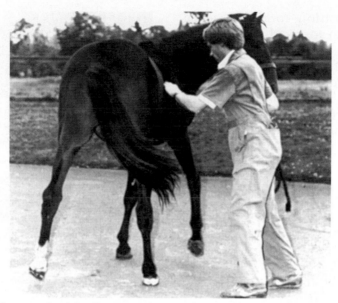

Fig. 11-8. Spinning the horse to the right. The horse shows wide circumduction of the left hindlimb, which is abnormal. (From Reed SM: *Vet Clin North Am Equine Pract* 3:255-440, 1987.)

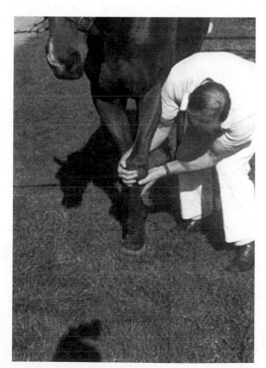

Fig. 11-9. Cross-legged placing response of the left forelimb. (From Speirs VC: *Clinical examination of horses*, St Louis, 1997, Saunders.)

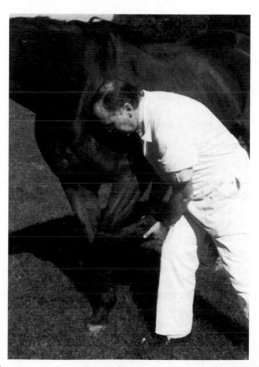

Fig. 11-10. Lateral hopping test. The left forelimb is elevated while pressure is applied to the shoulder to encourage hopping to the right. (From Speirs VC: *Clinical examination of horses*, St Louis, 1997, Saunders.)

(similar position to taking rectal temperature) to avoid being kicked (Fig. 11-11).

b. Patellar reflex/triceps reflex: The patellar tendon or triceps tendon is struck with a soft rubber mallet. This test is difficult to perform accurately in nonrecumbent animals and may elicit a kick in some individuals.

c. Withdrawal reflexes: A hemostat or blunt probe is used to press or pinch the skin of the limbs. The normal animal will withdraw (flex) the limb in response. The evaluator should avoid the path of the flexed limb as flexure may be forceful and rapid, producing injury.

7. Tail tone: Most horses resist elevation of the tail. A limp or weak tail may be abnormal.

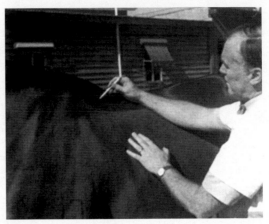

Fig. 11-12. Testing the cutaneous sensation of the trunk by gently pressing with a blunt instrument such as a ballpoint pen. (From Speirs VC: *Clinical examination of horses*, St Louis, 1997, Saunders.)

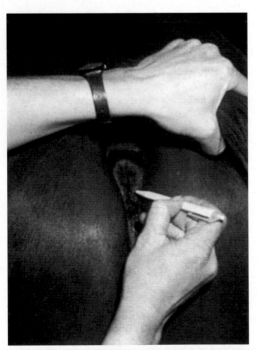

Fig. 11-11. The perineal reflex. (From Speirs VC: *Clinical examination of horses*, St Louis, 1997, Saunders.)

8. Cutaneous sensation
   a. Panniculus response: A blunt instrument is used to lightly stimulate (by pinching or pricking) the skin across the neck and body. Twitching of the cutaneous muscles in response is normal and should be brisk (Fig. 11-12).
   b. Limbs: The skin over the limbs is similarly stimulated, looking for areas of decreased or absent sensation.

Following the basic neurological exam, the clinician makes an initial assessment of the animal's condition and recommends treatment or further diagnostic tests. Box 11-4 and Fig. 11-13 cover special diagnostics.

GASTROINTESTINAL SYSTEM

The gastrointestinal (GI) system extends from the oral cavity to the anus and includes the accessory digestive glands (salivary glands, liver, and pancreas). The functions of the GI system are to (1) ingest and process nutrients and water and (2) excrete waste. The length of the GI tract in an average 1000 lb

BOX **11-4** Special Diagnostic Tests for the Neurological System

Cerebrospinal Fluid Collection and Analysis
Diagnostic Imaging

- *Plain film radiographs:* The head and cervical regions may be radiographed. Sedation or general anesthesia may be necessary. The thoracolumbar and sacral spine are difficult to image except perhaps in small individuals.
- *Contrast radiography (myelogram):* In large animals this procedure is used for cervical spinal cord evaluation. General anesthesia is required. The procedure is performed in lateral recumbency. Injection of contrast medium is performed at the atlantooccipital space. The head is elevated during and for approximately 5 minutes following injection of the contrast medium, to encourage caudal flow of the contrast material away from the brain. Owners should be warned of the risk of seizures and other possible reactions. Also, recovery from general anesthesia in neurologically affected animals presents additional patient risk (Fig. 11-13).
- *Computed tomography/MRI:* Currently available equipment limits imaging to the head and cranial cervical regions.
- *Nuclear scintigraphy:* This technology can be used to image the vertebral column.

Electrodiagnostics

The following are possible in large animals:
- *EEG:* electroencephalogram
- *EMG:* electromyogram
- *ABR:* auditory brainstem response testing
- *NCS:* nerve conduction studies

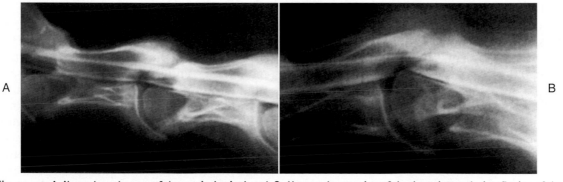

Fig. 11-13. A, Normal myelogram of the cervical spinal cord. **B,** Abnormal narrowing of the dye columns during flexion of the neck. (From Speirs VC: *Clinical examination of horses,* St Louis, 1997, Saunders.)

horse may exceed 100 feet. Horses are subject to a wide variety of diseases of the GI tract, many of which are affected by husbandry practices such as feeding, watering, exercise, parasite control, and dental care.

DENTISTRY

In 1995 the American Association of Equine Practitioners (AAEP) released a position statement on equine dentistry. It states, in part, that "Equine dentistry is the practice of veterinary medicine and should not be performed by anyone other than a licensed veterinarian or a certified veterinary technician under the employ of a licensed veterinarian."

The statement continues to define specific procedures that should be performed by veterinarians: "Any dental activity requiring sedation, tranquilization, analgesia or anesthesia and procedures which are invasive of the tissues of the oral cavity, including, but not limited to, extraction of permanent teeth, amputation of large molars, incisors and canine teeth, the extraction of first premolars (wolf teeth) and repair of damaged or diseased teeth, must be performed by a licensed veterinarian."

The role of the veterinary technician is also defined: "The rasping (floating) of molars, premolars and canine teeth and the removal of deciduous incisors and premolars (caps) may, provided a valid veterinary-client patient relationship exists, be performed by a certified veterinary technician under the employ of a licensed veterinarian."

The AAEP position statement should not be confused with state veterinary practice acts, and the technician should consult his or her state board of veterinary medicine for accepted veterinary practices in their state.

DENTAL EXAMINATION

Dental care should be part of a horse's routine health maintenance program. The oral cavity and teeth should be examined at least once a year by a veterinarian; twice a year is a better recommendation for most horses. Horses with special dental problems may need to be checked three to four times a year. Most dental abnormalities begin with no obvious external signs and develop gradually over time. However, the owner may report problems with chewing and eating such as dropping partially chewed food from the mouth (quidding), hypersalivation, and tilting the head while eating. Foul odor to the breath often accompanies tooth root disease. Owners may also report chronic weight loss. Finding whole, undigested grain particles in the feces is not necessarily an indication of a dental problem but should be an indication for a complete oral exam to rule out dental abnormalities.

The dental exam requires minimal equipment; a light source such as a penlight or flashlight and a dental speculum are all that are needed for many patients. A dose syringe to flush out the mouth is helpful. Physical restraint depends on the individual horse. Some uncooperative individuals require sedation to allow a thorough evaluation. The person performing the exam is in a vulnerable position and should stand to the side of the horse to avoid being struck by the front feet. Use of stocks or stacked hay bales may provide additional safety. Rarely, a fractious animal may have to undergo general anesthesia to allow an oral exam to be safely conducted.

The dental exam begins with an evaluation of the incisors. The lips are separated with the hands to reveal the incisors and gums (Fig. 11-14). The horse cooperates best if breathing is not obstructed during this maneuver. The incisors are checked for number and proper occlusion. The occlusal surfaces are checked for wear. The examiner then places the thumb into the interdental space and presses on the hard palate to encourage the horse to open the mouth (Fig. 11-15). The canines (if present) and rostral cheek teeth can be visually and manually examined, and the presence of wolf teeth (premolar 1) determined.

Full examination of the rest of the cheek teeth and oral cavity requires use of a speculum; in cooperative individuals, the tongue may be pulled laterally out of the mouth and held caudally against the commissure of the lips; in this position, the horse tends to hold the mouth open to avoid biting its own

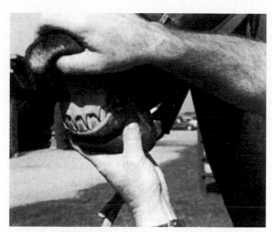

Fig. 11-14. Examination of the incisors. (From Speirs VC: *Clinical examination of horses*, St Louis, 1997, Saunders.)

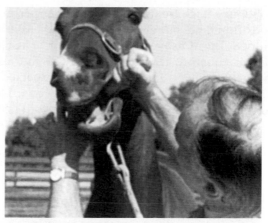

Fig. 11-16. Extruding the tongue against the commissure of the lip encourages opening of the mouth. (From Speirs VC: *Clinical examination of horses*, St Louis, 1997, Saunders.)

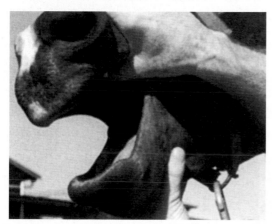

Fig. 11-15. Opening the mouth by use of pressure against the hard palate. (From Speirs VC: *Clinical examination of horses*, St Louis, 1997, Saunders.)

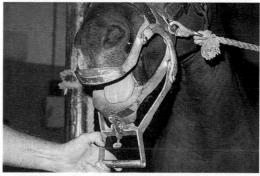

Fig. 11-17. MacAllen full mouth speculum. Incisor plates provide leverage to hold the mouth open. The speculum is adjustable. (From Baker GJ, Easley J: *Equine dentistry*, St Louis, 2002, Saunders.)

tongue (Fig. 11-16). Most individuals, however, require a mechanical mouth speculum to hold the mouth open for a thorough exam (Figs. 11-17 and 11-18). The cheek teeth are examined for number, sharp points, and occlusion. Visual examination alone may not be sufficient; manual evaluation is often necessary.

Radiographs are sometimes required as part of the dental exam, especially when involvement of tooth roots and accompanying sinus disease is suspected. Because radiographic cassettes and equipment are in close proximity to the patient's head and because of the prolonged exposure times needed for diagnostic quality films, sedation is almost always necessary. Common views include straight lateral (Fig. 11-19) and lateral oblique projections for the cheek teeth; lateral oblique views are used to decrease superimposition and better view the cheek teeth roots. The dorsoventral projection is used less frequently for the cheek teeth but is valuable when sinus disease is suspected. The incisors are usually radiographed with a dorsoventral (upper arcade) or ventrodorsal

(lower arcade) projection; superimposition of the incisors is alleviated by placing the film cassette between the incisors to create an intraoral or "bite plate" film. Grids are seldom necessary.

The results of the dental exam should be noted in the medical record. Dental charts are available for equines and provide an excellent format to record findings and describe procedures performed (Fig. 11-20). Digital photographs can enhance documentation of pretreatment and posttreatment results (Box 11-5).

REMOVAL OF CAPS

The deciduous premolars ("caps") are usually present at birth or by 1 to 2 weeks of age. They are normally shed when the underlying permanent premolar teeth erupt at $2\frac{1}{2}$ (PM2), 3 (PM3), and 4 (PM4) years of age (Fig. 11-21). Clients may find the caps on the stall floor or in feed buckets and call with concern about their horse losing a tooth, or they fail to recognize the "foreign object" as a tooth (Fig. 11-22).

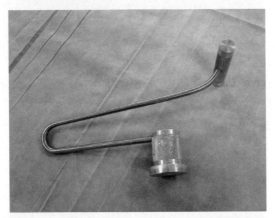

Fig. 11-18. Schoupe oral speculum. The rounded portion is inserted between the cheek teeth on one side of the mouth; the bar is handheld outside the cheek to stabilize the speculum.

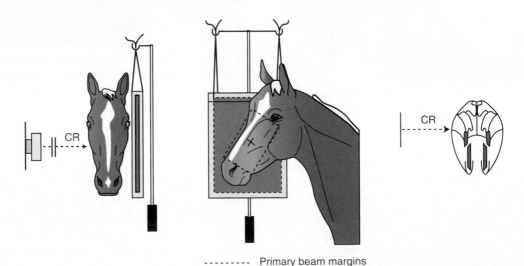

- - - - - - - - - Primary beam margins

Fig. 11-19. Film cassette orientation for a straight lateral projection of the maxillary cheek teeth. *CR*, Central ray. (From Baker GJ, Easley J: *Equine dentistry*, St Louis, 2002, Saunders.)

EQUINE DENTAL EVALUATION AND MAINTENANCE FORM

(SPACE ABOVE LEFT BLANK FOR ADDRESS OF DVM)
MEMBER AMERICAN ASSOCIATION OF EQUINE PRACTITIONERS

DATE _____ STABLES _____
OWNER _____ TRAINER _____
ADDRESS _____ _____
            _____
PHONE _____ PHONE _____

HORSE _____ BREED _____ COLOR _____ AGE _____ SEX _____
PROBLEMS _____
_____
_____

SOFT TISSUE	WOLF TEETH	INCISORS		CANINES			MOLARS
NORMAL	PRESENT	NORMAL	OVERBITE	NORMAL	NORMAL		FLOAT
LIPS	ABSENT	TILTED	UNDERBITE	UNERUPTED U L	HOOKS F R		CUT-FLOAT
TONGUE	UNERUPTED	SMILE	BROKEN TEETH	CUT	HIGH TEETH		CUT-FLOAT
PALATE	REMOVE	FROWN		BUFF	WAVE		CUT-LEVEL
GUMS	ROOT FRAGMENT	STEP		REMOVE TARTAR	STEPPED		CUT-LEVEL
BARS		CAPS		EXTRACT	SHEAR		CUT-LEVEL
CHEEKS		ALIGN			RAMP		CUT-LEVEL
		TOO LONG U L			RIMS		FLOAT
		SHORTEN			SEPARATION		BROKEN TEETH
		FLOAT			CUPPED OUT		
		DREMEL			CAPS REMOVED		
					TABLE ANGLES L____ R____		

FEE _____   FEE _____   FEE _____   FEE _____

SEDATION: DETOMIDINE _____ BUTORPHANOL _____ XYLAZINE _____ ACEPROMAZINE _____

FEE _____   FEE _____   FEE _____   FEE _____

OCCLUSION RIGHT _____
LEFT _____

111 110 109 108 107 106   105   104   103 102 101 201 102 103   104   105   206 207 208 209 210 211
                                            gum line

411 410 409 408 407 406   405   404   403 402 401 301 302 303   304   305   306 307 308 309 310 311

A = ABSENT   CH = CHIPPED   C = CUT   R = REDUCE   E = EXTRACT

TRIP FEE _____ COMMENTS _____

Fig. 11-20. Example of an equine dental chart. (From Baker GJ, Easley J: *Equine dentistry*, St Louis, 2002, Saunders.)

BOX 11-5	Dental Eruption Timetable (Equine)

Deciduous Teeth

First incisor	Birth to 1 week
Second incisor	4 to 6 weeks
Third incisor	6 to 9 months
Canine	(Absent)
First premolar	Birth to 2 weeks
Second premolar	Birth to 2 weeks
Third premolar	Birth to 2 weeks

Permanent Teeth

First incisor	I1	$2\frac{1}{2}$ years
Second incisor	I2	$3\frac{1}{2}$ years
Third incisor	I3	$4\frac{1}{2}$ years
Canine	C	4 to 5 years (rare in females)
First premolar	PM1	5 to 6 months (not always present)
Second premolar	PM2	$2\frac{1}{2}$ years
Third premolar	PM3	3 years
Fourth premolar	PM4	4 years
First molar	M1	9 to 12 months
Second molar	M2	2 years
Third molar	M3	$3\frac{1}{2}$ to 4 years

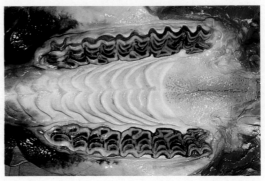

Fig. 11-21. Transverse skull section at the level of premolar 3 (PM3) in a $3\frac{1}{2}$-year-old horse. The short "caps" cover the oral aspect of each permanent PM3. (From Baker GJ, Easley J: *Equine dentistry,* St Louis, 2002, Saunders.)

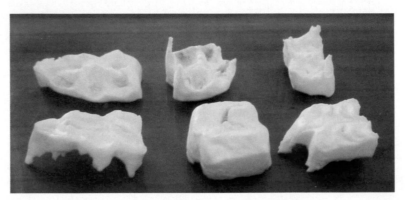

Fig. 11-22. Assorted caps. (From Allen T: *Manual of equine dentistry,* St Louis, 2003, Mosby.)

Occasionally, the caps are not shed and are referred to as *retained*. Retained caps are often loose and may cause pain and reluctance to chew, swallow, or accept a bit. Retained caps should be removed. Extraction of the cap begins with adequate physical restraint. If the area is painful or the patient is uncooperative, sedation may be required. As with any dental procedure, the operator should carefully position his or her body to avoid being struck by the front legs or a violently raised head. An oral speculum will facilitate the procedure. Removal is usually easily accomplished with an elevator to pry the cap loose and a grasping instrument such as cap-extracting forceps or wolf tooth forceps to remove the cap. The elevator is used to loosen any remaining tissue or tissue tags between the cap and the underlying permanent tooth. Once grasped with the forceps, the cap is gently rocked from side to side until it is removed. Bleeding is usually minimal, and no special aftercare is required.

WOLF TOOTH EXTRACTION

"Wolf tooth" is the layman's term for the first premolar (PM1). Wolf teeth are rudimentary and have no useful function. Mandibular wolf teeth are quite rare; maxillary wolf teeth are more common, and are usually visible above the gum line immediately rostral to the second premolars (Fig. 11-23). However, they may fail to erupt ("blind" wolf teeth) and may only be detected by palpation. Many horses have no wolf teeth. Unlike the other premolars, PM1 is typically small in size with a simple root. Because of its location, it may become sore from pressure from the bit and is often blamed for performance problems. It is common practice to remove wolf teeth before a horse begins training.

The procedure is performed in the standing horse and involves proper physical restraint and safety precautions. Tetanus immunity status should be determined and

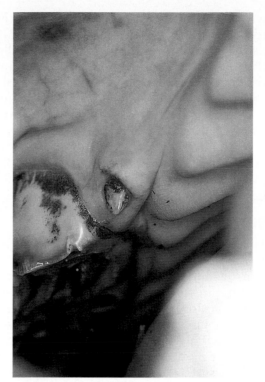

Fig. 11-23. A typically small maxillary wolf tooth (premolar [PM] 1) is present just rostral to PM2. (From Baker GJ, Easley J: *Equine dentistry*, St Louis, 2002, Saunders.)

prophylaxis administered before the procedure if necessary. Use of an oral speculum is desirable. Sedation is required; in addition, some clinicians also inject 1 to 2 ml of local anesthetic into the mucosa around each wolf tooth. The instruments required are a dental elevator and a pair of extraction forceps; wolf tooth elevators and wolf tooth forceps are made in a variety of sizes to accommodate different sizes of wolf teeth. A small scalpel blade is necessary to incise the gingiva over blind wolf teeth. The wolf tooth elevator is used to separate the gingiva and periodontal ligament from the entire circumference of the tooth, extending well below the gum line. The tooth is then grasped with the wolf tooth forceps and gently rocked and rotated until freed. Removal is usually straightforward, though occasionally the tooth root breaks off during extraction; this usually causes no problem and heals uneventfully. Following removal, bleeding is common; flushing the mouth with clean, warm water using a 60 ml catheter-tip syringe several times a day for 2 to 3 days is typical aftercare. The horse should not have a bit placed in the mouth for 3 to 5 days to allow healing of the gingival tissue.

DENTAL FLOATING

Filing or rasping of the teeth is known as *floating*. It is the most common dental procedure in horses and is part of the routine health care program. Several factors contribute to the need for floating. The cheek teeth (premolars and molars) advance slowly from their alveoli into the mouth continuously for most of the life of the horse. The occlusal surfaces are continually worn down by a natural side-to-side chewing motion, combined with sand and grit in the horse's diet—forming a "natural file" between opposing upper and lower teeth. However, the maxilla is approximately 30% wider than the mandible; this results in an "overhang" situation in which the upper and lower cheek teeth do not meet squarely. The buccal margin of the upper cheek teeth and the lingual margin of the lower cheek teeth are left without contact with an opposing surface. The natural file does not maintain these surfaces as well as the more central portions of the tooth, and these surfaces tend to become more prominent as the central portions are worn down. This results in formation of sharp edges, known as *points*, over time. Additionally, the upper and lower cheek teeth usually do not meet perfectly in the rostral-caudal plane; the upper cheek teeth are usually shifted slightly more rostrally, leaving the rostral margin of the upper PM2

and the caudal margin of the lower M3 without direct occlusion. Sharp points, referred to as *hooks (upper arcade)* and *ramps (lower arcade)*, tend to form along these surfaces (Fig. 11-24).

Points, hooks, and sharp edges can cause pain and discomfort to the horse, causing ulcerations and lacerations of the tongue and oral tissues, poor performance, and problems with mastication. In severe cases the horse may be unable to close the mouth completely. Severe cases often require cutting the teeth with special instruments to remove points before they can be filed smooth. Horses should be checked regularly for developing points and hooks and dental floating performed to prevent them from becoming problematic.

The age when floating begins depends entirely on the individual's need for the procedure, which is determined by oral examination (Fig. 11-25). Most horses need floating by the age of 3 to 4 years, but it is

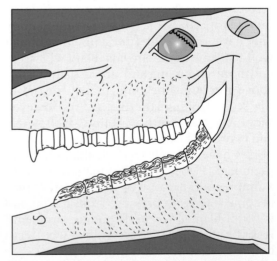

Fig. 11-24. Hooks on the upper premolar 2 and ramps on the lower molar 3. Note also the sharp points on the margins of the other cheek teeth. (From Allen T: *Manual of equine dentistry*, St Louis, 2003, Mosby.)

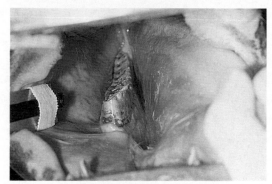

Fig. 11-25. Oral examination of the lower right cheek teeth, using a mouth speculum and good lighting. The cheek is retracted to the left; the tongue to the right. The lingual margins of the teeth have "points"; floating is used to remove and smooth the sharp edges. (From Baker GJ, Easley J: *Equine dentistry*, St Louis, 2002, Saunders.)

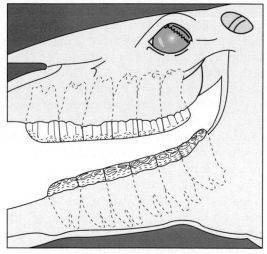

Fig. 11-26. Normal mouth after dentistry has been performed. (From Allen T: *Manual of equine dentistry*, St Louis, 2003, Mosby.)

not uncommon for horses as young as 2 years to have sharp points requiring treatment (note that when floating young horses, loose caps may dislodge and fall out of the mouth during the procedure). The frequency of floating also depends on individual need; most horses require it at least once a year, but many need it twice yearly. Some horses, especially geriatric horses and horses with missing cheek teeth, may need floating three to four times a year.

The primary goal of floating is to remove hooks, points, and any other sharp edges from the cheek teeth, restoring good occlusion and patient comfort (Fig. 11-26). Floating is also used to prevent overgrowth of a tooth when the opposing tooth has been lost. Much less commonly, the canines and incisors may be subject to overgrowth or prone to form sharp edges that must be filed to maintain occlusion and make the mouth comfortable.

The procedure is performed with the horse standing, except in intractable patients that may require general anesthesia. If horses are accustomed to the procedure at a young age by a patient operator, minimal physical restraint may be necessary. However, many horses dislike the noise and vibration associated with floating, and more aggressive physical restraint and/or chemical restraint must be used. The safety of personnel must be of primary concern, especially with the vulnerable position of the operator.

A minimum amount of equipment is required for floating. A mouth speculum is usually necessary, and a good light source is mandatory. In addition, a stainless steel bucket with water and disinfectant is useful for cleaning the instruments during and after use. A dose syringe for flushing the mouth before and after the procedure is also useful.

A wide array of dental floats is available. Float handles and float blades are usually purchased separately, allowing replacement of the blade when it becomes worn or when a different blade texture (fine, medium, or coarse) is desired. Carbide blades are usually preferred over steel for their durability. Individuals develop preferences for the shape and material of the handles and shafts.

The basic float set includes a long, straight float handle/shaft and blade for the lower cheek teeth and a shorter, angled float handle/shaft and blade for the upper cheek teeth. Additional handles and blades with specialized shapes can be added to the basic set (Fig. 11-27). Recently, motor-driven power floats have become popular. Floating teeth manually is a physical process requiring a good deal of stamina; power floats save the operator some "elbow grease" and may be more effective for individuals who lack strength. Power floats are expensive, however, and horses may resent the noise they create (Fig. 11-28).

Floating is not a simple procedure; it is as much an art as it is a science and is best learned from clinicians experienced in the procedure. Seminars with wet laboratories and several good texts are available to help the technician learn proper techniques.

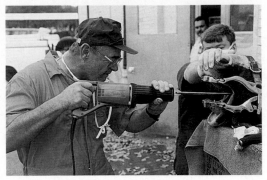

Fig. 11-28. Use of a power floating tool. (From Baker GJ, Easley J: *Equine dentistry*, St Louis, 2002, Saunders.)

COLIC EXAMINATION

Colic is a nonspecific term that means "abdominal pain." Although it is true that the overwhelming majority of colic in horses is caused by diseases of the GI system, other organ systems such as the urinary and reproductive tracts are also located in the abdomen and can cause colic when they are diseased. Some musculoskeletal conditions can also effectively mimic colic.

Horses with colic usually display easily observed signs of pain and discomfort. However, mild colic may be missed by inexperienced horse owners, and stoic horses may not show the full extent of their discomfort. Signs of colic pain may include one or more of the following:

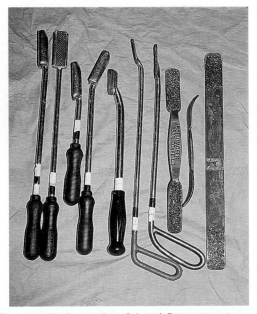

Fig. 11-27. Various styles of dental floats. (From Baker GJ, Easley J: *Equine dentistry*, St Louis, 2002, Saunders.)

- Sweating
- Pawing with the front feet: this may become so persistent that horses wear away areas of the hoof wall
- Frequent posturing to urinate but expelling little or no urine
- Looking back at the flanks
- Crouching as if preparing to lie down
- Lying down for prolonged periods of time
- Rolling on the ground
- Grinding the teeth (bruxism)
- Quivering upper lip

- Signs of self-trauma: accompanies severely painful conditions, and often is seen best on the head and face (especially the periorbital region) from repeatedly thrashing the head against the ground
- Increased respiratory and pulse rates
- Kicking at the abdomen with the hind feet
- Groaning
- Standing with the back arched ("hunched up")
- Playing with water but not drinking
- Lying on the back
- Dog-sitting: uncommon

In addition to signs of pain, various other clinical signs may occur depending on the underlying disease and severity of the underlying disease:

- Dehydration
- Cardiovascular shock
- Abdominal distension
- Abnormal mucous membrane color
- Abnormal feces or absence of feces
- Abnormal rectal temperature

Colic should be considered an emergency situation, and a veterinarian should be consulted immediately. The veterinarian will evaluate the situation, determine the urgency for a colic exam, and advise the client on how to manage the horse until it can be examined.

The goal of the colic exam is to diagnose the cause of the colic and then provide appropriate medical and/or surgical treatment to resolve it. Unfortunately, arriving at a specific diagnosis for the cause of colic is not often possible. This is due to the limitations of the tools used for the exam, relative to the size and anatomy of the equine abdomen. A large portion of the abdomen cannot be palpated rectally or visualized with radiographs, ultrasound, or even laparoscopy. Even exploratory abdominal surgery is limited in visualization and ability to exteriorize certain parts of the abdomen. Despite the infrequency of a specific diagnosis, successful

BOX	11-6 Classification of Types of Colic

1. Tympanic (gas) colic
2. Simple intestinal obstruction
3. Strangulating intestinal obstruction
4. Nonstrangulating intestinal infarction
5. Peritonitis
6. Enteritis/colitis
7. Gastrointestinal ulceration
8. Nongastrointestinal pain (urinary, reproductive, musculoskeletal)

Some cases may involve a combination of two or more of the above.

treatment of colic is often achieved. This is due in part to the commonly used strategy of categorizing colic based on clinical signs and laboratory tests; once categorized, rational treatment can be instituted (Box 11-6).

The technician performs a valuable role in assisting the veterinarian in the colic exam and should be familiar with the basic elements of the exam (Box 11-7). The veterinarian does not perform every component of the exam in each case and may alter the sequence of the exam based on the situation at hand. For instance, if shock is identified, treatment for shock may be instituted before continuing with the rest of the exam. The components of the colic exam include:

- Observation
  - Pain: The horse is observed for signs and severity of colic. Pain assessment can be the single most important piece of information obtained on a colic exam. Note that in severely painful patients, the rest of the exam may not be possible until pain is controlled.
  - Attitude
  - Environmental surroundings
- Obtain history (Box 11-8)
  - General husbandry and management practices

BOX **11-7**   Setup Checklist for Basic Colic Examination

Nose twitch
Thermometer
Stethoscope
Rectal sleeve
Lubricant (nonsterile)
Nasogastric tube (assorted sizes)
Stomach pump
Dose syringe
Stainless steel bucket and warm water
Adhesive tape, 1-inch width
Ethylenediamine tetraacetic acid (EDTA) and serum Vacutainer blood tubes
Vacutainer sleeve and 20-gauge (ga) Vacutainer needles
18-, 19-, and 20-ga $\times$ 1$\frac{1}{2}$-inch needles
3-, 6-, and 12-ml syringes
Clippers
Disposable razor
Latex examination gloves
Sterile latex gloves
Skin preparation materials (scrub, alcohol, gauze 4 $\times$ 4's)
Intravenous (IV) catheters/materials for IV catheterization
Local anesthetic
Sedative/Analgesic drugs

BOX **11-8**   History-Taking for Colic Patients

General Husbandry and Management

Environment/habitat
Feed types, sources
Feeding schedule
Water sources
Use of horse/daily routine
Routine/preventive health care program
Parasite control program
Medical/surgical history of patient

History Related to Current Colic Episode

Duration of colic (when first observed)
Progression of colic (pain increasing, decreasing, or static)
Recent feed consumption (what and when)
Recent water consumption
Recent medical problems/trauma
Recent medications
Possibility of exposure to foreign bodies or toxins
Pregnancy status
Previous colic episodes (diagnosis, treatments given, response)
Last defecation (character, volume, and time)
Response to treatment (if given)

- History of the current colic episode
- Basic physical exam
  - Temperature
  - Pulse rate and rhythm
  - Respiratory rate and character
  - Physical condition/evidence of self-trauma
  - Mucous membrane color
  - Capillary refill time
  - Abdominal auscultation and percussion
- Nasogastric intubation
- Rectal exam
- Diagnostic sampling
  - Abdominocentesis
  - Blood work
  - Fecal specimen
    - Parasite evaluation
    - Presence of sand
    - Fecal culture
- Diagnostic imaging (only in select cases)
  - Abdominal radiographs
  - Diagnostic ultrasound
  - Gastroscopy
  - Thermography
  - Laparoscopy

Nasogastric intubation is used as a diagnostic tool during the colic exam, and also as a treatment tool. Because horses cannot vomit, the stomach can become so distended with gas and ingesta that it can rupture internally.

Gastric rupture is a fatal condition, with or without surgery. Intubation can therefore be a life-saving maneuver, by providing an exit for accumulated gas and liquid. The stomach contents that are voided through the naso-gastric tube (NGT) are referred to as *reflux*. Reflux may be gas or liquid, or a combination of both. Gas reflux cannot be accurately measured, but liquid reflux can be collected into a bucket and measured (Fig. 11-29). As a diagnostic tool, the type and amount of reflux is very important information.

The NGT is also used in some cases to administer medications directly into the stomach. This can only be safely done in

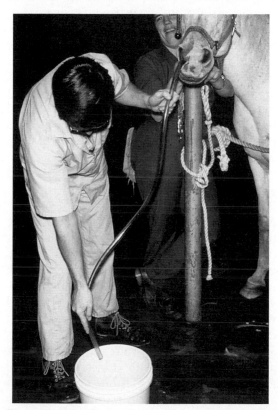

Fig. 11-29. Collecting gastric reflux into a bucket. Note that one hand is used to stabilize the tube near the nostril. (From Colahan PT et al: *Equine medicine and surgery*, ed 5, vol 1, St Louis, 1999, Mosby.)

horses that are not having gastric reflux. Small volumes are given through a dose syringe, and larger volumes are pumped directly from a bucket with a stomach pump. In colic cases, water is the most common treatment given by intubation. The water should be lukewarm in temperature. Substances such as electrolytes, bicarbonate, Epsom salts, activated charcoal, and mineral oil may be added to the water. Some of these substances are in powder form and should be dissolved well to prevent clogging the stomach pump. Mineral oil can be given with or without water (note that mineral oil stains clothing). After treatment, the NGT should be flushed thoroughly with warm or hot water and disinfectant; the outside of the tube should also be cleaned. Air can be flushed to clear the tube or it can be hung vertically to dry. The stomach pump should also be flushed with warm water and disinfectant. The pump should be regularly disassembled to allow cleaning and lubrication of the inside of the barrel. Also, there is a small rubber gasket ring inside the barrel of the pump around the plunger; it will wear out with use and should be checked for cracking and stretching. It is easily replaced.

The rectal exam is commonly performed in the diagnosis of colic. The procedure is potentially hazardous to both the clinician and the patient. The clinician is placed in a vulnerable position at the rear of the horse, and the equine rectum is easily torn. Rectal tears can be life threatening. Effective restraint is imperative and may need to be physical and/or chemical in order to control the patient. Equipment for the clinician is simple— a nonsterile, arm-length plastic sleeve and nonsterile lubricant are all that are required. Some clinicians prefer to add approximately 30 ml of local anesthetic to the lubricant to reduce patient straining. Some clinicians like to wear a latex exam glove over the plastic rectal sleeve. In addition, clinicians usually have a preference for performing the exam with the right or left hand.

Clients often view the rectal exam as a crystal ball, and sometimes it can be just that. However, although important information is usually obtained from the "rectal," its limitations must be understood. Some animals are simply too small or too uncooperative to safely be examined. The human arm can only reach about one third of the total area of the abdomen; many abdominal problems may be beyond the reach of the clinician. It is also obviously a blind procedure, and it can be difficult to determine precise anatomy when dealing with 100 feet of movable intestines in an abnormal animal. Still, it is one of the most valuable diagnostic tools of the colic exam.

The rectal exam usually provides an opportunity to collect fresh feces. With feces grasped in the hand, the rectal sleeve is turned inside-out. The hand is removed and the sleeve is tied shut to form a temporary container for the feces for transport to the clinic. It is standard to perform a gross exam for consistency, color, odor, blood, mucous strands, and parasites. If sand-related colic is suspected, feces can be mixed with a generous amount of water, mixed well, and allowed to settle in the rectal sleeve. The fingers are then used to check for a gritty feel of the settled material.

Abdominal radiographs are highly useful in foals. Their small size and lack of solid intestinal contents increases the possibility of diagnostic-quality films. Portable radiograph machines may be used, and lateral and dorsoventral projections are possible with sedation or general anesthesia. Radiography in adult horses is limited to lateral projections of the dorsal abdomen only, and portable machines do not have sufficient strength for this use. Very few diseases can be diagnosed in adults through abdominal radiographs.

Abdominal ultrasound is useful in equines of all sizes, though it is limited in its ability to penetrate deeply into the abdomen. It is best used to diagnose problems located close to the abdominal wall (outer circumference of the abdominal cavity).

After gathering information from the colic exam, the clinician formulates a treatment plan. Referral to a hospital setting may be recommended for surgery, intensive care, or further diagnostics not available in the field. Treatment plans vary considerably depending on the diagnosis, individual horse variables, available staff and facilities, and economic considerations. Severe pain is often an indication for surgical exploration of the abdomen or at least referral for further diagnostic evaluation, although there are exceptions. Common treatments for mild to moderate cases include restricted oral intake of food and water, fluid therapy, analgesic drugs for control of pain, hand-walking, and nonsteroidal antiinflammatory drugs. Patients are usually put on "colic watch" for frequent monitoring of pain and vital signs. Careful records should be kept to track the horse's progress and treatments, whether on the farm or in a hospital/clinic.

ABDOMINAL SURGERY

Abdominal surgery in the horse may be performed for the diagnosis and treatment of colic. Some abdominal problems can be treated with standing surgery through a flank incision, but this is usually not possible or feasible. Most abdominal surgery is performed with the horse under general anesthesia, in dorsal recumbency. The surgical team usually consists of at least four staff members— a primary surgeon, an assistant surgeon, a circulating operating room nurse, and an anesthetist. Teamwork is essential, especially in the preparation and induction phases of anesthesia, operating room setup, and patient positioning and surgical preparation. Because of the critical and involved nature

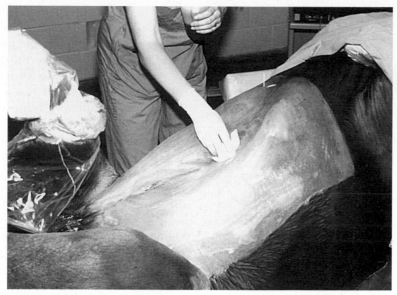

Fig. 11-30. Preparation for exploratory abdominal surgery. The patient is in dorsal recumbency under general anesthesia. The abdomen is clipped, the ventral midline is shaved, and the skin is sterilely prepared for a ventral midline incision. (From Auer JA, Stick JA: *Equine surgery*, ed 2, St Louis, 1999, Saunders.)

of the anesthesia, the anesthetist must be able to be totally devoted to the task of anesthesia, without distraction.

The surgical approach is usually through a ventral midline incision, which may reach 30 to 40 cm in length. Although it is preferable to clip the patient before surgery, often the emergency nature of the case does not allow time, and clipping will be done on the operating table. The standard clip is from xiphoid to the udder/prepuce, and laterally to each flank fold (Fig. 11-30). Additionally, the incisional area is usually shaved. The penis in males must be prevented from extending from the prepuce during surgery; therefore it is common to either purse-string suture or place several towel clamps to close the prepuce. Before closing the prepuce, an absorbent material such as a stack of gauze 4 × 4's is placed inside the prepuce to absorb any urine that may be passed.

The principles of asepsis and sterile surgery are no different from any other species and should be followed in every hospital or clinic performing equine surgery (Fig. 11-31). However, facilities differ considerably in their methods of anesthesia and recovery, patient preparation, surgical instruments and materials, and operating room protocol. The technician will need to "learn the ropes" at any hospital or clinic. Flexibility and patience are desirable traits for *everyone* on the surgical team.

OCULAR SYSTEM

Because of their pronounced lateral location on the skull, the eyes of the horse are predisposed to trauma; injuries to the orbit, eyelids, and globe are fairly common in equines. Lacerations of the eyelids, conjunctivitis, and corneal ulceration are some of the more

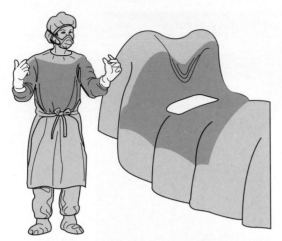

Fig. 11-31. The patient has been draped for abdominal surgery. Shaded areas indicate the sterile surgical field, which extends to include scrubbed personnel. (From Auer JA, Stick JA: *Equine surgery*, ed 2, St Louis, 1999, Saunders.)

common traumatic diseases of the equine eye. Intraocular diseases such as recurrent anterior uveitis ("moon blindness") and cataracts also occur. Abnormal growths such as sarcoids, melanomas, and squamous cell carcinoma may affect the periorbital tissues. Blockage of the nasolacrimal ducts also occurs with some frequency.

Eye problems are notorious for going unreported until it becomes obvious to the owner that the problem is not getting better on its own; unfortunately, this allows the disease to progress to a sometimes severe state. Owners do not realize the significance of certain clinical signs. For example, the combination of tearing (excessive lacrimation) and squinting (blepharospasm) can be especially significant and represents an urgent need for veterinary evaluation; these signs often indicate corneal ulceration or recurrent uveitis. Both conditions require urgent medical attention. Owners also tend to use scissors to snip off tags of tissue when eyelid margins have been lacerated, resulting

in permanent defects and chronic corneal ulceration. Another tendency of some owners is to try to treat eye problems with leftover eye ointments from other horses, not realizing that use of certain ointments can be disastrous for certain diseases. Veterinarians should be consulted promptly for *all* suspected eye problems, even when clinical signs may not be very impressive to the owners.

Most ocular problems are irritating or painful, and horses may try to rub the affected eye in response. It is *imperative* that this be prevented, since rubbing can cause even more trauma to the eye. Protective hoods and eye cups can be used to cover the affected eye (Fig. 11-32). In severe cases, crosstying the horse may be necessary.

OPHTHALMIC EXAMINATION

Examination and medication of the eyes are important in equine practice. Although referral to board-certified ophthalmologists is an option, most eye problems are diagnosed and treated in the field. The ophthalmic exam is usually performed in a dark environment. A penlight and ophthalmoscope are necessary for the basic exam; most field practitioners prefer a handheld direct ophthalmoscope (Fig. 11-33). The exam obviously requires good restraint of the head. Use of a nose twitch and sedatives may be necessary.

Depending on the extent of the exam, topical anesthesia of the cornea and conjunctiva may be required. Topical anesthesia is achieved with ophthalmic anesthetic solutions (0.5% proparacaine HCl or 0.5% tetracaine HCl). Dilation of the pupil may also be required for examination of the retina (1% tropicamide ophthalmic solution). Instilling topical medications into the eye must be done carefully; if the horse throws its head, the medication container can be jabbed into the eye, creating possibly severe trauma. To minimize this risk, the hand

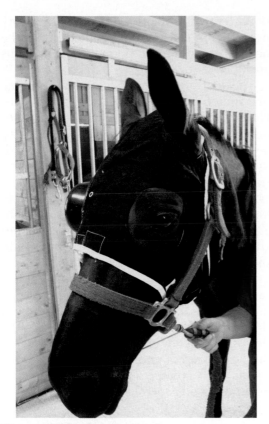

Fig. 11-32. Right eye cup and hood.

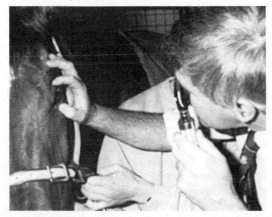

Fig. 11-33. Direct ophthalmoscope examination of the equine eye. (From Speirs VC: *Clinical examination of horses*, St Louis, 1997, Saunders.)

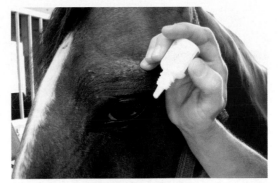

Fig. 11-34. Proper technique for medicating the eye. Note that the hand is stabilized against the horse's head.

holding the medication should always be rested against the horse's head so that if the head moves, the hand will move with the head (Fig. 11-34). Horses typically resist having the eyelids forced wide open; it is seldom necessary to do this to effectively place a topical solution. Simply everting only the lower lid and placing the solution or ointment into the lower conjunctival sac is effective and tolerated well by most patients.

Since blinking and squinting can interfere with the exam, it may be necessary to block sensation and motor control of the eyelids. Various nerve blocks in the periorbital region are available to desensitize and paralyze the eyelids to facilitate the exam. Whenever it is necessary to perform a skin prep in the area of the eye, surgical scrub soaps and alcohol must be used carefully or not at all. Soaps can be highly irritating if they run into the eye, possibly causing permanent damage. Rather, diluted surgical antiseptic solution (povidone-iodine solution diluted 50% with sterile saline) can be used in the same manner as scrub soap. Alcohol, which is also highly irritating, may be replaced with sterile saline solution for rinsing.

Because corneal lesions are prevalent in horses, it is often necessary to stain the cornea. Fluorescein stain strips may be

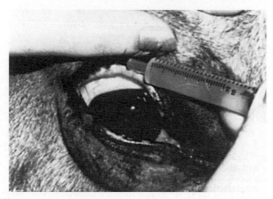

Fig. 11-35. Using a 3-ml syringe filled with fluorescein stain to irrigate the cornea. (From Roberts SM: *Vet Clin North Am Equine Pract* 8:427-668, 1992.)

placed directly against the eye, though many horses resist this. An alternative method of staining is to aspirate 2 to 3 ml of sterile saline (or sterile eyewash solution) into a 3 ml syringe, remove the plunger, and dip the dye strip to color the saline. The plunger is replaced, and the stained saline is given (with the needle removed!) by lifting the upper eyelid and gently irrigating the cornea. No more than 1 to 2 ml are necessary to effectively stain the cornea (Fig. 11-35). After applying the stain, 2 to 3 ml of plain saline are used to flush excess dye off the cornea. A penlight or ultraviolet light (Wood's lamp) is used to highlight and search for any areas of retained dye. Areas of staining indicate that the superficial layer of the cornea has been damaged.

NASOLACRIMAL DUCTS

Like other domestic mammals, horses have a nasolacrimal duct system that functions to drain fluid from the surface of the eye to the nasal cavity. The duct system begins at the eye with two lacrimal puncta, one dorsal and one ventral, both located in the palpebral (eyelid) conjunctiva at the medial canthus (Fig. 11-36, *A*). The duct courses through the skull to open in the floor of the nasal cavity near the mucocutaneous junction of the nostril, usually in the pigmented cutaneous area (Fig. 11-36, *B*).

The duct system may occasionally become obstructed with mucus or other debris. Flushing the nasolacrimal duct is sometimes necessary to restore patency. The duct can be flushed from either end. Flushing through the lacrimal puncta can be difficult in the standing horse. Either a 20- to 22-ga lacrimal cannula or a small-diameter flexible catheter (tomcat urinary catheter) can be inserted into a punctum and sterile fluid injected via an attached syringe. When unobstructed, fluid should flush from the nasal end of the duct.

Flushing from the nasal opening is much easier. A small 1- to 2-mm catheter is inserted into the nasal punctum, and sterile fluid flushed. Horses are usually startled when the fluid suddenly enters the eye, and throwing the head is a common response. Personnel should be prepared for this reaction and maintain good control of the head.

LONG-TERM OR INTENSIVE MEDICATION TECHNIQUES

Some ocular problems require long-term or frequent topical medication. Horses typically become resentful of ophthalmic treatments and are difficult to handle. Occasionally, with severe disease, it may be necessary to provide continual lavage of the eye. For reliable delivery of liquid ophthalmic solutions, indwelling lavage systems can be placed. Ointments, however, are too thick to be given by this method.

There are two main approaches for lavage systems. Subpalpebral lavage systems are placed through one or two incisions in the upper or lower eyelid; narrow rubber tubing is placed through the eyelid to open directly in the conjunctival sac, away from the cornea (Fig. 11-37). The tubing is sutured to

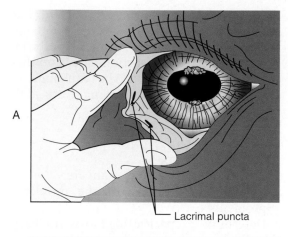

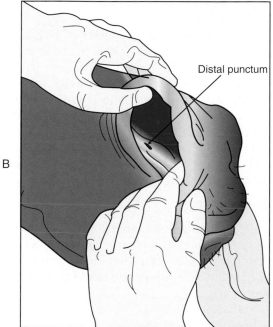

Fig. 11-36. **A,** The lacrimal puncta are located near the medial canthus of the eye. **B,** Nasal opening of the nasolacrimal duct on the floor of the nostril. (From Auer JA, Stick JA: *Equine surgery,* ed 2, St Louis, 1999, Saunders.)

the skin for stability; usually an intravenous (IV) extension set is attached to the tubing for easier access. Clinicians' preferences for types of tubing and methods of securing tubing to the skin vary.

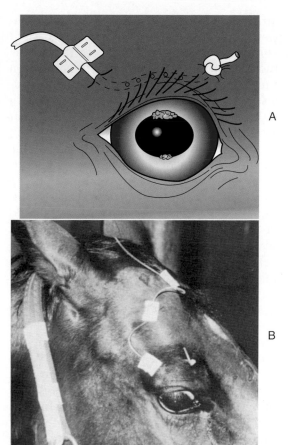

Fig. 11-37. **A,** Placing lavage tubing through the upper eyelid. **B,** A subpalpebral lavage system is sutured to the skin in several places for stability. It has been passed around the ear and taped to the halter over a tongue depressor. (From Auer JA, Stick JA: *Equine surgery,* ed 2, St Louis, 1999, Saunders.)

The other approach is the nasolacrimal lavage system, using tubing placed into the nasal punctum. A small stab incision through the nostril is often created so that the tubing can pass through the nostril and be secured to the skin. This helps protect the tubing from motion of the nostrils and possible nose rubbing by the patient.

When injecting through either type of system, the tubing should be cleaned before attaching syringes or fluid lines. The medication should be warm enough for patient comfort. The patient is often startled by the medication entering the eye; gentle injection pressure is preferred. After injecting a medication, the catheter should be cleared with either a saline or air flush, again noting that air hitting the eye can cause patient reaction. After treatment is complete, the lavage tubing should be capped or covered to prevent debris from entering the system; an injection cap can usually serve this purpose. Excess solution flowing down the horse's face should be dried thoroughly. Continual wetness can scald the skin and cause hair loss; applying petroleum jelly to the skin below the eye may provide some protection from "runoff."

MUSCULOSKELETAL SYSTEM

The musculoskeletal system consists of the skeleton and the associated structures that allow it to move. Bone, articular cartilage, ligaments, tendons, synovial structures, and muscles are the primary components. Injuries and disease of these structures are prevalent in horses; the musculoskeletal system is perhaps the most common body system that the equine practitioner evaluates and treats.

Swelling, discharge, and muscle atrophy are among the possible manifestations of musculoskeletal disease, but the most common clinical sign is an abnormal stance or gait, referred to as *lameness*. There are three reasons for lameness:

- Pain (inflammation): most common
- Mechanical interference, without pain: such as scar tissue restriction of a full range of motion
- Neurological lameness: caused by disease of the neurological system

Detecting the source of lameness can be a daunting task for the clinician. Many problems have no obvious external signs. Often, lame horses have more than one problem; there is usually one primary problem, but secondary problems often result from the horse's response to the primary problem. This creates a "chain reaction" situation that can be difficult to unravel. The temperament, size, and strength of the patient create additional challenges.

LAMENESS EXAMINATION

The goals of the lameness exam are:
1. Identify the location of the problem/problems
2. Determine a specific diagnosis for each problem
3. Plan therapy

The lameness exam consists of five basic steps. The veterinarian tailors the basic exam to accommodate patient variables, client considerations, and other variables such as facilities and weather. The technician may assist by taking take the history, providing restraint, and assisting in diagnostic techniques such as local anesthesia, sampling, and diagnostic imaging. The basic exam consists of the following:

HISTORY

Unless dealing with an experienced horse owner/trainer, it is best to guide the client through the history rather than letting him or her ramble. Questions should include the following:

- Signalment: What is the horse's age, breed, sex, and use/sport? Some diseases affect only certain ages or have increased incidence in particular breeds. Each equine sport has certain commonly associated lameness problems that help to direct the clinician to specific areas of the horse.
- Has the horse had previous health or lameness problems?
- How long has the horse been lame?
- Was the speed of onset sudden or gradual?

- Does the lameness get better or worse with exercise?
- Is there any known trauma or reason that the horse is lame?
- Has the owner given any treatment or medication?
- Is there any pattern to the lameness? Is the lameness associated with certain surfaces, gaits, or activities?

OBSERVATION

The horse is observed at rest (standing) and in motion.

At Rest

The horse is first observed from a distance for obvious problems like swelling and muscle atrophy. The conformation of the horse—how the horse is put together anatomically—is also noted. Conformation faults (abnormal conformation) can predispose the horse to certain lameness problems. How the horse stands may also have significance; some painful problems cause the horse to "point" a leg. As a generality, if the foreleg is held in front of vertical position (as viewed from the side), it indicates lower leg pain. If the foreleg is held behind vertical, it may indicate upper leg pain. Holding a hindleg in front of vertical may indicate upper leg pain.

In Motion

The horse is observed at various gaits. The usual method is to observe the horse moving directly away from and directly toward the clinician, and then from the side as the horse moves in both directions. The ground surface can affect the lameness; horses are usually more comfortable on soft surfaces and less likely to show lameness. Harder surfaces such as asphalt may be necessary to show the problem to the observer, especially with low-grade pain. The sounds heard when the hooves strike a hard surface can also be revealing.

Rough surfaces such as stone or gravel can make sound horses appear lame and should be avoided.

Horseshoes may also protect the affected leg from fully displaying pain, especially if the problem is in the hoof. It may be necessary to remove the shoes to fully evaluate the lameness.

The horse is an athletic animal that uses its head and neck as a "balancing arm" when in motion. The way that the horse uses its head and neck tends to change when the horse is in pain, and the clinician will need to observe the carriage of the head and neck. The handler should hold the head loosely so that abnormal head and neck movements can be seen.

Walk

- Walk in straight line
- Walk up and down an incline
- Backing up

Trot

- Trot in straight line
- Trot in circle (both directions)
- Flexion tests

The trot is usually the most informative gait. The trot has weight borne on two legs at a time, which is more than the other gaits. The increased weight-bearing helps to accentuate most lamenesses. The handler should encourage a slow trot (jog) from the horse rather than a fast trot; fast trotting obscures many lamenesses.

Trotting in circles may be done on a lead line or a lunge line. The lead line requires that the handler run in a circle with the horse. As an alternative, the horse can be placed on a lunge line (long lead line), if it is accustomed to it. The lunge line allows the handler to stand still while the horse circles around the handler; the length of the line controls the diameter of the circle. Circles accentuate the stresses on the inside aspects of the legs;

for instance, circling the horse to the right (clockwise) increases the stress on the lateral aspect of the right legs and the medial aspect of the left legs. The smaller the circle, the greater the force.

If circling is done on a hard surface, the horse may slip if the diameter of the circle is too tight. Bigger circles are therefore preferred on these surfaces.

The horse is observed for gait faults and lameness (Box 11-9). Especially significant are head-nodding and hip-hiking. Holding the head up distributes more weight to the hindlegs, and the horse takes advantage of this when in pain. When a front leg is painful, the horse can transfer weight to the hind end by elevating the head when the painful front leg hits the ground. The opposite effect occurs with hindleg pain; when the painful hindleg hits the ground, the horse lowers its head to shift more weight to the front leg. This head

BOX

BOX 11-9   Gait Faults

Gait faults refer to abnormal leg actions while the horse is in motion. They are usually related to abnormal conformation or the method of shoeing. Gait faults are not necessarily associated with lameness, but they can predispose a horse to certain lameness problems. Some examples of gait faults include the following:

- Paddling: the hoof is thrown laterally after it leaves the ground
- Winging: the hoof is thrown medially after it leaves the ground
- Interfering: hitting one limb with the other
- Plaiting: placing one hoof directly in front of the other
- Forging: hitting the sole of a front hoof with the toe of the back hoof of the same side
- Overreaching: stepping on the heel of a front hoof with the back hoof of the same side
- Scalping: striking the front of a back hoof with the front hoof of the same side

action is referred to as a *head-nod* or *head-bob* and is a valuable tool for the clinician.

Hip-hiking refers to the croup rising on one side when the hindlimb on the same side is painful, similar to a human's hip carriage when a leg is painful. It is a protective "splinting" type of motion, preventing full weight-bearing on the painful limb.

Flexion tests are done to evaluate joint pain. Sensory nerve endings for synovial joints are located in the joint capsule. For the test, one or more joints are manually flexed ("cramped") with moderate force to stretch the joint capsule (Fig. 11-38). The clinician maintains the flex for a time (which varies according to the size of the joint; <1 minute for small joints, 1 to 2 minutes for larger joints), and then asks for the horse to be immediately jogged away in a straight line. It is normal for the horse to take three to four "off" strides, but it should quickly return to soundness—a negative test. If the horse does not quickly return to a normal trot, the test is positive, and the joints tested by the flexion warrant further investigation.

1. Canter/gallop: not usually necessary.
2. Specific exercise: It may be necessary to see the horse exercise with a rider on its back, pulling a cart, jumping, etc., to observe the lameness problem.

After observing the horse in motion, the clinician grades the lameness. Different grading systems are available, but most clinicians use a five-grade system to describe the lameness (Box 11-10).

PALPATION

The horse is palpated, looking for areas of pain, heat, and swelling. The legs are palpated in a weight-bearing stance, then the leg is elevated and the palpation repeated. Knowledge of normal anatomy is essential. If the horse has shoes, the wear pattern on the shoes can be revealing; the shoe type and fit should also be noted. If barefoot, the wear

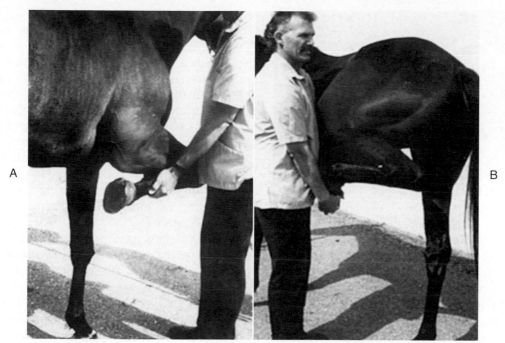

Fig. 11-38. A, Carpal flexion test. **B,** The hock flexion test also flexes the stifle because of the reciprocal apparatus. Note that the clinician elevates the leg beneath the horse, rather than pulling it out to the side or behind (which is often resisted by the horse). (From McIlwraith CW, Trotter GW: *Joint disease in the horse*, St Louis, 1996, Saunders.)

BOX 11-10	Lameness Severity Grading Scale

Grade 0 = Normal
Grade 1 = Difficult to see under any condition; obscure
Grade 2 = Difficult to see, except under certain conditions
Grade 3 = Consistently seen at the trot
Grade 4 = Obviously lame at all gaits
Grade 5 = Non–weight-bearing

pattern on the hoof wall can likewise provide information about weight-bearing. Hoof testers are used to find sources of pain within the hoof wall, since structures inside the hoof cannot be palpated (Fig. 11-39). A thorough palpation includes the neck, back, and hips; although primary problems in these areas are unusual, secondary pain is often created in these areas from abnormal weight-bearing in the legs.

LOCAL ANESTHESIA

"Nerve blocks" and "joint blocks" are often, but not always, necessary. They are used:
• To confirm the location of a suspected problem
• To assess the significance of a problem when more than one problem is found
• When the initial exam has failed to find a problem, to try to localize the problem to a smaller region of a leg

The goal of the procedure is to block pain perception. Local anesthetics can be deposited directly over nerves or directly into joints and other synovial structures to desensitize them.

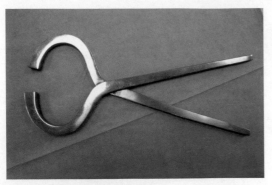

Fig. 11-39. Hoof testers.

By understanding which anatomical structures are supplied by individual nerves, the clinician can find the source or sources of pain in a leg through a process of elimination. In other words, if an area is blocked and the horse is still painful, then the problem must reside in another area. The clinician then chooses another area to desensitize, and so on, until the painful structure or area is located.

The clinician may block a specific structure if it is suspicious or start low on the leg and work proximally to find the anatomical level where the problem is located. Basically, a block is placed, and then the clinician watches the horse while in motion to see if the lameness has changed or disappeared. If the lameness is still present, then the source of pain has not been found, and another block is necessary to find the source. However, if the lameness is improved or disappears altogether, the clinician knows to look in the blocked area for the problem. "Looking" usually involves diagnostic imaging in order to obtain a specific diagnosis.

The procedure begins with cleaning the leg of dirt and debris. Skin preparation is different for nerve blocks and joint blocks. Synovial structures such as joints, bursae, and tendon sheaths must have a sterile skin prep. Clipping for synovial structure blocks is

preferable but not always possible, depending on the horse's circumstances; the owner should be consulted before any clipping is performed. The author recommends that after the skin has been prepped, povidone-iodine solution (not scrub) be dabbed to saturate the skin and allowed to air dry before the clinician performs the block. A clean prep technique using a standard scrub/alcohol prep is suitable for most peripheral nerve blocks unless the nerve is located in a location where there is a risk of entering a synovial structure. A standard sterile prep is used in these situations.

Veterinarians have preferences for where to perform the prep and block, the needle size/length, amount of anesthetic, and whether the block is performed with the leg weight-bearing or elevated. Most veterinarians prefer a fresh, previously unopened container of anesthetic for synovial structures to avoid the risk of possible contamination in previously opened bottles.

Restraint is extremely important; patient movement can cause injury to the patient or clinician. It is rare that blocks can be performed without some form of physical restraint such as a twitch. Insertion of the needle is painful, and the clinician should alert the restrainer when the needle is about to be placed. At that time, the strength of restraint is increased (tighten the twitch, grasp an elevated leg more firmly, etc.) until needle insertion is complete; the veterinarian may direct the technician to either maintain or loosen the restraint, depending on the patient's responses.

After the injection is completed, the block will need time to take effect. This time may range from 5 minutes for superficial nerves to 30 minutes for some joints. The horse may need to be walked during this time to help distribute the local anesthetic. The horse is then evaluated after the block has had sufficient time to take effect. The gaits and circumstances that showed the lameness best *before* the block are repeated after the block to best assess the results.

SPECIAL DIAGNOSTICS

Special diagnostics may include the following:

- Radiographs (plain films ± contrast techniques)
- Xeroradiographs
- Diagnostic ultrasound
- Thermography
- Nuclear scintigraphy
- Magnetic resonance imaging (MRI)
- Computed tomography (CT)
- Arthrocentesis
- Rectal exam (for fractured pelvis, sublumbar pain, etc.)
- Biopsy (muscle, bone, synovial membrane)
- Force-plate gait analysis
- High-speed cinematographic (video) gait analysis

SHOE REMOVAL

Horses are shod for several purposes. Preventive shoeing is most common and is used to support and protect the hooves. Modifications may be made to the trimming and shoeing to influence the way the hoof supports weight, how it behaves in motion, to improve traction on slick surfaces such as ice, or to improve performance for a particular sport. Therapeutic or prescription shoeing is used to treat specific problems and may be used on one or more hooves as necessary. Therapeutic shoes are often temporary, until the primary problem has healed (Fig. 11-40).

Horseshoes do not stop the hoof from growing. Hooves grow on average $1/4$ inch per month, though there is individual variation. Every 5 to 8 weeks, the shoes must be removed and the hooves trimmed to prevent overgrowth. The horse may be reshod after trimming. In some cases, the old shoes can be

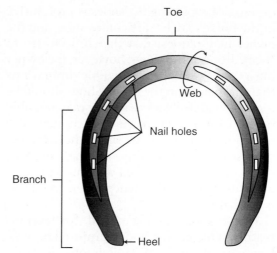

Fig. 11-40. Parts of the horseshoe.

reused (reset), but shoes eventually wear out and must be replaced. Bent shoes must also usually be replaced. Trimming and shoeing must be performed by knowledgeable professionals; farriers usually perform the trimming and shoeing for most horses. Trimming and shoeing are a regular expense for most horse owners and may be significant, especially when special shoeing is required. Many shoes must be handmade or carefully adjusted by the farrier, and the time required for the farm call and farrier's time and materials must be compensated. The owner must also schedule a time to be present for the shoeing, another potential inconvenience.

When it is necessary to remove shoes for veterinary purposes, several points should be kept in mind. First, unless it is an emergency, the owner should be consulted before removing shoes. When shoes are removed for a veterinary reason, the veterinarian is actually creating another bill (the farrier's) in addition to the veterinary bill because the farrier must be called to replace the shoe. A little client education as to why the shoes must be removed is wise. Sometimes the expense of replacing the shoes is prohibitive or the horse may be difficult to shoe, and the owner may request that the clinician try to "work around" the shoes; however, the owner must understand the possible limitations that this places on the exam. Shoes should be removed carefully so that they may possibly be used for a reset; resets save money. Also for this reason, removed shoes should never be discarded; in a clinic setting, removed shoes should be identified with marking tape and returned to the owner when the horse is discharged.

Horse shoes are removed for various reasons. Overgrown hooves, injured hooves, lameness exam, hoof radiographs, preparation for surgery, and recovery from general anesthesia are some of the indications for shoe removal. Additionally, horses may step or twist on their shoes and partially dislodge them; when shoes are loose or twisted, the potential for further damage to the foot and leg is high, and they should be immediately removed.

The horse should be adequately restrained; all steps of removal are done with the leg elevated. Shoe removal is a fairly straightforward procedure. In order to remove a shoe, one must understand how the shoe is held to the hoof. Shoes are usually attached with nails, though "glue-ons" have become popular for situations when nails cannot be easily used, such as for foals. It is sometimes necessary to add extra stability to the shoe; side clips or rims may be added to the shoe and positioned against the hoof wall (Fig. 11-41). Clips and rims supplement the lateral stability of the shoe but do not replace nails for holding the shoe on the hoof.

Horseshoe nails are shaped such that they follow a slightly curved path when driven with the hammer. Nails are driven from the bottom of the hoof wall, through the insensitive portion of the wall until they exit through the side of the hoof wall about $3/4$ to

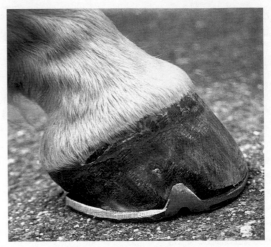

Fig. 11-41. Horseshoe with side clip. (From Colahan PT et al: *Equine medicine and surgery*, ed 5, St Louis, Mosby, 1999.)

1 inch from their point of entry (Fig. 11-42, *A* and *B*). Once the nail exits, the sharp point of the nail is removed and the remaining protruding portion is folded over 180 degrees and pressed flat against the hoof; this is referred to as *clinching* the nail. It is this folded portion (the clinch) that secures the nail and prevents it from backing out of the hoof. It is also this bent portion that must be removed or straightened in order to remove the nail, and therefore the shoe (Fig. 11-42, *C*).

Shoe removal involves three steps, as follows.

1. CLINCH REMOVAL

Counting the number of nail heads will confirm the number of clinches to be removed. There are two main methods for clinch removal. The first method is to file them off with a metal file or hoof rasp (Fig. 11-43). This must be done carefully to avoid removing large areas of periople (outer surface of the hoof). If the clinches are "buried" in the hoof wall, it can be difficult to file them off without creating much surface damage to the hoof wall. Rasping may be more comfortable

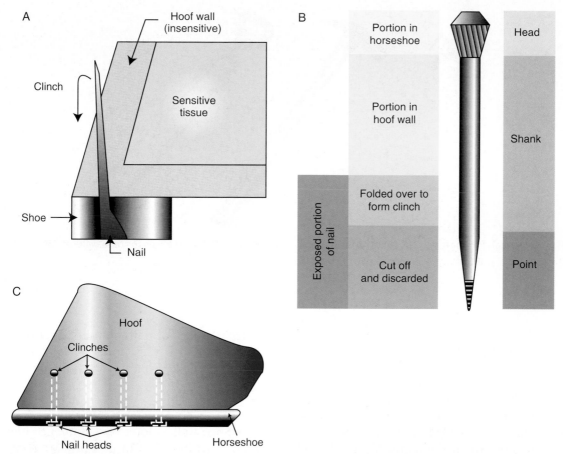

Fig. 11-42. **A,** Diagram of horseshoe nail driven properly through the hoof wall. **B,** Parts of the horseshoe nail. **C,** Diagram of horseshoe, nails and clinches.

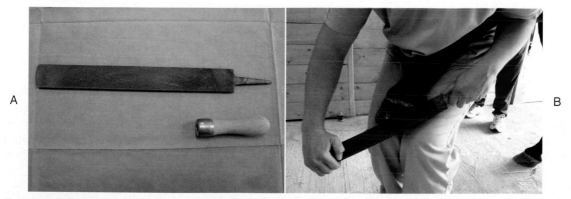

Fig. 11-43. **A,** Hoof rasp and optional handle. **B,** Use of a hoof rasp to file off the clinches of horseshoe nails.

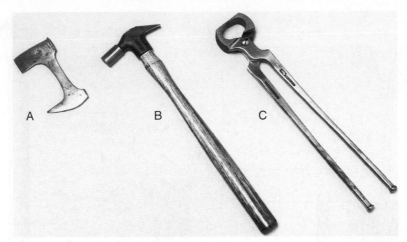

Fig. 11-44. Tools for shoe removal. **A,** Clinch cutter. **B,** Hammer. **C,** Shoe pull-offs. Note the knobs on the handles of the pull-offs. (From Colahan PT et al: *Equine medicine and surgery,* ed 5, vol 2, St Louis, 1999, Mosby.)

for sensitive hooves. The second method is to cut (or straighten) the clinches with a clinch cutter and hammer (Fig. 11-44). The clinch cutter has two blades, wide and narrow, each with a flattened top that can be struck with a hammer. The clinch cutter is positioned so that the selected blade is under the clinch and facing proximally along the hoof wall. The blade should be held as flat as possible against the hoof to engage the clinch but avoid gouging the hoof wall. The hammer is struck until the clinch is cut off or straightened enough to safely remove the nail (Fig. 11-45).

2. NAIL REMOVAL

Nail removal is done by pulling the nail out from the head. Crease nail pullers are designed to grasp the nail by the head and pull it from the shoe (Fig. 11-46). Pull-offs can be used to grasp nails with protruding heads. Individual nail removal is not always necessary; often, when the clinches have been removed, the act of pulling off the shoe pulls the nails out with the shoe, but this must be

carefully done. All nails should be retrieved from the area so that none are left on the ground to injure other horses or people.

3. SHOE REMOVAL

Shoe removal is done with shoe pullers ("pull-offs"). Shoe pullers look very similar to hoof trimmers ("nippers") but pull-offs are recognized by small knobs on the ends of the handles. Nippers should *never* be used to pull nails or remove shoes, as this will dull the cutting edges. Removal begins with elevation of the branches (heels) of the shoe and proceeds toward the toe (Fig. 11-47). The jaws of the pull-off are placed between one shoe branch and the hoof, and the handles are closed to push the jaws together. The handles are then rolled toward the midline of the toe, prying the shoe off the hoof (the toe should be well-supported before applying any leverage to the pull-offs). This is repeated on the other branch of the shoe, and then repeated as needed, progressing toward the toe and alternating sides until the shoe is free. The pull-off handles should *not* be rolled

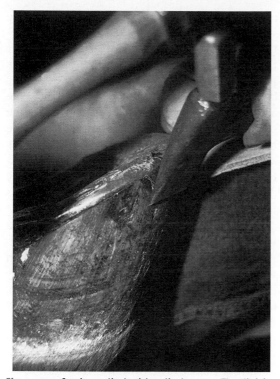

Fig. 11-45. Cutting a clinch with a clinch cutter. The clinician elevates the hoof and positions the clinch cutter blade beneath the clinch. A hammer is used to strike the clinch cutter and remove the clinch. (From Colahan PT et al: *Equine medicine and surgery,* ed 5, vol 2, St Louis, 1999, Mosby.)

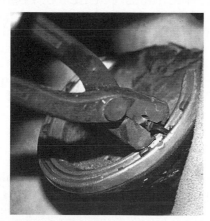

Fig. 11-46. Crease nail pullers are used to remove each nail. (From Colahan PT et al: *Equine medicine and surgery,* ed 5, vol 2, St Louis, 1999, Mosby.)

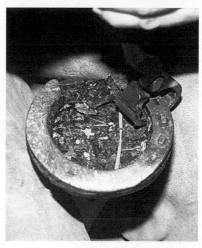

Fig. 11-47. Shoe pull-offs are used to pry the shoe away from the hoof, beginning at the heels and progressing toward the toe. (From Colahan PT et al: *Equine medicine and surgery,* ed 5, vol 2, St Louis, 1999, Mosby.)

toward the outside edge of the hoof wall; this tends to tear off pieces of the hoof wall.

Removal must be performed carefully to prevent damaging the hoof wall. Failure to remove clinches completely or to be aware of side clips can result in large chips and cracks, which will likely be problematic. Also, some methods of clinch removal (especially rasping) can scuff the outer layers of the hoof and damage the periople layer; this tends to bother pleasure horse clients more than racehorse owners and trainers. Although it is desirable not to bend shoes during removal, in case they can be reset, aluminum shoes are somewhat soft and commonly bend during removal. Most owners are aware of this.

After shoe removal, the unshod hoof is prone to chipping and cracking, especially if the horse is on hard surfaces. Chipping and cracking are unsightly and may interfere with the ability to replace a shoe (which makes farriers and owners quite unhappy). Hoof cracks can also extend into sensitive tissue and become a source of lameness.

To minimize this risk, a hoof rasp can be lightly used to round off any sharp edges on the bottom of the hoof wall where it meets the ground. Covering the hoof wall and sole with duct tape after shoe removal can also reduce the risk of chipping.

REPRODUCTIVE SYSTEM

Reproductive procedures may be a minimal portion of an equine practice, or they may be almost 100% of a practice in some parts of the country. Some large breeding facilities employ full-time veterinarians whose primary function is reproductive medicine and obstetrics. In the average equine practice, reproductive system diagnostics and therapeutics are among the more commonly performed procedures.

BREEDING SOUNDNESS EXAMINATION

Breeding soundness exams are used to evaluate the fertility of both males and females. They are usually performed near the beginning of the breeding season. A general physical exam is included as part of the exam. Breeding soundness examination of the male includes evaluation of the penis, prepuce, scrotum, and testicles and collection of an ejaculate for semen analysis. In the female, rectal palpation and ultrasound examination of the ovaries, uterus, and cervix are performed. A visual exam of the vagina and cervix is usually done, followed by uterine culture and possibly endometrial (uterine) biopsy. The results of the exam allow the veterinarian to assess fertility, identify potential conditions that might interfere with successful breeding, and diagnose venereal diseases.

MALE REPRODUCTIVE SYSTEM

The male reproductive system consists of the penis, testicles, epididymis/ductus deferens, and accessory sex glands. The reproductive system shares the penile portion of the urethra with the urinary system. The penis is of the musculocavernous type; the glans penis is housed within the prepuce. The prepuce is commonly referred to as the *sheath* in large animals. The testicles are housed within the scrotum between the hind legs. The horse has all four accessory sex glands: prostate (1), seminal vesicles (2), ampullae (2), and bulbourethral glands (2). The onset of puberty (age when able to impregnate a female) is between 18 and 24 months.

Examination of the external genitalia must be done carefully to prevent injury to the examiner. All males should be approached with caution, but breeding stallions especially can be unpredictable and difficult to control (a good rule of thumb is to never turn your back on a stallion). The horse must be adequately restrained, and the examiner is safest when positioned next to the horse's chest. Standing next to the hindquarters should be avoided if possible; even heavily tranquilized animals can kick with the hindlimbs.

Most males tend to resent handling of the genital areas. In order to evaluate the penis, it must be extended from the prepuce. Some males allow manual extension by inserting a gloved hand into the prepuce and gently grasping the penis; however, this is uncommon. Most males must be tranquilized to relax the retractor penis muscle and allow the penis to extend. Rarely, after tranquilization, the penis may remain extended for a prolonged period; this is more likely when phenothiazine-based tranquilizers are used for tranquilization. Regardless of the drugs used, if extension persists for longer than 2 hours, veterinary attention should be sought. Prolonged extension interferes with venous and lymphatic drainage of the prepuce and penis, resulting in rapid development of severe edema. Permanent damage to the penis (paralysis, paraphimosis, external

11-11 Penile Dysfunction Terminology

Penile paralysis: inability to retract the penis into the prepuce due to nerve or muscle (retractor penis muscle) disease.

Phimosis: inability to extend the penis from the prepuce, usually due to excessive swelling of the prepuce, which prevents the penis from exiting.

Paraphimosis: inability to retract the penis back into the prepuce, usually due to excessive swelling of the prepuce and/or penis.

Priapism: prolonged erection unrelated to sexual desire, usually due to failure of the blood to exit the erectile tissue of the glans penis. Swelling of the prepuce and penis develop within hours and result in paraphimosis in addition to the priapism.

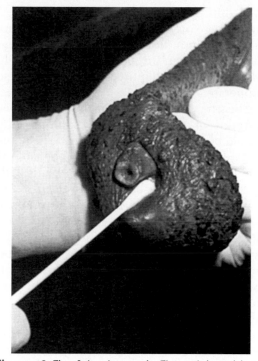

Fig. 11-48. Tip of the glans penis. The swab is positioned at the entrance to the urethral fossa. (From Speirs VC: *Clinical examination of horses,* St Louis, 1997, Saunders.)

trauma, priapism) may result if treatment is not instituted promptly (Box 11-11).

PREPUTIAL AND PENILE CLEANING

The prepuce and penis may accumulate a thick, foul-smelling, dark-colored material known as smegma. Smegma is the combination of secretions from sebaceous glands, sweat glands, dead cells, and dirt. Smegma tends to accumulate on the surface of the glans penis and inside the prepuce, causing crusting and irritation of the tissues. The tip of the penis also accumulates smegma in the urethral fossa (diverticulum), which is a 1-inch–deep "pocket" that completely encircles the urethral opening (Fig. 11-48). Smegma in the urethral fossa tends to harden into round balls that horsemen refer to as "beans" (Fig. 11-49). Horses may form multiple beans, and they may reach walnut size. The pocket shape of the fossa usually retains the beans, preventing them from falling out. The beans can compress the tip of the urethra and make urination difficult and painful. Because of these potential complications, it is part of the routine care of all male horses (castrated or not) to clean the penis and prepuce; this

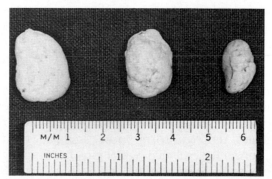

Fig. 11-49. Three masses of smegma ("beans") recovered from the urethral fossa. (From Colahan PT et al: *Equine medicine and surgery,* vol 2, ed 5, St Louis, 1999, Mosby.)

procedure is referred to as "sheath cleaning." Some horse owners perform sheath cleaning on their own horses, but many request the veterinarian to perform it, especially when sedation is required to make the horse cooperate.

Sheath cleaning begins with proper restraint of the horse. Gloves (nonsterile) should be worn for the procedure. The penis is extended manually or with the aid of tranquilization. While holding the penis with one hand, the other hand gently cleanses the penis and internal surface of the prepuce with warm water on either roll cotton or 4×4 gauze squares; vigorous scrubbing should be avoided. Crusts are softened with water and gently removed. The tip of the penis is then examined, and a finger inserted into the urethral fossa to remove any beans. The finger is swept 360 degrees around the fossa to assure thorough cleaning. In cases where crust removal leaves open sores, it may be beneficial to apply a small amount of nonirritating antibacterial ointment to the lesions.

Mild soap may be used during the cleaning procedure, although its use is optional. Some people believe that soap alters the normal bacterial flora and predisposes the horse to infectious problems; soap may also be irritating to the tissues (especially povidone-iodine). If soap is used, it is important to completely rinse all soap off the area to prevent tissue irritation. Rinsing is done with clean water—never with alcohol.

The frequency of sheath cleaning varies greatly among individual males. Most males benefit from cleaning several times a year, but some form more smegma and must be cleaned more frequently (monthly). Older males tend to form more smegma than younger males. Breeding stallions are routinely cleaned before breeding or semen collection. Owners of male horses should visually observe the penis when extended to urinate and have sheath cleaning performed as soon

BOX 11-12   Snow and Horse Urine

Clients in colder climates commonly report seeing a red or orange color after their horses urinate on snow (especially on a sunny day). Although this may be blood in the urine, it is far more likely to be pigments called porphyrins, which are normal components of plants in the horse's diet; sunlight activates the pigment in the urine, and the white snow highlights the color. Urinary tract problems are unusual in horses, and the occurrence of hematuria is therefore uncommon. If any doubt exists, a urine sample for urinalysis and the presence of blood quickly provides an answer.

as smegma build-up (flakes or deposits of smegma) is observed. Sometimes the male horse will not extend the penis from the prepuce to urinate; although this may be normal for an individual, it may also indicate pain and warrants consultation with a veterinarian. Similarly, preputial swelling, dribbling urine, or blood in the urine should also be evaluated (Box 11-12).

While the penis is extended, it should be examined for suspicious lesions. The penis and prepuce are susceptible to a variety of benign and malignant tumors, parasitic lesions (habronemiasis), and other growths. There is no typical appearance of these lesions; *any* abnormality is suspicious and is best evaluated by a veterinarian.

SEMEN COLLECTION

Semen may be collected for the following purposes:
- Breeding soundness exam: to determine the quality and quantity of sperm as part of the fertility evaluation of a breeding stallion
- Evaluate diseases of the male reproductive tract
- Collection and preparation of semen for artificial insemination

Although there are several ways to "collect a stallion," the most common is to collect semen into an artificial vagina (AV). Most stallions are collected into a handheld AV while the stallion mounts a mare in estrus ("jump" mare), but some can be trained to mount and ejaculate into an inanimate mounting dummy mare ("phantom"). Phantoms can be adjusted to a comfortable height for the stallion and reduce the risk of injury to the stallion from unwilling mares. The AV can be built into the phantom (Fig. 11-50).

There are several styles of artificial vagina, but all contain the same basic components. An outer casing provides for a secure grip on the device and protects the contents. An inner lining usually has a rubber bladder that can be filled with warm water; the stallion ejaculates into the inner lining. The inner lining leads to a collection bottle for containing the semen (Fig. 11-51).

The AV must be prepared for cleanliness and stallion comfort. The reusable rubber AV liner should be cleaned and flushed with clean hot water, then soaked in isopropyl alcohol for at least 2 hours, and air-dried. Soaps and disinfectants can build up residues in the rubber that may be spermicidal and are therefore seldom used. Some rubber liners can be gas sterilized with ethylene oxide but must be followed by 2 to 3 days of airing out; the manufacturer's instructions for cleaning options should be consulted. Disposable AV liners are available; these liners are nontoxic to sperm, but some stallions do not accept the plastic liners as well as the reusable rubber liners.

The optimal temperature inside the AV is approximately 45° C (113° F). Filling the AV with slightly warmer water allows for some heat loss before use but should not exceed 48° C (118.4° F). The liner should be checked for comfortable pressure; it should apply good contact around the penis and allow for full expansion of the penis, but overfilling may

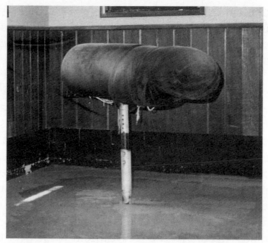

Fig. 11-50. Breeding phantom for semen collection. (From Colahan PT et al: *Equine medicine and surgery*, ed 5, vol 2, St Louis, 1999, Mosby.)

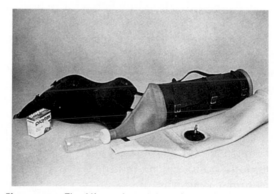

Fig. 11-51. The Missouri model equine artificial vagina consists of an outer leather case with handle, an inner rubber lining that can be filled with water and/or air, and a small collection bottle. (Accessories are visible in the background.) (From Colahan PT et al: *Equine medicine and surgery*, ed 5, vol 2, St Louis, 1999, Mosby.)

prevent the erect penis from entering the AV. The inner lining should be lubricated with a sterile nonspermicidal lubricant by placing the lubricant on a sterilely gloved hand and smearing the lubricant on the cranial two thirds of the liner. Finally, a gel filter is usually inserted into the AV to catch and strain out the gel fraction of the ejaculate and any impurities.

The stallion is prepared by washing the penis with warm water. The stallion is usually encouraged to have an erection by exposing him to a mare in heat, and the penis is cleaned while the erection is maintained. Gloves should be worn.

If using a jump mare, she also needs to be prepared. The tail should be wrapped or bandaged, and the perineal area washed with antiseptic scrub and clean water. Usually the mare needs to be restrained to prevent injury to the stallion and personnel; a twitch is commonly used, and sometimes hobbles are placed around the hindlimbs to prevent kicking.

The actual collection procedure is potentially dangerous. Breeding behavior in horses is usually aggressive and sometimes violent, and personnel are in vulnerable positions. Many facilities require personnel to wear helmets. The procedure requires a minimum of one person to handle the mare, one to handle the stallion, and one person to perform the collection into the AV. The usual method is to restrain the mare, then lead the stallion to approach the mare from her left side. The stallion is allowed to mount the mare, and the semen collector quickly moves in to grasp and divert the penis into the AV before it can enter the mare. The hands are then used to stabilize the AV alongside the mare while the stallion ejaculates. The AV is aimed slightly downward so that the ejaculate flows into the collection bottle (Fig. 11-52).

Following the collection procedure, the mare and stallion are quickly separated. The mare's perineal area is again cleansed, and the mare is examined for trauma to the legs and body. The stallion's penis is also cleansed, and he is examined for any evidence of genital or bodily trauma.

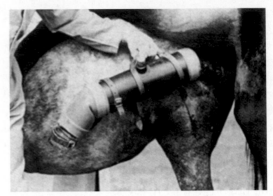

Fig. 11-52. After mounting the mare, the stallion's penis is diverted into an artificial vagina for ejaculation. (From Noakes DE, Parkinson TJ, England GCW: *Arthur's veterinary reproduction and obstetrics*, ed 8, London, 2001, Saunders.)

The collection bottle is taken rapidly to the laboratory for analysis. The container should not be shaken; it should be kept warm (37° C/98.6° F) in an incubator or water bath and protected from UV light until it can be analyzed, which should be as soon as possible. Semen analysis is performed on the gel-free fraction of the ejaculate, which contains the majority of the spermatozoa. Many good references on semen analysis that detail the laboratory procedures and normal/abnormal parameters are available. Generally semen analysis includes the following:

- Gross appearance: white, opaque (resembles skim milk); free of blood
- Volume (ml): usually measured by gradations on the collection bottle
- Sperm concentration: electronically, or manually with a hemocytometer
- Total number of sperm: multiply the volume (ml) by sperm concentration
- Sperm morphology: light microscope at 1000× magnification to examine air-dried, stained smears
- Live sperm percentage
- Sperm motility: estimate of number of sperm showing progressive forward motility
- pH: pH meter (pH paper lacks precision)

Semen may be prepared for artificial insemination of mares. Unlike semen from other species, equine semen does not freeze well and must be either used immediately (fresh semen) or stored in special refrigerated containers (cooled semen) for use within a short time (average 24 hours). The standard insemination dose for equines is 500 million progressively motile sperm per insemination; using the results of the semen analysis, a single ejaculate from a stallion can be split into several insemination doses for use on one or more mares. "Extenders" are commonly added to the semen; extenders are a combination of liquid and solid ingredients designed primarily to nourish the sperm and help them survive outside the stallion's reproductive tract. Extenders are also used to increase volume if the ejaculate is to be split into two or more aliquots. Most of the many recipes for extenders contain a source of protein and simple sugars. They are buffered for pH and add antibiotics to reduce the incidence of venereally transmitted bacterial disease. The benefits of extended semen are well documented.

Not all horse breed registries accept individuals that have been conceived by artificial insemination. Some registries allow artificial insemination, provided that it is performed with the mare and stallion on the same premises. If breed registration of offspring is desired, the horse owner should consult the breed registry for current regulations and restrictions.

CASTRATION

Castration (orchidectomy or gelding) is the most commonly performed equine surgical procedure; chemical castration, as performed in ruminants, is not currently available for equines. Removal of the testicles reduces or prevents sexual behavior and aggressive behavior and prevents reproduction by individuals judged to have inferior or undesirable genetic traits. Castration may also be necessary to treat certain malignancies, testicular trauma, or inguinal or scrotal hernias. The procedure can be performed at any age but is seldom done before 6 months of age. Most commonly it is performed between 1 and 2 years of age, when puberty begins and the accompanying behavior becomes objectionable. Some owners feel that castration at a young age retards the horse's skeletal and muscular growth, although others believe that castration before puberty results in greater growth in height. Some owners wait to see if the horse has a future as a breeding stallion and castrate later in life.

The procedure is almost always performed in the field, though some owners prefer to have it done in a hospital setting for cleanliness and in case of complications during or after surgery. When performed in the field, the operative area should be clean and free of wind or drafts. Noise and other distractions should be minimized. When the procedure is performed under general anesthesia, grassy areas are usually preferable to dirt surfaces; if a dirt surface is the only option, a large tarp or blanket should be placed beneath the hind end of the patient to minimize ground contamination.

The basic prerequisite for castration is the presence of two fully descended testicles. Because a simple visual assessment is unreliable, the veterinarian palpates the horse to ensure that both testicles are accessible before beginning the surgical procedure. Equines have a high incidence of retained testicles. Failure of one or both testicles to descend fully into the scrotal sacs is abnormal; such an animal is referred to as a *cryptorchid*. Testicles may be retained in the abdomen (abdominal cryptorchid) or in the inguinal canal (inguinal cryptorchid; "high flanker"). Retained testicles do not produce sperm, because the temperature adjacent to or within the body is too high. However, retained testicles produce testosterone efficiently, with resultant stallionlike behavior. Retained abdominal testes may also become tumorous. For these reasons, it is advisable to locate and remove retained testicles.

The surgical strategy for castrating a cryptorchid (cryptorchidectomy) is different from routine castration and usually general anesthesia is necessary. Retained testicles may be difficult to locate and difficult to surgically remove, especially if they are retained in the abdomen. Recently the use of laparoscopy to locate and remove abdominally retained testes has been advocated.

Castration is almost always performed using an instrument called an emasculator. There are several styles of emasculator; some crush and cut the spermatic cord at the same time with one set of jaws (Serra and White emasculators), and others have a two-jaw system (Reimer emasculator) that crushes the cord with one handle and cuts the cord with the other (Fig. 11-53). Surgeons usually develop preferences for a particular style of emasculator. The success of surgery depends in part on sharp, tight emasculators. To prepare the emasculators for surgery, they are disassembled and cleaned. Disassembly is necessary to thoroughly clean the recesses of the instrument jaws; a wing nut located on the instrument must be unscrewed to take the instrument apart. After cleaning, the instrument is reassembled, wrapped, and sterilized in an autoclave. Reassembly must be accurate, with the handles and jaws in proper orientation to the wing nut. The surgeon uses the wing nut to orient the emasculators when applying the instrument on the spermatic cord.

Patient Position

Castration can be performed with the horse standing or recumbent. A standing procedure may be preferred to avoid the risks of anesthetic recovery, or when patient factors such as large body size or history of anesthetic

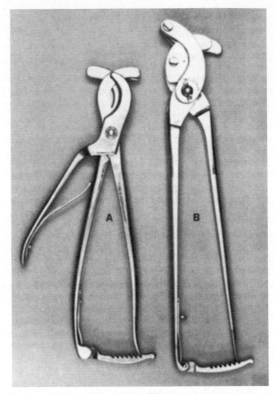

Fig. 11-53. Reimer **(A)** and Serra **(B)** emasculators. (From Auer JA: *Equine surgery,* St Louis, 1992, Saunders.)

problems increase risks of general anesthesia. Standing castration is preferred by most racehorse owners and trainers. The standing procedure is performed with a combination of heavy sedation and local anesthetic (deposited directly into the scrotal skin, testes, and spermatic cord). Because the horse is capable of responding to stimuli, including pain, there is increased risk of injury to both the clinician and the horse. The procedure is often performed with the horse standing next to a wall, to limit its ability to move. The surgeon and horse handler should stand on the same side of the horse. The tail should be wrapped or braided to keep it from contaminating the surgical field.

The recumbent procedure requires general anesthesia. Since the procedure is fairly quick

(15 to 30 minutes), short-acting IV anesthesia is usually adequate. The basic anesthetic protocol is heavy sedation with an alpha-2 agonist (xylazine or detomidine), followed by induction with ketamine or ultrashort-acting thiobarbiturate. Clinicians may add acepromazine or butorphanol to the sedative "cocktail." Some add the muscle relaxant guaifenesin to the induction agent. Many drug combinations are possible to try to improve overall analgesia and muscle relaxation, as well as duration of anesthesia. Some surgeons supplement general anesthesia with local anesthesia of the spermatic cord. Positioning for the recumbent procedure may be lateral or dorsal. In lateral recumbency, the upper hindlimb must be pulled cranially or flexed dorsally to give access to the scrotum; this is usually accomplished by placing a rope around the pastern and either tying the rope around the neck or having an assistant hold the rope for the duration of the procedure. In dorsal recumbency, the horse's body must be stabilized between hay bales or other supports. Clinicians have preferences for patient positioning.

Patient Preparation

The horse should have limited access to food before surgery in anticipation of depressed GI motility caused by the sedative and anesthetic drugs (see Chapter 8). IV catheterization for administration of anesthetic drugs is recommended but not essential. The patient should receive tetanus prophylaxis before (preferred) or immediately after surgery. Some veterinarians give antibiotics routinely before surgery; this is done for prophylaxis and is not mandatory. The patient should be groomed well before the procedure.

Procedure

Clipping is not usually necessary for routine castration. Surgical preparation of the skin is performed with surgical scrub and alcohol or clean water rinses of the prepuce and scrotum. The inner thighs should be included in the scrub area.

Draping is not performed for the standing procedure and is seldom performed for recumbent castrations in the field.

The surgical procedure involves two scrotal incisions, one over each testicle. The veterinarian exteriorizes a testicle and as much of its spermatic cord as possible, then applies emasculators to crush and cut the spermatic cord. The procedure is repeated for the other testicle. It is sometimes necessary to ligate the spermatic cord with suture material. After emasculation, the spermatic cord is checked for hemorrhage. Excess tissue and fat in the scrotal sac is removed, since it tends to hang from the incisions and serve as "fly food." The scrotal incisions may be sutured closed, but the common method is to manually enlarge (stretch) the incisions and leave them open to allow drainage.

Aftercare

The most common complications are hemorrhage and excessive swelling. Hemorrhage occurs commonly, and the source is usually skin vessels in the scrotum. This bleeding is not life threatening and stops within several hours. However, life-threatening hemorrhage may occur from the stump of the severed spermatic cord; ligation, application of hemostatic clamps, or reemasculation is required to stop the hemorrhage and prevent possible death. Following castration, the horse should be observed frequently during the first 24 hours for hemorrhage. A good rule of thumb for the bleeding horse is that if the drops of blood can be counted, it is probably not a life-threatening hemorrhage; the veterinarian should be alerted to the situation. If, however, the bleeding is a continuous stream, or drops occur so rapidly that they cannot be counted, the situation requires urgent veterinary attention. Stall rest for the first 24 hours after castration surgery is recommended to allow the severed blood vessels time to form adequate clots and to allow full recovery from anesthesia. Excessive activity in this initial postoperative period may dislodge clots that are trying to form.

Drainage from the incisions is expected after surgery, as is mild swelling of the scrotum and prepuce. The client is instructed on when and how to exercise the horse; it is believed that exercise facilitates drainage and minimizes swelling. Exercise is usually advised after the initial 24-hour postoperative period. Excessive swelling blocks the incisions and prevents external drainage; this leads to extreme swelling of the scrotum and prepuce, and the retained fluid is predisposed to infection. The veterinarian may need to inspect and manually reopen incisions that are not draining.

Hydrotherapy of the surgical area is sometimes prescribed to decrease edema in the scrotum and prepuce. Water should *never* be directed into the incisions; this risks driving debris and organisms into the scrotal sacs (the abdominal cavity has a direct communication with the inside of the spermatic cord). The water stream should be carefully applied to the sides of the prepuce and scrotum.

Because of the communication of the spermatic cord (via the vaginal process) with the abdominal cavity, evisceration of intestines may occur after surgery. This complication is rare but potentially fatal when it occurs. Evisceration is most likely in the first 4 hours after surgery but may occur up to 6 days postoperatively. The owner should inspect the surgical site with the veterinarian immediately after the surgical procedure to observe the normal postoperative appearance. Later, if any tissue protrudes from the incision that was not seen immediately following the surgery, the veterinarian should be notified immediately.

Horses castrated after onset of puberty should not have contact with mares for several weeks following surgery, to avoid arousal. It takes about 30 days for testosterone levels to subside following the procedure. Persistent stallionlike behavior may occur in geldings and is more likely when males are castrated later in life. Such individuals are referred to as "false rigs," and blame is usually placed on poor surgical technique by the veterinarian for failing to remove the epididymis and/ or enough spermatic cord ("proud cut"). However, the epididymis and spermatic cord cannot produce testosterone, and increased testosterone levels in false rigs are seldom documented. It is more likely that the persistent "sexual" behavior was learned before castration, or that it is part of the normal social interaction of horses (unrelated to sexual stimulation).

Healing of the scrotal incisions is usually complete in 3 to 4 weeks.

FEMALE REPRODUCTIVE SYSTEM

Some diseases of the female reproductive tract are unrelated to breeding and reproduction and require diagnostic procedures and medical or surgical treatment. However, the overwhelming majority of female reproductive system procedures are performed on breeding animals, with the ultimate goal being delivery of a live foal. Unlike their counterparts in other species, successful breeding and pregnancy in female horses is not often easy to accomplish. In order to produce a live foal, the following must occur:

• Successful breeding: Mares do not always readily accept the male. Also, timing of insemination (natural or artificial) must correspond to the time of ovulation; this may be difficult to determine. Also, the source of the semen (the stallion) may not be at the same location as the female, requiring that the semen be shipped to the mare or that the mare be shipped to the stallion's farm for breeding.

- Successful conception.
- Successful implantation: The period from conception to implantation is prolonged in horses; implantation begins approximately on day 35. Embryonic losses are high during the time before implantation.
- Successful gestation: Gestation in the horse averages 330 to 345 days.
- Successful parturition: The placenta begins to separate early during the delivery process; deprived of this oxygen source, foals rarely survive dystocias that last more than 1 hour.

After all of this, the foal must still survive the delicate neonatal period. Veterinary medicine is often involved in each of the above steps. Coupled with the economics of the breeding industry, breeding mares can be a tricky and expensive business (Table 11-1).

Frequently owners have additional concerns with getting mares bred early during the breeding season. Mares are seasonally polyestrous. They have estrous cycles from early spring to fall and are anestrus during the late fall and winter months. This means that, under natural conditions, horses usually breed and conceive in the spring and summer, and deliver about 11 months later—in spring or early summer. In certain horse breeds, all horses born in a calendar year are considered to be the same age and must compete against each other, regardless of the month they are born. It is advantageous to have foals born early in the year so that they will be bigger and stronger than foals born in late spring or summer of the same year. This is especially important in the racing breeds. Larger body size and muscle mass may also be a consideration in horse show halter conformation classes in some breeds that value heavier muscling (Quarter Horses, Paint Horses, Appaloosas, etc.). If a mare fails to breed successfully or has an early embryonic loss, it will be approximately 3 weeks before she cycles again. If she is bred again, it will be almost 2 weeks before an embryo can be detected with ultrasound. If there are several unsuccessful attempts to breed and conceive or if time out is required to treat a uterine infection or other disease, it is often May or June, and the resulting foal (if successful conception does occur) would be born "too late" the following year to be competitive.

One approach to compensate for the naturally short breeding season is to use artificial lighting. Artificial lighting during winter months can "fool" the mare's system by increasing the photoperiod to which she is exposed, resulting in winter estrous cycles. This is done to create a longer breeding season, usually so that foals can be born as early the following year as possible. A longer breeding season also allows more time for

TABLE 11-1	REPRODUCTIVE PHYSIOLOGY OF THE MARE	
	Average	*Range*
Puberty	18 mo	10-24 mo
Length of estrous cycle	21-22 days	19-24 days
Length of estrus	5-7 days	4-9 days
Length of diestrus	15-16 days	12-16 days
Ovulation	last 48 hr of estrus	
Length of gestation (light breeds)	333-342 days	305-365 days

repeated attempts to breed and conceive in case something goes "wrong." The artificial lighting is provided beginning in December, in gradually increasing increments until 16 total hours of light exposure per day is achieved. Most mares respond with estrous cycles beginning in January or February.

PREPARATION OF THE PERINEUM/VULVA

Many reproductive procedures in the mare begin with proper cleansing of the perineum and vulva, especially whenever the vagina is to be entered as part of the procedure. Cleansing is performed to prevent carrying feces and other debris inside the vagina, cervix, and uterus.

The tail should be bandaged or wrapped and either held or tied (around the mare's neck; *never* to an immovable object) to the side for the procedure (see Chapter 6). The mare should be properly restrained, although the amount of restraint may be minimal in mares that are accustomed to the procedure.

Cleansing is usually done with roll cotton soaked in warm, clean water. Povidone-iodine scrub, chlorhexidine scrub, or mild soap is usually used, depending on clinician preference. An initial cleansing of the anal area may be necessary to remove crusted feces and fecal water. Then, using scrub, the prep is begun on the lips of the vulva and gradually extended in circular fashion to include the perineum, anus, and inner aspect of the buttocks. Water is used in the same pattern to rinse the soap away. The process is repeated as many times as necessary until no residue is seen on the cotton.

Any water running down the horse's thighs and hocks should be wiped with dry cotton or a dry towel. Some mares are sensitive to the dripping of water on the hocks or running down the legs. This commonly occurs when water flows off the buttocks, causing some horses to kick. The technician should be careful to stand to the side of the hindquarters during cleansing of this area and be alert to possible kicks.

Once the area is prepped, the tail should not be allowed to contact the area. If defecation occurs, the entire cleaning process should be repeated. Following the veterinarian's procedures, it may be necessary to clean the area again to remove lubricant, blood, or other debris.

ESTROUS CYCLE DETERMINATION

It may be important to determine what stage of the estrous cycle a mare is in, in order to plan breeding dates or treatment of uterine infections. This is usually achieved by examining the ovaries for the presence and size of follicles. Follicles increase in size and become softer as the time of ovulation approaches. Secondarily, the cervix can be examined for consistency and/or appearance; the cervix relaxes (dilates) and becomes hyperemic during estrus. The methods available for estrous cycle staging may be performed at any time:

- Rectal palpation: The ovaries and cervix are evaluated. Because early follicles develop inside the ovary, they may be missed by palpation.
- Diagnostic ultrasound: This is the most accurate method for determining a mare's estrous cycle phase. A rectal exam is typically performed before the ultrasound to allow palpation of the uterus and cervix and clean out feces from the rectum so that the ultrasound transducer achieves good contact with the rectal wall. Ultrasound is superior to palpation of the ovaries in that it can visualize inside the ovaries to see structures such as small follicles, and it also allows precise measurement of follicle size. Follicle size is important, since most mares ovulate when follicle diameter is reaches 35 to 55 mm. Individuals usually establish a fairly consistent ovulation diameter, which can be followed year to year to help predict the time of ovulation.

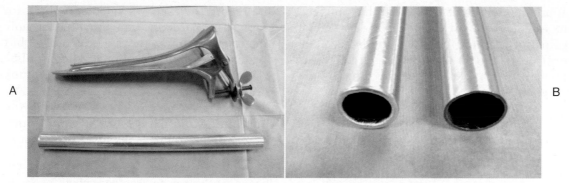

Fig. 11-54. A, Stainless steel reusable vaginal speculum *(top)* and disposable vaginal speculum *(bottom)*. **B,** The disposable vaginal speculum has a smooth, rounded edge *(left)* at one end designed to be inserted into the vagina. The sharper edge *(right)* is used as a handhold.

- Vaginal exam: This is usually a visual examination of the cervix, through a vaginal speculum. Preparation of the perineum/vulva should be performed. A vaginal speculum (disposable or reusable) and light source (penlight, flashlight) are required for a visual exam (Fig. 11-54). For a manual vaginal exam, the examiner needs a sterile obstetrical (OB) sleeve and sterile, water-soluble lubricant.

The cervix is observed; a relaxed, hyperemic cervix is consistent with estrogen influence (estrus), while a "high-dry-tight" cervix is consistent with progesterone influence (diestrus or "luteal phase"). Evaluation of the cervix is not as specific as other methods for staging the estrus cycle; it is typically used to supplement other observations.

PREGNANCY DIAGNOSIS

This procedure is used to identify the presence of an embryo or a fetus and to estimate gestational age of the embryo or fetus if the breeding date is unknown. It may be used to determine fetal viability, by confirming the presence and vigor of the fetal heartbeat. It is also used to identify twin conceptions, which are undesirable. The equine uterus is not designed to support and nourish more than

one fetus; competition for space and nutrition usually results in the death and abortion or stillbirth of both twin fetuses. Occasionally, one twin may be born alive but is typically weak and small, and it faces a high mortality rate. Birth of living twins is rare, and survival of both is even rarer. When twin embryos or fetuses are detected, the veterinarian needs to advise the owner of options to either terminate the pregnancy or to terminate only one of the embryos in hope that the other may survive.

The methods of pregnancy diagnosis include the following:

Rectal Palpation

Experienced clinicians can detect the presence of a pregnancy as early as 18 to 21 days; by 28 days, pregnancy is usually easy to confirm with rectal palpation. As pregnancy proceeds, the fetus enlarges and fluid accumulates around it, causing the uterus to gradually "fall" over the brim of the pelvis into the abdominal cavity. This leads to a time period from about day 90 to day 150 when it may be difficult to confirm a pregnancy, since the uterus is essentially out of reach of the palpator. After day 150, pregnancy determination is more consistent, and after approximately day 270 the fetus has enlarged to a size that can be reliably felt. Rectal palpation cannot be used to detect fetal heartbeat and can only detect a living fetus by detecting movement of the fetus in late pregnancy.

Diagnostic Ultrasound, per Rectum

Ultrasound can reliably detect the presence of an embryo as early as 10 to 12 days (Fig. 11-55, *A*) and is more reliable than rectal palpation for confirming twin conceptions (Fig. 11-55, *B*). The fetal heartbeat can be imaged as early as 4 weeks. Another advantage of ultrasound is the ability to show the client the examination on the viewing screen

and record the exam on video or as a photograph. The hardcopy can provide not only documentation for the medical record but also for the client—a popular client public relations tool (they can start a baby album). Ultrasound per rectum has the same time limitations as rectal palpation, with the timeframe from day 90 to 150 being somewhat difficult to image because of the uterus' position in the abdomen.

Diagnostic Ultrasound, Transabdominal

This method cannot be used while the uterus is contained within the pelvis, before approximately day 70 to 80 of pregnancy. From about day 80 until term, it is reliable. The exam

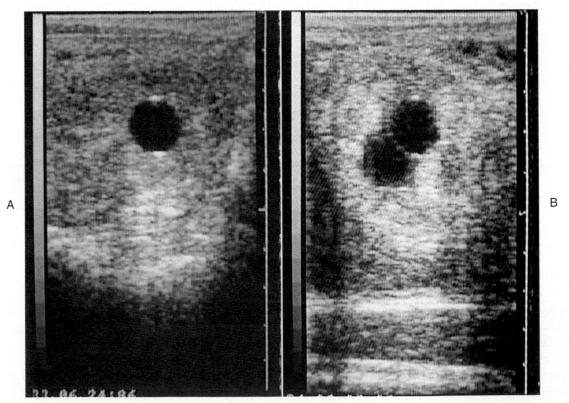

Fig. 11-55. A, Ultrasound examination of 13-day pregnancy. **B,** Twin embryos at 12 days. (From Colahan PT et al: *Equine medicine and surgery,* ed 5, vol 2, St Louis, 1999, Mosby.)

is performed through a clipped area on the ventrolateral abdomen, cranial to the mammary gland, using a transducer that can penetrate to a depth of 20 to 30 cm (2.5 to 3.5 MHz).

External Palpation ("Ballottement")

The examiner presses both fists against the lower flank area and rapidly presses inward; this is supposed to rapidly displace the pregnant uterus (if present), which then rebounds back into its original position and "bumps" the examiner's fists. This method lacks accuracy and has largely been replaced by other methods. External abdominal palpation as used in small animals is not possible in large animals.

Abdominal Radiographs

Although commonly used for pregnancy diagnosis in small animals, abdominal radiographs are not considered useful for this purpose in large animals.

Laboratory Tests

These tests are typically used when rectal examination is inconclusive or impossible to perform (on small females, wild or dangerous horses, etc.). They can be difficult to interpret and have limited usefulness. Many are not possible to perform or not reliable until later stages of pregnancy, well beyond the useful timeframe of the normal breeding season (should rebreeding be necessary).

- Progesterone assays: blood test. Normal levels are difficult to determine, since much individual variation exists. A "pregnant" level in one mare may be "nonpregnant" in another.
- Estrogen assays: Blood and urine tests are available for various analogs of estrogen but are generally not reliable until late pregnancy, after 150 days of gestation. A fecal test for estrogen is available and may be accurate after 120 days.

- Chorionic gonadotropin (pregnant mare serum gonadotropin, PMSG): blood test. Chorionic gonadotropin is produced by the endometrial cups from day 35 to 120. Mares that abort pregnancies after the endometrial cups have formed (day 35 to 38) may continue to test positive for pregnancy until approximately 120 days after conception because the endometrial cups may continue to secrete hormones until that time.
- Immunologic tests: newer tests (enzyme-linked immunosorbent assay [ELISA], Mare Immunologic Pregnancy test, Direct Latex Agglutination) that are being developed for pregnancy diagnosis after 35 to 40 days. The ELISA appears to be more accurate from day 35 to 90 than the other tests; after day 90, all tests are accurate.

FETAL SEX DETERMINATION

Ultrasound (per rectum) can be used to determine the sex of a fetus, with the optimum time between approximately day 60 and 75. It is accomplished by measuring the location of the developing genitals (genital tubercle) from the tail or umbilicus. In males the genital tubercle is closer to the umbilicus; in females, it is closer to the tail (Fig. 11-56). This method is 99% accurate when performed by experienced clinicians. Timing of the exam is critical, since the uterus begins to fall over the pelvic brim during exactly the same timeframe.

Sex can also be determined by transabdominal ultrasound scanning for specific male or female genitalia; the optimum time for this approach is from 100 to 220 days. After 220 days, the size and positioning of the fetus make sex determination by any approach difficult.

UTERINE CULTURE

The most common cause of infertility in the mare is uterine infection with bacteria.

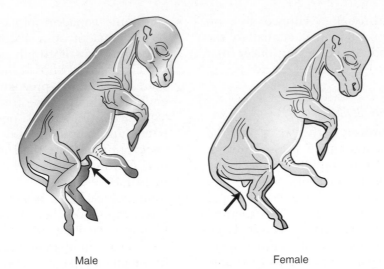

Male   Female

Fig. 11-56. Location of the genital tubercle in the male and female fetus. (From Reef VB: *Equine diagnostic ultrasound*, St Louis, 1998, Saunders.)

Mares with uterine infection generally have difficulty conceiving and supporting a pregnancy. Unlike other domestic species, uterine infections in horses are usually clinically "silent," with minimal or no external signs such as vulvar discharge or irritation. Systemic illness with signs of septicemia and fever is also unusual; most infections are fairly superficial in the uterine lining, and the bacteria do not gain entry into the bloodstream in significant numbers (the notable exception is uterine infection after foaling; after foaling, the separation of the placenta exposes many blood vessels in the uterine wall, and bacteria can gain ready entrance into the bloodstream). Therefore the only clue that a mare may have uterine infection is repeated unsuccessful breedings, either failing to conceive or conceiving and losing the embryo early in pregnancy. This usually prompts the client to call a veterinarian.

Performing a uterine culture can confirm the presence or absence of uterine infection. Sensitivity testing can also be performed to guide proper antibiotic therapy. Some breeders culture mares routinely at the beginning of the breeding season so that treatment of "dirty" mares can be pursued early on.

A uterine culturette is used to obtain the culture. Culturettes are commercially available and are generally about 24 to 30 inches in length. They consist of an outer protective plastic sleeve and an inner cotton-tipped swab. Most have a guarded tip, which is a "trap door" cap that prevents contamination of the swab as it is passes through the vulva, vagina, and cervix. Once in the uterus, the veterinarian presses forward on the swab and the tip opens to let the swab tip through.

Equipment
- ±Sterile OB sleeve or sterile rectal sleeve
- ±Vaginal speculum and light source
- Sterile water-soluble lubricant (KY Jelly)
- Uterine culturette
- Culture medium or transport tube

Procedure

The mare is restrained and the tail held or tied away from the perineum. The perineal/vulvar area is prepped routinely. The veterinarian may either pass the culturette manually, with the hand in a sterile plastic sleeve, or visually through a vaginal speculum. The uterine culturette is passed through the cervix and used to swab the lining of the uterus. Once the culturette is withdrawn, the cotton swab tip is collected and used for standard bacterial culture procedures; to avoid contaminating the swab, the guarded tip may be cut off or held out of the way. The cotton tip is commonly broken or cut free from the culturette stick and placed into a sterile glass tube or culture medium for transport to the laboratory. If transportation to the laboratory is delayed, the swab may dry, which will kill bacteria. Adding a small amount of sterile saline to the swab and refrigeration may delay drying.

Analysis of the sample commonly includes an air-dried smear for Gram's staining, as well as culture plating on blood agar and a gram-negative culture medium. Plates are incubated at 37° C (98.6° F) and checked daily for growth. Some practitioners request quantification (number of bacterial colonies) in addition to bacterial identification.

UTERINE INFUSION

Infusion is a method of delivering liquids into the uterus. There are several indications for the procedure:

- Treatment of uterine infection: Antibiotics are diluted in a sterile solution (such as sterile saline or LRS) and infused into the uterus. This may be repeated daily for several days.
- Routine flushing (lavage) of the uterus after an abortion or after foaling.
- "Postbreeding" infusion to prepare the uterus to receive an embryo.

The volume of liquid infused depends on the underlying reason for the infusion and may range from less than 100 ml for inseminations to several gallons in the case of postfoaling lavage. In the case of uterine lavage, the goal is to remove debris and exudates from the uterus; therefore the fluids are usually removed by siphon or internal massage. In the case of antibiotics and insemination, the goal is for the infused material to remain in the uterus. Mares often attempt to expel the infused material by assuming a urination stance and straining; if the infusion is intended to stay in the uterus, the mare should not be allowed to assume this position. Walking the mare briskly for several minutes after uterine infusion may help prevent this from occurring.

Equipment

- ±Sterile OB sleeve or sterile rectal sleeve
- ±Vaginal speculum and light source
- Sterile water-soluble lubricant
- ±Disposable uterine infusion pipette
- ±Fluid line (standard IV, arthroscopy, or bell IV)
- ±Sterile 60 ml syringes
- Infusion fluids

Procedure

The mare is restrained and the tail held or tied away from the perineum. The perineal/vulvar area is prepped routinely. The veterinarian gives the infusion by passing a uterine infusion pipette (or a fluid line) through the cervix into the uterus; infusion pipettes may be passed manually, with the hand in a sterile plastic sleeve, or visually through a vaginal speculum. Once the pipette or fluid line is in position, the fluids are delivered by attaching either a syringe or fluid line connected to the infusion fluids. Gravity flow or pressurized flow may be used. Immediately following the infusion, the mare is walked briskly for several minutes if the infused material is intended to remain in the uterus.

ARTIFICIAL INSEMINATION

Artificial insemination (AI) of the mare is basically performed as described earlier for uterine infusions, with a few alterations. All spermicidal chemicals must be avoided. Preparation of the perineum should be with mild soap (such as Ivory liquid), rather than surgical scrub solutions.

The semen should be protected from exposure to air, sunlight, and extreme heat or cold. Fresh semen is used immediately. Cooled semen is usually kept in plastic bags housed in a special insulated container (the Hamilton Equitaner is most popular). Cooled semen should be left in the container until it is ready to be used. It is not necessary to warm cooled semen; the warmth of the mare's reproductive tract is sufficient. After preparation of the mare, the plastic bags containing the semen are opened; the semen is aspirated into 35- or 60-ml syringes; at least 1 to 2 ml of semen should be left for semen analysis (to be performed immediately before or after the insemination procedure). Nonspermicidal syringes that do not have a rubber plunger are commercially available.

Frozen semen is stored in 0.5 to 5.0 ml straws in liquid nitrogen; the straws require brief thawing in a warm water bath just before use. Some of the straws are designed for insertion into special insemination guns, rather than aspirating the semen into a syringe.

The veterinarian or technician manually places an insemination pipette through the cervix into the uterus. The syringe containing the semen is attached to the pipette and slowly administered. To discourage straining and expulsion of the semen, it is common to walk the mare for several minutes after the procedure.

Performing multiple inseminations, every 24 to 48 hours, is common while the mare is in heat. Ultrasound exams are commonly used to follow development of the follicle and confirm ovulation so that inseminations may be optimally timed. This is especially useful when the volume of semen available is limited.

ENDOMETRIAL (UTERINE) BIOPSY

Biopsy of the lining of the uterus is done to evaluate the histological condition of the endometrium, usually as part of an assessment of a mare's fertility. The endometrium contains the endometrial glands, which support and nourish the embryo. The endometrium is also the site for implantation and development of the placenta. Uterine infections, trauma from foaling, and aging may cause abnormalities such as atrophy of the endometrial glands, fibrosis around the glands, and inflammation that can interfere with the ability to support pregnancy. Biopsy allows a histopathologist to examine the condition of the endometrium and assess the probability of the mare being able to support a pregnancy. The histopathologist usually assigns a grade of 1, 2, or 3 to the specimen, with grade 1 representing a normal or minimally abnormal specimen, grade 2 representing mild to moderate pathology, and grade 3 representing severe or irreversible pathology.

The endometrial biopsy is only one piece of information used to evaluate fertility; it is not used as the only criteria to assure or condemn a mare's future as a breeding animal. Some mares with grade 1 uteruses cannot maintain a pregnancy, and likewise, mares with grade 3 uteruses have been successfully bred. The biopsy is only part of the puzzle and is best used as a management tool for breeding.

The biopsy is obtained with a 70 cm length ($\approx$28 inch) stainless steel uterine biopsy forceps (Fig. 11-57). The forceps should be sterilized. The forceps have alligator jaws and can obtain a tissue sample approximately 1.5 mm long and 4 mm wide. It may be necessary to use a small syringe needle

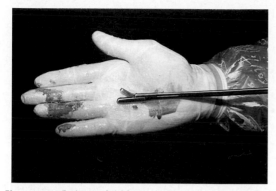

Fig. 11-57. Endometrial biopsy instrument, with the jaws open. (From Colahan PT et al: *Equine medicine and surgery*, ed 5, vol 2, St Louis, 1999, Mosby.)

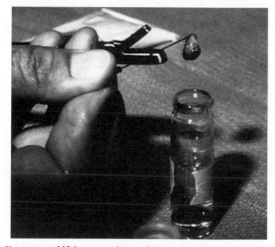

Fig. 11-58. Lifting an endometrial specimen from the biopsy forceps with a small-gauge needle. (From Colahan PT et al: *Equine medicine and surgery*, ed 5, vol 2, St Louis, 1999, Mosby.)

to carefully retrieve the sample from the forceps jaws (Fig. 11-58). Once retrieved, the sample is placed in a liquid fixative; the technician should consult the laboratory for the preferred method of fixation. Common fixatives include Bouin's fixative, 10% buffered formalin, and 70% alcohol. Samples should not sit in Bouin's fixative for more than 24 hours.

Equipment

- Sterile OB sleeve
- Sterile water-soluble lubricant
- Sterile uterine biopsy forceps

Procedure

The mare is restrained and the tail held or tied away from the perineum. The perineal/vulvar area is prepped routinely. This is a two-step procedure; the veterinarian first places the biopsy forceps through the vagina and cervix, into the uterus. The hand is then withdrawn from the vagina and reinserted into the rectum. With one hand in the rectum and the other hand controlling the biopsy instrument handles, the instrument is positioned against the uterine wall and the tissue sample obtained. The mare may experience temporary discomfort when the sample is snipped. The instrument is then withdrawn, and the tissue sample placed in the proper fixative. No special aftercare is required.

CASLICK'S SURGERY

The vulva forms an important protective seal for the vagina. Normally, when a female defecates, the fecal material and liquid fall directly to the ground; this is possible because the anus and vulva are aligned in a vertical plane. However, in some females, the anus is located more cranially than the vulva ("sunken anus"), resulting in a sloping perineum (Fig. 11-59). In extreme cases, a vulvar "shelf" exists below the anus. These abnormal conformations result in abnormal contact with fecal material when it is voided, and if the lips of the vulva do not form a perfect seal, the material can easily enter the vagina. Because the vagina leads to the cervix, and thereby the uterus, contaminants in the vagina can enter the uterus and cause uterine infection; this is one of the most common causes of uterine infections.

The lips of the vulva also guard against involuntary aspiration of air into the vagina.

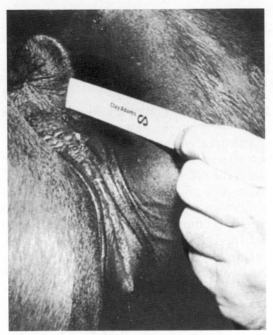

Fig. 11-59. Example of a sunken anus with sloping of the vulva. (From Auer JA, Stick JA: *Equine surgery*, ed 2, St Louis, 1999, Saunders.)

When air enters the vagina (pneumovagina or "windsucking"), it may carry dust, dirt, fecal matter, and other contaminants with it. Faulty conformation of the vulva and vulvar lips may result in pneumovagina.

Abnormal vulvar conformation may be inherited and is apparent at a young age. A sunken anus may also be acquired later in life and is a normal occurrence in old mares. Thin females also tend toward this conformation. Breeding and foaling injuries may tear the vulva and result in scarring, which prevents the lips from meeting and forming an effective seal.

Caslick's surgery is the most common reproductive surgery performed on females. It is done to treat pneumovagina and prevent contamination of the vagina. It is also commonly performed on racehorses when they enter race training due to the widely held belief that females running at top speeds aspirate air, even if the vulva has a good conformation.

Equipment

- Rectal sleeve/nonsterile lubricant
- Tail wrap or bandaging material
- Sterile surgical gloves
- Local anesthetic, 6- or 12-ml syringe, small-gauge needle (22-ga to 25-ga)
- Nonabsorbable suture, 2-0 (usually on reel)
- ±Nonabsorbable suture, 0, or sterile umbilical tape, for breeder's stitch
- Standard "laceration pack"
  - Needle holders
  - Thumb tissue forceps
  - Operating scissors
  - Surgical scissors (Metzenbaum and Mayo)
  - Scalpel handle and No. 10 surgical blade
  - Sterile 4 × 4 gauze squares
  - Surgical needles, cutting or reverse-cutting

Patient Preparation

Tetanus immunization status should be confirmed. The procedure is performed under local anesthesia of the vulva. The horse will need to be restrained, usually with a twitch; some horses require tranquilization. The surgeon may perform a rectal exam to remove feces from the rectum. The tail is then wrapped and secured out of the surgical field, and the perineum is prepped with surgical scrub soap and clean water. The surgeon anesthetizes the vulvar lips with several milliliters of local anesthetic, and a final scrub of the site is performed.

Procedure

A strip of vulvar mucosa is either split with a scalpel blade or removed with surgical scissors; this is done only across the dorsal aspect of the vulva. The ventral aspect must be left open so that the horse can urinate normally. The veterinarian uses several anatomical landmarks to determine the proper length of tissue to remove. The bleeding tissue edges are then brought together with suture, forming a side-to-side bridge of tissue that will heal with scar tissue.

Sometimes a single additional heavy-gauge suture may be placed across the most ventral aspect of the suture line. This single stitch, known as a "breeder's stitch," protects the integrity of the surgical site while it heals. Breeding or performing vaginal procedures on the female with the breeder's stitch in place is possible.

Aftercare

Antibiotic ointment may be placed on the incision line. The owner is instructed to keep the area clean. If material accumulates on the sutures, it may be gently removed by picking with clean gauze squares; however, wiping or scrubbing directly across the sutures should be avoided. Sutures are removed in 10 to 21 days.

If a pregnant mare has been "sewn down," the tissue should be "released" before foaling. If foaling occurs through the tissue bridge, it may tear severely and lead to more disfigurement of the vulva. Release of the site is done by cleansing the area and using scissors or a scalpel to separate the tissue on midline. Since the tissue is scar tissue, it is devoid of nerves and therefore does not require desensitization. However, as with any reproductive procedure, the horse should be properly restrained.

EMBRYO TRANSFER

A female horse cannot produce more than one foal per year with natural methods. Embryo transfer allows the possibility of multiple offspring from a single female each year, more than could be obtained naturally. Another advantage of embryo transfer is that the donor mare can remain in competition (racing, showing, etc.), without ever becoming pregnant herself. Embryo transfer consists of the following basic steps:

- Ovulation: The donor mare is monitored closely (via palpation or ultrasound) for time of ovulation or hormonally manipulated to induce ovulation.
- Breeding: The donor mare is bred by natural or (more commonly) artificial insemination.
- Embryo recovery: The donor's uterus is flushed 7 to 9 days after ovulation to recover an embryo (or possibly two embryos, if twin conception occurs); this is called *nonsurgical transvaginal recovery*. A two-way Foley catheter is positioned through the cervix and secured by inflating the cuff; several liters of specially prepared saline solution are infused (1 L at a time) and then drained by gravity flow into a special collection container that contains a filter cup to trap the embryo (Fig. 11-60).
- Embryo identification: The contents of the filter cup are poured into a sterile "search dish" and examined with a stereomicroscope (15×). Once identified, a special pipette is used to aspirate the embryo and place it in a special culture medium. The embryo is kept at room temperature until transferal, which should occur within 2 hours after recovery. Embryos may also be placed in a special embryo transport medium and stored (or shipped) for transfer within 12 to 24 hours.
- Embryo transfer: The embryo is transferred to a recipient mare that has been hormonally synchronized to prepare her reproductive tract for pregnancy. The embryo may be transferred surgically through a standing flank procedure (preferred) or ventral midline approach with general anesthesia, or it may be transferred nonsurgically through the vaginal/cervical route. The recipient carries the pregnancy and delivers and raises the foal. Parturition and lactation

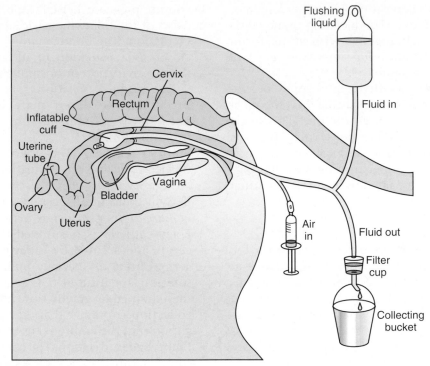

Fig. 11-60. Embryo flushing via a two-way Foley catheter. (From Reed SM, Bayly WM, Sellon DC: *Equine internal medicine*, ed 2, St Louis, 2004, Saunders.)

are no different from naturally conceived pregnancies.

Potentially, an embryo may be recovered from each estrous cycle; a single mare may therefore provide an average of six to eight embryos per breeding season. Some breed registries do not allow embryo transfer or limit the number of foals per year that can be registered to a single dam. Superovulation, which uses hormonal manipulation to induce ovulation of multiple eggs during a single estrous cycle, has been successful in cattle; it has not been perfected in the horse.

OBSTETRICAL PROCEDURES

Dystocia literally means "difficult birth." Parturition in the horse is rapid and somewhat explosive when compared to other species. Fortunately, the incidence of dystocia in mares is low compared to other large animal domestic species; however, the flip side is that when dystocia does occur in the horse, the consequences may be disastrous, and recovery of a live foal is not often achieved. This is due to rapid separation of the placenta from the uterus during delivery; foals cannot withstand being retained in the birth canal for long periods of time because their only means of oxygen—the placenta—ceases to function as separation proceeds. If a foal is not delivered and breathing on its own within about 45 to 60 minutes of the onset of stage 2 of labor (water breaking), it will likely be lost.

There are several causes of dystocia, which may be generally divided into fetal causes and maternal causes. Fetal causes are more common and include malformations of the fetus ("fetal monsters"; cannot conform to the shape of the birth canal), stillbirths (fetus cannot position itself for delivery), large fetal size compared to the size of the birth canal, and abnormal fetal presentation (fetal malposition). Maternal causes include a compromised birth canal in the mare (pelvic fractures, old injuries, etc.), uterine torsion, and ruptures of the supporting structures of the pelvis and abdominal wall.

The most common cause of dystocia in horses is fetal malposition. Normally, the fetus is mobile within the uterus during gestation. Just before birth, the fetus must orient itself to the normal head-first, forelegs extended, "head-diving" position that allows a normal delivery (Fig. 11-61). Any deviation from this position will likely result in inability to be expelled from the uterus (i.e., dystocia). Flexed legs, a flexed neck, "belly up" posture, breech (posterior) presentation, or a fetus that is dead and cannot reposition itself all lead to delivery problems.

Signs of malposition include appearance of the nose with no hooves or just one hoof showing, hooves that are not facing toward the ground, and failure of any part of the fetus to appear at the vulva within 20 to 30 minutes after rupture of the chorioallantoic sac ("water breaking").

Dystocia is a true emergency situation. The technician should be familiar with the procedures and equipment used to treat dystocias in order to provide assistance under what is usually a tense situation for everyone involved.

The first step in attending a mare in dystocia is to evaluate her for signs of urgent conditions such as hemorrhage and shock. Treatment for these conditions is necessary before beginning obstetrical manipulations. Once the mare's condition is stabilized, the veterinarian proceeds with examination of the dystocia. Physical restraint must be adequate

for the situation; behavior is unpredictable during delivery (stage 2 of labor), and mares may stand or lie down with little warning. Stocks are not recommended. It is preferable to perform the exam and treatment in an area where personnel can move easily to safety. Chemical restraint and/or caudal epidural anesthesia may be used to minimize straining by the mare; it is difficult (and dangerous) to examine the fetus or treat the dystocia while the mare is straining, often violently, to deliver the fetus.

Once the mare is restrained, a rectal exam may be performed, usually followed by a vaginal exam. The tail should be wrapped and the perineal area cleaned for the vaginal exam; these procedures must be performed thoroughly but promptly, since time is precious. The clinician either wears plastic sleeves or uses scrubbed hands and arms to enter the vagina, depending on personal preference. Sterile procedures are not necessary; parturition is not a sterile process, but it should nonetheless be kept as clean as possible.

Once the cause of the dystocia is diagnosed and the condition of the fetus determined, the veterinarian will advise the client of the options available and must proceed rapidly to save both mare and foal, if possible. There are three primary methods of treating dystocias:

• Mutation and delivery by traction
• Fetotomy
• Caesarean section

Mutation and Delivery by Traction

This is the most common procedure and is almost always the first method attempted to resolve the dystocia. Basically, mutation means to change the position of the fetus so that it can be delivered. It is extremely difficult to reposition a fetus while it is in the birth canal; the fetus is often wedged in the canal, and there simply is not enough room to maneuver. Therefore it is usually necessary

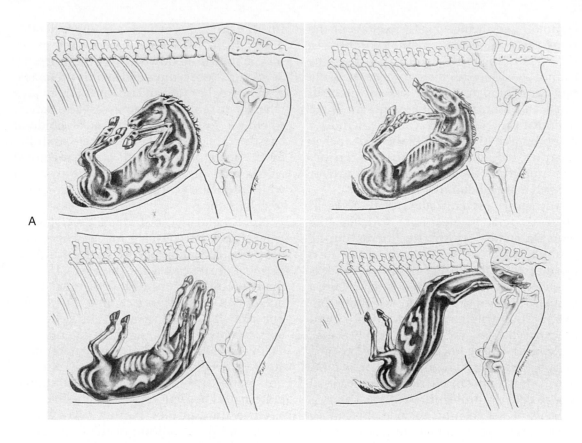

A

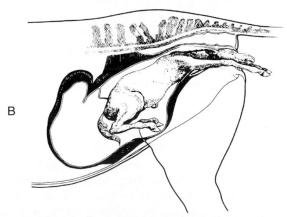

B

Fig. 11-61. A, Fetal rotation during early labor. **B,** Final normal fetal delivery posture, lateral view. (From Colahan PT et al: *Equine medicine and surgery,* ed 5, vol 2, Mosby, 1999.)

to repel (push) the fetus back into the uterus in order to have enough space to reposition it. Repelling the fetus can be difficult; sometimes the mare is placed on an incline, with her head facing downhill, to assist the fetus going back into the uterus. In extreme cases the mare may be anesthetized and her hindquarters lifted with a hoist.

Lubrication is essential for obstetrical maneuvers, especially if the fetus is to be repositioned and/or pulled from the birth canal. It is common to use an NGT and pump to instill several liters or even gallons of lubricant into the vagina and uterus; an adequate amount should be available. The lubricant should be clean but does not have to be sterile.

Once the malposition is corrected (if it can be corrected), attempts are made to deliver the fetus by traction. Traction (pulling) on the fetus may be applied directly with the hands or through various obstetrical instruments designed to get a firm hold on the fetus' limbs and/or head and neck. These instruments should be clean and may be disinfected before and during use by placing them in a stainless steel bucket with water and disinfectant solution. The most common instruments used are obstetrical chains (or nylon straps with "D" rings) and handles (Fig. 11-62). By placing the chains (or straps) around the limbs, the clinician can bring the fetus into the proper position; the handles can be attached and passed to assistants to help the clinician apply traction. If the fetus is dead, other instruments such as blunt eye hooks, double-action sharp-pointed Krey hooks, wire obstetrical snares, and rope nooses may be used. Fetal extractors, commonly known as "calf jacks," are routinely used in cattle but are not designed for use in horses; they may cause unnecessary trauma to the mare's reproductive tract.

The traction team should work together, applying force under the direction of the

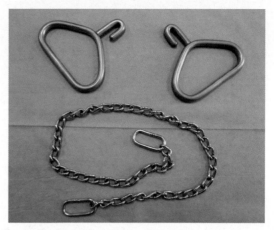

Fig. 11-62. Obstetrical chain and handles.

clinician. Traction is always applied with gradual, smooth motions; sharp, jerking motions should be avoided. The natural pathway of delivery is not in a straight line behind the mare; rather, it follows a curved path from the pelvis down toward the ground. In order to simulate the natural arc of delivery, traction is applied toward the ground at a 45-degree angle, if the mare is standing. If the mare is recumbent, the same path should be recreated as if the mare were standing. Liberal amounts of lubricant should be available to assist the delivery.

Fetotomy

If the fetus is dead and cannot be delivered by mutation and traction, a fetotomy may be performed. This involves making one or more cuts through the fetus to amputate portions of the limbs, head, or neck and then removing the severed portions. Doing so reduces the size of the fetus and also allows removal of parts that are rigid and unable to conform to the birth canal. One to three transections are generally sufficient and must be carefully performed to prevent lacerating the mare's reproductive tract. The mare is sedated and given a caudal epidural for the procedure.

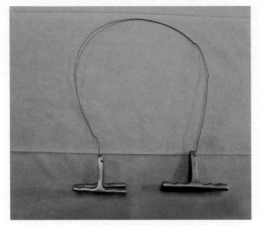

Fig. 11-63. Wire saw and handles. The wire is supplied on a spool and cut to the desired length. The handles are then clamped to secure the ends of the wire.

Transections are performed with special guarded, handheld fetotomy knives or by using obstetrical wire as a saw blade (Gigli's wire saw) (Fig. 11-63). In order to protect the mare's reproductive tract from the sawing action, the wire is passed through a rigid metal tube (fetotome) that extends from the vulva through the cervix. The wire is placed internally and looped around the part to be amputated, and the wire ends are brought outside the mare. Handles are attached to each end, and a to-and-fro motion on the handles is used to transform the wire into a cutting instrument. Once the necessary parts have been removed, traction is placed on the remaining portion to remove it. Because amputation may create sharp, exposed pieces of bone, removal must be carefully done to prevent puncturing or lacerating the reproductive tract. Again, liberal lubricant should be available.

Fetotomy avoids major abdominal surgery and has less aftercare, quicker recovery, and fewer complications than a caesarean section. However, the risk of lacerations and punctures of the mare's reproductive organs makes many clinicians reluctant to perform fetotomy. In addition, any prolonged obstetrical procedure tends to damage the lining of the vagina and cervix, resulting in scar tissue and adhesions that interfere with future attempts to conceive and carry a fetus. This risk is higher in horses than in cattle.

Caesarean Section

This is generally the last resort for removal of a fetus, due to the complication rate associated with the procedure. Unlike cattle, which tolerate caesarean section as a standing surgery through the flank, the procedure in horses is usually performed under general anesthesia in dorsal recumbency via a ventral midline incision. Infection (especially peritonitis), septicemia, laminitis, hemorrhage, and retained placentas are not uncommon following caesarean section. Recovery of a live foal from the procedure is unusual, due primarily to the time delay between the onset of the dystocia and the surgical treatment by caesarean section. However, a team of assistants should be prepared to receive and care for the foal if it is alive. If alive, the foal is usually depressed from the effects of the general anesthetic drugs, and resuscitation drugs and equipment should be available.

CARDIOVASCULAR SYSTEM

The cardiovascular system is evaluated primarily by history and physical examination, including careful auscultation of the thoracic cavity. It is common to evaluate the horse at rest and again following exercise. This is done because many questionable findings at rest may disappear at the higher heart rates associated with exercise, which increases the likelihood that the questionable finding is physiological (normal). When exercise accentuates the suspicious finding, such as a murmur that gets louder in intensity, it becomes more likely that the finding is, in fact, pathological, and closer investigation is warranted. The electrocardiogram, diagnostic ultrasound and echocardiography, thoracic radiography, and cardiac catheterization are available as special diagnostics for in-depth examination of the cardiovascular system.

ELECTROCARDIOGRAM (EKG OR ECG)

Because the body consists primarily of water and electrolytes, similar to saltwater, electrical currents are readily conducted throughout the body. It is possible to measure the changes in voltage between any two points on the surface of the body with electrodes and record the findings on paper. This produces a trace called an electrocardiogram (ECG).

The electrocardiogram is useful in determining cardiac rate and rhythm and identifying problems with electrical conduction (arrhythmias) in large animals. However, unlike small animals, it is not highly useful in calculating heart chamber enlargement in large animals because of differences in the anatomy and physiology of the Purkinje fiber system. Fortunately, echocardiography is readily available and more suitable than the ECG for assessing chamber size and myocardial function.

The standard ECG is performed on the standing animal at rest. However, some arrhythmias only occur occasionally or under special circumstances and may be missed by the standard 5- to 10-minute standing ECG exam. Long-term or ambulatory (Holter) ECG monitoring is readily available and useful for detecting intermittent problems. The procedure uses flat electrodes attached to a portable monitor, which is fastened to a surcingle (chest strap) that the horse wears. The ECG is recorded onto magnetic tape and then analyzed with computer software. Holter monitoring is useful for continuous data collection for up to 24 hours or during exercise and recovery but does not allow highly detailed evaluation of the waveforms. Simple heart rate monitors are available to monitor the heart rate only (no ECG trace) and are popular for race and endurance training.

PROCEDURE (STANDING ELECTROCARDIOGRAM)

The ECG machine should be plugged into a grounded circuit to prevent shocking the patient, and the ground beneath the patient should be dry (a dry rubber mat is optimal and reduces the chance of electrical interference). The ground electrode should always be attached to the patient. Patient lead cables 4 to 5 feet in length are desirable for large animal use.

Muscle activity interferes with the accuracy of the ECG; therefore the exam should take place in a quiet environment. The horse should stand squarely, bearing weight evenly on all four legs for the duration of each lead trace. Shivering, skin twitches, and weight shifts all decrease the quality of the trace.

The leads are attached to the animal with alligator clips, rubber straps, or adhesive pads. Alligator clips may pinch the skin too tightly for the comfort of some animals; filing down the serrated points of the alligator clips may increase their comfort. Also, grasping a maximal amount of skin with the clip is more comfortable than grasping a small area. The electrodes must contact the skin, not just the hair of the skin. The contact points should be moistened with an electrode gel or paste. If these are not available, alcohol or a salt-containing solution can be substituted; these tend to evaporate rapidly and may need to be repeatedly applied to maintain effective conduction.

The ECG lead systems used in large animals are basically identical to those used in small animals and are based on Einthoven's triangle. The standard bipolar leads (I, II, III) and the augmented unipolar leads (aVR, aVL, aVF) are used most often. The chest leads (CV6LL, CV6LU, V10, CV6RL, CV6RU) are less commonly used. As with other species, lead II is used most often to calculate heart rate and assess rhythm and waveforms. Lead placement is summarized in Fig. 11-64. For the forelimb leads, the electrodes are placed over the caudal aspect of the forearm, approximately 10 to 15 cm distal to the point of the elbow (olecranon). For the hindlimb leads,

the electrodes are placed over the cranial or lateral aspect of the stifle.

The base-apex lead is popular for monitoring during anesthesia because it is less affected by motion, seldom interferes with the surgical site, and produces large waveforms. The right arm (forelimb) electrode is attached to the skin over the right jugular groove in the caudal one third of the neck or just cranial to the withers on the base of the right side of the neck. The left arm (forelimb)

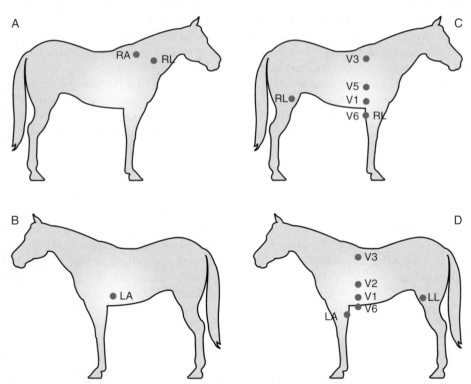

Fig. 11-64. Sites for lead placement for obtaining a base-apex electrocardiogram (ECG) **(A, B)** and a complete ECG **(C, D)** in a horse. The red circles represent the site of attachment for the electrodes. **(A)** Position of the electrode placement on the right side of the horse for obtaining a base-apex ECG using the electrodes from lead I. **(B)** Position of the electrode placement on the left side of the horse for obtaining a base-apex ECG using the electrodes from lead I. **(C)** Position of the electrode placement on the right side of the horse for obtaining a complete ECG. **(D)** Position of the electrode placement on the left side of the horse for obtaining a complete ECG. *LA*, left foreleg (left arm); *LL*, left hindleg (left leg); *RA*, right foreleg (right arm); *RL*, right hindleg (right leg). *V1*, first chest lead (CV6LL); *V2*, second chest lead (CV6LU); *V3*, third chest lead (V10). *V4*, fourth chest lead (CV6RL); *V5*, fifth chest lead (CV6RU). (From Marr C: *Cardiology of the horse*, St Louis, 1999, Saunders.)

electrode is attached to the skin of the chest wall at the level of the left olecranon, which is the area of the cardiac apex. The right leg electrode serves as the ground electrode and may be attached to the skin of the horse at any convenient location remote from the heart. The lead selector is positioned to lead I to complete the setup.

The paper recording speed is usually 25 mm per second in large animals, though 50 mm/sec can be used effectively. Sensitivity is set at 1 mV/cm. Because of the low heart rates in large animals, it is desirable to record leads for several minutes each. Labeling the tracing immediately to identify different leads is always wise.

Interpretation of the ECG uses the same techniques as for other species. The heart rate and rhythm are determined, and the amplitude and length of the waveforms can be measured. Data have been published giving approximate normal ranges of waveform amplitude and duration for both horses and ponies and have even been determined for some individual breeds. Several differences in waveforms should be noted in horses (versus small animals):

- The P wave in normal horses at rest is usually bifid (double-peaked).
- The T wave in horses is variable and should not be overinterpreted. T wave abnormalities seldom correlate with cardiac disease. The T wave in lead II and the base-apex lead is commonly biphasic (negative portion and positive portion).

- Wandering pacemaker (regular rhythm, with varying shapes of the P wave) is fairly common and is usually normal.
- Second-degree atrioventricular (A-V) block is present in a high percentage of horses at rest and is normal.

SUGGESTED READING

Allen T: *Manual of equine dentistry,* St Louis, 2003, Mosby.

Baker GJ, Easley J: *Equine dentistry,* St Louis, 2002, Saunders.

Butler KD: *The principles of horseshoeing II,* Maryville, Mo, 1985, Doug Butler Publisher.

Colahan PT et al: *Equine medicine and surgery,* ed 5, St Louis, 1999, Mosby.

McCurnin DM, Bassert JM: *Clinical textbook for veterinary technicians,* ed 6, St Louis, 2006, Saunders.

Noakes DE, Parkinson TJ, England GCW: *Arthur's veterinary reproduction and obstetrics,* ed 8, London, 2001, Saunders.

Orsini JA, Divers TJ: *Manual of equine emergencies,* ed 2, St Louis, 2003, Saunders.

Reed SM: Neurologic diseases, *Vet Clin North Am Equine Pract* 3:255-440, 1987.

Speirs VC: *Clinical examination of horses,* St Louis, 1997, Saunders.

Stashak TS: *Adams' lameness in horses,* ed 5, Philadelphia, 2002, Lippincott Williams & Wilkins.

White NA: *The equine acute abdomen,* Philadelphia, 1990, Lea & Febiger.

12

Equine Euthanasia and Necropsy Techniques

EUTHANASIA

Although the general public is less likely to look upon large animals as companion animals, those who work with large animals know differently. They can be companions in every sense of the word, and saying goodbye to a friend is never easy. The grief and bereavement that one may feel after loss of a special horse, cow, sheep, goat, or pig is every bit as real as grieving a cherished dog, cat, or bird. Even people who have a primarily economic relationship with large animals often develop a fondness for a few special individuals. But regardless of the individual's relationship with his or her animals—large or small, companion or business—it is the responsibility of humans to try to provide a humane ending when a life, for whatever reason, comes to its conclusion.

There are many ways to euthanize a horse; however, they are not all necessarily humane. People tend to form strong opinions about which methods are acceptable and which are not; oftentimes these opinions are based on rumors or observations made by well-meaning individuals who lack the medical knowledge to understand the response of an animal's body to the method of death. Sometimes the opinion is formed after watching a euthanasia that was improperly performed or had an unexpected complication. Veterinary technicians deal with euthanasia on an almost daily basis and should not hesitate to form their own independent thoughts and opinions about the various ways to euthanize a horse. While these opinions are (and should) be based largely on the technician's own experiences with equine euthanasia, it is wise to base these opinions on medically sound information.

It is legally advisable to have the owner or an agent for the owner sign a euthanasia consent form. These forms can even be signed in advance for gravely ill horses in a hospital setting or when an owner is traveling so that a suffering animal can be promptly euthanized without waiting to make contact with the owner. It is sometimes necessary for the veterinarian to consult with an insurance company before euthanasia is performed, though this is not necessary in an emergency situation when an animal is clearly suffering. In such an instance, the horse may be euthanized and the insurance company notified as soon as possible.

METHODS OF EUTHANASIA

When selecting an appropriate method of euthanasia, many factors must be considered (Box 12-1). According to the *2000 Report of the American Veterinary Medical Association Panel on Euthanasia,* the following are considered acceptable, humane methods for equine euthanasia:

- Intravenous (IV) injection of barbituric acid derivatives: This is the *preferred* method of euthanasia for horses. Pentobarbital or pentobarbital-containing solutions

12-1 Factors Affecting Euthanasia

The following factors are considered when selecting the best method for euthanasia:

Patient Factors
- Physical status/underlying diseases
- Degree of domestication and human handling
- Emergency euthanasia versus nonemergency euthanasia
- Possibility of infectious disease
- Patient size and weight

Human Factors
- Level of training of person administering euthanasia
- Availability and level of training of assistants
- Safety
- Owner's wishes
- Aesthetics

Facility/Equipment Factors
- Availability of drugs/injection supplies
- Availability of equipment for physical euthanasia methods (captive bolt pistol, firearms)
- Location of euthanasia procedure
- Method and availability of restraint
- Disposition of the body after euthanasia

---

are preferred. Because of the large volume of these solutions required, an IV catheter is suggested to facilitate the injection, though this may not always be necessary or practical. The solution should be injected rapidly; therefore a 14- to 16-gauge (ga) needle or catheter is required. The jugular veins are the safest locations for the person administering the injection; if the veins are thrombosed or inaccessible, other large veins such as the cephalic or lateral thoracic veins may be used, with caution. Barbiturates are controlled substances, subject to U.S. Drug Enforcement Administration regulations.

- Penetrating captive bolt: acceptable. This method is preferred over gunshot. The person performing the procedure should be trained in the proper anatomic location and technique. The horse should be properly restrained. Loss of consciousness is extremely rapid (instantaneous), but muscle activity may continue and be objectionable to observe.

- Inhalant anesthetics: acceptable. Administration of an overdose of anesthetic gases such as halothane, isoflurane, enflurane, sevoflurane, etc., is acceptable, but the large volumes required are costly and may be difficult to administer in some circumstances.

- IV injection of potassium chloride (KCl) combined with prior general anesthesia: acceptable. If the animal is in a surgical plane of anesthesia, KCl may be used to induce euthanasia. It must *never* be used in a conscious or lightly anesthetized animal. KCl causes cardiac arrest and is more rapid than an overdose of inhalant gas. It is also considerably less expensive and is not a controlled substance.

- Gunshot: conditionally acceptable, when other methods are not available. The person performing the procedure should be trained in the use of firearms and in the proper anatomic location and technique. The horse should be properly restrained. Loss of consciousness following a properly delivered projectile is extremely rapid (instantaneous), but muscle activity may continue and be objectionable to observe.

- IV injection of chloral hydrate: conditionally acceptable, but only after sedation. Chloral hydrate affects the cerebrum slowly; therefore the prior sedation is necessary to keep the animal restrained while the chloral hydrate takes effect.

Neuromuscular blocking agents are absolutely condemned in all species as euthanasia agents, but they may be used in emergency situations as *restraining* agents to gain control of a dangerous animal for euthanasia. Once the dangerous situation is under control, one of the acceptable euthanasia methods above should be used as soon as possible. Neuromuscular blocking agents should not be used to perform the actual euthanasia.

There are some logistical problems related to the euthanasia of large animals. Technicians can provide valuable information to clients, who seldom are prepared to deal with the specifics of the procedure. The actual location of the procedure should be carefully selected, if time allows. For instance, euthanasia inside a stall or building creates the question of how to remove the body from the building. (This usually means dragging the body manually or with machinery such as a tractor or truck winch.) The size and weight of most large animals makes removal difficult; therefore it is usually preferable to perform the procedure outside. This may not always be possible, especially when the animal's disease makes it impossible or dangerous to try to move it to an outdoor location.

When barbiturate solutions or other chemicals are used to euthanize animals, the chemical residues may be toxic to predator animals that eat the tissues of the deceased animal. If disposal of the body will be delayed, it may be prudent to cover the body with heavy plastic or tarp to discourage scavenging. This may be more of a factor when the body is outside in an open field setting, though many barns are readily accessible to dogs and other animals.

As with euthanasia of any species, the owner should be asked if he or she wishes to be present during the procedure. Time to say goodbye should be provided. Standing equine euthanasia tends to make more of an impression on people because of the visual effect of such a large animal falling to the ground, unlike small animals that can be held in the arms and cradled gently as they collapse. Combined with possible involuntary muscle activity and reflexes persisting for several minutes, whether or not to view it is a significant decision (especially where children are concerned). If the owner will view the procedure, the author strongly recommends that he or she be given the opportunity to be informed about the horse's physical responses to euthanasia *beforehand* so that they are not caught off guard by the natural reflex motions and muscle activity that often accompany death. This information should not be forced on the client; rather, simply asking "would you like for me to explain the procedure— how the drugs work, and what you're likely to see?" gives the client an option. Most clients say yes, but some may find the details disturbing and not wish to hear them. If a client does wish to hear the information, keep the explanation brief and simple, and avoid excessive use of medical terms.

Because of the possible dangers associated with a large, standing animal falling to recumbency, all untrained and nonessential people—owners included—should be instructed to maintain a safe, *specific* distance from the procedure until an "all clear" signal is given by the veterinarian. When the animal is recumbent and limb motion has ceased, it may then be suitable for the "family" to approach the animal.

It is thought best for other members of a species not to witness euthanasia of their own kind; the excitement, involuntary vocalizations, and body odors associated with the procedure may be stressful. However, it is not always possible or practical to completely separate other equines. It is considered acceptable, once the procedure is complete, to allow other horses to interact with the body unless contagious disease has been diagnosed or is a possibility. This is commonly done with mares when their foal dies naturally or by euthanasia. A brief time period (45 to 50 minutes) allows the mare to observe and prod the foal's body; it is believed that this interaction provides the mare a chance to better "accept" the foal's death. Of course, this has never been proven, but many horsemen believe in this practice. Because of the risk of infectious organisms, mares should *not* be allowed to contact or interact with aborted fetuses.

Another major decision concerns disposition of the body. Technicians should be familiar with the options available in their geographical area. These options are first limited by state and local laws, and then by availability. Most states have a time limit on carcass disposal after euthanasia, typically 24 to 72 hours. Burning and burial may be prohibited in some areas, or may be allowed only if special regulations are followed. Some jurisdictions may require a special permit to burn or bury. Clients should know what options are available so that they can select the one they are most comfortable with.

Burial will require excavation of a grave. This is usually done with a backhoe or bulldozer. It is useful to keep a list of local contractors who are willing to perform this service. Excavation may be affected by the time of year, especially in northern climates where the ground freezes in winter, making excavation difficult or impossible. Special considerations include whether the horse will be walked into the grave and euthanized there or whether the body will be pulled/pushed into the grave after death. The veterinarian likely will have a preference for his or her personal safety in each situation. Some people find it objectionable to force an animal to walk into its own grave. Others find it objectionable to watch the body be pushed into the grave by a bulldozer. Different situations call for different approaches.

General guidelines for burial include selecting a site away from any open water sources (such as ponds or creeks) or drinking water sources such as wells. The depth of the hole should be at least 8 feet or deeper but should not penetrate within 5 feet of the water table. If the water table is less than 8 feet, then soil should be mounded above ground to produce above-ground soil coverage. At least 3 to 5 feet of dirt coverage is necessary to prevent scavenging or exposure by weather factors. Covering the body with slaked (hydrated) lime is often required by law; this is done for sanitary reasons and to speed decomposition of the body. Again, local laws should be consulted for specific burial depths, soil types, water table requirements, and carcass coverage.

If burial of the total body is not allowed or not practical, it may be possible to offer the alternative of burying only selected body parts. Burial of the hooves and the heart is a traditional approach that may appeal to some owners. The veterinarian and/or technicians can remove these parts either on the farm or in the clinic (depending on where death occurs) and place them in a selected container for burial or return to the owner. Cremation of the entire body is usually not practical either, and cremation of the hooves and heart is a very acceptable alternative.

Cremation must usually be performed at a state-licensed incineration facility, where strict emission guidelines and temperature requirements must be followed.

If burial is not an option, then removal of the body will be necessary. The body is most often sent for rendering. Pickup is usually provided by a licensed livestock disposal hauler, which may be provided by the rendering company. If possible, euthanasia should be performed in an area that the hauler's truck can easily access. Some local regulations now require that animals euthanized with barbiturates be treated as biomedical waste, with subsequent labeling and handling requirements; livestock disposal haulers may refuse pickup of biomedical waste if they are not certified to transport biohazardous materials. Landfills may be an alternative for disposal in some states; landfills may accept large animal carcasses for a standard or weight-based fee. The phone numbers of rendering and hauling companies/individuals and approximate costs for pickup should be available to clients.

Another concern related to disposition is providing clients with remembrances of their animal. Clients should be asked if they want the halter removed for a keepsake or if they prefer the horse to be buried with the halter. Some clients may want to have the horseshoes. A lock of mane, tail, or forelock is sometimes requested. These are usually removed after death. The client's wishes should be respected, no matter how unusual the request, and any requested item or body part treated with respect.

NECROPSY

Large animal necropsy is performed for the same reasons as small animal necropsy, and the procedures are similar. Necropsy is used to determine or confirm the cause of death and any factors that may have contributed to death. The necropsy consists of a gross visual examination and may extend to include a sample collection for special laboratory examinations such as histopathology, toxicology, microbiology, parasitology, cytology, and chemistry.

Owner permission should always be obtained before the procedure begins. Owners are not always willing to have the procedure performed, and it is not always necessary to have a necropsy performed unless there is something to be gained by it. Likewise, it is not always necessary to perform a complete, total body necropsy procedure. Oftentimes the veterinarian will want to evaluate only certain organs or tissues or collect only specific samples. The procedure may also be affected by insurance coverage, which is common in the horse industry. The insurance company may require that a necropsy be performed and may also specify the samples to be taken.

The timing of the necropsy is of great importance. Autolysis (decomposition), which begins immediately following death, destroys cell architecture and alters many chemical and microbiological findings. Autolysis is accelerated by microorganisms; the gastrointestinal tracts of herbivores contain incredible numbers of microbes, which do not die when the herbivore dies. Other areas of the body such as the respiratory tract and skin also contain numerous microorganisms. Following death of the "host," the microbes can spread throughout the body without much resistance, disrupting tissues as they go. Heat also contributes to the speed of autolysis; heat may come from the external environment, as well as from internal heat created by microbial fermentation in the intestinal tract. Refrigeration of the carcass may delay (but not prevent) autolysis; however, refrigeration for large animals is only available at some clinic or hospital facilities. Therefore most large animal necropsies must be conducted promptly after death in order to yield meaningful results.

The location of the necropsy is important. It is preferable to perform the procedure in a setting that can be readily disinfected and can provide containment of any toxic or infectious materials. Obviously, this ideal setting is seldom available outside of a clinic or hospital. Large animal necropsies are usually messy procedures, especially when the intestinal tract is opened. In a field setting the procedure is ideally done in an area that can be restricted from other animals, away from water and food sources. Covering the ground with hydrated lime or saturating the ground with dilute bleach after the procedure is advised. The ability of the public to view the necropsy must also be anticipated; many laypeople may be disturbed or even offended by the sight or smell of the procedure. Blocking the view with vehicles or makeshift curtains may be helpful.

Documenting the necropsy findings is important. This should be done in the form of a written report of observations. Photographs of the necropsy findings may be advisable in certain circumstances to supplement written descriptions. The report must include an accurate description of the animal, including all identifying marks (natural and artificial); photographs may assist the animal identification. Digital photography can facilitate the recording and storage of photo images.

Before beginning the necropsy, all materials should be assembled. It is desirable to have supplies that are dedicated to necropsies, to minimize possible spread of microorganisms. Standard dissecting equipment for necropsies is used: an assortment of scalpel blades and handles, heavy tissue (Mayo) scissors, Metzenbaum scissors, operating scissors, hemostatic forceps, boning or necropsy knives, sharpening steel, thumb tissue forceps, utility scissors, and a ruler.

Special equipment for large animal necropsies may include large cutting shears (such as long-handled garden pruning shears) or a hand ax for opening the rib cage and a hand saw or Stryker saw for cutting bone. If the carcass is to be closed after the procedure, the closure material (suture, string, twine, etc.) should be readily available.

If samples are to be collected, appropriate culturettes, containers, and fixatives should be gathered. Containers should be labeled before the procedure. The laboratory that will run each test should be consulted for preferred fixatives and handling procedures. Tissues for histopathology are most commonly placed in 10% neutral buffered formalin for preservation; as with small animals, a ratio of 10:1 formalin-to-tissue volume should be maintained in the sample containers. Large animals do *not* require larger tissue samples than small animals; samples thicker than 0.5 to 0.7 cm may impede penetration of the fixative. Ideal samples are 1 cm × 1 cm × 0.5 cm; samples should not exceed 3 cm square.

Protective clothing is a must, especially where zoonotic disease is a concern. Plastic arm sleeves (rectal sleeves) are recommended for exploring the abdominal and thoracic cavities; latex examination gloves placed over the arm sleeve can provide an additional layer of protection for the hands, as well as a more secure grip on instruments. Coveralls are commonly worn for large animal necropsy, and a plastic apron gives additional protection. Rubber boots or disposable shoe covers should be worn. A cap, facemask, and eye protection are important when zoonotic organisms may exist. Whatever is worn during the necropsy should be covered, removed, or disinfected before attending other animals.

EQUINE NECROPSY PROCEDURE

There is no single, correct technique for performing a necropsy. The order that the organ systems are examined and the method of obtaining samples can be modified for individual preference and different situations. What is important is to be thorough, so that nothing is overlooked. Establishing a routine procedure is helpful, and checklists can help assure that the examination and sample collection are complete. A basic necropsy examination procedure is described below; in-depth methodology and techniques are well described in other references.

1. **Position:** The standard body position for equine necropsy is left lateral recumbency, though this can be modified for different situations.

2. **Examine the body for external lesions, parasites, and body condition:** Examine all mucous membranes and body openings, including the oral cavity. Examine any surgical incisions and veins that have been catheterized or used for injections.

3. **Skin incision:** A ventral midline incision is made through the skin and subcutaneous tissue from the xiphoid process extending caudally to the prepuce or mammary gland. The incision is directed toward the right inguinal canal to avoid the prepuce/penis in the male or mammary gland in the female, then returns to midline, and continues to the anus. Returning to the xiphoid process, extend the skin incision to the chin along ventral midline. Reflect the skin dorsally across the thorax and abdomen.

4. **Reflect the limbs:** Returning to the right inguinal canal, a knife is used to incise the joint capsule of the coxofemoral joint and the ligament of the head of the femur. The hindlimb is reflected dorsally. The right forelimb is reflected dorsally by dissecting along a plane medial to the scapula.

5. **Reflect the prepuce/penis or mammary gland:** Dissection just deep to

these structures will free them from the body wall and allow them to be reflected. The entire mammary gland may be removed if necessary for closer inspection.

6. **Examine the scrotum/testicles/spermatic cord:** If necessary, the scrotum may be opened and the testicles and spermatic cords examined and/or removed.

7. **Open the abdominal cavity:** Great care must be taken not to accidentally incise any abdominal organs; this is especially difficult if the abdomen is bloated. The abdominal wall and peritoneum are entered on ventral midline, through the linea alba. A small incision is carefully made to enter the abdominal cavity through the linea alba, and then either a hand or other instrument is used to form a barrier between the cutting instrument and the organs as the incision is extended cranially to the xiphoid and caudally to the pelvic brim. After completing the ventral midline incision into the abdomen, a second incision is made to connect the caudal aspect of the ventral midline incision with the junction of the vertebral column and the last rib. This forms a triangular flap based along the last rib that can be reflected craniodorsally over the caudal thorax.

   Once the abdominal cavity is exposed, the position of the organs is noted as normal or abnormal, and the volume and appearance of the peritoneal fluid is assessed. Normally the peritoneal fluid is clear and yellow, and the volume is approximately 200 ml. Samples of peritoneal fluid can be obtained at this time. If a urine sample is necessary, it can be aseptically aspirated from the bladder with a needle and syringe.

8. **Open the thoracic cavity:** First, palpate the abdominal aspect of the diaphragm for defects, and then make a small puncture

of the diaphragm to check for negative pressure in the thoracic cavity. The diaphragm should collapse, and the sound of air rushing in may be heard if negative pressure, which is normal, exists.

An ax or pruning shears is used to cut the ribs at the costosternal junctions, being careful not to cut the heart or lungs. Once all ribs have been cut along the sternum, they are cut again approximately 6 inches lateral to the vertebral column. Sever the diaphragm on the right side along its attachment to the last rib. This frees the right rib cage to be reflected dorsally.

The position of the organs is noted as normal or abnormal, and the volume and appearance of the pleural fluid is assessed. Normally the pleural fluid is clear and yellow, and the volume is approximately 100 ml. Samples of pleural fluid can be collected at this time.

9. **Remove the pluck (tongue, trachea, esophagus, heart, and lungs):** These are removed together in one piece, en bloc. First, the tongue is retracted ventrally through an incision between the mandibles; extend the neck and make an incision along the medial aspect of either mandible, being sure that the incision is deep enough to enter the oral cavity. Evert the free portion of the tongue ventrally through the incision, between the mandibles. The mandibular attachments of the tongue will need to be severed to allow complete eversion of the tongue. The hyoid apparatus is then transected with shears to allow the tongue to be freed completely from the oral cavity and pharynx. Once freed, the tongue can be used as a "handle" to elevate and provide tension on the other organs as they are removed. Elevate the tongue, and carefully transect the soft tissue attachments on the lateral and dorsal aspects of the larynx, then the trachea/esophagus,

proceeding caudally to the thoracic inlet, then through the thoracic inlet to the area of the carina. The attachments of the pleura run along the dorsal aspect of the thoracic cavity. The pluck is then attached only by the esophagus, aorta, and caudal vena cava where they penetrate the diaphragm. Cut along the thoracic aspect of the diaphragm to transect these structures where they contact the diaphragm. This will free the pluck. Remove the pluck, and examine the internal surfaces of the rib cage. Return to the head and evaluate the pharynx, guttural pouches, and oral cavity as needed.

10. **Examine the pluck:**
    a. *Tongue:* Make several transverse cuts through the tongue.
    b. *Pharynx:* Open the pharynx; examine the tonsils.
    c. *Esophagus:* Open the esophagus longitudinally along its entire length.
    d. *Thyroid glands*
    e. *Larynx/Trachea/Bronchi:* Open longitudinally.
    f. *Thymus gland:* (if present)
    g. *Lungs:* Palpate all lobes for deep lesions. "Book" the lung by making multiple parallel incisions through the lobes.
    h. *Heart:* Open the pericardial sac and examine the pericardial fluid for volume and appearance. Observe the surface and overall size and shape of the heart.
       Open the heart by first positioning the apex toward the examiner and the right side of the heart to the right side of the examiner:
       • Open the right side of the heart: Incise the right ventricle adjacent to the interventricular septum, along the right longitudinal coronary groove from its apex through the right atrioventricular (A-V) valve into the right atrium. A second

incision is made along the left longitudinal coronary groove from the apex through the right A-V valve and semilunar (pulmonary) valve into the pulmonary artery.

- Open the left side of the heart: Incise the left ventricle along the left coronary groove, continuing through the left A-V valve into the left atrium. The pulmonary vein is identified at its opening into the left atrium and is opened longitudinally. The aorta is opened longitudinally by inserting scissors under the medial cusp of the left A-V valve and cutting through the semilunar (aortic) valve.

Note the contents of each chamber. Rinse the interior surfaces with water, and examine all heart valve leaflets, chordae tendineae, papillary muscle, and endocardium.

i. *Lymph nodes*: Lymph nodes will be encountered in the pharyngeal and tracheobronchial areas. They should be evaluated.

11. **Eviscerate and evaluate the abdominal cavity:**
    a. Remove the omentum and spleen.
    b. Identify and remove the right adrenal gland: located cranial and medial to the right kidney.
    c. Identify and remove the pancreas: located in the mesentery between the base of the cecum and the duodenum, in the dorsal abdomen.
    d. Remove the intestinal tract in segments (stomach, small intestine, large intestine) or remove the entire intestinal tract by transecting the root of the mesentery, the distal small colon, and the distal esophagus just caudal to the diaphragm. It may be beneficial to tie off open segments with string before transection to prevent spillage of contents.
    e. Remove the liver by severing its attachments to the diaphragm.
    f. Identify and remove the left adrenal gland: located cranial and medial to the left kidney.
    g. Remove the kidneys, ureters, and urinary bladder en bloc: Each kidney is dissected free, and the ureter is dissected along its course to the bladder. The urethra is transected, and the attachments of the bladder are cut to free the entire urinary tract.
    h. Remove the ovaries and uterus by pulling them cranially and transecting caudally to the cervix. If the entire female reproductive tract is to be evaluated, skip this step and proceed to open the pelvic cavity.
    i. Remove or evaluate male accessory sex glands and vas deferens if necessary.
    j. Evaluate abdominal aorta: palpate and incise longitudinally with scissors.

12. **Open the pelvic cavity:** Remove the ventral wall of the pelvis by transecting (with a handsaw) the right and left pubic bones parallel to the symphysis pubis, and then continuing the cuts through the obturator foramen and ischium on each side. Evaluate the pelvic organs:
    a. Rectum/Anus
    b. Female reproductive tract (pelvic portion)
    c. Prostate gland (males only)

13. **Evaluate the abdominal and pelvic viscera:**
    a. *Liver:* observe size, shape and color. Palpate for deep lesions and to assess consistency. Book the parenchyma and observe for lesions.
    b. *Pancreas:* observe size, color, consistency.
    c. *Spleen:* separate from the stomach. Palpate for deep lesions. Book the parenchyma and observe for lesions.

d. *Stomach:* open along the greater curvature, including the pylorus. Observe stomach contents. Rinse gently with water and observe the gastric mucosa (excessive water pressure will alter the mucosa).

e. *Intestinal tract:*
   i. Small intestine: Beginning with a small incision into the duodenal lumen, open the small intestine by cutting the mesenteric attachment and tensing 2 to 3 feet of intestine; cut the intestinal wall with scissors (blunt tip inside the lumen). Evaluate the opened segment for content, then rinse and evaluate the mucosa. Repeat the procedure, opening 2 to 3 feet at a time, until the entire length of the small intestine is examined.
   ii. Mesenteric lymph nodes: located in the root of the mesentery
   iii. Colonic lymph nodes: Lay out the large colon and cecum. The lymph nodes are located adjacent to the bowel, within the mesentery.
   iv. Large colon, cecum, transverse colon, small colon: Open with scissors and evaluate contents, mucosa and intestinal wall.

f. *Kidneys/Ureters:* Observe size and shape. Open with a single sagittal incision through the entire parenchyma, from cortex to medulla to renal pelvis. Peel back the renal capsule and evaluate the outer cortical surface. Examine the renal pelvis for shape and contents. Extend incisions longitudinally to open the ureters.

g. *Urinary bladder:* Open and assess contents; examine mucosa and wall thickness.

h. *Adrenal glands:* Section sagitally; evaluate cortex and medulla. Handle gently to avoid creating crushing artifacts.

14. **Musculoskeletal system:** Several skeletal muscles should be incised and examined for color and consistency. Several joints should be opened and the synovial fluid and articular cartilage observed. If bone marrow is needed, the ribs are easily accessed; a saw is used to transect the bones, and rongeurs or a bone curette can be used to scoop out the marrow.

15. **Superficial lymph nodes:** Several superficial lymph nodes should be selected for examination of size and consistency, and sectioned to view the internal surfaces.

If the body is to be hauled away after the necropsy, the necropsy incisions should be closed to keep the viscera contained within the carcass. Many hauling companies will not accept the carcass unless the organs are removed or secured within the body. The incisions can be closed with heavy-gauge suture material or heavy string or twine. The closure material should pass through the skin and/or underlying fascia in order to gain adequate holding strength. It should pass at least 1 inch away from the edges of the necropsy incision to prevent ripping through the tissues. If string or twine is used, it is necessary to create small stab incisions in order to pass the string/twine through these tissues. The technician must be careful when making the stab incisions to avoid self-injury.

Removal of Brain and Spinal Cord

It is occasionally desirable to remove the brain and/or spinal cord for evaluation of neurological conditions. Neurological tissue autolyzes rapidly after death; if histopathological examination of nerve tissue is necessary, these tissues should be promptly harvested:

- **Aspiration of cerebrospinal fluid:** If cerebrospinal fluid is needed, it is aspirated from the atlantooccipital space before removing the head.

- **Removal of the head:** The head is disarticulated through the atlantooccipital joint, approaching from the ventral aspect of the neck. If the brain is to be submitted for rabies evaluation, most diagnostic laboratories will accept the entire head, and it should be properly packaged, labeled, and refrigerated.
- **Removal of the brain:** The head should be stabilized in a vice or against a solid object. The skin is incised from the angles of the mandibles dorsally across the poll and reflected cranially. A skull cap is then created by making three incisions into the bony calvarium with a handsaw:
  - Make a transverse incision across the frontal bones that connects the supraorbital foramen, just caudal to the orbits. Be sure to cut through the frontal sinus (Fig. 12-1).
  - Make two lateral incisions, from each supraorbital foramen to the occipital condyle on the same side. Be sure to cut into the foramen magnum posteriorly. Loosen the skull cap with a chisel and pry it off carefully to reveal the brain and meninges.

The brain is removed by incising the dura mater and reflecting it from the brain. Starting at the rostral aspect of the brain, lift the brain tissue and sever the cranial nerves. When the entire brain can be elevated, transect the brainstem. Remove the brain and process the tissues as necessary.

The pituitary gland will remain in the sella turcica. Forceps are used to elevate the gland and any attachments are gently divided to free it.

- **Removal of the spinal cord:** Reflect the skin, musculature, and other soft tissues lateral to the dorsal spinous processes of the vertebrae. The desired segments of the vertebral column are removed intact from the carcass. The spinal cord is then removed in segments or en bloc. It is easier to remove the spinal cord in multiple small segments, by cutting transversely across the middle of adjacent vertebrae to form individual segments, then grasping the dura mater and removing the spinal cord segments from the vertebral canal by severing the spinal nerves in the epidural space with scissors (Figs. 12-2 to 12-4). Each segment should be accurately labeled and packaged separately. Incising the dura

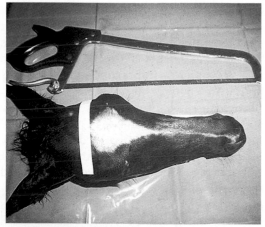

Fig. 12-1. Location of the transverse incision for exposure of the brain. (From Colahan PT et al: *Equine medicine and surgery,* ed 5, St Louis, 1999, Mosby.)

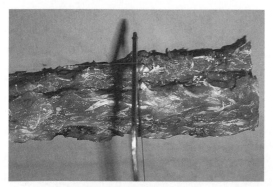

Fig. 12-2. The cervical segment of the vertebral column has been removed. A handsaw is used to cut through the center of adjacent vertebrae to form segments. (From Colahan PT et al: *Equine medicine and surgery,* ed 5, St Louis, 1999, Mosby.)

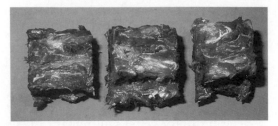

Fig. 12-3. The procedure produces adjacent segments of vertebrae. (From Colahan PT et al: *Equine medicine and surgery*, ed 5, St Louis, 1999, Mosby.)

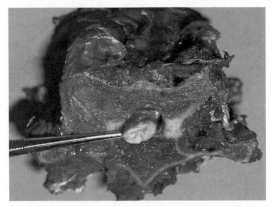

Fig. 12-4. The segments are viewed end on, and forceps are used to grasp the dura mater so that the spinal nerves within the epidural space can be cut with scissors. (From Colahan PT et al: *Equine medicine and surgery*, ed 5, St Louis, 1999, Mosby.)

mater of each segment longitudinally facilitates penetration of the fixative.

It is difficult to remove the entire spinal cord or long segments of the spinal cord in one piece. Use of hand tools (meat cleaver or axe) to split the vertebral column sagitally is possible but tends to be destructive. Power tools (especially a band saw) are preferred to perform sequential dorsal laminectomies through the vertebrae; this exposes the spinal cord. The spinal nerves must be severed to free and remove the spinal cord.

Necropsy of the Aborted Fetus

Aborted fetuses and tissues before 90 days of gestation are seldom found, especially in pasture settings. After 90 days, finding a fetus becomes more likely, and when an owner finds an aborted fetus, the veterinarian is usually asked to determine the cause of death. This requires examination and diagnostic testing of the mare, the placental tissues, and the aborted fetus. The client should understand that in spite of thorough examination of the mare, placental tissues, and aborted fetus, it is not always possible to diagnose the cause of an abortion.

Aborted fetuses and placental tissues, when found, are often in advanced states of autolysis; however, this should not prevent an attempt to necropsy and obtain samples. Any aborted fetus and its associated tissues should be placed immediately in a clean plastic bag and refrigerated (not frozen). It may be possible to submit the entire refrigerated fetus to a diagnostic laboratory for full examination. If submission of the entire fetus is not feasible, a necropsy can be done to collect appropriate specimens for submission to the laboratory.

Because of the possibility of infectious organisms causing abortion, the potential consequences of contagious disease must not be underestimated. Many contagious abortive diseases may be passed directly from mare to mare via direct or indirect contact. Also, it is the nature of large animals to "investigate" aborted fetuses and membranes by smelling and even licking them. Whenever a mare aborts, she should be separated immediately from other pregnant mares until the cause of abortion has been determined. The ground where the abortion occurred should be disinfected and roped or fenced off to access by other animals until the cause is known. If abortion occurs in a stall, the stall should be stripped and disinfected; the bedding should be handled as potentially contaminated and may possibly be burned if local laws allow. Isolation of the stall and areas where the mare traveled may be necessary. The veterinarian will advise the client on the best course of action. It is preferable not to open the fetus for necropsy in any area that could be accessed by other animals. The area of the necropsy should be disinfected and all clothing, instruments, and sample containers used in the procedure must be handled appropriately.

The procedure for necropsy of the fetus is as follows:

1. Identify sex, weigh, and measure crownrump length (distance from poll to tail base, measured along and against the dorsal midline). Note extent of hair growth. Note any obvious congenital or hereditary defects.
2. Place the fetus in right lateral recumbency.
3. Reflect or remove the left limbs. Skin the left body wall.
4. Incise the body wall behind the ribs into the flank area, and reflect the abdominal wall without touching the underlying viscera. Aspirate any available peritoneal fluid, and place it in a serum (red top) tube.
5. Using sterile instruments and aseptic technique, sample the abdominal organs in situ. Collect pieces of spleen, liver, and kidney for viral isolation (VI) and fluorescent antibody (FA) testing. VI samples may be pooled in one container. FA samples should be kept separate, in whirl-pak bags. A viral transport medium should be added to all VI and FA containers; use enough to just cover the tissues.
6. The thoracic cavity is entered through the diaphragm or by removing the left chest wall. Aspirate any available pleural fluid, and place it in a serum (red top) tube.
7. Using sterile instruments and aseptic technique, sample the thoracic organs in situ. Collect pieces of lung and thymus for VI and FA testing.
8. Collect bacterial culture samples from the lung and liver. Place the tissue samples in whirl-pak bags; do not add viral transport medium to the bacteriologic samples.
9. Make a small hole in the stomach wall, and sample the gastric fluid with a culturette for bacteriologic culture.
10. Once all microbiological samples have been obtained, histology samples are collected into 10% neutral buffered formalin:
    a. Liver: several sections
    b. Lung: several sections
    c. Kidney
    d. Spleen
    e. Heart
    f. Thymus
    Other desirable tissues are adrenal gland, stomach, small intestine, large intestine, skeletal muscle, tongue, eyelid, and brain (cerebrum, cerebellum, and brainstem).
11. If toxicologic analysis is to be performed, place a large piece of liver in a whirl-pak bag. Also aspirate fluid from the anterior eye chamber and place in a serum (red top) tube.

All samples are promptly shipped to the diagnostic laboratory. Microbiologic and toxicologic samples should be shipped frozen, on ice packs. Freezing of histopathology samples disrupts cell architecture and should *not* be done.

SUGGESTED READING

2000 Report of the AVMA Panel on Euthanasia, *JAVMA* 218(5):669-696, 2001.

Buergelt CD: Necropsy. In Colahan PT et al, editors: *Equine medicine and surgery*, ed 5, vol 1, St Louis, 1999, Mosby.

Taboada J: Euthanasia. In McCurnin DM, Bassert JM: *Clinical textbook for veterinary technicians*, ed 6, St Louis, 2006, Saunders.

part II

RUMINANT CLINICAL PROCEDURES

13

Ruminant Restraint and Basic Physical Examination

RESTRAINT

When working with any species, some understanding of their basic instincts and typical behaviors is essential (Table 13-1). Although ruminant species share many physiological traits, they do not share a common "mentality," and the behavioral differences among the various ruminant species should be understood. The methods of restraint used for cattle, sheep, and goats are quite different.

BOVINE RESTRAINT

Cattle (bovines) show different behaviors according to their breed, sex, and age. Breed usually determines the destiny of cattle by classifying them as either a beef or dairy breed. Beef and dairy life cycles, husbandry, and handling are dramatically different. Before entering the feedlot, beef animals are largely maintained in open range or field settings and only occasionally handled by humans; they do not often develop trust in humans and therefore resist handling and restraint. They are very suspicious of enclosures such as pens and chutes. Dairy animals, especially females, are handled more frequently; lactating cows are milked twice daily and receive most of their food in a controlled, sheltered setting. Dairy cows, therefore, tend to be easier to handle than their beef counterparts.

Regardless of breed, the size and strength of these animals cannot be overestimated, and even an apparently docile individual can become exceedingly dangerous to handle in some circumstances. Bulls of all breeds are typically unpredictable and aggressive and should never be trusted; "never turn your back on a bull" is good advice. Dairy bulls, in particular, are regarded as some of the most dangerous domestic animals to handle

TABLE

13-1 AGE AND SEX TERMINOLOGY FOR RUMINANTS

	Cattle	Sheep	Goat
Parturition (Freshening)	Calving	Lambing	Kidding
Neonate	Calf	Lamb	Kid
Male (<1 yr)	Bull calf	Ram lamb	Buck kid
Female (<1 yr)	Heifer calf	Ewe lamb	Doe kid
Immature female (has not given birth)	Heifer	Yearling ewe	Yearling doe
Mature female	Cow	Ewe	Doe (Nanny)
Mature male	Bull	Ram	Buck (Billy)
Castrated male	Steer	Wether	Wether

and restrain. Cows with calves are often aggressive in their efforts to protect their calves and can inflict serious injury. The herding instinct is strong in cattle, and when completely separated from others, as is necessary for some procedures, they may struggle violently to rejoin the herd. Cattle have little objection to trying to go over or through fences or other objects that stand in their way of rejoining the herd.

Most veterinary procedures require two stages of animal handling: first, the individual must be separated from the herd, and second, the individual must then be restrained appropriately for the procedure. Each farm presents a unique layout of fences, pastures, barns, and facilities for separating individuals from the herd. The usual method of separation is to first drive a group of cattle containing one or more desired individuals into a smaller working area such as a corral or pen. Leading from this small pen area is a cattle chute, a narrow walkway designed so that cattle must walk through it in single file. The cattle chute typically leads to a working chute, which provides head and body restraint for one animal at a time. A single animal enters the working chute, is restrained there while procedures are performed, and then released back to the group or herd. Although nice in theory, the reality is that the facilities available on some farms are in various states of repair and disrepair, and some small "backyard" farms may not have any special facilities at all. The ability to improvise, and remain safe, is essential.

Recumbent Animals

Cattle usually stand up when a human enters their immediate area. Occasionally, an animal may not rise or may have physical conditions that make it reluctant to rise. If it is necessary to get the animal to its feet, and the animal is capable, the handler should stand along the backside of the animal, never

between the legs or by the head. The back, rib, or thigh area can be tapped, slapped, or poked with the hand or a blunt item such as a stick or gently kicked with the foot. The handler may also thrust his or her knees into the animal's back and rib area. More severe instruments such as a whip or electric cattle prod should be reserved for cases where standing is absolutely necessary for assessment or treatment of serious or life-threatening situations and are best used by experienced personnel. Again, it should be determined that the animal has the physical capability to stand before using these devices.

Moving and Herding

Herding cattle must be done as calmly as possible. They should not be made to move any faster than a walk. The shoulder area is critical to moving cattle; if approached from behind the shoulder, they generally move forward. If approached from in front of the shoulder, they tend to move backwards. Loud noises and rapid motions should be avoided; once a group of cattle is suspicious of a situation, it can be difficult to gain control. Likewise, when moving groups of cattle toward enclosures and through gates, it is wise to keep unfamiliar vehicles, equipment, and personnel out of sight and quiet. Asking the farmer if assistance in herding the cattle is necessary and, if so, how the farmer wants to go about it is good practice; do not assume that help is needed or wanted.

Use of electric cattle prods is reserved for encouraging animals to move when other methods have failed. They should be used judiciously and briefly, and applied only to body areas with sufficient muscle mass. They should never be applied to the head. Sometimes just the noise of the activated prod will provide enough encouragment to move an animal without actually applying it to the animal.

Chute Restraint

The "working" chute is designed to hold one animal at a time. The animal is encouraged to enter the chute by giving the impression that it can walk all the way through it; as the animal tries to walk forward out of the chute, however, the end of the chute has a mechanism to trap the neck between two vertical bars called the head catch. These bars close down to a width that neither the head nor shoulders can fit through, thereby greatly limiting the ability of the animal to move forward or backwards. The head and neck can, however, move up and down, and side to side. This presents great danger to personnel and to the animal, since throwing the head violently becomes the primary method of defense. Until and unless the head is fully restrained, the operator should never place his or her body in a position to be struck by the animal's head; the power of a head strike can result in severe personal injury.

The method of applying the head catch bars depends on the chute design. Some chutes have self-closing head catch mechanisms that are activated by the animal's shoulders as it tries to walk through; others must be closed manually. The handlers must be aware of the metal levers attached to the chute; they may sometimes be triggered to move with tremendous speed and force, inflicting personal injury. In addition to the head catch, working chutes may have adjustable side panels that close inward to touch the sides of the animal (squeeze chute), greatly limiting the ability of the body to move laterally (Fig. 13-1). The side panels have bars that can be removed or folded down to allow access to the part of the body being worked on. The head catch is always applied first, then the squeeze is applied. To release

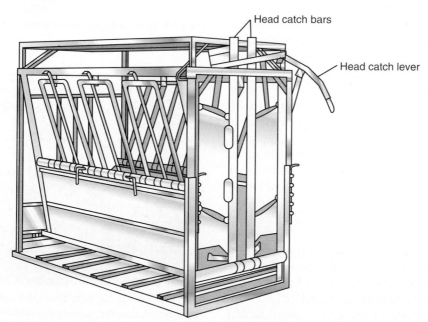

Head catch bars

Head catch lever

Fig. 13-1. Typical cattle squeeze chute with side bars that can be removed or lowered for access to the animal. Note the vertical head catch bars at the front of the chute.

the animal, the squeeze is released first, then the head catch; if there is a rear gate, it is not opened until the animal has exited the chute and materials are ready for the next animal.

Squeeze chutes and head catches are not designed for or suitable for use on calves or other large animal species. Also, careful attention must be given if an animal collapses or goes down in a working chute; the design of some chutes may occlude the trachea or blood flow to the head, and legs may be seriously injured if they become wedged in the bars or rails.

Head Restraint

Head restraint may be applied to cooperative animals without use of a chute, but most individuals must be placed in a chute first. Once the animal's body is secured within the working chute and head catch, further restraint of the head may be desired. Whenever applying head restraint, stay at arm's length from the head and avoid getting in a position to be struck by any part of the head.

Rope cattle halters are perhaps the safest method of head restraint. Cattle halters are used to control the head by tying or securing the head to an immovable object with a rope attached to the halter. However, unlike horses, few cattle are accustomed to being led by halter and lead rope; therefore leading is seldom possible. Cattle halters are typically made of one continuous piece of rope, with a "slip" portion that allows adjustment for individual animals. The halter has two loops: a smaller loop designed to fit around the nose (nose loop or noseband) and a larger loop that goes across the poll, behind the ears (crown loop or head stall). The nose loop is loosened and placed first, at a level about halfway between the eyes and the nostrils. Then, the crown loop is passed over and behind the ears; the free end of the rope is then pulled to take up slack and tighten the halter. Once positioned, the halter should not be on or

near the eyes, nor should the nose loop be so low that nostril breathing is occluded (Fig. 13-2). The free end of the rope may be used to pull or tie the head in position for the desired procedure (Fig. 13-3).

Nose leads (cattle nose tongs) are another common method of head restraint (Fig. 13-4). They apply blunt, pinching pressure to the nasal septum, which creates discomfort and

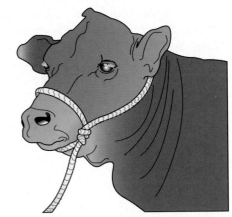

Fig. 13-2. Proper placement of a rope cattle halter.

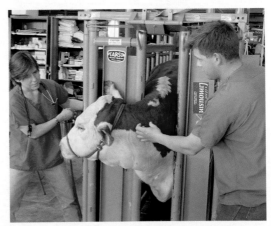

Fig. 13-3. The cow has been placed in a chute with a head catch; a rope halter has also been placed to allow further control of the head. (From McCurnin DM, Bassert JM: *Clinical textbook for veterinary technicians*, ed 6, St Louis, 2006, Saunders.)

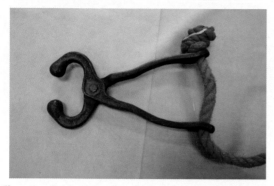

Fig. 13-4. Cattle nose tongs with ball tips and attached rope.

makes the animal reluctant to move. Nose tongs are not to be used as the only head restraint; they may be used to supplement a halter and/or head catch. Nose tongs usually have a rope attached to the handles; the rope can be used to pull or tie the head to either side for procedures. To apply the nose lead, it is helpful to take advantage of the animal's curiosity; open the jaws of the tongs, go slowly toward the animal's nose, slip one ball tip into one nostril, and then position the other ball tip in the other nostril and close the handles. This should be done as one rapid, smooth motion. With the handles closed, slack is taken out of the attached rope, which can then be used to handle and secure the instrument. This device must be carefully used; if the animal falls or resists violently, the nasal septum may be torn. It is best not to tie nose tongs to an immovable object, but if the rope must be tied, a quick-release knot should be used and closely attended. Nose tongs are not intended for use on calves.

Nose rings are placed through the nasal septum and are often used in bulls. Ropes or poles can be attached to the nose ring for additional control of the head, but, as with nose leads, the nasal septum can be torn. Nose rings should not be used to tie the head for head restraint.

Tail Restraint

The tail of the bovine is not as strong as the tail of the horse; the vertebrae are much smaller and are easily broken. The tail is never used to move or lift a recumbent bovine. The tail may, however, be used for restraint for short periods of time, through use of a tail hold (tail jack). The tail hold is used to supplement other forms of restraint and may discourage (but not prevent) kicking.

The handler should stand behind the cow, but off to one side to avoid being kicked. The tail hold is applied by using both hands to grasp the tail close to its base, in the proximal third of the tail. The tail is lifted directly up and over the back, and constant pressure is applied toward the head, keeping the tail on midline.

A variation of the tail hold, "tailing," is used to encourage cattle to move forward, especially to move forward in a chute. The middle of the tail is grasped and twisted forward to one side or the other over the back, off of midline. Firm pressure is applied, but excessive pressure can fracture the tail. This maneuver creates some discomfort, and the usual response of the cow is to walk forward, away from the pressure. Again, do not stand directly behind the animal while tailing it.

Tying the tail out of the way is sometimes necessary for cleanliness during some procedures, but is not used for restraint of the animal. The tail tie is performed similar to the horse, using the hair of the switch to fold over twine, roll gauze, or narrow rope. Care must be taken not to incorporate the tail's vertebrae into the tie. Tails should only be secured to the animal itself (as in horses), rather than to immovable objects. The tail can be tied around the neck or over the back and around the opposite upper forelimb (Fig. 13-5).

Leg Restraint

Cattle are as capable as horses are in delivering hard, fast kicks with the hind legs.

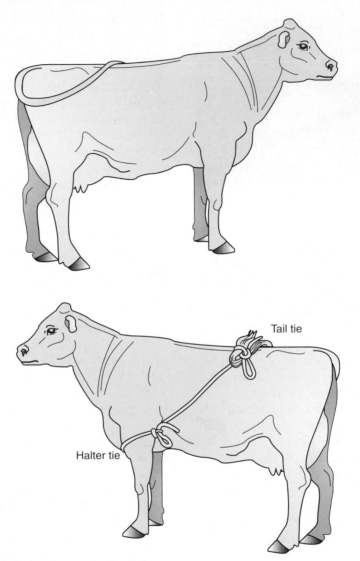

Fig. 13-5. Tail tie over the back to the opposite forelimb.

"Cow-kicking" refers to the common tendency of cattle to swing the kicking leg forward, then laterally, then out behind them. Even when standing by the shoulder, the handler can be struck with a hind leg kick. Also, it is a common misconception that cattle cannot simply kick straight behind (like a horse) or kick with both hind legs at the same time.

Hobbles (sometimes called hopples) are devices designed to prevent kicking. Various commercial and homemade devices are available to fasten to the hind legs, either around the pasterns or over the common calcaneal tendons just above the hocks. Milking hobbles are popular among dairy farmers; they consist of two U-shaped metal bands connected by a chain that passes across the front of the hindlimbs (Fig. 13-6). The metal bands are placed over the common calcaneal tendons by holding a band in each hand and reaching across the front of the rear legs to apply the first metal band to the opposite rear leg (Figs. 13-7 and 13-8). The band for the near leg is then quickly placed. The handler should be prepared to move quickly if the cow kicks during placement of the bands.

Another method of discouraging kicking is by use of pressure on the flank. This is most often done with a flank rope. A rope (with an eye on one end) is passed over the body of the animal just cranial to the udder (females) or the prepuce (males), encircling the body. The free end is passed through the eye and pulled tightly to place pressure on the flanks (Fig. 13-9). Be careful not to place the rope directly on the udder or prepuce.

Lifting legs is necessary to examine feet and trim hooves. Cattle seldom stand still to allow these procedures to be done. The animal should first be restrained in a chute or other appropriate manner. Occasionally, an animal may allow the leg to be lifted by hand, but most need the leg elevated with the use of ropes. For lifting a front leg, a rope with an eye on one end is used to form a loop or double loop around the leg at or just above the fetlock area; the free end is then passed over the back of the animal or over a top rail of the chute for leverage as it is

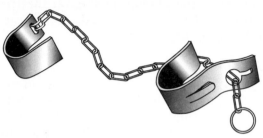

Fig. 13-6. Milking hobbles.

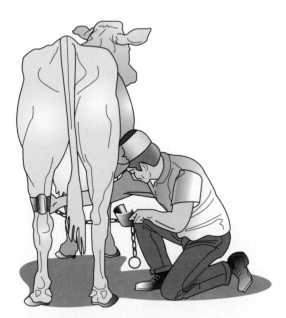

Fig. 13-7. Placing milking hobbles.

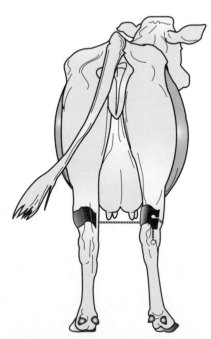

Fig. 13-8. Milking hobbles in place.

A

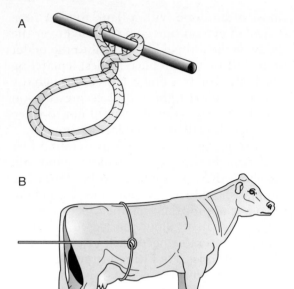

B

Fig. 13-9. A, Flank rope. **B,** Use of a flank rope on a cow in a cattle chute. (From McCurnin DM, Bassert JM: *Clinical textbook for veterinary technicians*, ed 6, St Louis, 2006, Saunders.)

pulled to elevate the leg (Fig. 13-10). The rope should not be tied but rather held by an assistant so that it can be immediately released if the animal goes down. A second rope may be added if the leg needs to be pulled laterally after it is elevated.

The hind legs must be extended and lifted to the rear of the animal. This requires a beam, pulley, or hook above and slightly behind the animal for leverage. The rope is passed around the fetlock or the hock and tightened, then the free end is passed over a beam or through a pulley or hook behind and above the animal. Pulling on the free end then elevates and extends the leg caudally (Fig. 13-11).

Casting

Casting is the method of forcing an animal to the ground, usually with ropes. Unlike horses, casting cattle is relatively simple, using ropes to apply firm, constant pressure to sensitive points on the body. The animal responds by lying down, usually with little struggling. Once down, the legs may be tied if necessary for the procedure.

Several configurations of casting "harnesses" have been described. It is important

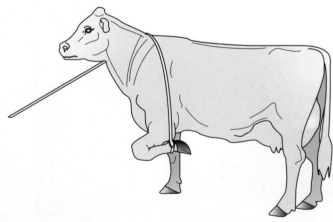

Fig. 13-10. Leg rope for elevating a front limb.

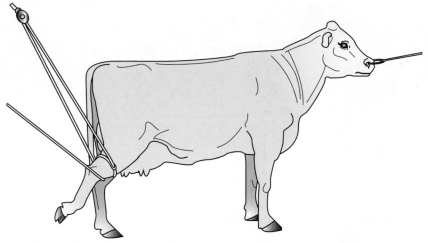

Fig. 13-11. Use of a rope around the hock and elevated hook to elevate a hind leg.

not to trap the udder, prepuce, or scrotum in the body ropes. Control of the head should be gained before applying any method of casting (Figs. 13-12 and 13-13).

Recumbent ruminants are susceptible to bloat of the rumen/reticulum. Risk of bloat can be minimized by placing the animal in sternal recumbency, though this position is seldom feasible for most procedures that require casting. If lateral recumbency is required, right lateral recumbency is preferred; this positions the rumen uppermost, where it can be observed for signs of bloat. All effort should be made to minimize the time spent in any recumbent position.

Calf Restraint

Young calves are naturally curious and usually easy to catch and restrain if the dam is not present. If the calf is with its dam, the calf will follow its mother into barns or small pens but also will use her as a shield to avoid capture. Separating the pair for the procedure or restraining the cow may be necessary. Be aware of the cow's protective instincts in these situations; cows may become aggressive in attempts to protect their young.

To hold or guide a calf, one arm should be placed around the front of the neck or chest. The other arm should wrap around behind the hindquarters or grasp the base of the tail if more control is necessary.

If it is necessary to put a calf into lateral recumbency, it may be placed on the ground by "flanking." Standing aside and facing the calf, the handler reaches both arms across the calf's back, down the side of the body, then under the calf's body to grasp the legs nearest the handler. The calf is then lifted off the ground and allowed to slide down the handler's legs to the ground. Do not throw the calf to the ground; use your legs to ease the descent (Fig. 13-14). Once down, the handler quickly places one knee over the neck and one over the back to keep the calf down while the procedure is performed (do not place the entire bodyweight on the calf, and do not occlude the trachea). Often, the legs are secured with rope loops above the pasterns and tied with a quick release knot; the procedure determines which legs need to be tied (Fig. 13-15).

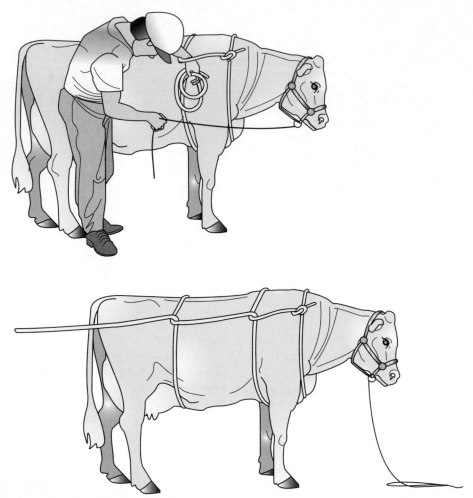

Fig. 13-12. One method of applying a casting harness. Pulling caudally on the free end forces the animal to lie down.

RESTRAINT OF SHEEP

Sheep are timid animals. They do not seem to enjoy being stroked or petted. They are easily frightened but seldom respond with aggression; aggression, when displayed, is in the form of head-butting or stomping the front feet. The usual response is to flee when frightened, and they may cause serious injury to themselves in their efforts to escape. They may even exhaust themselves to the point of collapse or hyperthermia trying to get away from perceived danger. Therefore unlike other large animal species where there is significant risk of injury to the handler in catching and restraining them, the primary concern when working with sheep is injuring the sheep themselves with efforts to catch and restrain them.

Sheep have *extremely* strong flocking instincts and tend to behave as a group. When one sheep becomes nervous or fearful, the entire flock tends to follow suit; it may

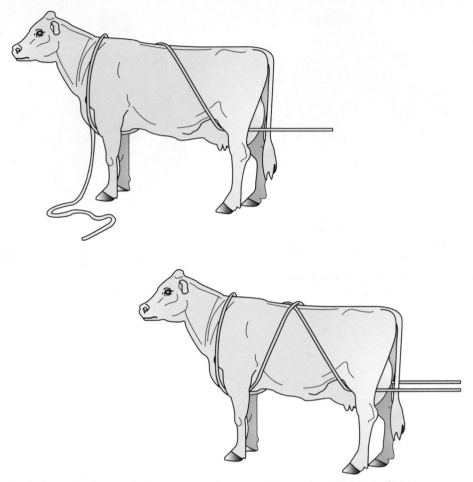

Fig. 13-13. The Burley casting harness. Pulling on the two free ends of the rope forces the cow to lie down.

be impossible to gain any control once the flock is upset. Using a calm, quiet, patient approach is essential with these animals.

When catching sheep, several points are key. Individual sheep need to be separated from the flock; this is often done by first driving the flock into an enclosure or pen, then cornering a single sheep against a fence or wall, where it can be handled. Hurdles (small, handheld wooden panels or sections of fence) are useful for limiting escape routes when trying to isolate an animal against a wall

or in a corner. The sheep may try to flee by going through the fence or climbing along the fence or wall; therefore these structures must be carefully chosen to minimize the risk of injury to the animal. It does not take much force to fracture the legs or vertebrae; therefore catching sheep by grabbing legs or throwing them to the ground should be avoided. Another common tendency to avoid is catching them by grabbing the wool; this can easily pull out the wool and bruise or rip the skin, which is fragile. Grabbing by the

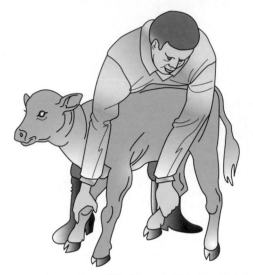

Fig. 13-14. One method of flanking a calf. The handler's legs are used to slide the calf to the ground.

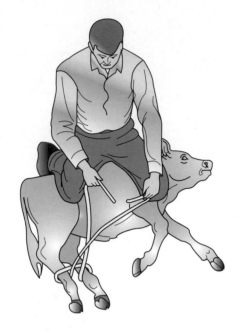

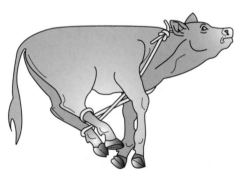

Fig. 13-15. After the calf is on the ground, the handler's knees are placed to keep the calf from rising. Ropes may be placed around the legs if desired.

horns (when present) must be done with care to avoid breaking them.

The value of the fleece must also be respected. Pulled-out clumps of wool lessens the value of the fleece, and separating the natural interlock of the wool fibers by improper handling also devalues the fleece. When handling sheep, the fleece should not be parted unless absolutely necessary. To part the wool, lay the hands flat on the wool and gently separate the fibers only enough to see the underlying skin (Fig. 13-16). If necessary to palpate the body, keep the fingers together to minimize disturbance of the wool fibers.

Sheep are held by circling the neck with one arm and placing the other arm around the rump (Fig. 13-17). The rear end may also be controlled by placing an arm over the back to grasp the skinfold of the lower flank. Many procedures can be done by simply backing the sheep into a corner, straddling the animal between the handler's legs, and squeezing the sheep's shoulders firmly

between the legs. The head or neck can be controlled in this position (Fig. 13-18).

Procedures such as examination of the hooves, shearing, and vaccination require immobilizing the animal with a technique known as "setting up" the sheep. This method essentially sits the sheep down on its rump; without contact of the feet with the ground, the animal cannot struggle and basically becomes submissive to the handler. There are

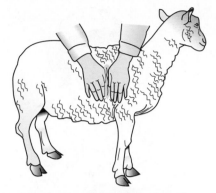

Fig. 13-16. Parting the wool to observe the body.

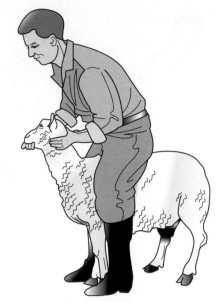

Fig. 13-18. Straddling a sheep for restraint.

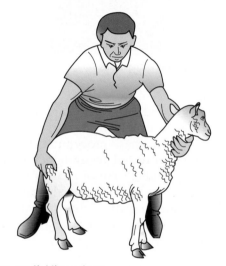

Fig. 13-17. Holding a sheep.

several methods of setting up sheep. The restraint is applied by standing to the side of the sheep, with one hand under the neck, and the other reaching across the back to grasp either the flank skinfold, the upper portion of the opposite hind leg, or reaching back under the abdomen to grasp the upper hind leg on the same side as the handler. Once the hold is secured, the head is turned to face the rump, the sheep is lifted slightly off the ground, and the sheep is set down

(not thrown) on its buttocks on the ground in front of the handler. The sheep is supported in a tilted-back sitting position against the legs of the handler, similar to a recliner chair back. In this position, the handler's hands are free to perform procedures or restrain the front legs. The animal can also be lowered from this position into lateral or dorsal recumbency if necessary (Figs. 13-19 and 13-20).

Shepherd's crooks are properly applied around a hind leg, at the level of the hock or above. Placing the crook below the hock risks fracturing the leg. Once the hind leg is caught, the handler quickly moves in to grasp the sheep as described above. The crook may cause trauma if placed around the neck, and it is not intended for this location.

Lamb Restraint

Small lambs are carried by placing one hand under the body and between the forelimbs to support the sternum, and the other hand around the neck (Fig. 13-21).

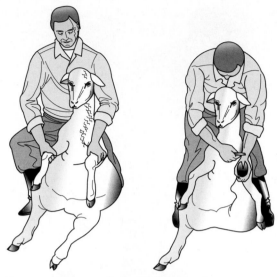

Fig. 13-19. Sheep may be "set up" for restraint.

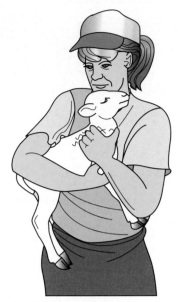

Fig. 13-21. Carrying young lambs.

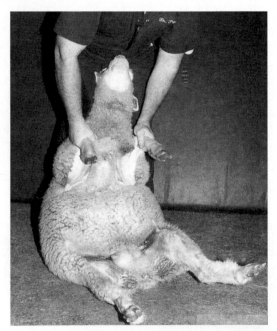

Fig. 13-20. Sheep in proper position on its rump. Note the reclined position of the sheep against the handler's legs. (From Pugh DG: *Sheep and goat medicine*, St Louis, 2002, Saunders.)

Castration and tail docking are performed at an early age, usually in the first to second week of life. For these procedures, the lamb is restrained in dorsal recumbency with its back in the handler's lap or against the handler's body. The head is placed against the handler's body, and the right limbs are held (above the fetlock) by the right hand, the left limbs by the left hand (Fig. 13-22).

RESTRAINT OF GOATS

Although similar to sheep in size, goats are entirely different in temperament and behavior. Goats are gregarious and seem to enjoy the company of other species of animals. They are inquisitive and often respond to human touch and affection. They do not have the same flocking instinct as sheep and show more of a tendency toward independent behavior. If herded like sheep or cattle, the group often fragments and scatters. Goats form a social hierarchy within a group, and dominant males and females can be identified. If the dominant goat in the group can be identified, leading that individual to the desired location often results in the others following.

Goats may show aggression, usually in the form of head-butting. This is usually preceded by raising the hair on the spine, stamping the front feet, and making a characteristic sneezing/snorting noise. Head-butting can cause significant personal injury, regardless of whether horns are present. Bucks (intact male goats) may be especially aggressive during the breeding season.

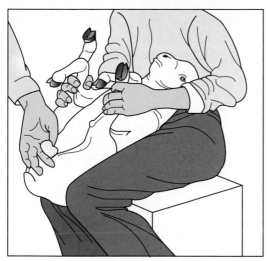

Fig. 13-22. Restraint of a lamb for castration and tail docking.

Head Restraint

Goats can be handled by the beard, if present. One hand is used to grasp the beard, while the other arm is placed around the neck to control the head. The beard may be handled firmly, and even used to lead the goat, but should not be used to apply unnecessary force or punishment (Fig. 13-23). If horns are present, they may be used for head restraint. Horns should be held near their base. Rough handling by the horns is often resented. Goats resent being held by the ears, and owners consider ear restraint to be abusive.

Goats readily accept neck collars or chains, which provide a convenient hold on the animal. They may be led by the collar and can be taught to stand while tied by the collar to a fence or wall.

Body Restraint

Most procedures are best performed by limiting the ability of the goat to move around. Backing the goat into a wall or corner, or positioning it alongside a wall or fence, is helpful. One arm can then be placed around the chest or neck for minor procedures. Lifting one front leg is another form of restraint for minor procedures. Straddling the goat and squeezing its shoulders between the handler's legs may also be useful; the hands can then be used for head restraint.

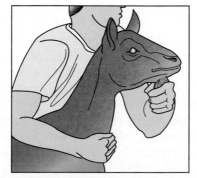 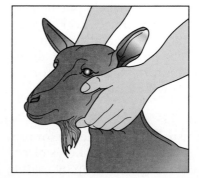

Fig. 13-23. Head restraint of a goat by grasping the beard and neck.

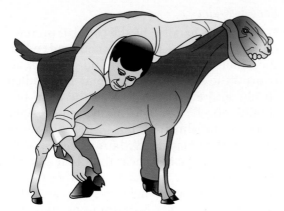

Fig. 13-24. Position for flanking a goat.

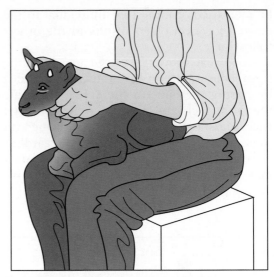

Fig. 13-25. Restraining a kid in the handler's lap.

Goats do not tolerate being set up like sheep. Rather, they are placed in recumbency on the ground by flanking. This may be done similar to a calf. Another method is to stand alongside the goat and hold the muzzle in one hand; the other hand reaches over the back and grasps the near hind leg. The leg is elevated, and the handler attempts to move the leg forward and the muzzle caudally as if to touch them together. This causes the goat to lose its balance and fall to the ground. Once recumbent, the handler's knees placed on the neck and back may discourage the goat from rising (Fig. 13-24).

Leg Restraint

Front legs are elevated by grasping the leg at the fetlock, lifting it so that it bends at the knee. The leg can be held in one hand or rested on the handler's knee. Rear legs are also lifted by the fetlock and brought out slightly behind the goat. Legs should always be lifted to a comfortable position for the goat; otherwise it will resist.

Kid Restraint

Small kids are usually held in the lap for procedures such as dehorning. The kid is placed in sternal recumbency on the lap by folding its front legs beneath it, and the handler's forearms are placed on the back and pressed down to keep the kid from rising. The hands can be used to control the head (Fig. 13-25).

Kids may also be held in dorsal recumbency in the lap or against the handler's legs, the same way as for lambs.

BASIC PHYSICAL EXAMINATION

The physical examination process always begins with taking the history and inspecting the animal's environment. Because ruminants are usually kept in herd situations, conditions affecting one animal may have consequences for the others on the farm. The history should focus not only on the individual but also on the management of the entire group. Food and water sources, pasture management, herd health programs, introduction of new animals, feeding practices, toxin exposure, and environmental stresses are among the factors that should be explored. Many farmers attempt treatment of animals before calling the veterinarian, and they should be asked about any treatments and/or medications that may have been given.

It is *essential* not to appear to pass judgment on the farmer's practices during the history taking and inspection of the facilities; simply record the facts, and allow the veterinarian to make any suggestions or assessments of management practices.

The physical examination of any animal should begin with an initial visual observation of the animal from a distance. The animal's posture, behavior, body condition, and alertness are easily observed. More specific signs such as breathing pattern and respiratory noises, body swellings, skin wounds, and muscle atrophy may also be noted.

The direct, hands-on physical examination typically includes temperature/pulse/respiration (TPR), heart/lung auscultation, abdominal auscultation and assessment of rumen function, hydration status, and examination of mucous membranes.

Temperature is taken rectally and is performed similarly to temperature taking of horses. When taking the rectal temperature of the goat, a dark brown, waxy material may be seen near the anus; this secretion is normal and is produced by sebaceous glands under the tailhead. The pulse can be palpated readily at the facial artery, but the coccygeal, median (forelimb), and great metatarsal (hindlimb) arteries are also available. The femoral artery is most convenient in sheep and goats. The respiratory rate is best taken by counting chest excursions from a distance, prior to herding or handling; the excitement and fear of herding or being restrained can cause dramatic increases in respiratory rate, especially in hot environmental temperatures, that do not reflect the true respiratory rate of the animal at rest. Ruminants are capable of open-mouth breathing, though it is usually considered to be a sign of distress or heat stress (usually when environmental temperature exceeds 85° F). An abdominal breathing pattern is normal. Normal values are given in Table 13-2.

Auscultation of the heart and lungs is performed as for the horse. Heart auscultation is performed using the same anatomical landmarks as in the horse: the shoulder joint and the olecranon for dorsal/ventral position and the caudal border of the triceps muscle for cranial/caudal position. This generally corresponds to the fourth to fifth intercostal space. Cardiac sounds are normally only S1 and S2 in cattle (unlike the horse, in which any combination of S3 and S4 may accompany S1 and S2). The borders for lung auscultation in the ruminant are between ribs No. 5 cranially and No. 11 caudally. If necessary to induce deep breathing for lung auscultation, the nostrils and mouth (since ruminants can mouth breathe) can be held closed for about a minute to stimulate deeper breathing and a higher respiratory rate.

Mucous membranes should be pink and moist, with a capillary refill time of 1 to 2 seconds. If necessary to fully open the mouth for examination, placing the fingers into the interdental space and pressing on the hard palate encourages opening the mouth; the tongue can be quickly grasped and brought to the side at the commissure of the lips, where

TABLE 13-2 **NORMAL TEMPERATURE, PULSE, AND RESPIRATION VALUES FOR ADULT RUMINANTS**

	Rectal Temperature °F	Heart Rate	Respiratory Rate
Cattle	101.5 (range 100.4-103.1)	40-80/min	10-30/min
Sheep	102.5 (range 102.0-104.0)	70-90/min	12-25/min
Goat	102.0 (range 101.5-104.0)	70-90/min	15-30/min

it encourages the animal to keep the mouth open. Alternatively, use of a mouth speculum may be indicated. The tongue of cattle is strong and has a single deep transverse groove across its dorsal surface; this groove is often mistaken for a laceration. The molars of ruminants may be sharp and jagged, and caution must be used whenever the hands are placed into the mouth. When examining the mouth and head, and especially with cattle, be aware of the possibility of being struck by the animal's head if it is not properly restrained.

When standing next to a ruminant, or when ausculting the thorax or trachea, occasional low-pitched fluttering sounds are heard; this is eructation (burping), which is normal in ruminants. Eructation rates are approximately 18/hour in cattle and 10/hour in sheep and goats.

Evaluation of the ruminant abdomen includes assessment of rumen contractions. The rumen occupies most of the left side of the abdominal cavity. The number of rumen contractions per minute may be counted by auscultation directly over the caudolateral rib cage or paralumbar fossa on the left side; contractions sound like a deep rumbling or "thunderstorm" noise that gets gradually louder as the contraction approaches the stethoscope. Rumen contractions can also be counted by ballottement (palpation) by pressing both fists firmly into the left paralumbar

fossa (use one fist in the sheep and goat); the fists are allowed to remain against the body wall for 1 minute. Each rumen contraction is felt as a wave passing under the hands, pushing the hands slightly outward. The normal animal has one to two contractions per minute. Hypomotility or absence of motility (ileus) are abnormal findings; hypermotility of the rumen is unusual. Auscultation of the right side of the abdomen usually reveals few sounds; this is normal in ruminants.

The shape of the abdomen is observed by standing behind the animal, facing the head. The overall shape of the right and left abdominal "silhouettes" should be similar, with the overall outline of the cow resembling a pear (wider at the lower flanks than at the paralumbar fossae). The paralumbar fossae should be normally flat or slightly sunken. Accumulation of gas within certain portions of the gastrointestinal (GI) tract (tympany or "bloat") can produce asymmetry and enlargement of the abdominal wall. Severe abdominal gas accumulation causes enlargement of the paralumbar fossa on both sides of the animal, changing shape from a "pear" to an "apple." The most common location for bloat, the rumen, appears as an enlargement of the left paralumbar fossa; this has been referred to as a "papple" shape, where the left side resembles an apple and the right side a pear (Figs. 13-26 and 13-27).

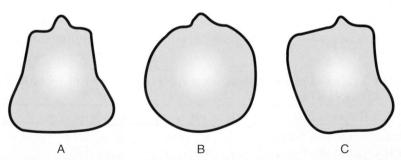

A   B   C

Fig. 13-26. Shapes of the ruminant abdomen, observed from behind. **A,** Normal pear shape. **B,** Abnormal apple shape. **C,** Abnormal "papple" shape.

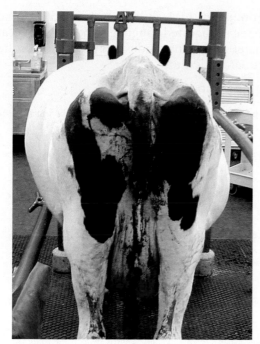

Fig. 13-27. Classic "papple" abdomen shape in a cow with ruminal bloat. (From Fubini SL, Ducharme NG: *Farm animal surgery*, St Louis, 2004, Saunders.)

Gas accumulations can also be detected by percussion and auscultation with the stethoscope. The stethoscope is held in place with one hand, while the other hand is used to snap a finger against the abdominal wall at several locations around the stethoscope head. Gas accumulations make a resonant "ping" sound, like a high-pitched drum. Pings generally indicate abnormal position or contents of one or more GI tract organs. Note that solid organs and non-GI organs cannot accumulate gas, and therefore do not ping (except the uterus, which is extremely rare). Pinging should be performed on both sides of the abdomen and may detect abnormalities before they are visible as external enlargement of the abdomen (Figs. 13-28 and 13-29).

The character of feces and urine, if available for observation, should be evaluated. Fecal character varies among the ruminants. Cattle defecate 12 to 18 times a day; the feces have a semisolid "cow-plop" consistency,

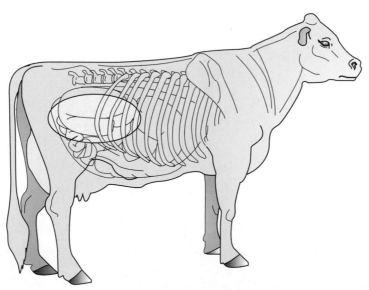

Fig. 13-28. Example of abdominal percussion or "pinging"; the shaded area indicates the location of resonance (ping) associated with accumulation of air in the cecum, due to cecal volvulus. (From Fubini SL, Ducharme NG: *Farm animal surgery*, St Louis, 2004, Saunders.)

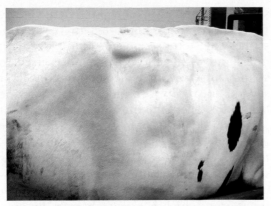

Fig. 13-29. Right side of a Holstein cow with cecal volvulus (rib cage visible to the right, tuber coxae and pelvis to the left). Observe the distension in the right paralumbar fossa, corresponding to the area of abdominal "ping." (From Fubini SL, Ducharme NG: *Farm animal surgery,* St Louis, 2004, Saunders.)

without a distinct form. Goats produce formed feces in the shape of small, solid pellets. Sheep feces are also pelleted. The color of the feces depends on the diet, ranging from green to dark brown. It is not normal to see undigested roughage fibers in the fecal material; this may indicate dysfunction of the rumen/reticulum.

SUGGESTED READING

Fubini SL, Ducharme NG: *Farm animal surgery,* St Louis, 2004, Saunders.

Leahy JR, Barrow P: *Restraint of animals,* Ithaca, NY, 1953, Cornell Campus Store.

McCurnin DM, Bassert JM: *Clinical textbook for veterinary technicians,* ed 6, St Louis, 2006, Saunders.

Pugh DG: *Sheep and goat medicine,* St Louis, 2002, Saunders.

Sirois M: *Principles and practice of veterinary technology,* ed 2, St Louis, 2004, Mosby.

Smith MC, Sherman DM: *Goat medicine,* Baltimore, 1994, Williams & Wilkins.

Sonsthagen TF: *Restraint of domestic animals,* St Louis, 1991, Mosby.

14

Diagnostic Sampling in Ruminants

Many diagnostic sampling procedures in ruminants are performed similarly to the procedures in horses and have been described in previous chapters. Only procedures that vary significantly or are unique to ruminants are discussed here.

VENOUS BLOOD SAMPLING

Collection of blood for diagnostic testing is one of the most common procedures performed on ruminants. Blood is usually submitted to a state/federal diagnostic laboratory for disease screening, which is especially important for herd health and control of disease in animals producing food (meat or milk) for human consumption. Blood can also be used to diagnose and guide treatment of individual animal diseases.

The location of venipuncture depends on the species, amount of blood needed, and the type of restraint to be used. Although theoretically any accessible vein can be used, several locations are preferred for anatomical and safety reasons.

The venipuncture site should always be cleaned before drawing a blood sample. Disinfection of the site with 70% isopropyl alcohol is sufficient. A common error is simply wiping off the hair. The site should be wiped down to and including the skin, and the area well soaked in the disinfectant. A simple check is to repeatedly apply the disinfectant and discard the applicator (gauze or cotton swabs) after each "scrub," until the applicator material remains white. Soaking the site with alcohol also helps visualization of the vein.

BOVINE VENIPUNCTURE

Venipuncture, like any diagnostic sampling procedure, begins with proper restraint of the animal. Cattle tend to resist venipuncture; it should never be attempted on an unrestrained animal. Simply placing a halter on the animal is not enough; the body must be restricted in movement, usually in a chute or head catch gate. Even when properly restrained, the technician should be prepared for a response by the animal when the needle penetrates the skin and avoid standing or kneeling where he or she may be injured.

Jugular Vein

The most common location for venipuncture is the jugular vein. It is the largest diameter and most accessible vein and is safest for the technician when the head is properly restrained. It is preferable to have the head pulled up and slightly to the opposite side from the technician; this requires use of a halter or nose tongs. If the head is pulled extremely to the side, it may make distension of the vein difficult to see.

Young calves may be restrained standing or placed in lateral recumbency. If standing, the head needs to be held tightly against the restrainer's body, being careful not to wrap the arms around the neck where they may interfere with access and distension of the jugular vein. If recumbent, the head needs to be restrained in the lap or against the restrainer's legs, taking care not to injure the eyes; the head should not be pressed into the ground.

After cleaning the site, the vein is distended by placing all of the fingers or a fist firmly into the jugular groove; the diameter of the jugular vein is quite large (1 to 2 inches), and using one finger or one thumb will not completely occlude it. Time is allowed for the vein to fill enough so that it can be readily seen. While maintaining distension with one hand, the other hand places a 16- or 18-gauge (ga), 1½-inch needle through the skin and into the vein at a 45-degree angle to the skin surface; this should be done in one swift, *committed* motion, noting that bovine skin is somewhat thicker than expected. The needle may be placed in either direction (cranially or caudally) for withdrawing blood, depending on personal preference. Likewise, the needle may be placed alone and then the syringe attached when placement in the vein is confirmed, or both may be placed as a single unit, depending on preference.

Distension of the vein is maintained while blood is collected into an attached syringe or Vacutainer tube. Once the sample is collected, the distension is released, and the needle withdrawn. Digital pressure is applied directly to the site for 15 to 30 seconds to discourage hematoma formation. The head restraint may then be released.

Coccygeal (Tail) Vein

The tail vein is easily accessed if the animal is limited in its side-to-side mobility and if the technician can be safely positioned to avoid a kick. Cattle are generally more tolerant of venipuncture in the tail than in the neck. Tail restraint is applied with one hand, using the vertical tail hold or "jack"; this also positions the tail for venipuncture (note that venipuncture cannot be performed with the

tail twisted). The other hand is used to clean the site with alcohol and perform the venipuncture.

Because the diameter of the vein is considerably smaller than the jugular vein, needles larger than 18-ga should not be used. An 18-, 19-, or 20-ga, 1- to 1½-inch needle is used; it is usual to leave the syringe attached during the procedure. Experienced operators may use Vacutainer tubes (Fig. 14-1).

The procedure is best performed in the proximal third of the tail, directly on ventral midline of the tail. The coccygeal vertebrae in this area have hemal processes (arches), which are bony canals on the ventral aspect of the vertebral bodies. The hemal processes protect the coccygeal artery and vein, which run through the canal; therefore venipuncture must be done between the vertebrae, where there are no hemal processes. The hemal processes are easily felt on ventral midline as firm, bony protrusions; the soft space between any two hemal processes is palpated, and the needle is directed into the space at a 45- to 90-degree angle to

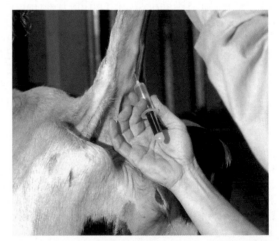

Fig. 14-1. Coccygeal venipuncture. (From Dyce KM, Sack WO, Wensing CJC: *Textbook of veterinary anatomy*, ed 3, St Louis, 2002, Saunders.)

the skin. The needle is advanced while aspirating *gently* on the syringe; the vessels are generally encountered ½ to 1 inch beneath the skin. If the needle contacts bone, slowly retract the needle and continue to aspirate. Once the needle bevel is in the lumen of the vein, the position is maintained while the blood sample is withdrawn.

The needle is withdrawn, and the tail is lowered. Digital pressure is kept over the site for approximately 15 seconds to discourage hematoma formation. Occasionally, the coccygeal artery may be entered accidentally during the procedure; this usually presents no problem other than hematoma formation. If the artery is entered, digital pressure over the site should be maintained for 45 to 60 seconds.

Subcutaneous Abdominal (Milk) Vein

The right and left milk veins course along the ventrolateral body wall of the thorax and abdomen. They provide major venous drainage of the udder, especially during lactation. They are easily identified as large-diameter tubular structures just beneath the skin, with a pronounced tortuous (twisty) course (Fig. 14-2).

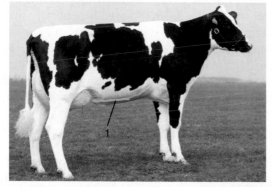

Fig. 14-2. The right milk vein (1) is readily visible in this Holstein cow. (From Dyce KM, Sack WO, Wensing CJC: *Textbook of veterinary anatomy*, ed 3, St Louis, 2002, Saunders.)

The milk veins appear inviting for venipuncture because of their large size; however, they are very prone to prolonged (sometimes pronounced) bleeding and large hematoma formation, and are therefore used only when no other vein is available or suitable for sampling.

The animal should be securely restrained, preferably in a chute or stanchion, and possibly with tail or leg restraint to discourage kicking. Two positions can be taken by the technician: (1) standing close to the flank, facing cranially, or (2) standing next to the shoulder of the cow, facing caudally. In either case, the technician should be prepared for a kick with the hindleg when the needle is placed. It is best not to kneel or squat; rather, bend over and keep the head as far above the level of the ventral abdomen as possible to avoid getting kicked.

The skin is prepared (prepped) with alcohol. It is not necessary to distend the vein; it stays in a distended state due to blood pressure and volume. However, it is frequently necessary to stabilize the vein with one hand because of its tendency to "roll." Venipuncture is performed preferably in the cranial half of the vein, where its course is straighter and more stable. An 18-, 19-, or 20-ga, 1½-inch needle is used; the needle may be inserted in either direction (note that the blood flows cranially). Redirecting the needle must be carefully and sparingly done, since it increases the risk of hematoma formation. Attachment of the syringe or Vacutainer tube may be done once the needle's location is confirmed.

Once the sample is obtained, the needle is withdrawn. Prolonged digital pressure must be applied over the puncture site for at least several minutes.

OVINE/CAPRINE VENIPUNCTURE

The jugular vein is most often used for venous sampling. In sheep it may be accessed with the animal standing or in the "set-up" rump position. In goats the standing position is used. For the standing procedure in either species, the animal is straddled and squeezed between the legs; it is helpful to back the animal against a solid object. It is possible for one person to access the vein, or two people may be used if desired (Figs. 14-3 and 14-4).

It is also possible to use the cephalic vein on the forearm or the femoral vein on the hindleg. Goats can remain standing for cephalic vein access, similar to the procedure in dogs. Backing the goat against a solid object is helpful. One person restrains the animal by circling the animal's neck with one arm, while the other hand is used to roll the vein laterally and occlude it. The person

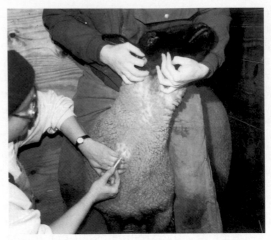

Fig. 14-4. One person restrains the sheep by straddling the shoulders and holding the head, while the other person obtains a jugular vein sample. (From Sirois M: *Principles and practice of veterinary technology*, St Louis, 2004, Mosby.)

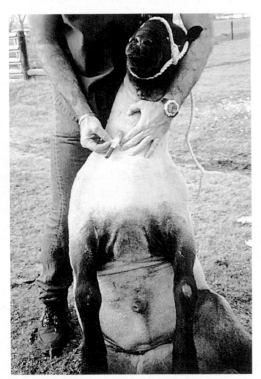

Fig. 14-3. One person can set up a sheep and obtain a jugular vein blood sample. (From McCurnin DM, Bassert JM: *Clinical textbook for veterinary technicians*, ed 5, St Louis, 2002, Saunders.)

drawing the sample needs to hold the distal limb to steady it. The cephalic vein in sheep may be accessed in the set-up rump position. Lateral recumbency is required for access to the femoral vein.

The animal is appropriately restrained. If wool is present, it is parted over and along the selected vein. Alcohol is suitable for disinfecting the skin. An 18-, 19-, 20-, or 22-ga, 1- to 1½-inch needle is used, depending on the size of the animal; 20-ga is generally preferred. Vacutainer systems may also be used. The procedure is performed as described for cattle. Firm occlusion of the vein is necessary, and the vein should be well distended before placement of the needle.

ARTERIAL BLOOD SAMPLING

Arterial sampling is difficult in awake animals, even when well restrained. Blood may be drawn from the brachial and femoral arteries on the limbs, or from the auricular (ear) arteries. The auricular arteries and palpable peripheral limb arteries may be accessible in anesthetized patients.

ABDOMINOCENTESIS

Abdominal (peritoneal) fluid is collected from the most dependent portion of the ventral abdomen. However, the procedure in adults is performed slightly to the right of ventral midline (3 to 5 cm) to avoid the rumen. Sometimes the location of the procedure is altered based on the suspected abdominal disease; in these cases the clinician will indicate where the abdomen should be prepped.

The site should be clipped and sterilely prepped. A needle or cannula at least $1\frac{1}{2}$ to 3 inches long must be used to penetrate the abdominal wall of cattle; 1- to $1\frac{1}{2}$-inch length is sufficient for most small ruminants. Needle diameter may range from 18- to 20-ga. The milk veins (subcutaneous abdominal veins) must be avoided.

RUMEN FLUID COLLECTION

Rumen fluid analysis can aid in diagnosis of diseases of the forestomachs. The sample can be obtained by the orogastric (otherwise known as *ororumen*) route, via passage of an orogastric tube (see Chapter 15) or directly through the lower left abdominal wall via rumenocentesis.

Rumenocentesis is performed with a 14-ga needle for cattle and a 16- or 18-ga needle for small ruminants through a site caudal to the xiphoid process and left of ventral midline. The site should be clipped and sterilely prepped. The clinician inserts the needle through the skin, into the rumen, and aspirates the rumen fluid with a syringe (Fig. 14-5).

Rumen fluid may be analyzed for color, pH, odor, identification and assessment of microbial organisms and numbers, and electrolyte levels. Normal rumen fluid is green, has a "sweet pungent" fermented odor, and

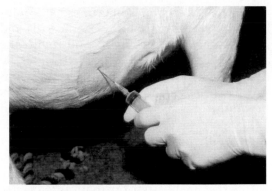

Fig. 14-5. Percutaneous rumenocentesis performed through the ventral left abdomen. (From Pugh DG: *Sheep and goat medicine*, St Louis, 2002, Saunders.)

should have a mixed population of actively motile protozoa. The pH generally ranges from 6.5 to 7.5.

URINE COLLECTION

Urine is collected by either catching a voided sample or by bladder catheterization via the urethra. Cystocentesis is possible in small ruminants and calves but is seldom performed.

VOIDED URINE SAMPLING

In cattle, females may be encouraged to urinate by "titillating," which is a method of stimulating the perineal area. The skin beneath the vulva is lightly stroked with the fingers or with straw until urination occurs. The tail should not be held during the procedure, to avoid distracting the cow. If this method does not work, repeated parting of the lips of the vulva may be effective. The initial urine stream is not collected, since it contains more "contaminants" (debris and bacteria). A midstream sample is preferred and is collected into a clean container. If bacterial culture is to be performed, the container should be sterile.

Female sheep can sometimes be stimulated to urinate by holding the nostrils and mouth shut for up to 45 seconds (with the animal standing). The hold should be released when the animal indicates discomfort by struggling; urination usually follows promptly. This maneuver is best performed with two people; one occludes the nostrils, and the other collects the urine specimen.

Female goats must usually be collected with the "patience" method (wait patiently with a specimen cup for urination to occur); holding the nostrils is seldom effective. Goats often urinate upon standing after spending time in recumbency. Sometimes urination may be encouraged by placing the animal in a new stall or pen area.

Male ruminants are difficult to stimulate to urinate. Manual stimulation of the prepuce is sometimes effective. Male goats tend to urinate more frequently during breeding season as part of their natural mating behavior.

BLADDER/URETHRAL CATHETERIZATION

Female

Catheterization of the female urethra is performed similarly to that of the mare and as sterilely as possible. The animal must be properly restrained. The tail must be held or tied out of the way for the entire procedure. The vulva is prepped with warm water and antiseptic soap or solution. The clinician wears sterile gloves and uses sterile lubricating jelly to pass a hand or the fingers into the vestibule of the vagina. The urethral opening is generally within 5 to 10 cm of the vulva (depending on the size of the animal) and opens on ventral midline. A small animal vaginal speculum and light source may be helpful in does and ewes to allow visualization of the urethral opening. A suitable catheter is placed into the urethral entrance and advanced into the bladder.

Female ruminants have a small blind "sac" extending from the ventral aspect of the urethra (suburethral diverticulum) that will prevent passage of the catheter if it accidentally enters the sac. If resistance is encountered, the catheter is simply withdrawn slightly and redirected in a more dorsal direction. Once in the bladder, urine may be collected by gravity flow or by aspirating with a sterile syringe.

Adult does and ewes may be catheterized with a No. 10 to 12 French catheter. Small females may require slightly smaller diameters. Adult cows may be catheterized with the same urinary catheters (rigid or flexible) as used in the mare; a No. 12 to 20 French diameter is suitable. Urinary catheters should always be sterile.

Male

The anatomy of the urethra of male ruminants makes bladder catheterization difficult to impossible to perform. In sheep and goats, the urethra opens 1 to 2 cm beyond the tip of the glans penis through the urethral process; this narrow structure can be difficult to enter with a catheter and may have to be amputated before a catheter can be introduced into the urethra. Even after successful introduction of a catheter, advancing the catheter into the bladder is often impossible. All domestic ruminants have an S-shaped curvature of the penis and urethra (sigmoid flexure) that often hinders passage of a catheter beyond that point. Yet another anatomical obstruction, the urethral diverticulum, is a blind sac near the ischial arch; this usually presents a final roadblock to the catheter tip, keeping it from entering the bladder (Fig. 14-6).

Extending the penis in many males for urethral catheterization may be difficult. In sheep and goats, the male can be "set up" and rocked backward slightly on the rump; sedation greatly assists the procedure. The sigmoid

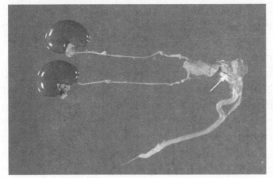

Fig. 14-6. Dissected urogenital tract of a buck. The *arrow* points to the urethral diverticulum in the area of the ischial arch, distal to the neck of the bladder. Note also the S-curved sigmoid flexure of the shaft of the penis and the small urethral process extending from the tip of the glans. (From Pugh DG: *Sheep and goat medicine*, St Louis, 2002, Saunders.)

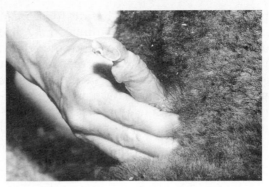

Fig. 14-7. Exteriorization of a ram's penis. Note the urethral process. (From Pugh DG: *Sheep and goat medicine*, St Louis, 2002, Saunders.)

flexure can be palpated through the prepuce; the penis is grasped with one hand (through the preputial skin) just caudal to the flexure. The penis is pushed cranially, while the other hand retracts the prepuce caudally. This maneuver exteriorizes the glans penis and helps to partially straighten out the S-shaped sigmoid flexure. If desired, the glans can be grasped with a gauze sponge and used to keep the penis extended (Fig. 14-7). The restrainer maintains this position, while another person cleans the glans and performs the urethral catheterization. Note that extending the penis of young males (prepubertal) may be difficult.

Bladder catheterization in male cattle is virtually impossible by the urethral route.

CEREBROSPINAL FLUID SAMPLING

Cerebrospinal fluid samples may be collected from either the atlantooccipital space (i.e., cisterna magna) or the lumbosacral space, using the same landmarks as described for horses. The animal must be heavily sedated

or under general anesthesia for use of either location. The atlantoccipital space is only accessed with the animal in lateral recumbency, with the head ventroflexed as much as possible. The lumbosacral space is also accessed in lateral recumbency with the spine ventroflexed. In older calves and adult cattle, the lumbosacral tap may be performed in a standing, sedated animal if very secure restraint is available.

Regardless of patient positioning, attention must be given toward keeping the spine in a straight alignment, since any lateral deviations make the procedure difficult. Needle diameter for either location may be either 18- or 20-ga. The depth of the lumbosacral space is not as deep as in the horse, and a $3\frac{1}{2}$-inch length spinal needle is suitable for most ruminants (including adult cattle).

MILK SAMPLING

Mastitis, or inflammation of the mammary gland, causes an estimated loss of more than 1 billion dollars to the dairy industry in the United States each year. Diagnosis and treatment of mastitis is critical for the health of dairy animals and for the successful production of milk that is safe for human consumption. Non–dairy animals may also develop mastitis and suffer from the related pain and inflammation. Mastitis is almost always caused by bacterial infection (septic mastitis), but inflammation *without* infection may occur if a teat or udder is traumatically injured (e.g., laceration, getting kicked or stepped on).

Mastitis is divided into two major categories on the basis of clinical signs. "Clinical mastitis" means there are clinical signs that need no special equipment to detect—palpation of a hard, hot mammary gland or visualization of abnormal milk (clumps of exudates or foul odor). "Subclinical mastitis" has no obviously visible clinical signs in the udder or in the milk and must be detected by special diagnostic testing. The definitive diagnosis of mastitis is made through sampling and testing milk.

MILKING PROCEDURE

Obtaining milk from the udder should be done as cleanly as possible; milk only teats that are clean, dry, and free of dirt and debris. The milker's hands should be clean and dry. Usually, only the teats are washed in preparation for milking; this is due to the risk of actually *causing* mastitis by washing the entire udder before milking. When the entire udder is washed, the water and contaminants (caked feces, mud, urine, etc.) flow with gravity down the sides of the udder and off the teat ends. During milking, the teat orifice (streak canal) must open, and this provides a route for bacteria to ascend up into the mammary gland. This is the route by which virtually all septic mastitis occurs: microorganisms ascending into the gland through the teat orifice. Mastitis does *not* occur by seeding of the mammary gland through the blood, as is commonly thought. Since the teat orifice cannot be completely sterilized, it is very important to keep contamination of the area around the orifice as low as possible, especially while the orifice is open. It is also important to realize that the orifice does not snap shut when milking is over; rather, it closes gradually over the following 1 to 2 hours. This is the rationale for using teat dips and teat guards after milking—to try to provide some residual germicidal action during this period when the teat orifice is open and susceptible to bacterial entry (Boxes 14-1 and 14-2).

Milking should be done in a clean, dry, stress-free environment. Milk letdown requires the pituitary hormone oxytocin. Epinephrine, released as part of the stress response, counteracts the effects of oxytocin. Loud noises, barking dogs, and unfamiliar personnel may all reduce milk letdown.

Farmers vary in the products they use to clean udders and teats, as well as the methods they use to rinse and dry teats in preparation for milking. Milk sampling for mastitis is done by hand milking. The basic procedure for hand milking is as follows:

1. Palpate the udder and teats. The classic clinical signs of mastitis are a hard, hot, and often painful, quarter (cattle) or half (sheep and goats).
2. Wash teats with a sanitizing solution.
3. Dry teats thoroughly with individual paper towels.
4. Grasp the teat at its base, by gently but firmly "pinching" it between the thumb and first or second fingers.
5. While maintaining the "pinch," slide the pinch down the teat, toward the teat end. Any milk in the teat canal has only one way out—the teat orifice—since the finger pinch prevents it from moving backwards.
6. The "sliding pinch" may be repeated as many times as needed to collect the desired volume of milk. The pinch must be totally released when the fingers are returned to the base of the teat.

14-1 Organisms Causing Mastitis in Cattle

Definitions

- Contagious mastitis: can be spread directly from cow to cow, usually at milking time (milking machines or contaminated hands or towels).
- Environmental mastitis: spread to individual cows through environmental contamination of bedding, soil, standing water, feces, etc.
- Gangrenous mastitis: severe infection that results in destruction of the affected quarter, with necrosis and sloughing. Severe *Staphylococcus* infections and wounds that allow *Clostridium* sp. to become established may result in gangrenous mastitis.
- Clinical mastitis: visible signs of disease in the milk and/or the affected quarter.
- Subclinical mastitis: no visible signs of disease. Causes the greatest economic loss to dairy farmers because of lowered production. Requires special diagnostic testing of the milk to diagnose.

Main Two Organisms Causing Mastitis

Approximately 95% of mastitis is caused by the following two organisms. These bacteria tend to cause local infections of the mammary glands and seldom cause systemic illness:

- *Streptococcus agalactiae:* can be spread from cow to cow (contagious mastitis). Relatively easy to treat with antibiotics and good sanitation practices.
- *Staphylococcus aureus:* can be spread from cow to cow (contagious mastitis). Tends to form microabscesses that resist penetration by antibiotics, making infection difficult to treat.

Other Organisms Causing Mastitis

- Coliforms (especially *Escherichia coli*, *Klebsiella* sp., *Enterobacter aerogenes*): release endotoxins, which enter the bloodstream and can cause endotoxemia and even death. Acute septic mastitis is characterized by fever, anorexia, rumen atony, dehydration, and diarrhea. The affected milk is watery and has a "Gatorade" appearance. Treatment involves systemic antibiotics, nonsteroidal antiinflammatory drugs, possible fluid therapy, and stripping of all milk every 2 to 4 hours.
- Corynebacteria: The milk is thick and creamy, sometimes called "mayonnaise mastitis." Difficult to impossible to treat successfully.
- Leptospirosis: The milk is thick but has no clots or blood, and affected quarters are not hard and hot. Sometimes called "cold mastitis." Leptospirosis is a fastidious bacterium that is difficult to culture.
- Mycoplasma: Rarely causes mastitis. No cure.
- Environmental streptococci: *S. uberis*, *S. bovis*, *S. dysgalactiae*, *Enterococcus* sp.

MASTITIS TESTS

Strip Cup (Plate) Examination

The strip cup is a special milk collection cup with a black lid. The first milk that is expressed from the teat, called the foremilk, should be squirted onto the black lid and observed for abnormalities and odor. Normal milk should be watery, chalky colored, and free of solid clumps; it should not have a sour or fetid odor. Clumps, clots, flakes, abnormal color, blood, and bad odor are all indicators of possible mastitis. Strip cup examination is an important screening test but only detects "clinical mastitis" (obvious clinical signs); subclinical mastitis (without visible clinical signs) will not be detected. Further testing is necessary to confirm the disease.

BOX 14-2   Organisms Causing Septic Mastitis in Sheep and Goats

- *Staphylococcus* sp.: the most prevalent cause of mastitis. *S. aureus* and *S. epidermidis* predominate. *S. aureus* may cause "bluebag," a form of mastitis in which altered blood flow causes the affected gland to appear cyanotic in color. Bluebag causes systemic illness (toxemia) with fever, anorexia, and depression. The condition may progress to a gangrenous mastitis with eventual sloughing of the affected half. Without treatment, mortality is high.
- Coliform mastitis: less common in small ruminants than in cattle. *Escherichia coli* and *Klebsiella* sp. predominate.
- *Pasteurella haemolytica:* more common in sheep than in goats. May cause bluebag.
- *Streptococcus* sp.: less common in small ruminants than in cattle.
- *Pseudomonas aeruginosa*
- *Mycoplasma* sp.: no truly effective treatment. Affected animals are usually culled.
- Viral mastitis: uncommon. Associated with ovine progressive pneumonia in sheep and caprine arthritis/encephalitis (CAE) in goats. The udder becomes firm due to chronic fibrosis of the mammary glands; farmers refer to the disease as "hard udder." Affected animals should be culled.
- *Bacillus* sp.: a common cause of subclinical mastitis.

California Mastitis Test

The California Mastitis Test (CMT) is one of the most commonly used field tests to identify individual cows (or does or ewes) affected with mastitis, and it specifically identifies which quarters (or halves) are affected. This is important because mastitis seldom involves an entire udder; it is much more common that only one or two quarters are diseased. The test is sensitive enough to detect subclinical mastitis and roughly quantifies the severity of inflammation. Inflammation in the udder stimulates migration of white blood cells (WBCs) into the affected gland and also causes the death of some of the epithelial (milk-producing) cells of the affected gland. These sloughed epithelial cells and WBCs, referred to as *somatic cells,* enter the milk, where they may be detected. The California Mastitis Test basically uses detergent chemicals to lyse somatic cells in the milk, which releases their DNA. The test then detects the released DNA by changes in the consistency of the tested milk. The consistency reflects the "somatic cell count," or SCC, of the milk; the higher the count, the more severe the inflammation.

The test uses a white plastic test "paddle" with four cups labeled A to D. The test should not be performed on the foremilk, which typically contains higher SCC, even in normal milk. The udder is cleaned, and the foremilk is discarded. Then, each quarter is milked into a separate paddle cup; only enough milk to cover the bottom of the cup is necessary (≈2 to 3 ml). One way to be sure of the proper milk volume is to fill all of the cups with several squirts of milk, then tilt the paddle briefly vertically; excess milk spills from the cup. The test reagent is then added, using an equal volume of reagent as milk in each cup. The paddle is kept horizontal and gently moved in a circular path to produce a swirling of the cup contents. The test is read after about 10 seconds of mixing, *while continuing to swirl the paddle.* Interpretation must be prompt because mild positive reactions tend to disappear after 20 to 30 seconds.

Accurately recording the results is important for identifying which quarters are affected and need to be treated. The paddle has a handle, which should be consistently pointed in the same direction (relative to the cow) so that the technician can always be sure which teats correspond to which sample cup. For instance, if the handle is always pointed toward the cow's head, then the results can be accurately recorded no matter which side of the cow the technician stood on to take the samples.

Interpretation of the CMT involves two variables: changes in consistency and changes in color. Consistency changes correspond to the SCC and are placed into one of five possible categories (Tables 14-1 and 14-2). Color changes correspond to the pH of the mixture; the test reagent contains brom-cresol purple, a pH indicator that remains purple when alkaline and turns yellow in acidic conditions (pH < 5.2). A grade of "+" is given for alkaline milk, and "Y" for acidic milk. Acidic milk is unusual. Normal milk has a pH of 6.4 to 6.8.

False positives may occur in late lactation, during estrus, and if the foremilk is tested; the SCC tends to be naturally high in all of these situations. Also, trauma to the udder or teat elevates SCC, indicating inflammation but not necessarily infection.

TABLE

14-1 CALIFORNIA MASTITIS TEST: GRADING TEST REACTIONS

Symbol	Suggested Meaning	Description of Visible Reaction	"Quickie" Description
N	Negative	Mixture remains liquid with no evidence of formation of a precipitate	Water
T	Trace	A slight precipitate forms and is best seen by tipping the paddle back and forth and observing the mixture as it flows over the bottom of the cup. Trace reactions tend to disappear with continued movement of the fluid.	Slime
+1	Weak positive	A distinct precipitate forms, but there is no tendency toward gel formation. The precipitate may disappear with continued movement of the paddle.	Thick slime
+2	Distinct positive	The mixture thickens immediately with some suggestion of gel formation. As the mixture is swirled, it tends to move in toward the center of the cup, leaving the bottom of the outer edge of the cup exposed. When the motion is stopped, the mixture levels out again and covers the bottom of the cup.	Gel
+3	Strong positive	A gel is formed, causing the surface of the mixture to become convex. Usually there is a central peak that projects above the main mass after motion of the paddle has stopped. Viscosity is greatly increased so that there is a tendency for the mass to adhere to the bottom of the cup.	Jelly

TABLE

14-2   CALIFORNIA MASTITIS TEST: INTERPRETATION OF RESULTS

Test Score	Interpretation in Cattle	Interpretation in Goats
N	Normal (0-200,000 cells/ml)	Normal (0-480,000 cells/ml)
T	Normal (150,000-500,000)	Normal (0-640,000)
+1	Suspicious (500,000-1,500,000)	Suspicious (240,000-1,440,000)
+2	Mastitis (1,500,000-5,000,000)	Mastitis (1,080,000-5,850,000)
+3	Mastitis (>5,000,000 cells/ml)	Mastitis (>10,000,000 cells/ml)

Positive quarters are usually treated by intramammary infusion (see Chapter 15).

Milk Culture and Sensitivity

Milk culture is seldom necessary to confirm the diagnosis of mastitis, but it may be helpful for screening a herd for subclinical cases or identifying the bacteria in cases that are severe or refractory to routine antibiotic therapy. Samples may be collected individually from each quarter, or all four quarters may be pooled together for a screening sample for each animal.

Samples should be collected into sterile tubes; glass tubes with screw caps are preferred. Tubes should be labeled and paperwork finished before the procedure. The procedure for collecting the samples is as follows:

1. Wash hands thoroughly.
2. Wash teats in a sanitizing solution and dry teats with individual paper towels.
3. Strip and discard one to two squirts of milk from each teat.
4. Dip teats in germicidal teat dip, and allow 30 seconds of contact time. Dry each teat with an individual paper towel.
5. Thoroughly clean the teat orifice with a cotton swab soaked in alcohol. Begin with the far teats, then the near teats (prevents contaminating the near teats when reaching across to swab the far side).
6. Open the sterile tube and hold it at a 45-degree angle so that debris cannot fall into the tube. Do not allow anything to touch the opening of the tube. Collect one to two squirts from each quarter. Begin with the near teats, then collect the far teats.
7. Cap the tube immediately.
8. Tubes should be refrigerated (4° C or 39° F), not frozen, until they can be processed in the laboratory. Processing should occur within 24 hours, by swabbing on a blood agar plate, and should be followed using routine microbial culture methods. In rare cases when processing cannot be done within 24 hours, the samples should be frozen as soon as possible.

SUGGESTED READING

Fubini SL, Ducharme NG: *Farm animal surgery*, St Louis, 2004, Saunders.

McCurnin DM, Bassert JM: *Clinical textbook for veterinary technicians*, ed 6, St Louis, 2006, Saunders.

Pugh DG: *Sheep and goat medicine*, St Louis, 2002, Saunders.

Sirois M: *Principles and practice of veterinary technology*, ed 2, St Louis, 2004, Mosby.

Smith MC, Sherman DM: *Goat medicine*, Baltimore, 1994, Williams & Wilkins.

15

Medication Techniques in Ruminants

Medicating ruminants is often complicated by the production of meat and milk products destined for human consumption. In order to prevent certain drugs and other chemicals (such as pesticides) from entering the human food chain, withdrawal intervals ("withdrawal times") have been established for many of the substances used in food-producing animals. The withdrawal interval is the time between administration of a known dose of a drug or chemical to an animal and the time that the animal's meat, milk, or eggs are presumably safe for human consumption. The Food and Drug Administration (FDA) is the agency responsible for drug approval and for establishing withdrawal intervals for drugs approved for use in food animals, based on scientific evidence. Withdrawal intervals are printed on the labels of approved substances. Residue-contaminated meat or milk has *significant* economic and legal consequences for the farmer, and sometimes the farmer may see the veterinarian (and veterinary staff) as being responsible for contamination by failing to follow proper procedures or giving inaccurate advice.

Many drugs are not approved for use in food animals, but may be desirable or necessary to use in certain situations. This is referred to as "extralabel drug use." Withdrawal intervals are not printed on the labels of such drugs. In order to guide veterinarians in the extralabel use of drugs in food animal species, FARAD (Food Animal Residue Avoidance Databank) is a convenient source of information. FARAD is the primary resource for recommendations for withdrawal times after extralabel drug use in food animals. It is a computer-based "decision support system" that provides current label information on withdrawal times of approved drugs, a database of scientific articles with data on drug residues and pharmacokinetics on nonapproved drugs, and official tolerances of drug and pesticide residues in meat, milk, and eggs. (FARAD may be contacted at www.farad.org or by phone at 1-888-USFARAD. FARAD is administered through the US Department of Agriculture [USDA]).

Accurate record keeping is essential. Treatment records should accurately identify each animal treated, the type of medication, the dose and route that the medication was given, and the withholding time (if any) that was recommended to the farmer. Recording the drug lot numbers is also advisable.

ORAL MEDICATION

Some oral medications may be placed in the water source or mixed with food; this can be done for individual animals or on a herd basis. However, this is not a reliable method of delivering most medications. When it is necessary to ensure delivery of medication to individual animals or control doses for each animal, medication techniques for individuals will be required.

BALLING GUN

The balling gun is an instrument used to deliver medication that is in capsule or bolus (large tablet) form. Balling guns are available in different sizes and are made of metal, plastic, or a combination of metal with a plastic tip (Fig. 15-1). The instrument should be checked for sharp edges before use. Severe trauma (laceration, abscessation) to the pharynx, epiglottis, and oral cavity of the animal may result from poor technique.

Head restraint is essential. Cattle are best placed in a head catch. With cooperative cattle, the operator can stand next to the head, facing in the same direction as the animal. One arm is placed across and over the bridge of the nose, and that hand can be used to reach in the interdental space to place pressure on the hard palate or to grasp the nostrils. The other hand operates the balling gun. Small ruminants may be backed into a corner or wall and straddled; one hand is used to elevate and restrain the head, and the other hand operates the balling gun (Fig. 15-2). The head of any species should not be elevated beyond a natural position (nose should not be higher than the top of the head), to decrease the risk of accidental aspiration of the medication into the trachea. If the animal is reluctant to open the mouth, pressing on the hard palate

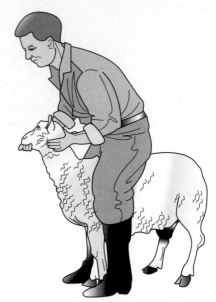

Fig. 15-2. Position for restraint and oral medication of sheep and goats.

through the interdental space or putting a finger/thumb in each nostril and elevating the nose may provide encouragement.

The balling gun (loaded with medication) is introduced into the side of the mouth through the interdental space, above the tongue. It is then redirected caudally and advanced over the base of the tongue; failure to deliver the medication over the tongue base likely results in the animal spitting it out. However, the gun should not be placed so far back that it wedges in the pharynx/larynx, where it can cause significant damage. The plunger of the instrument is pressed to "eject" the tablet into the mouth, and the balling gun is carefully removed with a smooth motion. In small ruminants, the mouth can be held shut until swallowing occurs. The animal is observed to be sure that all medication is swallowed.

The balling gun is not a suitable instrument for very young animals or for horses.

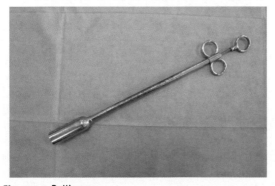

Fig. 15-1. Balling gun.

DRENCHING

Delivery of liquid oral medication directly into the oral cavity is referred to as *drenching*. Liquid medications can be delivered with an oral dose syringe or 60-ml catheter-tip syringe using a technique similar to passage of the balling gun; the tip of the syringe should be positioned over the base of the tongue to prevent spillage from the mouth. The tip of the nose should not be held higher than the top of the head, to minimize the risk of aspiration into the trachea. The liquid should not be injected with unnecessarily high pressure, since this might "shoot" medication into the trachea. Rather, deliver the liquid slowly, allowing the animal time to swallow. If coughing occurs, the procedure should be stopped until the animal has a chance to "clear its throat" and settle down.

FRICK SPECULUM

The Frick speculum is a rigid metal tube that may be used as an oral or vaginal speculum in cattle (Fig. 15-3). It is placed in the mouth in exactly the same fashion as a balling gun. Held in this position, it can be used to deliver boluses and liquids or assist passage of an orogastric (stomach) tube (Fig. 15-4).

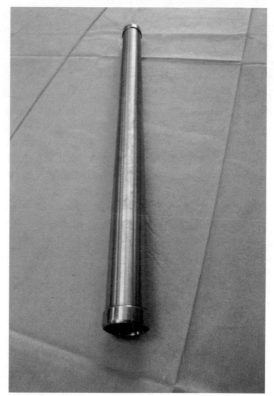

Fig. 15-3. Frick speculum for cattle.

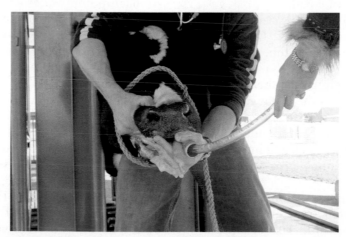

Fig. 15-4. A Frick speculum has been placed to allow passage of a stomach (ororumen) tube. (From McCurnin DM, Bassert JM: *Clinical textbook for veterinary technicians*, ed 6, St Louis, 2006, Saunders.)

The stainless steel construction allows the Frick speculum to be disinfected and/or sterilized.

RUMEN (GASTRIC) INTUBATION

Large quantities of fluids can be delivered directly into the rumen/reticulum by passage of a stomach tube. Intubation is also used to relieve rumen bloat and can be used to withdraw samples of rumen fluid for analysis or transfer to other animals (rumen inoculation). The tube can be placed through the nasogastric or orogastric (ororumen) route. The nasogastric route, used in horses, is not commonly used in ruminants; the nasal passages of cattle are of smaller diameter than in horses, and this significantly limits the tube diameter that can be used. Therefore the oral route is used most often.

The mouth must first be held open with a speculum, to keep the animal from damaging the tube. There are a variety of speculums available commercially, and many can be easily homemade. In cattle, the Frick speculum is popular. In small ruminants, a block of wood with a circular hole cut in it, a short piece of polyvinyl chloride (PVC) pipe, or a tape roll can be placed between the lower incisors and the dental pad.

The stomach tube must be sized appropriately for length and diameter. The length of most commercially available tubes is sufficient to reach the rumen; the necessary length can be estimated by holding the tube outside the animal and simulating the distance from the mouth to the rumen. The outer diameter of the tube should be approximately 5/8 to 1 inch for adult cattle; small and medium foal stomach tubes are suitable for calves, sheep, and goats.

The tip and first portion of the tube should be lubricated with either water or water-soluble lubricant. The speculum is placed and may need to be held by an assistant. The stomach tube is placed through the speculum and advanced to the pharynx. Once the tube reaches the back of the pharynx, resistance is felt; the animal usually swallows at this time, and the tube is advanced into the esophagus with the swallow. It may be necessary to withdraw the tube slightly, rotate it slightly, and advance it again if the initial attempt fails. Coughing often indicates entry into the trachea, but this is not always 100% reliable. Feeling air pass out of the tube when the animal exhales may also indicate improper placement in the trachea, although this is also not always reliable. Proper placement in the esophagus is confirmed by palpating or observing the tube in the esophagus; feeling mild resistance as it is passed; and finally confirming its location in the rumen by the strong smell of rumen gas, aspiration of rumen fluid, or by having an assistant listen with a stethoscope over the rumen (left paralumbar fossa) while the operator blows air through the tube; a gurgling sound should be heard with the stethoscope. No material should be delivered through the tube until it is absolutely certain that the tube has reached the rumen.

Liquids can be given by gravity flow through a funnel, by dose syringe, or with a stomach pump; water or air is then used to "clear" residual medication from the tube. Before removing the tube, the end should be kinked off or occluded to prevent accidentally spilling its contents into the trachea and nasal passages as it is withdrawn. Removal should be done in a single, smooth motion.

Ruminants are capable of regurgitation. Passage of the tube may stimulate regurgitation. Regurgitation may occur through and around the stomach tube. Aspiration of the regurgitated liquid into the lungs is a real concern. For this reason, the head should not be forced into an elevated position during passage of the tube or while the tube is in the rumen.

Neonatal sheep and goats do not require use of a speculum. Small rubber urinary catheters or infant feeding tubes (10- to 18-French) may be used.

PARENTERAL INJECTION TECHNIQUES

INTRAMUSCULAR INJECTIONS

Research has shown that intramuscular (IM) injections usually cause scar tissue formation at the injection site. The scar tissue is visible and causes toughness in the meat, which may extend as much as 3 inches from the injection site. There is also the risk of abscessation. These "injection site blemishes" must be trimmed out of the meat when it is processed, thus decreasing the value of the carcass. This has resulted in a trend of avoiding IM injections into the muscles that yield valuable cuts of meat (hindlegs) and the development of subcutaneously injectable drugs (when possible) to replace intramuscular medications.

Recommendations include the following:
1. Use subcutaneous (SQ) products whenever possible (must be FDA-approved for SQ administration).
2. Use sharp, single-use, sterile needles from 16- to 20-gauge (ga), 1- to 1½-inch length (depending on the size of the animal, size of the muscle, and the "thickness" of the medication). Generally cattle require a 16- to 18-ga needle; small ruminants and calves, an 18- to 20-ga needle; and lambs/kids, a 20- to 22-ga needle.
3. Do not inject more than 10 ml per IM injection site in cattle or 5 ml in small ruminants.
4. Keep IM injection sites separated by at least 4 inches.
5. The preferred IM injection site is in front of the shoulder (lateral cervical area).
6. Avoid injecting through wet or dirty skin.

Intramuscular Injection Sites

IM injection locations and techniques are similar to those used in the horse (see Chapter 4).

Appropriate restraint should always be applied before injection. The site should always be cleaned (down to and including the skin) with 70% alcohol or other suitable antiseptic. In sheep, part the wool down to the skin to allow proper cleaning of the injection site. IM injections should not be performed until the needle has been aspirated to confirm that the needle bevel is not in a blood vessel.

Clinicians vary in their preferences for use of certain muscle groups. Commonly used sites include the following:
- Gluteal muscles: This site is becoming less popular due to potential scarring of the valuable meat cuts. Dairy cattle, sheep, and goats have very thin gluteals; therefore these muscles are usually avoided; if necessary to use the gluteals in these animals, a short needle (<1 inch) should be used, and only small quantities of medication (<10 ml per site in cattle, <5 ml in goats) should be given.
- Semitendinosus/semimembranosus muscle: This site is used more often in young cattle and the small ruminants. A tail jack may be applied for additional restraint. The sciatic nerve, which lies in the sciatic groove, must be avoided.
- Triceps muscle: This site is appropriate for small volumes of medication.
- Lateral cervical muscles: This site is used mostly in cattle and occasionally in goats and is preferred to the gluteals in meat-producing animals. This location is generally avoided in show goats because of the possibility of a tissue reaction being mistaken for an abscess of the prescapular lymph node, which mimics the caprine disease of caseous lymphadenitis. In small animals such as goats, needle length should not exceed 1 inch. The landmarks are similar to those described for the horse—a triangular area bounded by the cervical vertebrae ventrally, the shoulder

(scapula) caudally, and the nuchal ligament dorsally. Injections should be given well within these boundaries.

- Longissimus muscle: this muscle lies over the back, along either side of the vertebral column. The lumbar portion of this muscle may be used for injections in goats, if the hide is not to be marketed. Injections (of any kind) into any area of the back often devalue the hide due to scarring and other blemishes. Only small volumes (<5 ml) should be injected.

INTRAVENOUS INJECTIONS

The jugular vein is the preferred site to administer intravenous (IV) medications and fluids. The cephalic vein, caudal auricular vein (cattle), and coccygeal (tail vein) may also be used for small volumes of drugs. The coccygeal vein should not be used for any drug that causes irritation if accidentally given perivascularly. The coccygeal artery, which is the only arterial supply to the tail, lies adjacent to the vein; any tissue reaction (swelling, scarring) could compromise blood flow and possibly result in necrosis and sloughing of the tail.

Venipuncture sites and techniques have been described (see Chapter 14).

SUBCUTANEOUS INJECTIONS

SQ injections can be given anywhere that skin can be lifted with the fingers. In ruminants, the common locations are over the lateral cervical region, over the thorax several inches caudal to the shoulder, in the axilla, in the ventral aspect of the flank ("flank fold"), and in the pectoral area (brisket). The area over the scapula, just caudal to the scapular spine, is less often used. Injections into the back area are possible but usually avoided because of devaluing the hide.

Needle diameter may range from 14- to 20-ga in adult cattle and 18- to 22-ga in small ruminants. A 1-inch needle length is sufficient, but 1½ inches may be used with care.

Maximum injection volume is also determined by species and location. Injected volumes are usually small, but up to 250 ml can be given at one site in adult cattle, and up to 50 ml in calves and adult small ruminants. Large volumes may tend to experience some leakage of the medication through the needle hole after the needle is withdrawn; pinching or putting pressure over the needle hole may minimize this occurrence.

Restraint depends on the species and the location of the injection. Sheep may be set up for easy access to the axilla and flank fold. The skin should be cleaned with 70% alcohol or other antiseptic. The skin is pinched and elevated to form a "skin tent," and the needle is inserted into the "tent," being careful not to go all the way through the "tent." Before injection, the syringe should be aspirated to be sure that it is not within a blood vessel. After injection, the needle is withdrawn and the "tent" released.

INTRADERMAL INJECTIONS

Injections into the dermis are more often used for diagnostic, rather than treatment, purposes. In ruminants, tuberculosis testing is the primary indication for intradermal (ID) injections. The standard location for routine tuberculosis testing is in the caudal tail fold. The right and left caudal tail folds are best seen by elevating the tail; this puts tension on the tail folds, which are located at the base of the tail. Intradermal skin testing for allergic reactions is performed in the lateral cervical or flank area.

If hair is present, it must be clipped before injection. ID injections are performed by first cleaning the skin; depending on the material to be injected, antiseptics may or may not be used. Antiseptic residues may cause tissue reaction if injected intradermally, which can confuse proper interpretation of skin tests. The skin should be allowed to dry before injecting.

A 25- or 26-ga needle is used for the injection, though a 22- or 23-ga may be necessary in cattle for the thicker skin of the neck and flank. The skin is pinched firmly; the needle bevel should face outward toward the operator. The needle is held parallel to the pinched skin and advanced into the dermis. Injection should produce a small bleb within (not beneath) the skin; if not seen, the needle is likely placed too deeply, and the injection procedure should be repeated.

INTRAVENOUS CATHETERIZATION

The jugular vein is the preferred site for IV catheterization in all ruminant species. If the jugular veins are not usable, the cephalic veins may be used. The caudal auricular vein (ear vein) in adult cattle may accept a small-gauge catheter, but this is rarely feasible because of difficulties in stabilizing a catheter at that location. The subcutaneous abdominal veins (milk veins) are not suitable for indwelling IV catheters. Catheter diameter may be 10- to 14-ga for cattle (18- to 20-ga for the ear vein), and 14- to 18-ga for calves and small ruminants. Small individuals may use catheters that are 2 to 3 inches in length.

Insertion technique and principles of maintaining the catheter are identical to those described for horses (see Chapter 4). Head restraint with a halter and nose tongs is desirable for catheterizing the ear vein.

INTRAMAMMARY INFUSION

Medications may be deposited (infused) into individual teats to treat or prevent diseases of the mammary glands. Antibiotics are by far the most common type of medication given by this route; they are most commonly used to treat active cases of mastitis in lactating cows ("wet cow treatment") or to treat or prevent mastitis in cows that are completing a lactation cycle ("dry cow treatment"). Mastitis primarily affects dairy cows and

dairy goats, but all milk-producing females are susceptible.

Mammary infusions are usually purchased in disposable plastic syringes that are designed to treat a single teat and its associated gland. The syringe may come with an attached infusion tip, or a teat cannula or disposable plastic infusion tip will need to be placed on the end of the syringe. Bovine cannulas and infusion tips are too large for small ruminants. A small ⅛-inch infusion tip is now commercially available for these smaller animals, and sterile tomcat catheters may also be used for goats and sheep with small teat orifices. Infusion tips, cannulas, or catheters should never be used on more than one teat unless thoroughly cleaned and sterilized. Single-use, disposable plastic infusion tips are preferred and are inexpensive.

The standing position is preferred for all species. Dairy animals usually require minimal restraint, but occasionally the pain associated with some mastitis cases causes the animal to resent handling of the affected gland. Applying a tail hold may be helpful in these cases. Non–dairy animals should be approached with caution and will require more secure restraint, typically using some form of chute restraint for cattle. The technician should not sit or get in a position where he or she could be injured by a kick.

Because contact time must be maximized in order for the antibiotics to have their best effect, treatment is usually done after milking. Expressing all of the milk in the affected gland also helps the infusion to distribute within the gland. "Mastitis milk" is contaminated with bacteria and should be collected in a container where it can be safely discarded to prevent environmental contamination.

Infusion of any material into the udder must be done as cleanly as possible. The hands should be washed with soap and water before the procedure. The teats and udder are washed with warm water and mild antiseptic soap, and each teat is dried with an individual cloth towel or paper towel (preferred) to prevent cross-contamination of the teats. Any residual milk is stripped from the teat. Each teat to be treated is dipped in a liquid germicidal teat dip and allowed 30 seconds of contact time before drying with an individual towel. Each teat orifice to be treated is then thoroughly cleaned with a cotton swab soaked in alcohol; teats on the far side of the udder from the technician are swabbed first (to prevent contamination by the technician's arms when reaching across the udder). The alcohol is allowed to air dry. Infusion is performed in reverse order from cleansing (i.e., treat the near teats first, *then* reach across to treat the far teats) to prevent contaminating the clean teat ends.

With one hand stabilizing the end of the teat, the infusion tip is inserted through the teat orifice. Driving the tip deeply into the teat canal is not necessary, and attempting to do so may cause injury and increase risk of contamination. Simply advance the tip just beyond the teat opening ($\approx\frac{1}{8}$ to $\frac{1}{4}$ inch). The stabilizing hand is then used to gently pinch the teat orifice closed around the infusion tip, to prevent leakage of medication. The plunger is slowly depressed to deliver the medication. After delivering the desired volume, withdraw the syringe and tip, and gently squeeze the teat end closed with one hand. Use the other hand to gently massage the medication up into the associated gland to help its distribution. The teat should be dipped again in a germicidal teat dip and allowed to air dry.

Whenever antibiotics or other medications are delivered by intramammary infusion, the milk is subject to a withdrawal time to allow for clearance of drug residues. The required withdrawal time varies with different antibiotics and should be printed on the package insert and on the individual infusion syringes. Placing a temporary marking on all treated animals is common practice to prevent accidental milking and contamination of the milk supply destined for human consumption.

INTRANASAL ADMINISTRATION

Some vaccines and a small number of medications are available for intranasal administration. They are administered similarly to small animals. Head restraint is necessary. The nasal passage to be used should be cleared of any nasal exudates. The nose should be slightly elevated. The medication syringe (without needle!) is inserted just inside the nostril, and the plunger depressed in one rapid motion. A common response of the animal is to throw its head upward; therefore the technician should avoid positioning his or her body anywhere above the animal's head. Another common response of the animal is to sneeze, which expels some of the medication; this is usually of little consequence, since pharmaceutical companies compensate for this by adding extra volume to the dose syringes.

SUGGESTED READING

Fubini SL, Ducharme NG: *Farm animal surgery*, St Louis, 2004, Saunders.

Jaffe TJ: Diagnostic sampling and therapeutic techniques. In McCurnin DM, Bassert JM: *Clinical textbook for veterinary technicians*, ed 6, St Louis, 2006, Saunders.

Leahy JR, Barrow P: *Restraint of animals*, ed 2, Ithaca, NY, 1953, Cornell Campus Store.

Pugh DG: *Sheep and goat medicine*, St Louis, 2002, Saunders.

Sirois M: *Principles and practice of veterinary technology*, ed 2, St Louis, 2004, Mosby.

Smith MC, Sherman DM: *Goat medicine*, Baltimore, 1994, Williams & Wilkins.

Sonsthagen TF: *Restraint of domestic animals*, St Louis, 1991, Mosby.

16

Ruminant Surgery and Anesthesia

The advances in large animal surgical and anesthetic procedures are not limited to horses. Essentially all of the technology available to equines—surgical lasers, endoscopy and laparoscopy, arthroscopy, and internal fixation—are available to ruminants. However, the economic value of these animals seldom justifies the expenses involved in surgical treatment of many diseases. Essentially, the production animal usually must be able to "pay its way." Notable exceptions are high-producing dairy females and registered breeding stock of all species, which may have considerable value. Also, pet animals often engage an owner's emotions, and the bond formed between them may increase the likelihood of paying for costly procedures.

As with equines, surgical procedures can be divided into two main categories:
1. Standing surgery procedures
2. General anesthesia (recumbent) procedures

A third option which is sometimes used in ruminants is to combine heavy sedation with forced recumbency (casting); this method is often used to treat conditions of the limbs and feet.

STANDING SURGERY

The overwhelming majority of ruminant surgeries are performed in the standing position, using a combination of sedation/tranquilization and local or regional anesthesia. Cattle generally seem to tolerate standing procedures better than horses. Standing procedures are often used to repair traumatic injuries such as lacerations and punctures. Castration, caesarean section, correction of gastrointestinal (GI) tract abnormalities, enucleation, dehorning, and treatment of distal limb injuries are some of the more common standing surgical procedures. The indications and considerations for standing surgery in ruminants are identical to those in horses (see Chapter 8).

Surgical procedures may be accompanied by medications such as antibiotics, anti-inflammatory drugs, local anesthetics, and muscle relaxants. Concern for drug residues is always a concern for the practitioner. Females must have their pregnancy status determined in order to anticipate possible drug effects on the fetuses. All medications should be carefully recorded with dose, route of administration, location of administration, and any instructions or advice given to the client regarding drug use.

PREPARATION FOR STANDING SURGERY

Preparation (prepping) for standing surgery is usually straightforward. The location where the procedure is to be performed should ideally be clean, dry, and free of drafts; however, field situations are usually less than ideal. When this occurs, one must improvise to try to create the best possible conditions for the given situation.

Equipment and supplies should be assembled beforehand. It is preferable to keep surgical instruments elevated above ground level; they should be convenient to the surgeon but out of reach of the animal if it moves.

The form of restraint depends entirely on facilities available; personnel availability and experience; expected duration of the procedure; and patient factors such as species, age, temperament, anatomical location of the procedure, anticipated level of pain, and general health of the animal.

If sedation or tranquilization is to be used in adult ruminants, it is sometimes preferable to withhold food and water before the administration of these drugs, especially for intraabdominal procedures. Sedatives and tranquilizers depress GI motility, which increases the risk of rumen tympany (bloat). Additionally, ruminants occasionally regurgitate when heavily sedated and risk aspiration of the regurgitated material. Decreasing the volume of rumen contents may reduce these risks. Food may be safely withheld for up to 12 to 24 hours before the procedure, and water up to 6 hours. Since many standing procedures are performed on an emergency basis, without time for fasting, equipment should be available to deal with these complications, should they occur.

CONTROL OF PAIN

Local anesthesia is used alone or to supplement the analgesic effects of some sedatives and tranquilizers. Lidocaine, mepivacaine, and bupivacaine are the most commonly used local anesthetic drugs. Because lidocaine is the least expensive and least toxic (comparatively) of these drugs, it is most commonly used in farm animals. Note, however, that none of the local anesthetic drugs are approved for use in food animals in the United States, and clients must be advised of withdrawal times. Sometimes large volumes of these drugs are injected to produce large areas of desensitized tissue, and it is possible to reach toxic doses. Lidocaine has a toxic

(total) dose of 13 mg/kg bodyweight in cattle and sheep; goats are more sensitive (10 mg/kg total dose). Signs of toxicity from this family of local anesthetics (amides) include hypotension, drowsiness or sedation, muscle twitching, respiratory depression, and possibly convulsions. Treatment is supportive, since no specific antidote exists. Intravenous fluids, respiratory support, and anticonvulsants can be given as needed. To minimize the risk of toxicity, it is recommended to use local anesthetic concentrations no stronger than 2%. Especially in goats, dilution to 1% or less solution is advisable; dilution of 2% solution with an equal part of sterile saline achieves a 1% solution. In kids, many clinicians advocate dilution to a maximum 0.5% solution.

Local anesthesia in ruminants can be performed in several ways. Usually the anatomical location and expected level of pain dictate the method of local anesthesia used. Specific nerve blocks and field blocks may be used, similar to those described for equines. Common techniques used in ruminants include the following:

L Block

L block is a type of field block used to desensitize the flank for standing flank laparotomies. Local anesthetic is deposited in an inverted "L" configuration in the flank (Fig. 16-1). The anesthetic must be deposited in several layers (i.e., the subcutaneous tissue and all muscular layers of the abdominal wall). Large volumes of local anesthetic are required; often up to 100 ml of 2% solution are necessary in adult cattle. The anesthetic is deposited with an 18-gauge (ga) × 1½- to 3-inch needle (cattle) or 18- to 20-ga × 1- to 1½-inch needle (small ruminants). At least 10 to 15 minutes should be allowed for the anesthetic to diffuse and take effect before beginning the surgical procedure. The inverted "L" essentially forms a wall of anesthesia that protects the surgical field.

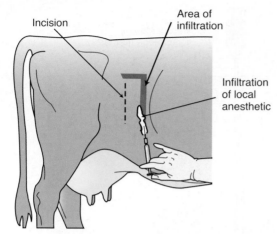

Fig. 16-1. Technique for the inverted "L" flank block for standing abdominal surgery. (Modified from Turner AS, McIlwraith CW: *Techniques in large animal surgery*, Philadelphia, 1982, Lea & Febiger.)

It is the simplest technique for desensitizing the flank and therefore is commonly employed.

Paravertebral Block

This technique uses multiple specific nerve blocks to create a large region of flank anesthesia. Innervation of the flank arises from the spinal nerves of T13, L1, and L2 spinal segments. These nerves can be blocked near their exit from the vertebral column at a "paravertebral" location. There are two main ways to approach these nerves: from a dorsal approach near the intervertebral foramina (Cambridge, Farquharson, or proximal paravertebral method) or from a lateral approach near the tips of the transverse processes of the lumbar vertebrae (Magda, Cornell, or distal paravertebral method) (Fig. 16-2). Cattle require a 16- to 18-ga × 3- to 6-inch length needle for the proximal paravertebral (dorsal) approach; note that some clinicians prefer to first place a 14-ga × 1-inch needle as a trocar through the skin and muscle layers, then insert an 18-ga needle

through the 14-ga needle to actually deliver the anesthetic. An 18- to 20-ga × 1½- to 3-inch spinal needle (no trocar needed) is sufficient for small ruminants. Up to 20 ml of anesthetic is necessary for each of the three injection sites in cattle, and 2 to 5 ml per site in sheep and goats.

For the distal paravertebral (lateral) approach, an 18-ga × 1½- to 3-inch needle is sufficient for cattle; a 20- to 22-ga × 1-inch needle is used in the small ruminants. Ten to 20 ml of anesthetic is deposited at each of the three injection sites in cattle, and 2 to 4 ml in sheep and goats.

The paravertebral block desensitizes all layers of the flank, from skin down to the peritoneum. Note that with the proximal paravertebral approach, once the block takes effect, paralysis of the longissimus muscle along the spine may cause temporary lateral curvature of the spine (bowing or scoliosis) toward the side of the block. This curvature may create some gaping of the skin incision, making suture closure more difficult. The distal paravertebral approach should not create scoliosis.

Cornual Nerve Block

The cornual nerve block is used for desensitization of the horn and horn base for dehorning surgery. The block is performed differently for cattle and goats, since the innervation is different.

Cattle

Cattle have a single nerve supply to each horn. The cornual nerve emerges from the orbit and ascends toward the base of the horn just below the temporal ridge of the frontal bone. Local anesthetic (≈3 to 5 ml in calves, 5 to 10 ml in adults) is deposited with an 18- to 20-ga × 1- to 1½-inch needle just ventral to the temporal ridge at a site approximately halfway between the horn base and the lateral canthus of the eye. The nerve is covered

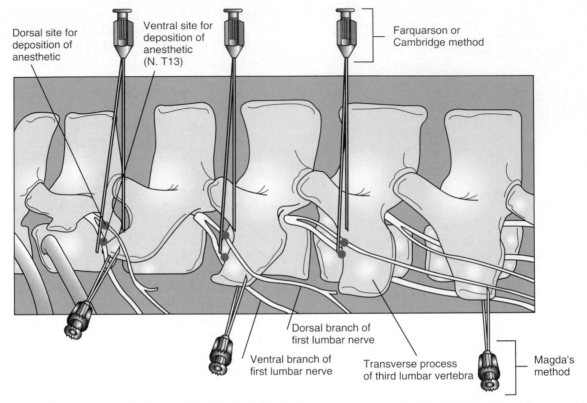

Fig. 16-2. Two approaches for the paravertebral block of the flank. (Modified from Turner AS, McIlwraith CW: *Techniques in large animal surgery*, Philadelphia, 1982, Lea & Febiger.)

only by skin and a thin layer of muscle at this location; depth of needle penetration is 1 cm in calves to 2.5 cm in large adults (Fig. 16-3).

Adult cattle with well-developed horns may require a second injection of several milliliters of anesthetic at the base of the horn, along the caudal aspect, just beneath the skin.

Goats

Goats have a dual nerve supply to each horn; therefore two sites must be blocked:

- The cornual branch from the lacrimal nerve is blocked just behind the caudal ridge of the supraorbital process, at a depth of approximately 1 to 1.5 cm. A 22- to 23-ga × 1-inch needle is used, and local anesthetic (0.5 to 1 ml for kids, 2 to 4 ml for adults) is deposited.
- The cornual branch of the infratrochlear nerve is blocked at the dorsomedial margin of the orbit, at a depth of approximately 0.5 cm. A 22- to 25-ga needle is used, and local anesthetic is deposited (0.5 ml for kids, 1 to 3 ml for adults) (Fig. 16-4).

Sheep are rarely dehorned. The nerve supply is only from the cornual branch of the lacrimal nerve; it is blocked using the same protocol as for blocking the cornual branch of the lacrimal nerve in goats.

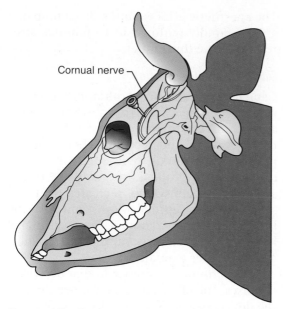

Cornual nerve

Fig. 16-3. Needle placement for desensitizing the cornual nerve in the bovine. The cornual nerve follows the temporal ridge to the base of the horn. (Modified from Muir WW III et al: *Veterinary anesthesia,* ed 3, St Louis, 2000, Mosby.)

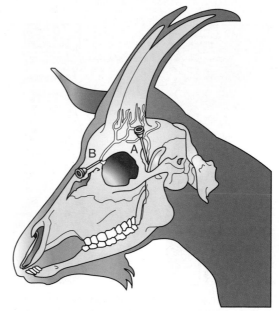

Fig. 16-4. Anesthesia for dehorning in the goat. **A,** Needle placement for desensitizing the cornual branch of the lacrimal nerve. **B,** Needle placement for desensitizing the cornual branch of the infratrochlear nerve. (Modified from Muir WW III et al: *Veterinary anesthesia,* ed 3, St Louis, 2000, Mosby.)

Intravenous Regional Analgesia (Bier Block)

Intravenous (IV) analgesia is considered superior to specific nerve blocks and ring blocks for most surgical procedures on the distal limbs. The technique uses an IV injection of local anesthetic, distal to a previously placed tourniquet. The anesthetic diffuses out of the veins and blocks the nerves in the area. Although it is seldom performed on standing animals, it is a common method of local analgesia for surgical procedures on awake, sedated animals in lateral recumbency.

The animal is restrained, sedated, and cast (placed in recumbency) to administer this form of regional anesthesia. A tourniquet is applied at the desired level on the limb, which is determined by the location of the surgical procedure. For procedures on the feet, the tourniquet is placed at midcarpus

or midtarsus. For more proximal procedures, the tourniquet is placed just proximal to the carpus or tarsus. Rubber tubing or other elastic strapping material is suitable for the tourniquet. Cotton or foam padding should be used beneath the tubing for additional protection of underlying tissues, especially where the tourniquet crosses superficial tendons. Proximal to the tarsus, the grooves in front of the common calcaneal tendon should be "filled in" on both sides of the leg with a roll gauze or other soft padding before placing the tourniquet; this is necessary to achieve complete arterial occlusion.

Any large superficial vein may be used; generally the dorsal metacarpal (metatarsal) or palmar (plantar) metacarpal (metatarsal) veins are used (Fig. 16-5). The site should be clipped and prepped. Lidocaine *without*

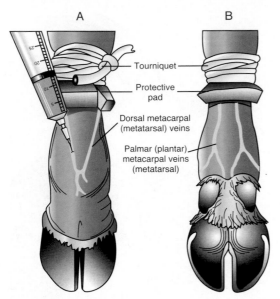

Fig. 16-5. Intravenous regional anesthesia. **A,** Dorsal aspect of the distal limb. **B,** Palmar (plantar) aspect. (Modified from Turner AS, McIlwraith CW: *Techniques in large animal surgery,* Philadelphia, 1982, Lea & Febiger.)

epinephrine (2%) or mepivacaine (2%) is injected intravenously, with the needle directed distally; the back pressure creates some resistance to injection. An 18- to 20-ga needle is used for cattle, and a 22- to 25-ga needle for small ruminants. Up to 10 ml of anesthetic is used in small ruminants, and up to 30 ml in cattle. After withdrawing the needle, digital pressure should be placed over the injection site for longer than normal to prevent hematoma formation.

Anesthesia is sufficient for surgery in 10 to 15 minutes and persists as long as the tourniquet is kept in place. Tourniquets may cause complications such as tissue necrosis, pain, and swelling if left in place longer than 2 hours. Release of the tourniquet should be gradual to prevent a bolus release of local anesthetic drug into the general circulation and possible resulting hypotension.

The anesthetic effects on the distal limb disappear rapidly within 5 to 10 minutes after release of the tourniquet.

Caudal Epidural Analgesia

Caudal epidurals are commonly used in ruminants, especially for obstetric procedures and treatment of prolapses of the uterus, vagina, and rectum. When properly performed, the anus, perineum, vulva, caudal vagina, and caudal aspects of the thighs are desensitized, which decreases pain and straining by the animal. Motor control of the hind legs is usually retained, but occasionally hind limb ataxia may occur if excessive anesthetic diffuses cranially.

The technique is similar to that described in horses. The procedure is performed through the dorsal aspect of the tail base, at the first intercoccygeal space (the sacrococcygeal space is also possible but is more difficult to identify and less commonly used). To identify the first intercoccygeal space, the tail is manipulated up and down while palpating the dorsal aspect of the tail base for the first obviously movable articulation (joint) caudal to the sacrum (Fig. 16-6). The area is clipped and sterilely prepped, and aseptic technique is used for the procedure. Generally it is unnecessary to block the skin and subcutaneous tissue, but a small bleb of subcutaneous anesthetic can be placed with a 25-ga needle if desired. For placement of the epidural anesthetic, cattle require an 18-ga × 1½- to 3-inch needle; small ruminants require an 18- to 21-ga × 1- to 1½-inch needle. The needle enters on dorsal midline at a 45-degree angle, and anesthetic is deposited into the epidural space. Lidocaine 2%, *without epinephrine,* is most commonly used (1 ml/100 kg bodyweight, or ≈5 to 6 ml in adult cattle). Mepivacaine 2% is also suitable. Because of sensitivity to local anesthetics, the dose should not exceed 0.5 to 1 ml of 2% solution per 50 kg bodyweight in sheep and goats.

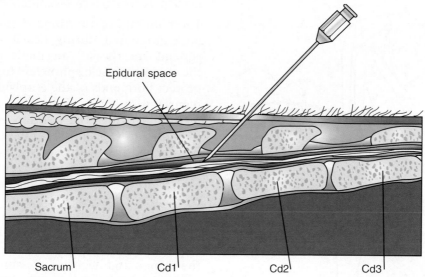

Epidural space

Sacrum   Cd1   Cd2   Cd3

Fig. 16-6. Location of first intercoccygeal space for bovine caudal epidural anesthesia. (Modified from Turner AS, McIlwraith CW: *Techniques in large animal surgery*, Philadelphia, 1982, Lea & Febiger.)

The anesthetic generally takes effect in 10 to 20 minutes and lasts 1 to 2 hours on average.

If prolonged anesthesia is necessary, it is possible to place a small-diameter epidural catheter (commercially available) or similar sterile medical tubing into the epidural space to provide continuous caudal epidural anesthesia. The catheter is inserted at the same location as described on p. 362 and threaded cranially along the epidural space (Fig. 16-7). The catheter is placed and maintained aseptically; the end of the catheter is protected with an injection cap, and the exposed portion of the catheter should be secured to the skin. Small doses of lidocaine can be given every few hours, as needed for pain or straining. A protective gauze bandage is advisable between uses. This technique spares the discomfort and tissue trauma from repeated standard epidurals. Disadvantages include kinking of the catheter and plugging of the tip with tissue or fibrin. Continuous caudal epidural anesthesia is also used successfully in equines.

Cranial epidurals are infrequently used in small ruminants and are generally avoided in cattle. They are performed at the lumbosacral space, using landmarks similar to lumbosacral cerebrospinal fluid (CSF) centesis. Cranial epidurals are technically more difficult to perform and have more potential complications than caudal epidurals, including accidental injection into the subarachnoid space/CSF. Posterior paralysis, including the hindlimbs, occurs and produces recumbency. Animals may require assistance standing as the anesthesia begins to wear off and are prone to "splay-legged" recoveries with overabduction of hindlimbs and resulting damage to the pelvis and inner thigh muscles.

GENERAL ANESTHESIA

Most surgical procedures in ruminants can be performed as standing procedures. General anesthesia is required when the technical/anatomical aspects of the procedure or the ability to control pain and motion exceed

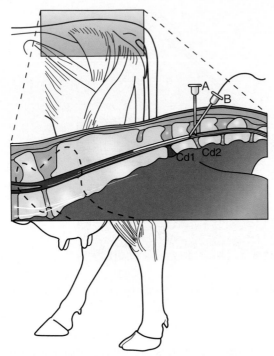

Fig. 16-7. Comparison of placement of standard caudal epidural **(A)** and continuous caudal epidural **(B)** in cattle. (Modified from Muir WW III et al: *Veterinary anesthesia*, ed 3, St Louis, 2000, Mosby.)

the capability of sedative drugs and local anesthesia. The techniques used to perform general anesthesia in ruminants are similar to those used in horses. However, there are some important differences: (1) The physiology of ruminants creates the potential for several unique complications during the induction and maintenance phases of anesthesia, and (2) in sharp contrast to equines, ruminants tend to have uneventful recoveries that seldom require special assistance.

ANESTHETIC RISKS FOR RUMINANTS

For preparation and administration of general anesthesia to the ruminant patient, the following risks should be considered:

Ruminants Are Prone to Regurgitation

The contents of the rumen/reticulum may be regurgitated during heavy sedation or general anesthesia. Anesthetic drugs relax the smooth muscle sphincters that normally protect both ends of the esophagus, making regurgitation more likely. The amount of regurgitated material is often voluminous; in adult cattle, gallons of rumen liquid may be expelled in a matter of seconds. The primary risk associated with regurgitation is aspiration of some of this material into the trachea and lungs, leading to aspiration pneumonia.

In order to minimize this risk, the most important principle is to reduce the size of the rumen and decrease pressure inside the organ. In adult cattle, food is withheld for 12 to 36 hours, and water for 6 to 12 hours before general anesthesia. In small ruminants, food is withheld for 12 to 24 hours; it is not necessary to withhold water. In calves, lambs, and kids that are consuming solid food material, fasting for 2 to 4 hours is sufficient (withhold food only; water is permitted). In very young ruminants, the rumen/reticulum has little function, and the risk of regurgitation is minimal. Fasting of neonates may cause hypoglycemia and is not recommended.

Other precautions include the following:
- A cuffed endotracheal tube is *essential* to protect the trachea from aspiration, and it should be inserted *as soon as possible* after anesthetic induction. Endotracheal intubation should be the priority of the anesthetic team at this time. Materials for intubation (oral speculum, appropriately sized endotracheal tube, sterile lubricant, laryngoscope, air syringe, etc.) should be assembled beforehand and readily available.
- Stimulation of the pharynx/larynx, which occurs during intubation, may induce a gag reflex and cause regurgitation, especially in light planes of anesthesia.

Intubation technique should be rapid and minimize stimulation of this area. The cuff should be inflated as soon as the tube is properly inserted.

- Ruminants should never be rolled under anesthesia, unless a cuffed endotracheal tube is in place.

Ruminants Are Prone to Distension of the Rumen (Bloat) During General Anesthesia

The combined effects of drug-induced depression of GI motility and the ongoing fermentation in the rumen/reticulum creates gas, which may accumulate and cause bloat. The distension of the rumen may press on the diaphragm and lungs and contribute to hypoventilation. Some degree of bloat is expected in all anesthetized ruminants; the key is to minimize it. Precautions include the following:

- Fasting as discussed on p. 364 to decrease the contents and weight of the rumen.
- Be prepared to treat bloat, especially after the procedure. A stomach tube, oral speculum, rumen trocar, etc., should be readily available in the surgery and recovery areas.

Ruminants, Like Horses, Are Prone to Hypoventilation and Inadequate Arterial Oxygenation

The size and weight of the rumen/reticulum and other GI organs compress the lungs and compromise diaphragm function. Anesthetic drugs depress the respiratory centers in the brain. The combined effect is likely to produce hypoventilation. Fasting is essential to reduce the size and weight of the GI tract. Anesthetic depth should not exceed what is necessary for the surgical procedure.

Ruminants Are at Risk for Development of Compartment Syndrome

Large bodyweight places adult cattle at greatest risk for developing postanesthetic myopathy and neuropathy; small ruminants are at considerably less risk. The risk factors and preventative measures are similar to those described in equines (see Chapter 8). Proper patient positioning and padding are essential during general anesthesia.

PREANESTHETIC PREPARATION AND ANESTHETIC MANAGEMENT

Preanesthetic Evaluation

A basic physical examination should always be performed. The extent of blood work and other laboratory tests depends on the health status of the animal and the nature and length of the procedure.

Preanesthetic Drugs

Most of the anesthetic drugs used in ruminants are not approved for use in food animals; drug residues must be considered and the client advised accordingly. Withdrawal times may not be established for many of these drugs, since their use is "extra-label." The Food Animal Residue Avoidance Databank (FARAD, *www.farad.org* or 888-USFARAD) is a valuable resource for current information on pharmacokinetics and withdrawal recommendations. Some of the drugs in use include the following:

Acepromazine

Acepromazine helps calm nervous cattle but does not have a strong tranquilizing effect at recommended doses. Males experience a prolonged period of penile relaxation, which increases risk of injury to the penis. The tranquilization effects last 2 to 4 hours; the prolonged time of elimination may be undesirable. Acepromazine should be avoided in dehydrated patients because of the tendency to produce hypotension by dilation of peripheral blood vessels.

Xylazine

Xylazine is the most commonly used preanesthetic sedative drug. It is useful for casting animals for recumbent procedures and for sedation during standing surgical procedures. Low doses (0.05 to 0.1 mg/kg IV) (0.1 to 0.5 mg/kg intramuscular [IM]) provide excellent sedation; moderate doses may result in recumbency.

It is *very* important to note that *ruminants are highly sensitive to xylazine*. It takes approximately *one tenth* of a "horse dose" to produce similar sedative effects in cattle. Some breeds such as Herefords and Brahmas may be even more sensitive, and goats and sheep may be more sensitive than cattle. Only low-concentration xylazine (20 mg/ml) should be used in ruminants to prevent accidental overdosing.

Clinical effects include the following:
- Bloat often develops from depression of rumen motility
- Bradycardia: dose-dependent cardiovascular depression
- Decreased ventilation: dose-dependent respiratory depression
- Hyperglycemia: leads to increased urine output
- Uterine contractions: may cause premature labor in late pregnancy
- Passes, unchanged, into milk: may affect nursing neonates

The sedation, cardiovascular, respiratory, and muscle relaxation effects may be reversed with either yohimbine or tolazoline. Rapid IV injection of alpha-2 antagonists should be avoided.

Detomidine/Medetomidine

Clinical indications, effects, and sensitivity are similar to xylazine.

Anticholinergics (atropine, glycopyrrolate)

Ruminants produce copious amounts of saliva, which continues under anesthesia. However, anticholinergic drugs do not significantly reduce saliva production and are not used for this purpose in ruminants. Patient positioning with the nose below the level of the pharynx and use of a cuffed endotracheal tube are used to prevent aspiration of saliva (a "spit bucket" under the patient's mouth is useful!). Anticholinergics increase the incidence of bloat because of their depressant effects on GI motility.

Induction Drugs

There are many possible induction and maintenance drug regimens. As with equines, injectable drugs can be used for induction and maintenance, or injectable drugs can be used for induction followed by inhalant gases for maintenance.

Inhalant gases

In animals weighing less than 150 lb, face-mask induction is possible. Small animal anesthesia machines can be used. Adult sheep and goats may resist facemask induction unless sick or sedated. Oxygen (3 to 5 L/min) is given for 1 to 2 minutes before introducing the anesthetic gas. Recommended gas concentrations are: halothane 3% to 4%, isoflurane 3%, and sevoflurane 4% to 6%. Intubation is performed as soon as depth of anesthesia allows.

Thiobarbiturates

Thiobarbiturates are not for use in animals younger than 3 months of age. Thiobarbiturates can cross the placenta and cause adverse effects on the fetus.

Ketamine

Ketamine is used in combination with a sedative such as xylazine or acepromazine. Diazepam combinations are useful in small ruminants.

Guaifenesin

Guaifenesin is combined with thiobarbiturates, xylazine, ketamine, etc., for induction and sometimes for maintenance. It is used for its muscle relaxant effects and to decrease required doses of other anesthetic drugs.

Guaifenesin can immobilize an animal, but it is *not* an anesthetic or analgesic drug. It is given intravenously "to effect." Solutions for IV use in ruminants should not exceed 5% solutions; significant hemolysis may occur at stronger concentrations.

One popular guaifenesin combination is the "triple drip," a mixture of xylazine/guaifenesin/ketamine given intravenously (note that ruminant "triple drip" formulations are different from equine "triple drip" doses because of ruminant sensitivity to xylazine; they should never be substituted for each other). An initial loading dose is given to produce recumbency, then the infusion rate is decreased for maintenance anesthesia. However, there is potential for excessive cardiovascular and respiratory depression. An alternative "double drip" formulation, using only IV guaifenesin/ketamine, is a safer alternative for induction of anesthesia in calm or sedated animals and may be used effectively for maintenance of anesthesia for 1 to 2 hours.

Telazol

Telazol may be used for induction in calves and small ruminants. It may also be used for maintenance of short-term surgical anesthesia.

Propofol

Propofol may be used for induction in calves and small ruminants. A single dose produces approximately 10 minutes of surgical anesthesia, which facilitates intubation and other short procedures. A continuous drip can be used to maintain anesthesia for slightly longer periods of time.

Endotracheal Intubation

After induction, rapid intubation and inflation of the cuff are essential. All necessary intubation equipment should be assembled before inducing the patient, and appropriately sized cuffed endotracheal tubes should be selected and lubricated with sterile lubricating jelly. Two common methods of intubation are used:

Direct visualization

A long-blade laryngoscope is useful for calves and small ruminants (Fig. 16-8). Intubation is easiest to accomplish with the patient in sternal recumbency, with the head and neck held in extension. Tubes less than 12 mm (internal diameter) may be easier to insert using a long plastic or metal stylet as a guide. The stylet is placed inside the endotracheal tube such that 15 to 20 cm of the stylet tip is exposed at the distal end of the tube. The laryngoscope is placed in the mouth, and the epiglottis is visualized; the tip of the scope is used to depress the epiglottis. The stylet tip is placed just beyond the larynx into the trachea. Keeping the stylet steady in this position, the endotracheal tube is passed over the stylet into the trachea and the cuff inflated. The stylet is withdrawn (Fig. 16-9).

Palpation

This method is only suitable for cattle and perhaps larger sheep and goats. An oral speculum is positioned to open the mouth. The head and neck should be extended so that the trachea, throat, and nose form a straight line; sternal recumbency is preferred but not essential. One hand is cupped over the end of the endotracheal tube and inserted into the mouth and pharynx. The epiglottis is palpated

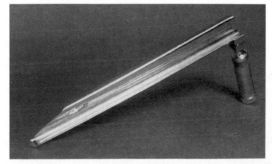

Fig. 16-8. Endotracheal intubation of calves and small ruminants is assisted by visualization with a long-blade laryngoscope. (Modified from Muir WW III et al: *Veterinary anesthesia,* ed 3, St Louis, 2000, Mosby.)

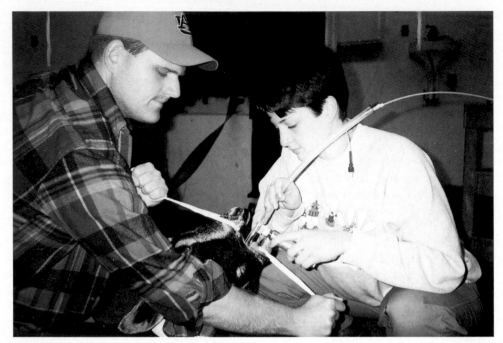

Fig. 16-9. Endotracheal intubation in a goat. Note that the head and neck are held in extension to create a straight line from mouth to trachea. An assistant uses gauze strips to open the mouth. A long-blade laryngoscope is used to visualize the larynx and depress the epiglottis. The stylet is placed into the proximal trachea, and then the endotracheal tube is advanced over the stylet and into the trachea. (From Pugh DG: *Sheep and goat medicine,* St Louis, 2002, Saunders.)

and depressed with one or more fingers while manually guiding the tip of the tube into the trachea. The arm is withdrawn, and the cuff is inflated. This method allows rapid identification of the tracheal entrance and insertion of the tube, rather than repeated attempts to blindly pass the endotracheal tube, which may stimulate regurgitation before the tube has been successfully inserted. Be sure to remove all jewelry before performing this technique (Fig. 16-10).

As with other species, appropriate endotracheal tube size is estimated by palpation of tracheal diameter through the skin of the neck.

Approximate tube sizes (internal diameter):

10-12 mm	adult sheep and goats
10-14 mm	calves
15-18 mm	older calves (≈200 kg)
20-25 mm	cows
25-30 mm	bulls

Maintenance of Anesthesia

Anesthesia may be maintained with injectable drugs or with inhalant gases. Generally inhalation is preferred for longer (>60 minutes) procedures. Small animal anesthesia machines may be used for animals weighing up to approximately 150 kg.

Inhalant gas	Induction %	Maintenance % (surgical anesthesia)
Halothane	3-5	1-2
Isoflurane	2-4	1.5-2.5
Sevoflurane	4-6	3-4

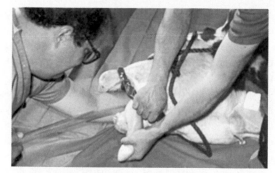

Fig. 16-10. Intubation of an adult cow by palpation of the larynx. A mouth speculum is used to keep the mouth open. (From Hubbell JAE et al: *Comp Cont Ed Pract Vet* 8(11):F92-F102, 1986.)

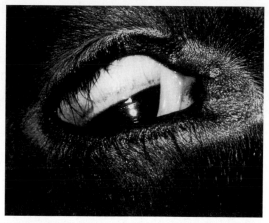

Fig. 16-11. Ventromedial rotation of the bovine eye during light anesthesia. (From Muir WW III et al: *Veterinary anesthesia*, ed 3, St Louis, 2000, Mosby.)

Nitrous oxide gas is not recommended for use in ruminants, primarily because of its poor solubility in blood. This creates a tendency for nitrous oxide to diffuse out of the blood into gas-filled organs such as the rumen, thus contributing to the development of bloat.

Monitoring of Anesthesia

Anesthetic monitoring is similar to that used for equines. An anesthetic record should be maintained for each anesthetic episode. As with equines, hypotension, hypoventilation, and bradycardia are the most commonly encountered complications. The following parameters may be monitored:

Depth of anesthesia

- Ocular reflexes: As with other species, the corneal reflex should always be present. The palpebral reflex may be delayed but should be present.
- Eyeball position: The eye tends to roll ventromedially in light surgical anesthesia and returns to a central position in deep surgical anesthesia (Fig. 16-11).
- Pupil size: The pupils dilate when an overdose of inhalant gas occurs. A central eyeball position *with* dilated pupils usually indicates that excessive anesthesia has

been administered, and immediate evaluation and action is indicated to prevent possibly severe complications.
- Lack of muscle movement in response to the surgical procedure.

Ventilation

- Respiratory rate and depth (tidal volume). A respiratory rate of 20 to 40 is desirable in adult ruminants.
- Mucous membrane color.
- Blood gas monitoring.

Circulation

- Peripheral pulse strength: may be taken at the coccygeal, median, median auricular, or femoral arteries. Subjective; may be misleading.
- Mucous membrane color.
- Capillary refill time.
- Heart rate: depends largely upon the anesthetic drugs used. Generally, desirable heart rates under anesthesia:
  - Sheep and goats: maintain 80 to 150 beats/min
  - Cattle: maintain 60 to 120 beats/min

- Blood pressure monitoring
  - Indirect: cuff placed over the coccygeal artery
  - Direct: catheter placed in the median auricular artery
  - Mean arterial pressure should be maintained above 70 mm Hg. Mean arterial pressure less than 60 mm Hg is hypotension requiring immediate treatment.

Body Temperature

Body temperature is especially important in young animals.

Intravenous Fluids

IV fluids are recommended for systemically sick animals, for procedures in which significant hemorrhage occurs, or for routine procedures lasting longer than 1 hour. Placement of an IV catheter before any general anesthetic episode is advisable for emergency access and fluid administration if needed. Lactated Ringer's solution is most often used, at a rate of 5 to 10 ml/kg/hr. Neonates may require a dextrose solution (5% dextrose) or addition of a glucose-containing solution to supplement IV fluids.

Oxygen Supplementation

When patients are maintained with injectable anesthesia, it may be desirable or necessary to deliver supplemental oxygen. Ambu-bags are helpful in assisting breathing in small ruminants. Supplemental oxygen can also be delivered directly from a gas anesthesia machine or directly from an oxygen tank by placing insufflation tubing directly into the endotracheal tube.

RECOVERY

Ruminants are allowed to breathe 100% oxygen for as long as possible from the anesthetic machine before being disconnected. After being disconnected, oxygen from a tank source may be given in the recovery area by placing insufflation tubing into the endotracheal tube while it is in place.

Ruminants are recovered in sternal recumbency if possible; this position improves ventilation and facilitates eructation (necessary to alleviate the bloat that usually develops to some degree during anesthesia). They may be propped sternally between support pads or hay bales. The front legs are folded beneath the chest. If lateral recumbency is necessary, right lateral recumbency is less likely to cause regurgitation (less weight on the rumen).

Regurgitation and aspiration are still possible during recovery. Leaving the endotracheal tube in place with the cuff at least partially inflated is important until the swallowing reflex is observed. The tube should be removed with the cuff partially inflated. The head should be placed such that any regurgitated material can flow freely from the mouth; this requires that the head be slightly "downhill."

Equipment for treatment of bloat should be readily available. An oral speculum, stomach tube, rumen trocar, and skin prepping materials are recommended.

Cattle are generally "sensible" in the recovery stall and seldom try to stand prematurely. Assistance is not often required. However, the recovery period should still be closely observed, and personnel should be available to assist should an emergency occur.

SUGGESTED READING

Fubini SL, Ducharme NG: *Farm animal surgery*, St Louis, 2004, Saunders.

Muir WW et al: *Handbook of veterinary anesthesia*, ed 3, St Louis, 2000, Mosby.

Pugh DG: *Sheep and goat medicine*, St Louis, 2002, Saunders.

Turner AS, McIlwraith CW: *Techniques in large animal surgery*, Philadelphia, 1982, Lea & Febiger.

17

Ruminant Neonatal Care

Except for the relatively few ruminants that are kept as pets, the overwhelming majority of ruminants are kept for production of meat, milk, hide, hair, or breeding/genetic potential. The economics of production are such that successful business depends largely on successful reproduction, from conception to delivery of the newborn. The neonate must then survive to an age where it can contribute economically to the business. Any loss of life from conception until economic contribution represents a significant loss to the producer.

The neonatal period is a time of significant losses to the producer, through morbidity and mortality. Neonates are susceptible to various conditions as they adapt to their new environment. Starvation and hypothermia are among the leading causes of mortality in the first 3 days of life. Caring for the very young involves not only knowledge of routine care but also recognition of abnormalities. Early identification and treatment of problems offers the best chance for success.

The basic needs of neonatal ruminants are the same as those of neonatal foals. Some important species differences exist, however.

BOVINE

GESTATION AND PARTURITION

Gestation in the bovine lasts 283 days on average (range 276 to 295 days). Clinical changes associated with impending parturition are softening of the muscles and ligaments of the hindquarters and tailhead, giving the tailhead an elevated appearance 24 to 48 hours before labor. Other signs include swelling of the vulva, thick mucus discharge from the vulva, and enlargement of the udder and distension of the teats. The cow may tend to separate from the herd and become defensive of her "personal space." A slight fall in rectal temperature (0.6° C) is reported to occur as long as 54 hours before birth but is not a reliable predictor of labor.

The preparatory stage of labor (stage 1) typically lasts about 6 hours. During this time, there is restlessness and little interest in food; there may be occasional kicking at the belly and straining. Delivery of the fetus (stage 2 of labor) occurs in 30 minutes to 4 hours, with approximately 75 minutes being the average. Heifers generally take longer than cows to deliver the fetus. Because the placenta detaches slowly, the fetus can continue to receive oxygen for much longer than the equine fetus, and live deliveries may occur up to 6 to 8 hours after stage 2 begins. Calves are normally delivered in anterior presentation, with the front legs extended and the head between the front legs ("head-diving" posture) (Fig. 17-1). If no progress is made after 1 hour of straining to deliver, or if abnormal fetal posture is observed, the delivery should be treated as a dystocia, and immediate veterinary consultation is advisable.

After delivery, the placenta continues its slow detachment from the uterine wall, and cows typically take about 4 to 6 hours to

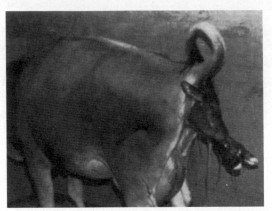

Fig. 17-1. Normal anterior presentation of fetal calf in stage 2 of labor. (From Noakes DE, Parkinson TJ, England GCW: *Veterinary reproduction and obstetrics*, ed 8, St Louis, 2001, Saunders.)

expel the placenta (stage 3 of labor); up to 12 hours is not uncommon. If the fetal membranes are not passed within 24 hours, veterinary assistance is warranted. Cows, unlike mares, may eat the afterbirth.

ROUTINE CARE OF THE NEONATAL CALF

Once delivery is complete, the needs of the newborn that must be addressed are as follows:
1. Oxygenation/Pulse assessment
2. Temperature regulation
3. Care of the umbilical cord and umbilicus
4. Nutrition (nursing)
5. Bonding of cow and calf
6. Passage of meconium
7. Adequacy of passive transfer of antibodies
8. Physical examination of the calf

Oxygenation/Pulse Assessment

The most immediate need is to be sure that the airway is cleared of fetal membranes and fluid. The fetal membranes can be manually removed if they are blocking the nostrils. A bulb syringe or suction tubing may be used to aspirate liquid from each nostril. Most of the fluid in the lungs will be reabsorbed gradually by the lymphatic system; suspending the calf by the hindlimbs to assist drainage is unnecessary, and suspending the calf may interfere with normal function of the diaphragm. Breathing can be stimulated by placing the calf in sternal recumbency and briskly rubbing the body with towels. Calves normally take the first breath within 30 seconds of birth and develop an irregular rate that gradually becomes regular at 45 to 60 breaths per minute.

The pulse should be assessed for rate and quality. A heart rate of 90 to 110 beats/min is normal in neonatal calves. The pulse should be strong and have regular rhythm.

Mucous membranes should be moist and pale pink to pink. Capillary refill time (CRT) should be less than 2 seconds.

Temperature Regulation

All neonates are susceptible to hypothermia in the postnatal period. Drying the animal and providing a draft-free area, deep bedding, and supplemental heat sources when the environmental temperature is low help maintain body heat. Following an initial period of low rectal temperature immediately after birth, the temperature of the newborn calf should be 37° C to 38° C (100° F to 102° F).

Care of Umbilical Cord and Umbilicus

The umbilical cord usually ruptures naturally without complication. Excessive hemorrhage is uncommon but can be controlled by placing hemostatic clamps across the bleeding stump for several hours. If necessary to manually cut or rupture it, the same methods as described for foals should be used (see Chapter 10). Topical treatment of the umbilical stump with 3% povidone-iodine solution or dilute chlorhexidine solution (1:4) is recommended. Continued treatment once or twice daily for the first several days of life is desirable; however, this is not always practical in a farm setting.

The umbilicus should be observed for swelling, discharge, moisture, and pain. Umbilical hernia, omphalophlebitis, and umbilical abscessation are conditions that require medical and/or surgical treatment, and should be evaluated by a veterinarian. Umbilical herniation is the most common congenital defect in cattle. Umbilical infections usually develop in the first 2 weeks of life. Patent urachus, which is common in foals, is uncommon in cattle.

Nutrition (Nursing)

Calves typically achieve sternal recumbency several minutes after birth and try to stand within 15 to 30 minutes; most calves are standing and nursing within 1 to 2 hours (range, 1 to 4 hours). The average time to nursing is 81 minutes in beef breeds; dairy breeds typically take longer. Calves may have some difficulty locating and nursing teats on large, distended udders where the teat ends are close to the ground. Observing the newborn from a distance to assess and confirm nursing behavior is important.

As with other species, colostrum ingestion and absorption is *essential* for natural passive transfer of antibodies. A general guideline is that the newborn should ingest 10% to 15% of its bodyweight in colostrum within the first 12 to 24 hours of life. However, this recommendation is affected by the concentration of IgG in the colostrum and assumes that the colostrum is of good quality (adequate IgG level). Colostrum quality may be assessed with a colostrometer; a specific gravity above 1.050 corresponds to an adequate IgG level in the colostrum of approximately 50 g/L. The concentration of IgG in the colostrum of dairy breeds is considerably lower than beef breeds, and it may take more volume of colostrum from dairy cows (compared to beef cows) to achieve adequate levels of protection in the calf. A common recommendation is that calves should receive at least 4 L of colostrum (dairy cow origin) before 12 hours of age, compared to 1 to 2 L for beef cow colostrum.

If the calf's nursing intake is in question, colostrum can be bottle-fed or tube-fed, by dividing the desired total colostrum volume into smaller portions given every 2 hours, preferably within the first 12 hours of life. Some farms routinely administer colostrum by stomach tube several hours after birth to ensure adequate intake. To avoid over-distension of the abomasum, no more than 2 L of liquid should be given per feeding. Sick neonates may not tolerate this feeding volume, requiring more frequent feedings of smaller amounts. Note also that sick neonates metabolize IgG faster and therefore may require more IgG for protection than healthy calves.

Nutritional management of beef and dairy calves is vastly different. Beef calves normally remain with the dam and suckle naturally until they are weaned at several months of age. Dairy calves, however, are typically separated from the dam after they suckle colostrum or are removed sometime in the first few days of life. They are fed twice daily on bucket- or bottle-fed milk or, more commonly, milk replacers (powders reconstituted with water). The general recommendation is to feed milk replacer at 5% to 6% of bodyweight twice daily, though different milk replacer formulations may have different feeding recommendations. The label should always be consulted. The composition of milk replacement products has been the subject of much research and debate, especially with regard to the amount, digestibility, and source of protein (milk-derived versus plant-derived versus animal-derived) used in the formulation.

The maintenance and growth energy requirements for healthy calves have been estimated. The maintenance requirement is approximately 50 kcal/kg/day. The growth requirement is approximately 300 kcal/100 g bodyweight gain. These requirements would be expected to be significantly higher for sick neonates. Whole milk contains approximately 70 kcal/100ml; an average calf would need to consume 3 L for daily maintenance plus 4 to 5 additional liters to gain 1 kg of bodyweight.

Hypoglycemia is a life-threatening condition and may develop rapidly (within hours), especially in sick or weak neonates that are unable to nurse normally. Hypoglycemia alone causes weakness and depression as early clinical signs. Blood (serum) glucose may be measured and should ideally range from 90 to 120 mg/dl; portable glucometers are convenient for field use. Treatment with supplemental oral or parenteral glucose solutions is indicated when glucose levels fall below 90 mg/dl; below 60 mg/dl is immediately life threatening.

Bonding of Cow and Calf

Human interference should be minimized in the neonatal period to allow maternal bonding to occur. Rejection of calves is uncommon but is more likely to occur with first-calf heifers, twin births, and calves delivered by caesarean section.

Passage of Meconium

Meconium, the first feces, is typically dark in color and may range in consistency from hard to pasty. It should be passed in the first 24 hours of life. If it is not passed, or if colic signs are observed, veterinary consultation for meconium impaction is recommended. If digital examination of the rectum or insertion of a rectal thermometer is not possible, or if there is only mucus in the rectum, a genetic defect of the intestinal tract such as incomplete colon, rectum, or anus (atresia coli, atresia recti, and atresia ani, respectively) should also be considered in the differential diagnosis.

Adequacy of Passive Transfer of Antibodies

Routine testing of blood antibody levels is seldom performed in ruminants, primarily because of the economic costs associated with testing and treatment. Even if testing confirms a low level of antibodies in the calf, treatment with intravenous (IV) plasma transfusion is seldom economically justified. However, in valuable calves, blood may be analyzed for immunoglobulins with a serum IgG level, radial immunodiffusion, refractometry using serum, or latex agglutination tests performed at approximately 24 hours of age. Although still the subject of some debate, a minimum level of 1000 mg/dl serum IgG is considered adequate by most clinicians (sample drawn between 24 and 48 hours of age). After 24 hours of age, when the gastrointestinal (GI) tract can no longer absorb orally administered IgG, failure of passive transfer (<1000 mg/dl IgG) may only be treated with IV plasma products or IV hyperimmune serum. Commercially prepared bovine plasma is available but expensive. Alternatively, fresh plasma may be collected on the farm, preferably from the dam or other animal on the same farm so that immunity to the local environmental microorganisms is high.

Physical Examination of the Calf

A complete physical examination begins with observation from a distance. The neonate is observed for mental alertness and behavior, suckling activity, and gait. Respiratory rate and effort are also best observed from a distance because the rate and effort usually increase with restraint. After the visual examination, the calf is restrained for the "hands-on" examination, which may range from a simple temperature, pulse, and respiration check to a thorough evaluation using a body systems approach (Table 17-1).

TABLE

17-1   NORMAL PHYSICAL EXAMINATION PARAMETERS FOR CALVES

Parameter	Normal
Cardiovascular System	
Mucous membrane color	Pale pink to pink; no petechiae or icterus
Capillary time	<2 sec
Pulse rate	90-110 beats/min
Heart auscultation	Absence of murmurs
Respiratory System	
Respiratory rate	40-60 breaths/min
Respiratory effort	Absence of nostril flare
Respiratory noise	Regular
Respiratory rhythm	Regular
Lung auscultation	Moist sounds immediately after birth
	Easier to hear sounds than in adults
	Audible sounds over all lung fields
Gastrointestinal System	
Suckling reflex	Vigorous
Oral cavity	Absence of cleft palate
Gastrointestinal auscultation	Borborygmus in all quadrants
	Absence of tympany (pings)
Passage of meconium	Within 24 hours of birth
Abdominal contour	Absence of distention
Urinary System	
Urination	Within 12 hr of birth
	Volume ≈34 ml/kg/day
	Absence of straining
Umbilicus	
Appearance	Dry, nonpainful, small size
Ophthalmic System	
Corneas	Clear
Sclera	Bilateral hemorrhages normal
Eyelids	Absence of entropion
Musculoskeletal System	
Gait	No lameness
Joints	No effusion

Continued.

TABLE

17-1   NORMAL PHYSICAL EXAMINATION PARAMETERS FOR CALVES—CONT'D

Parameter	Normal
Musculoskeletal System—cont'd	
Limbs	Straight or mild carpal valgus
Ribs	Absence of fractures, crepitus
Neurological System	
Mental attitude	Bright, alert, responsive
Gait	Lacks coordination in initial attempts to stand
Stance	Initial base-wide stance after birth
Head carriage	Absence of head tilt

IDENTIFICATION AND CARE OF THE SICK NEONATAL CALF

Many conditions affecting neonatal foals also affect neonatal calves. Neonatal bacterial septicemia is a similar disease in both species, with failure of passive transfer of colostral antibodies being the primary risk factor. Environmental conditions and management practices also play a role. As with foals, initial clinical signs are vague and often include depression, dehydration, and diarrhea. Lethargy, decreased suckling, weakness, and increased recumbency time may also occur. As the disease progresses, signs depend on the organ systems that are affected. Mortality without treatment is high. Gram-negative bacteria account for most cases of septicemia, and *Escherichia coli* is most often isolated.

Specific therapy for neonatal septicemia involves antibiotics, using blood culture and other body fluid samples to confirm bacterial identity and sensitivity to antimicrobial drugs. Other therapy is supportive, based on the organ systems affected. IV fluid therapy, parenteral nutrition, respiratory support, management of recumbency issues, control of seizures, and treatment of failure of passive transfer are all possible in neonatal calves. Methods are similar to those described in Chapter 10. However, such measures are seldom economically feasible, and the veterinarian must communicate with the client to find the best solutions to the animal's problems. Blood work and diagnostic imaging studies, which are all highly desirable clinical tools, are not essential for low-level "practical" management of the disease. Broad-spectrum antibiotics, minimal fluid therapy via stomach (ororumen) tube or drenching, administration of colostrum, and keeping the calf warm and dry can often be successful if instituted early in the course of disease. Recumbent animals with multiple organ system involvement have a poor prognosis, even with aggressive treatment.

Diarrhea may occur in the absence of septicemia, especially in calves older than 4 days of age. "Calf scours" is a common condition of calves that may have a high morbidity with significant fatalities. Scours has numerous causes, including the following:

- Bacteria: *E. coli*, *Salmonella*, *Clostridium perfringens* type D

- Viruses: rotavirus, coronavirus, bovine viral diarrhea (BVD)
- Protozoa: *Cryptosporidium, Eimeria*
- Nutrition: milk replacers, milk "overload"
- Management: overcrowding, stress, etc.

Since the etiological agents are usually infectious, it is common to have a herd problem with the disease. Multiple factors may be involved. The veterinarian must work closely with the owner to identify risk factors and management factors, identify the specific cause, and plan treatment and prevention strategies. The most common cause of death in calves with diarrhea is dehydration and associated metabolic acidosis. The cornerstone of treatment is to correct and prevent further dehydration through use of oral (stomach tube) or parenteral fluids; bicarbonate is often added to fluids to correct acidosis. Hypoglycemia and electrolyte imbalances may also need to be treated through fluid therapy. Total removal of milk from the diet during the diarrheal episode has historically been a common recommendation but is now currently debated; research has demonstrated improved survival and less weight loss when milk feedings are continued and alternated with oral electrolyte/bicarbonate fluids. Segregation of sick calves in a "sick pen" or barn is recommended, along with proper cleaning and disinfection procedures. All personnel should remember that *Salmonella* and *Cryptosporidium* are zoonotic etiological agents and take precautions to prevent possible human infections.

Calf pneumonia is primarily a disease of calves older than 4 weeks of age and is a common condition in this age group. It is caused by a combination of management factors (stress, overcrowding), environmental factors (temperature, stress, poor ventilation), and infectious bacterial, viral, and/or mycoplasmal agents. High morbidity with some mortality is typical. Treatment relies on early identification of the sick individual, segregation of affected animals, and antibiotic therapy. High fever (>104.0° F); depression; tachypnea; and a soft, moist cough are the hallmarks of the disease.

In contrast, neonatal pneumonia at younger than 4 days of age is uncommon. When it occurs, neonatal pneumonia is more likely the result of neonatal septicemia/bacteremia. Neonatal pneumonia is uncommon as a primary disease but may be caused by several of the viruses that affect bovines (Bovine Respiratory Syncytial virus, Infectious Bovine Rhinotracheitis virus, Bovine Viral Diarrhea virus, Bovine Coronavirus). *Mycoplasma* spp. may also cause neonatal pneumonia.

OVINE

GESTATION AND PARTURITION

Gestation in the ewe lasts an average of approximately 149 days (range 145 to 150). About 3 to 4 weeks before lambing, crutching is commonly performed. Crutching, the shearing of wool from the vulva and udder, is important because it allows the farmer to observe swelling of the vulva and udder, helps control passage of infectious fecal organisms to lambs, and helps the lambs find the udder. Facing, shearing the wool from around the eyes in breeds with facial wool, is also done to improve the dam's vision of her newborn lambs. Vaccination of the ewe to boost colostral antibody levels is also done at this time, as is deworming.

Clinical signs of approaching parturition include swelling of the vulva, mucoid vulvar discharge, relaxation of the pelvic ligaments, and enlargement of the udder. Ewes are often moved to lambing pens or stalls (known as "jugs") when these signs are seen. Most births occur during daytime hours.

In the preparatory stage of labor (stage 1), the ewe becomes restless, may urinate frequently, and may lie down repeatedly as contractions begin; she may separate from the flock if she has not already been segregated into a designated lambing area. Stage 1 usually lasts approximately 1 to 4 hours. The duration of stage 2 of labor (delivery of the fetus) is variable but typically lasts 1 to 2 hours, depending on the size of the fetus and its presentation. Most births (95%) occur in anterior "head-diving" presentation, with the head and front legs appearing first; however, successful breech births are possible, especially if the fetus is small and the hind feet are presented first. Twin births are common in sheep, and triplets are not unusual. The interval between delivering each fetus in a multiple birth may vary from several minutes to an hour. Straining for an hour without producing a fetus is an indication for assistance. Stage 3 (passage of the placenta/placentas) usually occurs within 2 to 3 hours but may take up to 6 hours after delivery. If the ewe shows no signs of toxemia or septicemia, no treatment is necessary until 12 hours postpartum.

ROUTINE CARE OF THE NEONATAL LAMB

Routine care of newborn lambs is similar to that of calves. The immediate needs of the newborn include the following:

Oxygenation/Pulse Assessment

Fetal membranes should be cleared from the nostrils. Briskly rubbing the lamb with towels helps to stimulate breathing and dries the body. Sternal recumbency facilitates breathing. If spontaneous breathing does not occur in 20 to 30 seconds after birth, artificial respiration through the nostril may be attempted. A respiratory resuscitation rate of approximately 20/min is desirable.

The heart rate should be 90 to 150. If a pulse cannot be palpated, cardiac massage can be performed by compressing the lamb's ventral chest wall just behind the elbows, using the thumb and two to three fingers.

Return of a palpable pulse and improvement in mucous membrane color indicate that effective resuscitation has occurred, and chest compressions may be stopped. Close monitoring of the cardiovascular and respiratory systems is essential following any resuscitation effort.

Temperature Regulation

Lambs are especially susceptible to hypothermia in the first 36 hours of life. Heat lamps and other devices may be used if environmental temperatures are cold. Lambs with rectal temperature below 100° F should be warmed immediately; heat lamps, blow dryers, blankets, and warm water bottles are useful.

Care of the Umbilical Cord and Umbilicus

Treatment of the navel with iodine or chlorhexidine solutions is advised. The umbilicus should be observed for signs of infection (heat, pain, swelling, exudates), which is most likely to occur in the first 2 weeks of life.

Nutrition (Nursing)

Lambs may attempt to stand as soon as 10 to 15 minutes after birth, and most stand successfully in approximately 30 minutes. Successful nursing should occur within 1 to 2 hours (average 90 minutes). Lambs may need assistance finding the udder.

Bonding of Ewe and Lamb

The ewe vigorously licks the newborn and will usually eat the fetal membranes. Fetal fluids are an essential part of recognition and bonding of the ewe with her lambs; maternal bonding is mediated by the sense of smell, with an olfactory attraction to the amniotic fluid. The maternal bonding period is short, with the first 6 to 12 hours being most critical, and minimal human interference is advisable during this time. It is usual to manually assist ewes having difficulty delivering and clear membranes from the newborn's nostrils, but further contact is minimized unless an emergency situation occurs.

Passage of Meconium

Meconium should be passed within 24 hours.

Adequacy of Passive Transfer of Antibodies

Lambs should consume a total of 10% to 15% of their bodyweight in colostrum in the first 24 hours of life. It is important to provide colostrum soon after birth, and if nursing intake is questionable, a goal of 50 ml/kg in the first 2 hours is desirable. Bottle- or tube-feeding may be necessary to ensure ingestion of colostrum. Ewe colostrum is preferred, but goat colostrum may be substituted. Cow colostrum has questionable efficacy. Commercial "colostrum substitutes" typically are unacceptably low in immunoglobulins.

Physical Examination of the Lamb

Examination of the lamb using a body system approach is possible and is indicated especially in any sick or weak lamb. The same approach as described in calves is used, with an initial observation from a distance, followed by restraint and a hands-on systemic evaluation.

IDENTIFICATION AND CARE OF THE SICK NEONATAL LAMB

Starvation and diarrhea are the primary causes of neonatal death on most farms. Starvation occurs when a lamb fails to ingest sufficient calories; rejected lambs and weak lambs (due to hypothermia, prenatal or postnatal infections, prematurity, congenital defects, etc.) are most susceptible. Diarrhea in the first few days of life is generally caused by *E. coli* and less often by *Clostridium perfringens* type C. Starvation, hypothermia, and diarrhea can all result in weakness; conversely, weakness can result in starvation

and hypothermia, creating a cycle that can be fatal to a lamb within hours.

It is essential to address hypoglycemia and hypothermia in any sick or weak lamb. Sick lambs must be kept warm and dry and must be given nutritional support. Tubing 2 to 4 oz of warm colostrum (from ewe or goat source) improves survival. Dextrose 5%, approximately 20 ml, may be given subcutaneously for an additional energy source. Milk replacers are available for lambs and may be helpful for raising orphaned or rejected lambs. Milk replacers cannot, however, substitute for colostrum in providing immunoglobulins in the immediate neonatal period.

Bottle feeding using a commercial lamb nipple on a bottle works well. The nipple is placed in the lamb's mouth, and the lamb's jaw may be moved to simulate a chewing motion. This often stimulates the nursing reflex. If the neonate is too weak to nurse, tube feeding is required. A small, approximately 8-French (Fr) red rubber urethral tube or 14- to 18-Fr infant feeding tube can be attached to a 60-ml catheter-tip syringe and used as an ororumen tube for lambs. Alternatively, commercially available stainless steel lamb probes are available for passage into the esophagus (Fig. 17-2). The lamb is placed in right lateral recumbency, with the head and neck extended. An oral speculum is not required; pressure on the jaw opens the mouth. The tube or probe is inserted into the mouth and gently advanced to the pharynx; rather than forcing the tube into the esophagus, it is best to allow the lamb to swallow and advance the tube "with the swallow." If correctly passed, the tube can easily be felt in the esophagus, dorsolateral to the trachea; there should be a small amount of resistance as the tube is advanced. If the tube is in the trachea, it cannot be palpated and the lamb will likely cough. When confirmed to be in the esophagus, the tube is advanced and the dosing

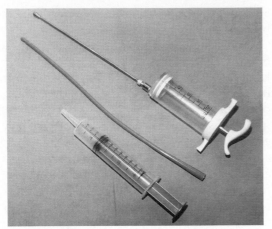

Fig. 17-2. A stainless steel, blunt-tip lamb probe with attached dose syringe *(top)* and a flexible rubber tube and catheter-tip syringe. (From Teeple TN: Nursing care of food animals, camelids, and ratites. In Sirois M, editor: *Principles and practice of veterinary technology*, ed 2, St Louis, 2004, Mosby.)

syringe is attached. Any liquid given by tube should be warmed, and the fluid should be delivered slowly either by slowly depressing the syringe plunger or by using gravity flow from the syringe barrel (with the plunger removed).

Although intensive care medicine is available to treat sick lambs just as in other species, the value of a neonatal lamb seldom justifies the expense associated with diagnostic testing, IV fluids, respiratory support, plasma transfusions, medications, and other treatments. A practical, economical "on-the-farm" approach is almost always used.

CAPRINE

GESTATION AND PARTURITION

Gestation in the doe lasts from 147 to 155 days, with an average of 150 days. Twins and triplets are more common than singleton births. About 4 weeks before birth, the doe is vaccinated and dewormed. As the time of parturition approaches, clinical signs include swelling of the vulva, mucoid vulvar discharge, relaxation of the pelvic ligaments, and enlargement of the udder. Dairy does are commonly moved into special pens for kidding, and the hair around the udder and perineum may be clipped. Goats that give birth in the field should have access to a shelter or sheltered area. In natural conditions, does typically "hide" their kids after they are born. The doe leaves her kids hidden while she browses for food; however, she remains within an audible distance and responds to distress calls from the kids. Whether in a pen or in the field, it is important to provide an area for the doe to "hide" her kids; small boxes may be constructed in pens for artificial cover.

The stages of labor and associated behaviors are similar to those described for sheep. Goats tend to separate from the herd, become restless, paw, and show nesting behavior in stage 1. Stage 1 may last up to 12 hours, especially in first-time (primiparous) mothers. Stage 2, with passage of all fetuses, is usually completed within 2 hours. If obvious contractions fail to produce a fetus in 30 to 60 minutes, dystocia may be occurring and veterinary assistance should be sought. The large majority of births occur in anterior presentation. Stage 3 is complete within 4 hours.

ROUTINE CARE OF THE NEONATAL KID

Routine care of newborn kids is similar to that of lambs and calves. The immediate needs of the newborn include the following:

Oxygenation/Pulse Assessment

Fetal membranes, fluid, and mucus should be cleared from the nostrils. Briskly rubbing with towels helps to stimulate breathing and dries the body. Sternal recumbency facilitates breathing. If spontaneous breathing does not occur in 20 to 30 seconds after birth, artificial respiration through the mouth or nostril may be attempted.

The heart rate may be 90 to 150 in neonates. If a pulse cannot be palpated, cardiac massage can be performed as described on p. 378 for lambs.

Temperature Regulation

Kids are especially susceptible to hypothermia in the first 36 hours of life. Heat lamps and other devices may be used if environmental temperatures are cold. A rectal temperature below 100° F indicates the need for immediate warming; heat lamps, blow dryers, blankets, and warm water bottles are useful.

Care of the Umbilical Cord and Umbilicus

Treatment of the navel with iodine or chlorhexidine solutions is advised. The umbilicus should be observed daily for signs of infection (heat, pain, swelling, exudates).

Nutrition (Nursing)

Kids may attempt to stand soon after birth, and most stand successfully in approximately 30 minutes. Successful nursing should occur within 1 to 2 hours. Palpation of the abdomen for "fullness" after observing the kid on the doe's teat may help to confirm that nursing has successfully occurred. Commercial goat milk replacers are available but are not substitutes for colostrum.

Bonding of Doe and Kid

The doe vigorously licks the newborn and eats the fetal membranes. This behavior is considered essential for maternal bonding. Does should not be frightened or disturbed during the critical first hour after birth. Dairy kid management, like dairy calf management, often involves removal of the kids shortly after birth and hand-raising them; obviously maternal bonding is not of concern in these circumstances.

Passage of Meconium

Meconium should be passed within 24 hours.

Adequacy of Passive Transfer of Antibodies

Kids should consume a total of 10% to 15% of their bodyweight in colostrum in the first 24 hours of life. This amount may be divided into several feedings. Kids should consume at least 50 ml/kg of colostrum within the first 2 to 4 hours of life. If nursing intake is questionable, bottle- or tube-feeding may be necessary to ensure ingestion of colostrum. The same methods and instruments may be used for kids as for lambs.

Physical Examination of the Kid

Examination of the neonate using a body system approach is indicated especially in any sick or weak kid. The same approach is used as described in calves, with an initial observation from a distance, followed by restraint and a hands-on systemic evaluation.

IDENTIFICATION AND CARE OF THE SICK NEONATAL KID

Normal kids are strong and vigorous, especially in their efforts to nurse. Weakness and depression are the most common clinical signs of illness in the neonatal period. Hypothermia and hypoglycemia are the most common causes of weakness and depression, and they commonly coexist. Neonates are especially susceptible to both conditions. Hypothermia and/or hypoglycemia may cause weakness and depression or may be caused by weakness/ depression from other diseases. The deadly cycle that can develop between these conditions may lead to rapid mortality. A rectal temperature below 100° F warrants immediate treatment; clinical signs of hypothermia begin at approximately ≤98° F. Affected animals must be kept warm and dry, out of wind or drafts. The hypoglycemic animal must have nutritional needs provided by supplementing glucose, and perhaps electrolytes and other fluids as well. The route of fluid administration depends on the severity of dehydration and hypoglycemia, as well as practical concerns such as person-nel and cost. Subcutaneous fluid therapy is commonly used because of effectiveness and practicality in animals that cannot be bottle- or tube-fed (lack GI function).

Similar to lambs and calves, neonatal septicemia and neonatal diarrhea (scours) are among the more common diseases of newborns. The principles of diagnosis and treatment are similar. Intensive care medicine and diagnostic testing may be provided for valuable or valued individuals.

SUGGESTED READING

Hafez ESE: *Reproduction in farm animals,* ed 6, Philadelphia, 1993, Lea & Febiger.

Hunt E: Neonatal disease and disease management. In Howard JL, Smith RA, editors: *Current veterinary therapy, food animal practice,* ed 4, St Louis, 1999, Saunders.

Noakes DE, Parkinson TJ, England GCW: *Arthur's veterinary reproduction and obstetrics,* ed 8, St Louis, 2001, Saunders.

Pugh DG: *Sheep and goat medicine,* St Louis, 2002, Saunders.

Smith BP: *Large animal internal medicine,* ed 3, St Louis, 2002, Mosby.

Smith MC, Sherman DM: *Goat medicine,* Baltimore, 1994, Williams & Wilkins.

18

Common Clinical Procedures in Ruminants

RUMINAL DISTENSION

Ruminal distension is a clinical sign, not a specific disease. The rumen may distend with fluid, gas, or both. Gas distension is also referred to as ruminal tympany or bloat. Fluid distension is sometimes referred to as "splashy rumen." Causes of ruminal distension are numerous and include the following:

- Dietary: inadequate roughage, overconsumption of grain ("grain overload"), ingestion of foreign bodies, toxin ingestion
- Mechanical: esophageal obstruction that prevents eructation, stenosis of outflow tracts from the rumen/reticulum or abomasum
- Derangement of motility: dysfunction of the vagus nerve, hypomotility or atony secondary to many other diseases, drugs, and advanced pregnancy

An often used term, "vagal indigestion," is somewhat confusing ("vague indigestion"). It has been used as a synonym for chronic indigestion, from any disease that disturbs outflow from the forestomachs or abomasum. Outflow disturbance may be caused by a variety of conditions, including true dysfunction of the vagus nerve. However, primary vagus nerve problems are uncommon; emptying defects of the forestomachs are more prevalent than vagus nerve disease. Emptying defects may be caused by mechanical obstructions (foreign bodies, such as sheets of plastic

or placentas), anatomical obstructions (pyloric stenosis, compression by tumors or abscesses), or physiological alterations in motility.

Bloat (ruminal tympany) is properly used to refer to distension of the rumen with the gases of fermentation. Gas may exist in two forms: free gas and foamy gas (froth). Ruminants produce large amounts of gas as a result of fermentation of plant material in the rumen/reticulum. Rumen gas may only exit via one route—the cardia and esophagus—by the process of eructation. Ruminants have the capability to eructate several times more gas than can be produced in the rumen; therefore overproduction of gas is not the problem. The real problem is inability of the gas to exit the rumen, either because something is interfering with eructation or the gas is trapped inside bubbles (foam).

Bloat is classified as frothy bloat or free-gas bloat. Passage of a stomach (ororumen) tube is usually necessary to differentiate them. *Frothy bloat* is often associated with legume pastures or greenchop, especially when they are lush. Legumes contain high levels of soluble proteins that tend to form foam with "stable" bubbles that cannot be eructated and are not easily broken down. Accumulations of "nonbubble" gas are referred to as *free-gas bloat*. Free-gas bloat has many possible etiologies, such as obstruction of the esophagus (choke), obstructions of the cardia (abscesses, tumors, foreign bodies, fluid buildup in the rumen above the level of the cardia), hypomotility (from hypocalcemia, hyperacidity of rumen contents, or drugs), and positioning in lateral recumbency. Bloat is more common in cattle than in small ruminants.

Ruminal distension may be mild, moderate, or severe and may occur acutely or chronically. Diagnosis is by observation of the abdominal contour (silhouette), abdominal auscultation, ballottement of the rumen, and rectal examination. The rumen occupies most of the left side of adult ruminants; distension tends to cause enlargement on the left side of the animal. Gas distension produces primarily distension of the upper left abdominal quadrant (especially visible in the left paralumbar fossa), and fluid distension produces primarily distension of the lower left abdominal quadrant. Severe fluid distension can enlarge the rumen such that the distension also affects the right lower abdominal quadrant (Fig. 18-1).

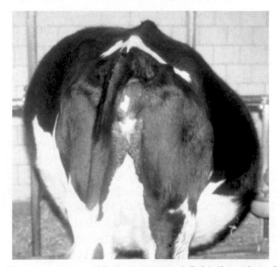

Fig. 18-1. A cow with severe gas and fluid distension of the rumen. The left upper, left lower, and right lower abdominal quadrants are distended in a classic "papple"-shaped abdomen, caused by vagal indigestion. (From Fubini SL, Ducharme NG: *Farm animal surgery*, St Louis, 2004, Saunders.)

Auscultation typically reveals hypomotility or complete atony of the rumen, although hypermotility may occur early in the disease in some cases. If a gas cap develops in the rumen, it may be detected by percussion ("pinging") over the upper left abdominal quadrant; however, left displacement of the abomasum may also produce a "ping" in this area, and this test is not specific for bloat. Rumen ballottement may be used to count rumen contractions and assess its fluid content. Rectal examination in large ruminants is useful for assessing rumen size and contents. Radiographs may be helpful in identifying metallic foreign bodies.

Distension can produce other clinical signs. Anorexia is common. Discomfort is often indicated by repeated rising and lying down. Heart rate tends to increase as the distension increases. Severe distension may press on the thoracic cavity, compromising lung expansion and resulting in shallow, rapid, frequently open-mouth breathing. Severe distension may also compromise venous blood flow returning to the heart, with development of shock.

Treatment options are medical and surgical, depending on the cause and severity of the ruminal distension. Mild cases often resolve on their own; keeping the animal up and moving may help. On the other hand, acute, severe gas bloat can be life threatening within 1 to 4 hours, due to the respiratory and cardiovascular compromise. Decompression can be life saving and is the most critical treatment. Passage of a stomach (ororumen) tube is the simplest and quickest method of decompression; however, it is effective for free gas, but foam does not readily exit through or around the tube. When gas cannot be relieved by a tube, an exit for the gas must be created through the abdominal wall. This may be done by use of a trocar or surgical incision into the rumen.

Trocarization of the rumen may be done with a large-bore hypodermic needle or commercially available rumen trocars. The site for trocarization is determined by auscultation and "pinging" of the left side of the abdomen for the point of maximal tympany, typically at a location in the left paralumbar fossa. The thoracic cavity must be avoided. The site is clipped and sterilely prepared (prepped); local anesthetic may be deposited in the subcutaneous and muscle layers of the abdomen. The clinician wears sterile gloves and places the trocar through the skin into the rumen. Some of the larger trocars may require a stab incision through the skin and abdominal wall. Most trocars are used to alleviate the gas and medicate the rumen, and then are withdrawn. A few trocars are designed to be indwelling for longer periods of time and may be self retaining (Fig. 18-2).

Surgical rumenotomy or rumenostomy may be necessary to decompress the rumen, explore the rumen, or remove rumen contents and foreign objects. Rumen surgery is usually performed in the standing animal through a left flank approach, using sedation and local anesthesia. Use of a rumen board assists rumenotomy. The rumen board is designed to support a portion of the rumen outside the abdomen so that any spillage of rumen contents from the open rumen does not contaminate the abdominal cavity (Fig. 18-3).

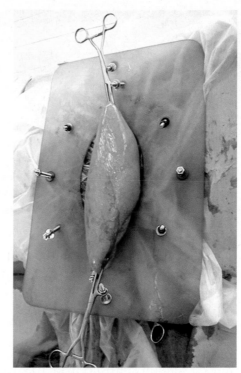

Fig. 18-3. A portion of the rumen has been exteriorized through the left flank and stabilized with a rumen board. The rumen can be safely opened with a vertical incision. (From Fubini SL, Ducharme NG: *Farm animal surgery*, St Louis, 2004, Saunders.)

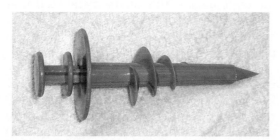

Fig. 18-2. Corkscrew-style (Buff's rumen screw) self-retaining rumen trocar. (From Fubini SL, Ducharme NG: *Farm animal surgery*, St Louis, 2004, Saunders.)

After evacuation and exploration of the rumen through the rumenotomy, the rumen incision is closed and returned to the abdomen. Closure of the abdominal wall is performed in several layers.

A permanent opening of the rumen through the abdominal wall, a rumenostomy (also known as *rumen fistula*), may be surgically created for selected cases; this technique is helpful for chronic bloaters. The opening of the rumenostomy is protected by a commercially available plastic, lightweight fistula with a removable cover (Fig. 18-4).

When frothy bloat is detected, various oral medications may be used to try to break

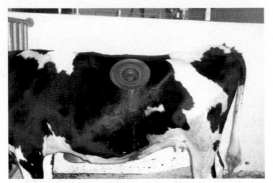

Fig. 18-4. Cow with a surgically placed commercial rumen fistula. (From Fubini SL, Ducharme NG: *Farm animal surgery*, St Louis, 2004, Saunders.)

up the foam bubbles. These anti-foaming medications are primarily surfactants, which reduce the surface tension of the bubbles and encourage their breakup. They may be given through a stomach tube or, if rumen trocarization is performed, given directly into the rumen through the trocar. Poloxalene and dioctyl sodium sulfosuccinate (DSS) are popular surfactants. Mineral oil is also used in some cases. Animals should be removed from the offending pasture or feeds.

IDENTIFICATION

Identification is an essential management tool, especially for production animals. It is obviously necessary for establishing ownership, but it also allows for tracking and evaluation of an animal's productivity and performance. Herd health and reproductive programs can also be monitored and managed more effectively when records of individual animals are kept. Most identification methods are optional, and the farmer may choose the numbering/lettering systems. However, specific forms of identification may also be required to identify participation in federal disease eradication programs and may be required by breed registries for registered animals. In these cases, the numbers, letters, and symbols are dictated by

the governing agency. Animals may therefore carry several identification markers, serving different purposes.

Identification methods may be temporary or permanent. Methods include the following.

NECK CHAINS WITH TAGS

Tags may be colored, be numbered, or even contain microchips. Chains are usually made of plastic so that they can break free if entanglement occurs. Because of the tendency to catch on vegetation and fencing, neck chains are seldom used in free-ranging animals. Neck chains are a form of temporary marking. They are used mostly on dairy cattle and goats.

EAR TAGS

Flexible plastic ear tags are popular for temporary marking. Tags come in a variety of colors and may be prenumbered or blank; blank tags may be written on with waterproof marking pens. Ear tags may be purchased with impregnated insect repellent to minimize flies and other insects around the head area; the effects of the repellent may last 3 to 4 months.

The tag is placed between the middle cartilage ribs of the ear pinna, using an applicator gun (Fig. 18-5). The head is restrained, and alcohol is used to clean the skin of the pinna. The process is essentially ear piercing; the tag comes with a sharp metal stud that is "fired" through the ear with the applicator gun; the gun simultaneously applies a button backing to the stud.

Ear tags are removable, which is why they are considered temporary marking. They may be pulled out accidentally or removed intentionally by removing the stemmed button backing from the metal stud. If the tag is to be replaced, and the original ear pinna hole is still intact, the new tag can be directed through the old hole with the gun, thus sparing the animal some discomfort.

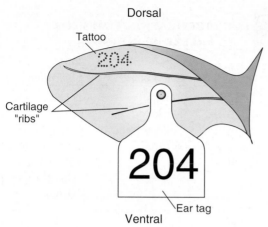

Fig. 18-5. Proper location of ear tag between the cartilage "ribs" of the ear pinna.

Metal ear tags, rather than plastic, are sometimes used for identification. They are placed with an applicator gun. Official orange metal ear tags, designed by the federal government, are used to identify bovine animals that have been vaccinated for brucellosis. Cattle (female) are usually vaccinated against brucellosis as calves (4 months to 1 year) and are referred to as "official calfhood vaccinates." By law, the official metal ear tag must be placed in the right ear. The vaccinated animal must also receive an official ear tattoo.

TATTOOS

Tattoos are commonly used for permanent identification. The location in ruminants is in the inner aspect of the ear pinna, in an area that is nonpigmented and free of hair (La Mancha goats, which genetically lack ear pinnae, are tattooed on the tail fold). The main types of tattoos are (1) those used for individual farm identification systems (optional), and (2) those used for breed registration or participation in federal disease control programs (required). In cattle, official calfhood vaccinates for brucellosis are required to be tattooed in the right ear.

The official tattoo consists of the U. S. Registered Shield and the letter "V," plus a series of letters and numbers as required by current regulations. Farm-origin identification tattoos should be placed in an area of the ear where they will not be altered by ear tags or required tattoos.

Tattoos are applied with a plier-type press applicator. The applicator is preloaded with the desired numbers and/or letters, which are made of sharp, needlelike projections that are pressed into the ear with the applicator. If multiple animals are being tattooed, the applicator gun and symbols should be disinfected between each use. Care must be taken to insert the proper numbers and letters, since the mark is permanent. Double-checking the characters by pressing the gun on a piece of paper is recommended.

The head must be securely restrained. The skin is cleaned with alcohol. Tattoo ink is rubbed on the ear pinna, then the applicator gun is positioned and pressed. The needlelike projections puncture and carry the ink below the skin. Additional ink may be rubbed in by hand over the punctures. The skin heals over the top of the ink, permanently trapping it just beneath the skin. In growing animals, the tattoo enlarges as the animal grows; however, the procedure is not performed on very young animals because of possible distortion from rapid growth. Most animals are tattooed around the time of weaning.

The main disadvantage of tattoos is that they cannot be seen from a distance and require head restraint in order to be read. Therefore they are commonly combined with other marking methods that can be seen from a convenient distance.

FREEZE BRANDING

This method uses liquid-nitrogen cooled branding irons to destroy the pigment-producing cells (melanocytes) associated with the hair follicles. The hair follicle itself is not permanently damaged; therefore hair regrows, but without pigment, resulting in white hairs.

Equipment for the procedure includes liquid nitrogen; approximately 1 quart liquid nitrogen/four animals is necessary. Leather gloves, preferably with a long cuff (welding gloves), should be worn for protection when handling liquid nitrogen. Eye goggles are advisable for protection from liquid nitrogen splashes. Clippers fitted with a No. 40 blade are used to remove hair from the branding site. A Styrofoam cooler or other insulated container is used to hold the liquid nitrogen and "dunk" the branding irons. Isopropyl alcohol (95%) is also required.

The procedure begins with proper restraint of the animal, preferably in a squeeze chute. The hair is clipped and brushed to remove debris. The branding irons are cooled in 3 to 4 inches deep of liquid nitrogen. When the liquid nitrogen stops bubbling, the branding iron is at proper temperature. The skin of the branding area is soaked thoroughly with 95% isopropyl alcohol, and then the branding iron is firmly applied with constant pressure. The animal experiences temporary discomfort, but the numbing effect of the cold provides relief in about 10 seconds.

The length of time of application of the branding iron is determined by the age and coat color of the animal. Table 18-1 shows the recommended times.

Branding white animals must use a slightly different principle, since white-hair brands obviously cannot be read. The goal in white animals is to completely destroy regrowth of hair, rather than just pigment, leaving a "bald brand." This requires complete destruction of the hair follicles, through prolonged application of the branding iron. When properly performed, the resulting brand is easily read.

When the branding iron is removed, the area is initially frozen and hard to the touch. Swelling occurs over the first several days.

TABLE 18-1 APPLICATION TIMES FOR FREEZE BRANDING

Age	Coat Color	Brand Application
Weaning	Black	45 sec
Weaning	Dark red	1 min
Weaning	Yellow (cream)	1 min, 15 sec
Weaning	White	2 min, 15 sec
Yearling	—	Add 15 sec to the above times

The site scabs over, and then the scab peels off in 2 to 3 weeks. Hair (white) will regrow in 6 to 8 weeks.

Several factors affect the success of the brand. Animals younger than weaning age (≈4 months) are poor candidates for the procedure because this age is a rapid growth phase that tends to distort the brand. Branding in either spring or fall is recommended because this is a time when the melanocytes are most active and therefore more easily destroyed. Finally, flat muscular areas produce the most readable brands; the side of the hindquarters (rump) is the most commonly used site in cattle. The neck may also be used.

Freeze branding does not cause permanent injury to the animal, and since the effects of the freeze are superficial, no significant damage to the hide occurs.

HOT BRANDING

Hot branding is the oldest branding method and is still widely used in some parts of the country. It has become controversial with the increasing presence of animal rights activism; however, the pain associated with the procedure is transient, and most people who are experienced with hot branding do not feel that the discomfort is significantly different from that caused by freeze branding. The goal of hot branding is total destruction of the hair follicle, such that no regrowth of hair will occur. The damage associated with the brand may devalue the hide.

HORN BRANDING

In animals with mature horns, heat may be used to mark a horn for animal identification.

EAR NOTCHING

This method involves removing small wedge-shaped pieces of cartilage from the margins of the ear pinna, producing permanent defects that are not affected by growth of the animal. The procedure can therefore be done at a very early age. An ear notcher, a plier-type instrument with a V-shaped cutting edge, is used to create the notches. The location of the notches corresponds to a standard numbering system. This method is commonly used in swine and is being used increasingly in small ruminants and cattle.

MARKING CHALK AND PAINT

Temporary marks may be placed anywhere on an animal with marking chalk and paint. This is commonly done to identify animals in heat, on medications, and animals to be separated or culled. Only nontoxic chemicals should be used; a variety of chalks and paints for livestock are commercially available.

INTEGUMENTARY SYSTEM

DEHORNING (CORNUECTOMY)

Ruminants may be horned or polled (genetically lacking horns), depending on species, breed, and sex. Horns grow continuously throughout the life of the animal, unless they are removed at their base. Horns are often removed, for several reasons. Horns are potentially dangerous weapons, even potentially fatal, to humans and to other animals. Great damage can be done by fighting using the horns. Feedlots typically pay less money for horned animals because of the additional expense of having the horns removed before the animal can be safely placed in a drylot group. Horned animals are more likely to cause damage to facilities and require more space in transportation vehicles. Horns may also become tangled in fences, branches, and other objects, resulting in great trauma to the animal, including death by hanging. In the United States dairy goats cannot be registered or shown if they have horns. Still, some owners desire that horns be left intact on animals kept on range conditions or tethers (for self-defense), or for personal cosmetic preference. Dehorning is a common procedure in cattle and goats but is seldom performed on rams.

It is in the best interest of the animal to remove the horns at the earliest possible age. Removal of mature horns has a higher complication rate, including increased hemorrhage, risk of infection (sinusitis and possible brain abscessation), and incomplete removal. It is also requires more sedation and local anesthesia, and technical skill. Removal of horns at an early stage is greatly preferred.

In horned animals, each horn grows from a separate horn bud (horn button), located on top of the head between the ears. The horn buds may be present at birth or become palpable as two hard lumps under the skin in the first couple of weeks. An irregular whorl of hair often covers each developing horn bud. Removal of the horn buds, before actual horn growth begins, is referred to as "disbudding." At this early stage, the horn buds are not yet attached to the skull, and therefore the frontal sinus is not exposed when they are removed. Disbudding can be done using several methods.

CHEMICAL CAUTERY

Various chemical pastes are available to cauterize and kill the germinal epithelium that eventually generates the horn. Best results are obtained if the procedure is performed in the first week of life, generally from day 3 to 7. Clipping the hair around the horn bud may increase contact with the paste and produce a more reliable result. Applying a liberal petroleum jelly "ring" around the area (before treatment) may help prevent the chemicals from running into the eyes and other tissues, which could cause severe trauma. The chemicals are also caustic to the tissues of other animals and humans; great care must be taken. The paste should be allowed to dry completely before allowing the animal to nurse. This method is not highly reliable in producing a complete kill of the germinal tissue and often results in a small, deformed, partial horn growth or "scur" that will have to be removed later by other methods. This procedure seems to cause more persistent pain than other methods, and the animal may rub the area in response, possibly spreading the paste to other areas and causing damage. The animal should be kept out of the rain for several days. Due to the potential risks, chemical cautery cannot be highly recommended for disbudding.

HEAT CAUTERY

This fast and almost bloodless method is popular, especially in goat kids. Electric disbudding irons are preferred, but fire-heated irons are still occasionally used in field situations. Clipping the hair from the area is advised, and tetanus prophylaxis should be given.

Kids may be held in the lap with the head held securely (Figs. 18-6 and 18-7). Some form of analgesia is desirable in all species. Local anesthesia is recommended for all patients, using a cornual nerve block. Sedation at this age is also possible but seldom necessary.

The tip of the disbudding iron is shaped in an open circle. When the iron is sufficiently

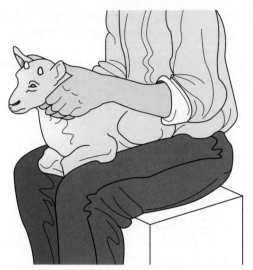

Fig. 18-6. Manual restraint for disbudding kids. The thumbs are placed behind the ears.

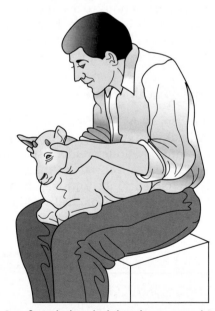

Fig. 18-7. Once the horn buds have been removed, pressure is applied with the thumbs above the eyes to help control hemorrhage from the cornual artery or placed in a holding or "disbudding" box for the procedure. (Modified from Leahy JR, Barrow P: *Restraint of animals*, Ithaca, NY, 1953, Cornell Campus Store.)

heated (cherry red in color), the tip is centered over the horn bud and applied with a circular "rocking" motion with light pressure. The goal is to completely kill the horn corium of the horn bud. Afterward, antibiotic powder or ointment should be applied to the area. The primary risk of the procedure is overheating the area, possibly resulting in heat-induced meningitis and malacia of the brain. Heat meningitis is recognized by sudden failure to nurse and lack of response to external stimuli. Treatment is supportive and rarely successful.

SURGICAL REMOVAL

It is possible to surgically excise the horn buds. General anesthesia may be used.

After several weeks of age, horn growth has begun, and removal is now referred to as "dehorning." Dehorning is usually performed on a conscious, sedated animal with local anesthesia for control of pain. Sedation with xylazine and local anesthesia with a cornual nerve block (see Chapter 16) and/or ring block at the base of the horn is most often used for these procedures. The animal must be physically restrained and the head securely held or tied. General anesthesia may be used, especially for adult animals with large horns. Clipping and surgical preparation of the skin are performed before the procedure. Tetanus vaccination status should be confirmed, and prophylaxis should be provided as needed.

Several dehorning methods are available. They are generally selected by the size of the horns.

Tube or Spoon Dehorners

Very small horns can be removed with tube or spoon dehorners (Fig. 18-8). These are small handheld "gouges" that are placed over the developing horn. They are twisted in a circular motion to cut away the horn and horn base. Bleeding is minimal and can be controlled with pressure.

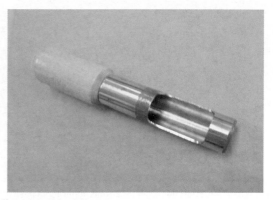

Fig. 18-8. Tube dehorner.

Lever-Type Dehorners

The Barnes dehorner is the most popular style of scoop-type dehorner for small and medium horns. It consists of two long handles, each with an extremely sharp metal cutting edge (Fig. 18-9, *A*). The handles are held together while the circular opening is placed over the horn and horn base (Fig. 18-9, *B*); spreading the handles apart actually closes the cutting edges together, producing a scooping-type cutting action that cuts under and removes the horn and its base in one piece (Fig. 18-10). Different sizes are available for different sizes of horns.

The Keystone dehorner is a larger instrument for larger horns. Pulling the lever handles together closes the cutting jaws of the instrument, removing the horn. Hemorrhage is often considerable and must be controlled by pulling the cornual arteries or cautery. Skull fractures are more likely to occur with this method than with others.

Surgical Saws

Large horns are removed by making a circular skin incision around the base of the horn, and then removing the horn and horn base with either a dehorning saw or Gigli wire saw (Figs. 18-11 and 18-12). An assistant is useful to stabilize the head while the sawing

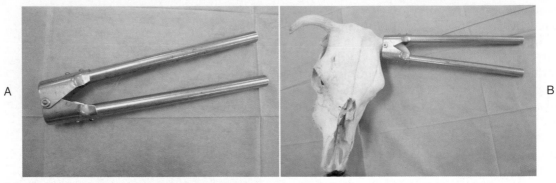

Fig. 18-9. **A,** Barnes dehorner. **B,** Barnes dehorner in position over a bovine horn.

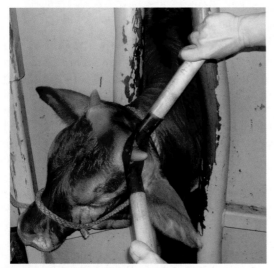

Fig. 18-10. **Dehorning a calf with a Barnes dehorner.** (From McCurnin DM, Bassert JM: *Clinical textbook for veterinary technicians,* ed 6, St Louis, 2006, Saunders.)

is performed. Hemorrhage occurs and must be controlled. It is sometimes possible for the surgeon to close the skin over the exposed sinuses with sutures ("cosmetic dehorning"); this is rarely possible with large horns (Fig. 18-13).

Complications of dehorning must be considered and owners well informed. Hemorrhage from removal of developed horns is expected and may be considerable.

The frontal sinus develops within the horn base and is exposed by dehorning; the resulting hole may be impressively large (Fig. 18-14). This exposure makes bacterial infection and parasitic invasion (myiasis— fly maggots) of the sinus possible. Rarely, infections may extend through the sinus and calvarium into the meninges and brain tissue. To minimize complications, blood clots should be removed from the exposed sinuses. Antibiotic ointment may be applied to the skin edges, and bandages may be applied to the head to cover the open sinuses. Bandages can be made from small stacks of sterile 4 × 4 gauze squares and held in place with elastic tape placed carefully in a figure eight around the head and ears (Fig. 18-15). Some clinicians do not advocate the use of bandages, preferring to heal the area as an open wound.

Antibiotic sprays and powders placed directly into the sinus may be irritating and delay healing, though they have historically been used successfully. Use of insect repellent is essential if dehorning is performed during fly season. Some clinicians advocate systemic antibiotics and nonsteroidal anti-inflammatory drugs. Healing normally occurs in 6 to 8 weeks for smaller horns. Large horns may require several months for healing and occasionally may fail to heal completely.

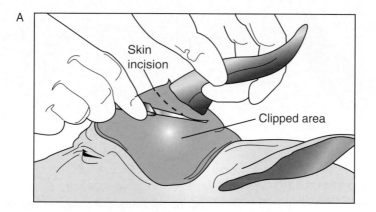

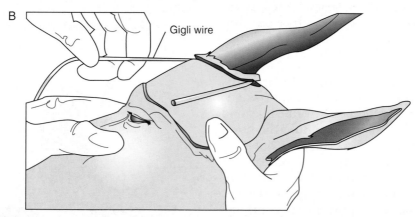

Fig. 18-11. A, Skin incision around the base of the horn. **B,** Placement of Gigli wire saw for dehorning in the goat. (Modified from Turner AS, McIlwraith CW: *Techniques in large animal surgery,* Philadelphia, 1982, Lea & Febiger.)

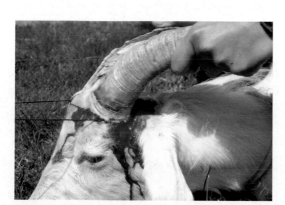

Fig. 18-12. Removal of a horn from an adult goat, using a **Gigli wire.** (Courtesy Dr. Mary Smith, Cornell University.)

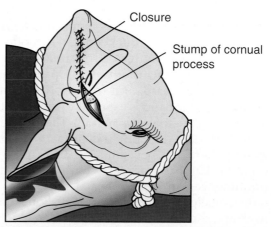

Fig. 18-13. Primary closure used in cosmetic dehorning **surgery.** (Modified from Turner AS, McIlwraith CW: *Techniques in large animal surgery,* Philadelphia, 1982, Lea & Febiger.)

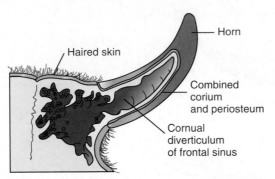

Fig. 18-14. Longitudinal cross-section of a horn, showing extension of the frontal sinus of the skull into the horn. Dehorning, which is performed at the base of the horn, **exposes the sinus.** (Modified from Frandson RD, Wilke WL, Fails AD: *Anatomy and physiology of farm animals*, ed 6, Philadelphia, 2003, Lippincott Williams & Wilkins.)

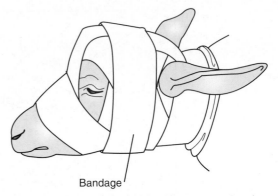

Fig. 18-15. Example of a head bandage after dehorning a goat or with elastic orthopedic stockinette with eyeholes. (Modified from Turner AS, McIlwraith CW: *Techniques in large animal surgery*, Philadelphia, 1982, Lea & Febiger.)

Removal of only the tips of the horns ("tipping") may be requested by some owners. The procedure should be performed beyond extent of the frontal sinus within the horn, to prevent creating a permanent opening. Radiographs may be taken to confirm the extent of the frontal sinus. Wire or dehorning saws may be used to remove the tip. Tip removal does not prevent the continual growth of the horn.

DESCENTING

Intact male goats are infamous for their offensive smell, or "buck odor." The odor actually has two sources. First, intact male goats urinate on themselves, primarily on their head, beard, and forelegs. This is a normal behavior and is especially prominent during the breeding season (fall). The second source of odor is from the primary scent glands; there is one gland situated at the caudomedial base of each horn (or horn prominences in polled goats) (Fig. 18-16). Other smaller glands are scattered about the neck and shoulder area. The scent glands are responsive to testosterone, which increases

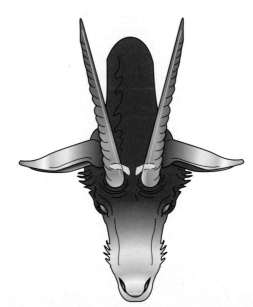

Fig. 18-16. The crescent-shaped scent glands are located caudomedially to the base of each horn. (Modified from Dyce KM, Sack WO, Wensing CJG: *Textbook of veterinary anatomy*, ed 3, St Louis, 2002, Saunders.)

during breeding season. The glands secrete a sebaceous material with a fetid odor. Owners frequently complain about the smell and request treatment.

Several approaches can be used to reduce and eliminate buck odor. Keeping the hair at the base of the horns clipped and frequently scrubbing the area may reduce, but not eliminate, the odor from the scent glands. Castration removes the primary sources of testosterone and therefore most of the noticeable odor from the scent glands. However, castration may not completely eliminate the self-urination behavior, especially if castration is performed after maturity. Surgical removal of the scent glands may also be done; it definitely ends the primary scent gland secretions but does not alter the self-urination behavior, if it exists. It is important to provide good client communication, since many pet goat owners think that descenting is the total answer to buck odor. They must realize that self-urination is not affected by descenting, and that only castration may eliminate, with occasional exception, self-urination.

Descenting may be done at any age. It is easiest to do it as a combined procedure with disbudding at an early age. Heat cautery is used to remove the horn buds as described earlier, and an additional overlapping area just caudomedial to each horn bud is also cauterized (Fig. 18-17). In the adult, the glands are recognized as a small hairless area with pores, just caudomedial to each horn. They may be removed during the dehorning procedure by extending the skin incisions to include them. They may also be removed at any time without dehorning the goat, as a separate procedure, under sedation and local anesthesia. The glands are identified and removed through surgical incisions. Sutures can be used to close the skin.

Descenting breeding bucks may have significant effects on breeding behavior. The identifying odor from the glands is used to attract females, and rubbing the top of the head on other animals and surfaces helps to

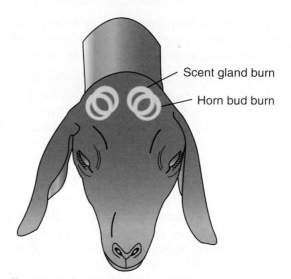

Fig. 18-17. Overlapping cautery circles are created by a disbudding iron, used to disbud and descent kids. (Modified from Ensminger ME: *Sheep and goat science*, ed 6, Danville, Ill, 2002, Interstate Publishing.)

"mark" a male's territory. Breeding females may reject males that lack this scent.

TAIL AMPUTATION (TAIL DOCKING)

Amputation of the tail may be done as an elective procedure or sometimes as a necessary procedure following severe injury. Elective tail amputation is commonly performed in sheep and sometimes in dairy cattle and is referred to as *tail docking*.

In dairy cattle, tail docking has historically been done to facilitate udder hygiene and improve the comfort and health of milking personnel (by reducing getting "swatted" with urine- and feces-soaked tails). However, the beneficial health claims have not been substantiated, nor have the claims of improved udder and milk hygiene. Potential animal welfare issues have been also identified, such as pain and discomfort related to the procedure and especially the inability to remove flies from the hindquarters.

The American Veterinary Medical Association (AVMA) Animal Welfare Committee released the following position statement in 2004:

> The AVMA opposes routine tail docking of cattle. Current scientific literature indicates that routine tail docking provides no benefit to the animal, and that tail docking can lead to distress during fly seasons. When medically necessary, amputation of tails must be performed by a licensed veterinarian.

In sheep, tail docking is performed to reduce the accumulation of feces/diarrhea which commonly occurs on natural-length tails. The fecal material tends to attract flies, leading to "fly strike" and maggot infestation, which is a potentially devastating condition for the animal. Long tails may also interfere with breeding. Removal is almost always performed in young lambs between 2 and 3 days to 2 weeks of age. At this young age pain appears minimal, and local anesthesia is considered optional. In fact, injecting local anesthetic is, in itself, a painful

procedure, sometimes causing as much discomfort as simple removal of the tail. The tail can be removed by several methods:

- Emasculator
- Emasculatome (Burdizzo)
- Heat cautery (electric "hot docker," hot chisel, or similar instrument)
- Sharp excision (scalpel or knife blade)
- Elastrator band (controversial; causes gradual ischemic necrosis)

The lamb is restrained off the ground or in the lap, with the hindquarters facing the clinician. The right legs are held in one hand, and the left in the other (Fig. 18-18). Clipping the hair is not necessary. The skin should be cleaned. The proper level of removal is at the mid to distal extent of the caudal tail fold; cutting the tail too close to the anus is believed to increase the incidence of rectal prolapse. Healing is complete in 2 to 3 weeks, regardless of the method used, unless complications occur. Hemorrhage and infection are the most common complications, though they are rare when the procedure is

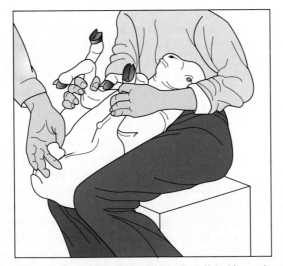
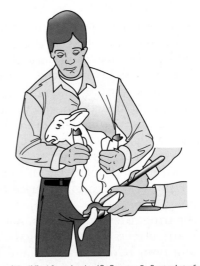

Fig. 18-18. Two methods of restraint of lambs for tail docking and castration. (Modified from Leahy JR, Barrow P: *Restraint of animals,* Ithaca, NY, 1953, Cornell Campus Store.)

properly performed. Hemorrhage is usually minimal at this early age. Instruments should always be thoroughly cleaned and disinfected between animals. Tetanus prophylaxis should be administered if it has not already been provided.

Injury to the tail may be severe enough to necessitate amputation in any species. Depending on the animal and the circumstances, the procedure may be done under general anesthesia or with sedation and local anesthesia (caudal epidural or subcutaneous ring block). The tail is clipped and sterilely prepped. A tourniquet at the base of the tail may be used for hemostasis. The clinician decides on the level of amputation, depending on the injury. The vertebral column is usually severed through an intervertebral space, leaving enough skin to suture over the remaining stump. Medication for pain control, antibiotics, and insect repellent may be necessary after surgery.

HOOF TRIMMING

Ruminants have cloven hooves, meaning that each limb has two weight-bearing digits, each with its own individual hoof (Fig. 18-19). The digits are commonly referred to as *claws*.

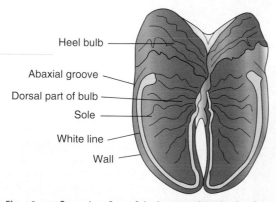

Fig. 18-19. Ground surface of the hooves of the bovine fore-foot. (Modified from Dyce KM, Sack WO, Wensing CJG: *Textbook of veterinary anatomy*, ed 3, St Louis, 2002, Saunders.)

Labels on figure:
Heel bulb
Abaxial groove
Dorsal part of bulb
Sole
White line
Wall

Hooves grow continuously during the life of the animal; the bovine hoof wall grows an average of 5 mm/month. Normal movement of the animal wears away the hoof wall at various rates, depending on the nature of the ground surface and activity level of the animal. Overgrowth may occur and require trimming to prevent potentially harmful deviations of the hoof such as "corkscrew claws" and "scissor claws." Uneven growth can also cause friction between the digits in the interdigital cleft, resulting in sores and abscesses and possible development of foot rot (Box 18-1).

Hoof trimming may be done on an as-needed basis or as part of a regular herd health program. Trimming may also be an essential part of the treatment of certain diseases such as foot rot. Sheep and goats are easiest to trim because of the minimal restraint needed. Sheep are trimmed in the "set-up" position (Fig. 18-20). Goats are usually trimmed in the standing position, with the operator standing to the side of the goat and lifting each leg individually (Fig. 18-21). The operator may reach across the back of the goat or stand alongside the goat and pick up the legs in a manner similar to horses. Uncooperative goats may need to have the head tied; an assistant may need to provide additional restraint; or the goats may need to be placed in lateral recumbency, with an assistant providing restraint of the neck and legs. A rump position similar to setting up sheep may be effective in some goats, though they generally resist this position.

Cattle seldom allow the legs to be manually lifted and manipulated, and restraint can be a major problem. They must usually be restrained in a chute, and the legs lifted with ropes (see Chapter 13). Alternatively, they may be placed on a special mechanical or hydraulic "tilt table," which elevates the animal off the ground and tips them into varying degrees of lateral recumbency.

BOX 18-1 Infectious Foot Rot (Interdigital Pododermatitis)

Infectious foot rot is a contagious and common disease of cattle and sheep and, to a much lesser extent, goats. All ages are susceptible, but the very young are rarely afflicted. The condition is painful, and animals in pain do not thrive. Major economic losses result from weight loss, low production, and costs of treatment.

Etiology

Often a mixed infection involving two primary bacterial organisms. The predominant organism may depend on the species of ruminant. *Dichelobacter* (formerly *Bacteroides*) *nodosus* is an anaerobic bacterium with the ability to destroy keratin. *Fusobacterium necrophorum* is an anaerobic bacterium thought to be necessary for *D. nodosus* to invade, by causing dermatitis between the claws, which *D. nodosus* can then use as an entry point.

Corynebacterium (Actinomyces) pyogenes may be involved, especially in the formation of deep abscesses.

The development of foot rot is largely influenced by management and environmental factors. These organisms are favored by moist or wet ground conditions. Trauma to the interdigital area from lacerations, abrasions, punctures, or softening from continual moisture allows the organisms to gain a foothold and cause disease. Foot rot is uncommon in dry environments and in animals with healthy, intact skin in the interdigital cleft.

Transmission

Infected animals shed the organism directly from wounds into the soil, where other animals may pick it up by foot contact with the soil. Untreated animals can be a source of herd infections for months to years.

Clinical Signs

One or more feet may be affected. Cases may be mild or moderately lame, but severe lameness affecting multiple individuals in a herd is the common presentation. There is inflammation and necrotic tissue in the affected interdigital clefts, which often produces an exudate and characteristic bad odor. Local swelling is common and may cause the claws to spread apart. A skin fissure often develops, with swollen, necrotic skin edges and purulent exudate. The infection may extend to undermine the hoof walls in the areas adjacent to the interdigital infection. The pain causes lameness, with limping or holding the leg up in an attempt to avoid bearing weight. Fever may develop, especially with deep tissue infection. Deep abscesses and infection of the coffin and pastern joints and associated tendons may develop.

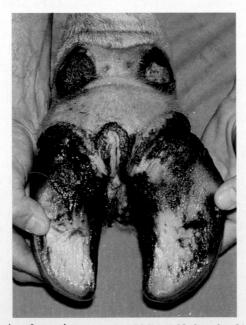

Interdigital pododermatitis (infectious foot rot). (From Petersen DC, Nelson DR: *Comp Cont Ed Pract Vet* 6(10):S566, October 1984.)

BOX **18-1** Infectious Foot Rot (Interdigital Pododermatitis)—Cont'd

Diagnosis

Generally by clinical signs and number of animals affected. Gram's stain of exudates may demonstrate the organisms, but this is usually not necessary. Culture of the primary organisms is difficult.

Treatment

The most important treatment is debridement of affected skin and hoof trimming to remove as much infected tissue as possible and "open up" infected areas to contact with air. Topical antibacterial agents, either antibiotics or antiseptics/astringents (copper sulfate, zinc sulfate, or 4% to 5% formalin) are commonly applied to all affected areas after trimming and debriding. Temporary bandages may be necessary after extensive debridement is performed. Foot baths may also be strategically placed so that animals must travel through them; these may help provide long-term treatment of a herd. Zinc sulfate is preferred for foot baths, since it does not stain like copper sulfate and does not irritate and burn tissue like formalin. Systemic antibiotics are sometimes used and are always indicated in cases of deep-seated infection. Drug residues must be considered.

Management practices must be assessed, especially with the goal of eliminating constant moisture conditions. Affected animals should be separated from the herd as soon as they are noticed to prevent further contamination of the environment.

Prevention

Regular hoof trimming, regular use of footbaths, and management to eliminate moist ground conditions are the most important preventative measures. Vaccinations against foot rot have been developed; however, the short duration of protection and the incidence of local injection-site reactions have led to limited use of the vaccines. Still, in herds where foot rot is a continual problem, vaccination may reduce the number and severity of infections. Chronically infected animals should be culled.

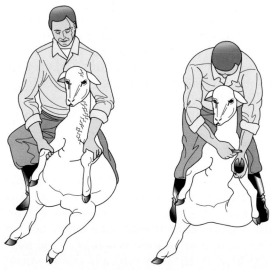

Fig. 18-20. Restraint of sheep for hoof trimming. (Modified from Leahy JR, Barrow P: *Restraint of animals*, Ithaca, NY, 1953, Cornell Campus Store.)

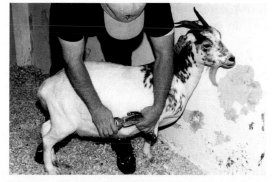

Fig. 18-21. Simple restraint of the goat for hoof trimming. The handler is pressing the goat against his legs with the arms. The left hand holds the foot while trimming with the right hand. (From Pugh DG: *Sheep and goat medicine*, Philadelphia, 2002, Saunders.)

Small tilt tables are available for calves and small ruminants. Tilt tables provide secure strapping for the body, head, and legs. Sedation is sometimes required to "table" the animal. If lateral recumbency is anticipated to last longer than 30 minutes, it is advisable to withhold food and water for several hours to reduce the risk of bloat and regurgitation. A final option if none of the previously mentioned methods is available is to cast the animal with ropes.

A variety of hoof knives, rasps, hoof nippers, hoof trimming shears, and curettes are available for trimming hooves. Hoof knives and trimming shears are usually sufficient for sheep and goats. Motorized rotary burrs may be helpful in cattle; motorized equipment must be used carefully to prevent excessive heating of the internal tissues in the hoof. Instruments should be disinfected between animals to prevent spreading infectious bacterial and fungal organisms.

The goal of hoof trimming is to provide a flat, level weight-bearing surface on both digits of each foot so that the digits bear weight evenly between them. The outer hoof walls of each digit should be the primary weight-bearing structures (Fig. 18-22). After cleaning off the bottom of the foot, any excessive toe is removed. The outer wall of each hoof is trimmed to parallel the coronary band; no portion of the wall should overlap or cover the sole. The inner hoof wall of each digit should be trimmed similarly but slightly shorter than the outer hoof wall (Fig. 18-23). As in horses, the hoof wall is the weight-bearing portion of the hoof, *not* the sole; therefore the walls should not be trimmed so short as to place the soles in a position of primary weight-bearing. The soles require careful removal of the thin outer layers; when the sole appears pink, it indicates that trimming is approaching the blood supply and should not go farther. Overgrowth of the sole provides crevices for possible development

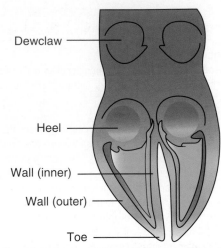

Fig. 18-22. The bottom of the sheep's or goat's foot. The toe should be cleaned out, and the outer hoof wall should be cut to remove all overgrowths, bring the wall down to the sole, and make the outer wall parallel with the coronary band. The inner hoof wall is then cut, with more inside wall than outside wall being removed. The heel should not be cut unless it is badly overgrown. (Modified from Pugh DG: *Sheep and goat medicine,* St Louis, 2002, Saunders.)

of foot rot; therefore paring out the sole is an important part of the hoof trimming procedure. Heels seldom need trimming unless they are overgrown. The hooves should be inspected for bruising and lesions around the coronary bands and lesions and growths in the interdigital cleft such as interdigital fibroma (hyperplasia or "corns") (Fig. 18-24). The clinician should be alerted if these are seen.

SUPERNUMERARY TEATS

Extra or accessory teats are found occasionally in small ruminants and cattle. They are usually small in size and may arise directly from the udder or from the side of a main teat. The most common location is caudal to the main teats (Fig. 18-25). They typically communicate with their own small, but functional, mammary gland tissue. Extra teats may interfere

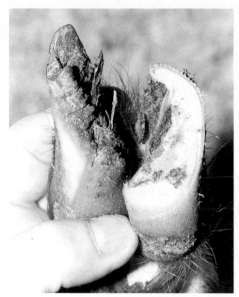

Fig. 18-23. Overgrown hoof before trimming *(left claw)* and after trimming *(right claw)*. After cleaning the toe, the operator trims the toe and outer wall. The inner wall is then trimmed slightly shorter than the outer wall. The procedure is repeated on the other hoof. (From Pugh DG: *Sheep and goat medicine*, St Louis, 2002, Saunders.)

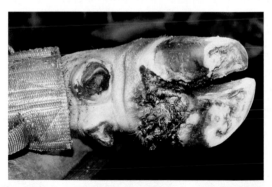

Fig. 18-24. Interdigital fibroma (corn) on a cow's foot. (From McCurnin DM, Bassert JM: *Clinical textbook for veterinary technicians*, ed 6, St Louis, 2006, Saunders.)

with proper fit of the milking machine cups and may become affected with mastitis. Therefore they are commonly amputated.

Tetanus prophylaxis should be provided. The amputation technique depends on the age

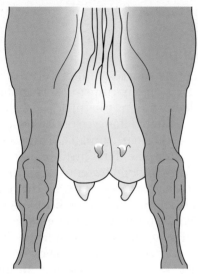

Fig. 18-25. Supernumerary teats on the caudal surface of the bovine mammary gland. (Modified from Dyce KM, Sack WO, Wensing CJG: *Textbook of veterinary anatomy*, ed 3, St Louis, 2002, Saunders.)

of the female. In young kids and lambs, serrated scissors are used to remove the teats at their base, by cutting in a craniocaudal direction, rather than laterally across the udder. Alternate methods using an emasculatome (Burdizzo) or emasculator to crush the base of the extra teat (for hemostasis) have been described for animals older than 6 months. In older (mature) animals with more developed teats and gland tissue, removal requires sedation and local anesthesia, skin incision, and dissection of the teat and its associated gland tissue. The incision is closed in layers with suture.

REPRODUCTIVE SYSTEM

INTERSEXUALITY

Intersexuality implies an individual with genital anatomical features of both sexes (hermaphrodite). Intersex conditions occur rarely in cattle and sheep and somewhat more often in goats.

FREEMARTINISM

In cattle the most common form of intersexuality is freemartinism. A freemartin is a female born twin to a male, with normal-appearing external female genitalia but grossly abnormal internal genitalia. The condition results when the fetal membranes of the twins form blood vessel communications (vascular anastomoses) between them, allowing testosterone and other hormones from the male to influence development of the female (Fig. 18-26). Reports indicate that the condition affects 92% of females born twin to a male. A persistent hymen, prominent clitoris, and abnormally small (hypoplastic) ovaries are common, as well as various degrees of development of testicles, epididymis, vesicular glands, and other internal male structures. The condition manifests internally in many ways, but the result is a sterile individual. There are several ways to diagnose freemartins based on clinical signs and chromosome analysis (karyotyping), but measuring vaginal length between 1 and 4 weeks of age and confirming the absence of a cervix are inexpensive and often used. Freemartins have an abnormally short vagina.

Freemartin goats and sheep are rare.

POLLED INTERSEX

In goats of many European breeds, infertility and the intersex condition are linked to the polled (hornless) genotype. The gene for polledness is dominant in these breeds; unfortunately an infertility gene (autosomal recessive) is linked to the polled gene. Therefore goats may have one of three possible genetic combinations (H = polled gene, h = horned gene):

HH = polled
Hh = polled (H is dominant)
hh = horned

Homozygous polled (HH) males are not intersex but have up to a 35% infertility rate due to abnormalities of the testicles and/or epididymis (Fig. 18-27). Homozygous polled (HH) females are intersex (male pseudohermaphrodites), with various degrees of development of both male and female reproductive organs and testosterone-producing tissue, usually in the form of hypoplastic testicles. They are sterile. They often show male behavior from testosterone production, including aggression and increased odor during breeding season; however, they do not produce sperm.

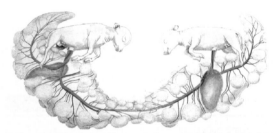

Fig. 18-26. Diagram of twin bovine pregnancy with conjoined circulations; freemartinism is possible. (From Dyce KM, Sack WO, Wensing CJG: *Textbook of veterinary anatomy*, ed 3, St Louis, 2002, Saunders.)

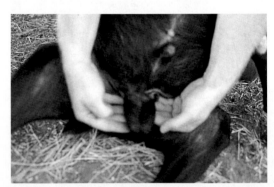

Fig. 18-27. Small, hard, hypoplastic testicles on a homozygous polled yearling buck. (From Pugh DG: *Sheep and goat medicine*, St Louis, 2002, Saunders.)

Heterozygotes have normal fertility. Although they do not produce horns, they may be recognized by prominent frontal "bumps" where the horns would have been; these "bumps" are typically oval in shape and lie close together in a "V" formation.

Infertility is not an issue for people not interested in breeding goats, but it is a major concern for producers and purebred breeders. In order to prevent homozygous polled offspring and the associated intersex/infertility, one of the breeding pair should be genetically horned (hh). Surgical removal of horns does not change the genetic makeup of an individual. Polled intersexes are extremely rare in Angora and Nubian goats, indicating a different heritability of the traits. There is no relationship of the presence or absence of horns with the occurrence of freemartinism.

MALE REPRODUCTIVE SYSTEM

BREEDING SOUNDNESS EXAMINATION/ SEMEN COLLECTION

Reproductive efficiency is absolutely essential for the success of any livestock operation. Owners must continually evaluate the reproductive performance of breeding males and females in the herd. The primary goal of a breeding soundness examination is to evaluate the current state of fertility of an individual, realizing that many factors can affect fertility. Animals with fertility problems are often candidates for culling, since they would cause an economic loss. The breeding soundness examination is only one piece of information used in formulating a farm's breeding management program.

The breeding soundness examination is usually performed just before the breeding season. The components of a basic breeding soundness examination of the male are similar in the ruminant species. The following parameters are evaluated.

Physical Examination

In addition to a general health evaluation, the examination emphasizes the physical ability to breed females (especially eyes, legs, and feet). A rectal examination of the internal accessory sex glands may be done in the bull.

Examination of external genitalia

- Prepuce and penis: ability to extend penis, extension of the penis in a straight line, skin lesions of prepuce or glans penis. Visualization of the penis of bulls is usually done during the semen collection procedure. Rams are set up on their rump; the external preputial ring is pushed caudally and down toward the abdomen to reveal the glans penis, which is gently grasped with a gauze square and pulled into extension.
- Scrotum and testicles: shape, size, consistency.
- Measurement of scrotal circumference: circumference correlates with the amount of sperm-producing tissue and, therefore, usually with actual sperm production. Many factors such as age, breed, and time of year can affect the circumference. Scrotal measuring tapes can be commercially obtained. Measurement is made by pulling the testicles fully into the scrotal sacs and measuring snugly around the largest circumference point (Fig. 18-28).

Semen quality evaluation

Semen is evaluated for sperm count/concentration, percentage of live spermatozoa, the motility of the spermatozoa, and sperm morphology. Care must be taken to prevent temperature-shock of the sperm, which can drastically affect the results of the semen evaluation. All surfaces that the semen contacts must be kept within the appropriate temperature range, from the semen collection container to the slides and microscope stage. This may require some planning, especially

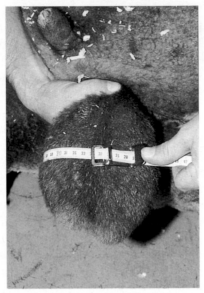

Fig. 18-28. Measuring the scrotal circumference of a ram. The procedure is the same for bucks. The tape measure should slightly indent the skin, and the examiner should firmly push the testicles into the scrotum with the free hand. Care should be taken to read the measurement at the correct location on the measuring tape. (From Pugh DG: *Sheep and goat medicine*, St Louis, 2002, Saunders.)

has also been described. Otherwise, electroejaculation with the buck standing is used. The buck is placed in a chute or pressed against a wall for restraint. Feces are removed from the rectum, and the electroejaculator probe is lubricated and inserted. Sterile gauze should be used to grasp the glans penis and direct it into the collection container, being sure that the urethral process is well within the margins of the container (Fig. 18-29).

Ram. Electroejaculation is most commonly used. The same electroejaculators used in bucks are suitable for the ram. The ram is collected standing or placed in lateral recumbency; the penis is manually extended from the prepuce. The collection container should be prepared and held ready, since some males may ejaculate at this time. If not, the rectum is cleared, and the lubricated electroejaculator probe is inserted and used to massage the accessory sex glands and apply a brief electrical current. The procedure is repeated until

in cold climates. Semen collection is accomplished by different methods in different species.

Bull. Electroejaculation is most commonly used. After manually evacuating the rectum, an electroejaculator is lubricated and inserted into the rectum. This device emits a mild electrical current that causes erection and ejaculation to occur. Vocalization during the procedure is common, and extension of the hindlegs may occur. While the penis is extended, it can be examined for lesions such as deviation, penile warts, scars, and hair rings. Trained bulls may be collected using a female in estrus and an artificial vagina.

Bucks. Some bucks are trained to collection via an artificial vagina. A technique for massage of the glans penis through the prepuce

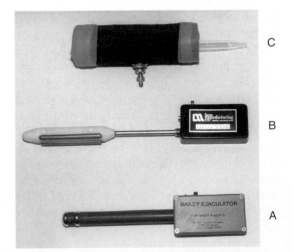

Fig. 18-29. The two electroejaculators shown here are the Bailey **(A)** and Lane **(B)** electroejaculators. Both contain batteries and require no external power source. Other models are available. An artificial vagina also is shown **(C)**. (From Pugh DG: *Sheep and goat medicine*, St Louis, 2002, Saunders.)

ejaculation occurs. As with the buck, the tip of the glans penis and urethral process should be held within the margins of the collection container, using sterile gauze pads to handle the penis. Vocalization and muscle contractions are typical during the procedure. Trained rams may be collected using an artificial vagina; the ram mounts a female in estrus or a mounting dummy.

Breeding behavior

Demonstrating breeding behavior is not always possible at the time of veterinary examination; owners often must make these observations under natural conditions. The libido and mounting behavior of the male are observed. Intromission into the vagina and ejaculation should be confirmed.

CASTRATION

Castration is one of the most commonly performed surgical procedures in ruminants. Although it can be done at any age, the complication rate and difficulty of the procedure increase with age; therefore early castration is usually in the best interest of the animal. Preferably, castration is performed at a time of year when flies and other insects are at a minimum. The environment should be clean and dry. Tetanus prophylaxis must be provided either with protection from the dam's colostrum or injection of tetanus antitoxin or tetanus toxoid.

Castration may be performed with strict attention to aseptic technique and anesthesia. Sterile gloves and instruments may be used, and proper skin preparation may be done. In reality, however, following these surgical "principles" requires extra time and expense, and they are not often adhered to in field situations. In these settings, instruments should always be cleaned of blood and debris and disinfected between each animal. Skin preparation is minimized to a brief but thorough scrub. The operator's hands should

be washed and disinfected thoroughly between each animal. Despite appearances, these field methods have been used successfully for many years.

There are a variety of ways to castrate an animal. Castration methods are selected on the basis of species, age, management, and environmental factors. Although all methods have been used successfully, some are used less often because of associated complications. The common practice of performing castration without local anesthesia or sedation has become controversial. However, the immature metabolism of very young animals limits the selection of drugs that can be safely used, and the restraint and pain caused by injecting local anesthetic may be as stressful and painful as the castration itself. Use of drugs also increases the time and cost of the procedure. However, as animal welfare awareness increases, the use of anesthesia will also undoubtedly increase.

The two basic categories of castration methods are open and closed. Both are used in ruminants. Open castration methods involve incision through the skin of the scrotum to expose the testicles. The incisions are left open to drain and heal by second intention. Although it is surgically possible to close the incisions with suture, this is almost never done because closure prevents drainage from the wound and requires more time and expense to perform. Closed castration techniques are performed without skin incision. Closed techniques are usually bloodless when performed correctly, which is an advantage during insect season. However, closed techniques are not without potential complications. (Note that closed castration [without skin incision] is never used in horses. In horses, the terms "open" and "closed" castration refer to whether or not the *vaginal tunic* is incised. Thus use of these terms may be confusing.)

Before any castration procedure, the presence of both testicles in the scrotum should be confirmed. Cryptorchidism is rare in ruminants, but castration of only one descended testicle should be avoided.

Bovine

Calves younger than 1 month are typically held in lateral recumbency, since they are too small for cattle chutes. Older calves are candidates for standing castration in a cattle chute or stocks, with tail restraint. The commonly used methods of castration in the bovine include the following.

Surgical "knife" castration

This is most commonly performed before or at the time of weaning, at approximately 3 to 4 months of age. However, it can be performed at any age. The first step of the procedure is to incise the scrotum to expose the testicles. A scalpel blade or castrating knife is used to cut laterally across and remove the entire bottom third of the scrotum, which exposes the testicles. Another method of incising the scrotum is with a Newberry knife, which is placed in the middle of the scrotum and pulled quickly, distally, to produce a vertical scrotal incision between the testicles.

The second step of the procedure is to remove the testicles. A testicle is grasped with sterile gauze 4 × 4's and pulled out of the scrotum to expose the spermatic cord. In young calves, the testicle can simply be pulled until the cord stretches and ruptures; the separation causes the smooth muscle in the wall of the testicular blood vessels to spasm shut ("vasospasm"), providing hemostasis. Alternatively, in older animals with more development of the spermatic cord, the cord can be ligated with absorbable suture and then cut to remove the testicle. The procedure is repeated on the other testicle. The scrotal incision is left open for drainage and heals as an open wound. After the procedure, antiseptic or antibiotic spray is usually applied to the scrotal incisions.

During insect season, repellent should be applied directly to the areas around the incision, but not in the incision itself.

Emasculators

This method is necessary for animals with more developed spermatic cords, in order to provide more reliable hemostasis. The scrotum is incised as described earlier on this page. After exposing the testicle and spermatic cord, emasculators are applied across the spermatic cord; the emasculators simultaneously crush and sever the cord. The emasculators are left in place for a brief time, depending on the size of the spermatic cord. The procedure is repeated on the other testicle. Antiseptic/antibiotic topical medications and insect repellent are used as described earlier on this page.

Emasculatome (Burdizzo)

This "bloodless" castration method is popular for castration during fly season. The emasculatome is a crushing "pincer"-type instrument that is used to crush the spermatic cord above the testicle, through the skin, without an incision. The spermatic cord is identified beneath the skin by palpation, and the instrument is applied across it (usually two applications, 1 to 2 cm apart). The procedure is repeated for the other cord. The instrument is never applied across the entire width of the scrotum, to preserve some blood flow to the scrotum and allow it to survive. The testicles subsequently atrophy within the scrotum, but usually do not slough. This method is less reliable, since it is performed "blindly" through the skin; incomplete destruction of the cord may result.

Elastrator

This "elastic castrator" is an instrument used to apply a special rubber band around the base of the scrotum, proximal to (above) the testicles. The band is so tight that it acts as a tourniquet, resulting in necrosis and sloughing of the testicles and scrotum in 2 to 3 weeks. Although no incision is used, the necrotic tissue may attract insects; repellent must be used during insect season. Elastrators are only suitable for animals younger than 2 weeks of age. The instrument and band should be soaked in disinfectant before use.

Chemical castration

This method has been used for very young males weighing less than 150 lb. Each testicle is injected with a castration solution containing a chemical that gradually destroys the testicular tissue and a local anesthetic for pain relief. The method is bloodless, and normally no tissue sloughing occurs. Castration is complete in 60 to 90 days. Proper injection technique is essential for the success of the procedure; otherwise, incomplete castration and other complications may result. The commercial availability of the solution has not been reliable.

Vaccination

A vaccine against the hormone GnRH (gonadotropin-releasing hormone) has been recently developed.

Complications of castration

Hemorrhage and infection are the primary postoperative complications. Hemorrhage is a complication of open (incisional) castration methods; animals should be observed for hemorrhage for 24 hours after open castration procedures. Infections usually occur from 5 to 15 days after open castration and are often associated with a failure of the incisions to drain; marked swelling, fever, and inappetence are common clinical signs. Antibiotics are given prophylactically by some clinicians in the hope of reducing postoperative infections.

Small Ruminant (Ovine/Caprine)

Routine castration of sheep and goats is usually done in the first week of life. In animals

that are to be kept long term, such as pets, it is advisable to wait until 5 to 6 months of age; early castration may retard the full development of the penile urethra, resulting in a narrow urethra that is prone to blockage with urinary calculi. Clients should understand that delayed castration has no effect on the formation of calculi and does not guarantee that obstructions of the urethra will never occur, but it may reduce the incidence of obstructions of the urethra.

Castration of the adult ram and buck has a higher incidence of complications. The mature testicles of these species are quite large for the size of the animal and have a well-developed blood supply; this increases the risk of hemorrhage. These animals should always be sedated for the procedure, since the stress of the procedure in a fully awake animal may cause shock and possibly death. Clients should understand the importance of castrating before sexual maturity is reached.

Restraint is age dependent and also depends on the clinician's preference. Lambs and kids may be restrained on their back in a handler's lap or held upside down by the hindlegs with the body resting against the handler's thighs (Fig. 18-30).

Small ruminants are especially sensitive to tetanus. Tetanus prophylaxis from either colostrum, tetanus antitoxin, or tetanus toxoid must be provided.

Methods of castration include the following:

Surgical "knife" castration

Sedation and local anesthesia may be used, but when castration is performed at several days of age it is common practice to perform the procedure without use of either. Older animals, especially mature males, should be sedated, and use of local anesthesia should be considered.

The scrotum is incised using one of the methods described above, and the testicles are exteriorized. Removal of the testicle is by

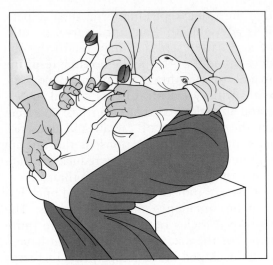

Fig. 18-30. Restraint of a lamb in the handler's lap for castration and tail docking.

traction in animals less than 4 months of age. Older animals with more development of the spermatic cord require measures to control hemorrhage, by use of an emasculator or ligation of the cord with suture. The scrotal incisions are left open to heal. Animals should be watched for hemorrhage during the immediate postoperative period, and for signs of infection in the days that follow. Use of insect repellent during fly season is essential to prevent fly strike and maggot infestation.

Elastrator

The elastrator technique is popular among farmers and technically simple to perform. It is for use on animals between 1 and 3 weeks old; after that time, it is considered an inhumane technique due to lingering signs of pain. Necrosis and then sloughing of the entrapped tissues occurs in less than 2 weeks. The risk of tetanus, which may occur following the period of necrosis and sloughing, may be more than with other methods. Repellent should be used during insect season.

Emasculatome (Burdizzo)

This method is used for older lambs and kids. Anesthesia is rarely used. The instrument is applied twice to each spermatic cord, through the skin, without incisions. Postoperative complications, including discomfort, have led to reduced popularity of this method.

Chemical castration

The same commercial solution used on calves has been successfully used in lambs and kids, at reduced dosages. Availability of the solution is questionable.

FEMALE REPRODUCTIVE SYSTEM

ESTROUS CYCLE DETERMINATION

Although females may be bred by simply turning out a male to run with the herd, most producers use planned breeding programs. Planned breeding may use either "hand-mating," where one male is allowed to naturally breed one selected female at a time in a controlled setting, or artificial insemination. Regardless of the method, planned breeding is more efficient, generally safer for the animals, and allows better record keeping than pasture breeding.

Successful breeding programs depend on knowledge of the estrous cycle and what stage of the reproductive cycle each breeding female is in. Table 18-2 reviews the reproductive physiology of females of the ruminant species. Various methods are used to determine the stage of a female's estrous cycle.

Rectal Palpation

This method is limited by size of the animal; therefore it is used primarily in cattle. The follicles and corpus lutea of cattle are more superficial on the ovary than in the horse; therefore palpation is more informative in cattle. Chute or headcatch restraint is generally used.

TABLE 18-2 REPRODUCTIVE PHYSIOLOGY OF FEMALE RUMINANTS (AVERAGE STATISTICS)

	Cattle	Sheep	Goats
Breeding season	Year-round polyestrous	Seasonally polyestrous* (short photoperiod)	Seasonally polyestrous* (short photoperiod)
Puberty†	7-18 mo	6-9 mo	6-9 mo
Length of estrous cycle	21 days	17 days	21 days
Length of estrus	18 hr	24-48 hr	24-36 hr
Ovulation	12-18 hr after estrus	Near the end of estrus	Near the end of estrus
Gestation	283 days	148 days	150 days

Variable, depending on breed. Some breeds cycle year-round.
†*Variable, depending on breed and body condition. In sheep and goats, the time of year when born has a marked effect; females born late may not mature in time for that year's breeding season and therefore will not begin cycling until the following year's breeding season.*

Ultrasound per Rectum

Although this is possible in cattle, it is seldom necessary because of the ease of palpation of the ovaries.

Observation of Standing Heat

Physical signs such as a swollen vulva, vaginal discharge, increased vocalization, frequent urination, and restlessness may be seen in ruminants in estrus. However, the most reliable indicator of estrus is observing a female allowing other animals to mount her. This is often simply performed by routine visual herd checks. Animals may be observed being "ridden" or may be checked for signs of having been mounted such as ruffled hair or hair loss in the tailhead area, or mud and dirt on top of the hindquarters. The number of the animal is recorded, and breeding planned accordingly.

Other methods exist to detect standing heat, without direct observation of the behavior. Heat mount detectors or chemical marking patches ("rump patches") are adhesive patches with chemicals contained in a flexible, clear plastic sleeve. The patch is placed on top of the hindquarters, over the sacral spine. If mounted, the weight of the mounting animal crushes the plastic sleeve, allowing the chemicals to mix, resulting in a color change. The herdsman simply checks the herd for activated rump patches, indicating standing heat.

Teaser animals may also be used to mark estrus females. Teaser animals are prepared in several ways; each method has advantages and disadvantages. Intact males may be vasectomized or have the penis surgically translocated to prevent entry into the vagina. Teaser females may be prepared by treatment with hormones, with or without spaying. Castrated males may be treated with testosterone. Once the teaser animal has been prepared, it is fitted with a marking device. The device is often a chin-ball halter or marking collar, which contains a dye reservoir. When the teaser mounts the estrus female, the riding activity applies the dye to-and-fro across the back of the estrus female. The herdsman checks the herd for the dye marks left by the teaser, indicating the females in standing heat.

Vaginal Cytology

Although cyclic changes do occur in the epithelial cells lining the vagina, the changes are not as specific as in small animal species. Cytology has limited practical application in ruminants.

ESTRUS SYNCHRONIZATION

For breeding management of large numbers of females, especially when artificial insemination is used, it may be advantageous to "synchronize" the herd so that labor and planning can be maximized for efficiency. This process is known as *estrus synchronization*.

Synchronization is usually accomplished by hormonal treatment with prostaglandin, progesterone, or estrogen compounds. The hormones may be used alone or in combination, depending on the desired effect. They are delivered either by injection, subcutaneous implant, or intravaginal drug-releasing sponges. Some hormones may be delivered orally as a feed additive. The regimen used depends largely on the species of ruminant and the management needs of the farm operation.

Subcutaneous hormone implants are used commonly in cattle and less often in small ruminants. The implants are placed on the outer (dorsal) aspect of the ear pinna, between the skin and the cartilage. Implants are injected using a special injection "gun" designed by the manufacturer for its individual brand of implant. The skin of the ear pinna should be cleaned before the injection.

PREGNANCY DIAGNOSIS

Confirming pregnancy has several important roles in a managed breeding program. It allows for planning of labor, feeding, veterinary, and space needs, and estimated budgeting for associated costs and potential profits. It also allows early identification of females with fertility problems so that diagnosis and treatment can be instituted in the hope of subsequent breeding and successful pregnancy without missing a breeding season. Failure to produce offspring each breeding season represents economic loss to the producer.

In reality, many herdsmen simply use the failure to return to heat as the primary pregnancy "test." However, failure to return to heat may indicate conditions other than pregnancy, such as a pathologically persistent corpus luteum or cystic ovaries. A variety of tools are available to diagnose pregnancy with greater precision. The accuracy of the many methods of pregnancy determination varies depending on the species, stage of pregnancy, and skill of the clinician. The cost of the procedure is usually a necessary consideration. Accurate breeding records are helpful in selecting the best diagnostic test for a suspected pregnant animal, based on the suspected length of the pregnancy.

Rectal Palpation

This is the most common method used in cattle. Experienced clinicians can detect pregnancies reliably as early as 25 to 30 days (Fig. 18-31). A method of rectal palpation with a hollow plastic "palpation rod" (Hulet's rod) has been described in sheep; the ewe is placed on her back (a submissive position for sheep), and the lubricated rod is inserted into the rectum and used to gently elevate and hold the uterus against the abdominal wall, where it can be palpated with the free hand. Developed fetuses may be felt through the abdominal wall. With experience, detection of pregnant ewes may be highly accurate after 60 days of gestation. Palpation rods may be used in goats but are difficult to use, since goats resent being restrained on their backs and often struggle; rectal tears and abortions have resulted.

Diagnostic Ultrasound, per Rectum

Ultrasound can detect pregnancy as early as 12 days in cattle and 18 days in small ruminants.

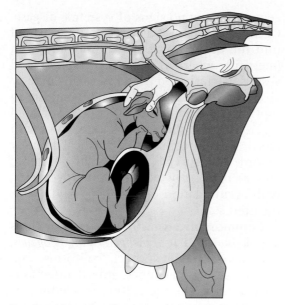

Fig. 18-31. Detection of pregnancy in the cow by rectal palpation. Pregnancy approaching term. (From Noakes DE, Parkinson TJ, England GCW: *Veterinary reproduction and obstetrics*, ed 8, London, 2001, Saunders.)

It is highly effective for early pregnancy diagnosis. However, it is seldom necessary to confirm pregnancy at this stage, and the added cost of the procedure is seldom justified. Ultrasound has the ability to perform accurate measurements and therefore may be used to estimate fetal age and determine fetal sex. Fetal sex is best determined between days 60 and 70, with high accuracy when performed by experienced clinicians. The distance between the genital tubercle and the umbilicus and tail is measured; in males, the tubercle is closer to the umbilicus, and in females it is closer to the tail.

In small ruminants, a linear array probe used in horses can be modified by taping it (and its cord) to an insemination/infusion pipette or small polyvinyl chloride pipe for advancement into the rectum.

Diagnostic Ultrasound, Transabdominal

Ultrasound through the abdominal wall is commonly used in small ruminants. The procedure may be done as early as day 30 to 45, but accuracy rates of greater than 95% are possible after day 60 of pregnancy. Most animals can be scanned while standing; clipping a small window may be necessary for proper contact of the transducer. A 5.0 MHz transducer may be suitable for early pregnancies, but with increasing abdominal size a 3.5 MHz transducer is preferred. The ultrasound transducer is placed near the front of the udder, to the right side of the udder, or high in the right inguinal region, depending on the stage of pregnancy. It is aimed first toward the pelvic inlet and slowly rotated cranially to produce a sweeping scan of the abdomen. Accurately counting fetuses with ultrasound is difficult, but the best chance for visualization of multiple fetuses occurs between days 45 and 90. Measurement of length of a fetus may allow estimation of fetal age. Fetal heartbeat may be seen by day 30 to 35.

Doppler Ultrasound, per Rectum and Transabdominal

This method has been used in small ruminants after day 35 to 40 of gestation. A rectal Doppler probe is used to "hear" the fetal heart rate, which is roughly twice the maternal heart rate. After approximately 50 days, Doppler may be used transabdominally and is highly accurate after 75 days. Counting fetuses with Doppler ultrasound is difficult.

Doppler ultrasound has also been used in cattle. The fetal heart can be heard via rectal Doppler by week 6 to 7.

Radiographs

Although possible in small ruminants, there is little indication for the procedure. However, it is highly reliable for pregnancy diagnosis, and it can be used to count the number of fetuses, since the incidence of twins and triplets in small ruminants is high. Mineralization of the fetal skeleton, which occurs as early as day 65 to 70, is necessary for viewing the fetus on a radiograph. Best results may occur after day 90. Fasting the female may improve visualization of fetuses.

Abdominal Ballottement

This method requires a fetus of sufficient size to be 'bumped' with the hands through the abdominal wall. One or both fists are placed over the right lower paralumbar fossa and pressed rapidly inward toward the uterus; this thrust displaces the fetus and fetal fluids momentarily, and then they rebound and give a characteristic "bump" back against the operator's hands, which are left pressed against the body wall. Sheep and goats should be beyond 100 days of gestation; cattle should be beyond 6 to 7 months of gestation. This method is not highly reliable.

Hormonal Assays

Assays for progesterone and estrogen compounds (estrone sulfate) in blood, urine, and milk are available. Pregnancy-specific protein B can also be detected in blood for early pregnancy diagnosis. Tests must be carefully selected on the basis of thorough knowledge of pregnancy physiology. All tests have potential pitfalls and limited timeframes during gestation when they are useful. The expense of hormonal tests is seldom justified in ruminants.

UTERINE CULTURE, BIOPSY, AND INFUSION

Uterine infections are common in cattle after calving because of the high incidence of retained placentas and dystocias. The most common type of uterine infection is endometritis, an infection of the lining of the uterus. It is characterized by a whitish to yellowish mucopurulent vaginal discharge in a cow that has recently given birth. Because the infection is superficial, cows generally show no signs of systemic disease. Occasionally, bacterial infections may extend into the deeper layers of the myometrium (metritis), where there is access to blood vessels. Bacteria and bacterial toxins may be absorbed into the bloodstream, resulting in septicemia, endotoxemia, and associated severe systemic illness and shock. Cows with metritis require intensive medical therapy in order to survive. Chronically, bacterial endometritis may develop into pyometra, with accumulation of purulent exudates in the uterus.

Common organisms in uterine infections are *Actinomyces (Corynebacterium) pyogenes*, streptococci, staphylococci, coliforms, and gram-negative anaerobes; mixed infections are common. Uterine culture is seldom performed in cases of endometritis; aerobic cultures often grow a "mixed bag" of organisms that may or may not be actual pathogens, and anaerobic culture is difficult to perform. Uterine biopsy is also rarely used. However, both procedures can be done in cattle, using the same instruments and methods as in the horse.

Uterine infusion and lavage are often used for treatment of uterine infections. Lavage is performed to "wash out" the uterus, by instilling large volumes of fluid and then siphoning out the fluid and debris. In order to accommodate the fluids and debris, large-bore tubing such as an equine stomach tube is often used. This is not a sterile procedure, but it should be performed as cleanly as possible. Similarly, uterine infusion is used to place liquid medications into the uterus, generally in smaller volumes that are intended to remain in the uterus to maximize contact time with the bacteria. Antibiotic solutions are most often used for infusions. Infusion and lavage fluids should be warm.

Preparation of the female for any uterine procedure is similar to that described in the horse. The tail is tied or held out of the way, and the vulva and perineum are washed thoroughly with warm water and disinfectant scrub. Clinician preference dictates the specific materials and equipment used for the procedures.

Metritis, endometritis, and pyometra are not common in sheep and goats but may occasionally follow cases of retained placenta or dystocia. Females of these species normally have a brownish-red, thick, nonodorous vaginal discharge for up to 4 weeks after birth; this normal fluid is called *lochia* and requires no treatment. However, the discharge associated with infection is also brownish-red but watery, with a bad odor. Clostridial organisms may sometimes be involved in severe cases. Uterine lavage and infusion are more difficult to safely perform in these species, but a 12- to 14-French Foley catheter may be passed through an open cervix with care.

Many clinicians treat uterine infections with hormones such as prostaglandins or oxytocin to cause contraction of the uterus and expulsion of the contents. This is sometimes used as the only treatment in small ruminants.

OBSTETRICAL PROCEDURES

Dystocias are fairly common occurrences in cattle and sheep but uncommon in goats. Many factors influence the incidence of dystocias, including breed of the sire, breed of the dam, age of the dam, number of fetuses, and bodyweight of the dam. Dystocias occur more frequently in first-time (primiparous) mothers and are less likely to occur with each subsequent pregnancy. One of the most common factors is breeding females to males that are considerably larger or are known to sire large birthweight offspring, as is commonly done in cattle, in hope of increasing calf size. Unfortunately, the larger birthweight size often exceeds the size of the dam's birth canal (especially in first-calf heifers), resulting in inability of the fetal

shoulders or hips to pass without assistance. Fetal malposition is another common cause of dystocias, especially in sheep and goats.

In any species, attending a dystocia begins with restraint of the animal, with a premium on safety for the clinician and assisting personnel. Personnel handling instruments or assisting the delivery should wear disposable gloves because of the possibility of zoonotic diseases, which may affect the reproductive tract and/or fetus and fetal membranes. A clean area should be established for equipment, and instruments should be sterilized or disinfected. If the tail is long enough to compromise cleanliness of the vulva, it should be held or tied to the side. Obstetrical maneuvers are not sterile, but every effort should still be made to keep the perineal area clean.

The examination of the patient begins with an evaluation of general physical status. Conditions such as cardiovascular shock may necessitate emergency therapy before treatment of the dystocia can begin. It is common in cattle to perform a caudal epidural to minimize straining during the vaginal examination and attempts at manipulation.

The approach to treatment of dystocias is the same as that used in horses. There are three main methods of treatment.

Mutation and Traction

This is by far the most common treatment. Liberal amounts of lubricant are essential for repositioning the fetus and helping it pass through the pelvic canal. Obstetrical chains/straps and handles are commonly used to facilitate manual traction on the fetus; various obstetrical hooks and snares are also used (Fig. 18-32).

When manual traction cannot deliver the fetus, it is common in cattle to use devices that create extra leverage on the fetus. In general, the reproductive tracts of cows appear to tolerate obstetrical maneuvers better than

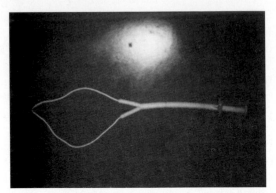

Fig. 18-32. Plastic head snare for traction delivery in small ruminants. (From Noakes DE, Parkinson TJ, England GCW: *Veterinary reproduction and obstetrics*, ed 8, London, 2001, Saunders.)

horses, with less trauma and inflammation, *when properly performed by experienced clinicians.* In general, more force may be used to extract a calf than a foal. The most often used device to increase traction and leverage on a fetus is the calf jack or calf puller. There are several brands and styles of these devices, and all have similar components: a long central metal rod, a metal rump support, and a handle on the central rod that operates a ratchet mechanism similar to a car tire jack. These mechanical traction devices are not for use on mares or small ruminants.

Malpositions must first be corrected; the calf jack is not a substitute for proper repositioning. After correcting the position of the fetus, obstetrical chains or straps are strategically placed on the fetus, most commonly on the front legs. The calf jack is then positioned with the rump support against the cow for stability and the central rod directed caudally behind the cow (Fig. 18-33). The obstetrical chains are then attached to the ratchet device on the central rod. Repeated pumping action on the handle, like a car jack, places increasing traction on the chains and, therefore, on the fetus. The central rod can be aimed slightly up or down to alter the forces on the fetus during the extraction.

In sheep and goats the most common cause of dystocia is abnormal presentation of the fetus. Manual mutation and/or traction are highly successful in treating simple malpositions in these species. Caudal epidurals are helpful in sheep and goats to decrease discomfort and straining. Attention to cleanliness of the patient and instruments is essential, and generous amounts of lubricant are necessary. Clipping the wool around the vulva may be necessary to cleanse the area thoroughly.

Fetotomy

In cases where the fetus has died, removal of selected parts of the fetus may be necessary in order to extract it. The clinician tries to use as few amputations as possible to decrease trauma to the female's reproductive tract. Once the amputations have been made, the actual delivery is performed with traction. Clinicians are more likely to perform fetotomy in cattle than in horses, because the complication rate is lower when the procedure is performed properly. Fetotomy is rarely needed in sheep and goats but may be performed if deemed necessary; generally only removal of the head is necessary. The procedure is described in more detail in Chapter 11.

Caesarean Section

Caesarean section is a fairly common surgical procedure in ruminants. In many cases it is faster and safer than fetotomy. In small ruminants, the clinician is limited by the size of the female's pelvis and reproductive tract, making treatment of complicated dystocias difficult. In cattle the trauma caused by attempting to deliver a calf vaginally may outweigh the benefits of trying to avoid the surgery. Fortunately, caesarean section in these species is a straightforward procedure with good survival rates for both dam and offspring. An additional "plus" is that the

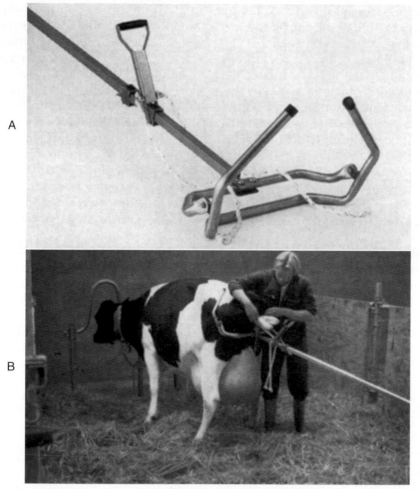

Fig. 18-33. A, The Vink calving jack is one model of commercially available calf puller. The rump support, central supporting rod, and ratchet handle are shown. **B,** The calving jack in place on a dystocia patient. The rump support rests on the pelvis, and the central supporting rod extends directly caudally behind the patient. The front feet and pasterns are seen extending from the vulva. The clinician has placed an obstetrical chain around each front leg of the fetus and attached the chains to the ratchet mechanism. (From Noakes DE, Parkinson TJ, England GCW: *Veterinary reproduction and obstetrics,* ed 8, London, 2001, Saunders.)

procedure can usually be done using local anesthesia, with or without sedation, therefore avoiding general anesthesia. Occasionally, general anesthesia may be necessary and may be safely used.

Caesarean section may be indicated in the following circumstances:
- Fetus too large for vaginal delivery
- Size of female prohibits vaginal manipulations by the clinician
- Failure of the cervix to dilate
- Cases of vaginal prolapse
- Fetal emphysema (dead, partially autolyzed fetus)
- Fetus too malformed for vaginal delivery (fetal "monsters")

• Planned termination of pregnancy, before term, to save the life of the dam (e.g., pregnancy toxemia in sheep and goats)

In small ruminants surgery is typically performed through the left flank with the female in right lateral recumbency. The legs can be restrained in extension with cotton ropes or with nylon ropes and padding. Tying the head may be stressful; having an assistant restrain the head is preferable. The head should not be restrained in an elevated position in case regurgitation occurs. Placing a towel over the eyes is helpful. Local anesthesia is performed with an "inverted-L" line block (Fig. 18-34). The flank area is clipped and surgically prepped for surgery. After the surgeon enters the abdomen and exteriorizes the uterus, sterile towels or laparotomy pads are helpful for packing the skin incision to prevent contamination of the abdominal cavity. An assistant (nonsterile) should be available to receive the fetuses and remove them from the surgical area. If they are alive, they are treated as any neonate delivered naturally. Clearing the airways, confirming breathing and pulse, and instituting drying

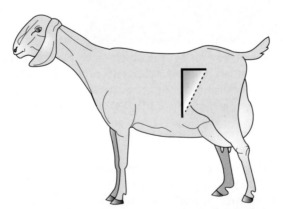

Fig. 18-34. Caesarean section via a left-flank approach in small ruminants. The dotted line indicates the surgical incision; the solid line indicates the location for the local anesthetic "inverted-L" block. (Modified from Pugh DG: *Sheep and goat medicine*, St Louis, 2002, Saunders.)

and warming procedures is necessary; the umbilical cord should be treated with antiseptic. After delivery of the fetuses, the uterus must be sutured closed, and a multilayer suture closure of the abdominal wall is performed. The surgeon determines the use of postoperative antibiotics and antiinflammatories.

Cattle are commonly operated on in the standing position, using a left flank incision. However, lateral or dorsal recumbency may be used, depending on the circumstances of the case, temperament of the animal, facilities, and surgeon's preference. For standing surgery, a cattle chute or stocks are desirable for body restraint but may not always be available. The head should be haltered and may need to be tied. The technician should be aware that although the procedure is intended to be performed with the animal standing, there is always the possibility that the animal may lie down during the procedure. Therefore if the head is tied for restraint, a quick-release knot should be used.

Sedation may not be necessary when a standing caesarean section is performed. It is often possible to place the local anesthesia with only physical restraint; additionally, use of sedatives may increase the likelihood of the cow lying down, and sedatives may have undesirable effects on the fetus. Local anesthesia for the surgery depends on the location of the incision. For anesthesia of the flank, the inverted-L or paravertebral blocks are most often used (see Chapter 16). Intravenous fluid support is not usually required for the surgery.

Because of the large size of calves, assistants must help the surgeon deliver the fetus, and then provide appropriate care if it is alive. Sterile obstetrical chains and handles should be available as part of the surgical instrumentation. The surgeon places the chains on the fetus and passes them off to assistants to hold. The assistants must be careful not to contaminate the surgical field during this maneuver. The surgeon then supports the uterus while verbally directing the assistants on how to best apply the direction and force of the traction. The umbilical cord is usually clamped with hemostatic forceps and cut by the surgeon during the delivery. After delivery is complete, the surgeon continues to close and lavage the uterus and close the abdominal incision (Fig. 18-35).

Materials for resuscitation, support, and care of a live calf should be available. Oxytocin is usually given postoperatively to speed involution of the uterus and passage of the placenta. Antibiotics and antiinflammatories may also be given.

Postoperative care includes close observation during the initial 48 hours after surgery for fever, anorexia, depression, and fecal consistency. Dry feces are not uncommon after the surgery. The incision should be kept clean and observed for signs of infection. Skin sutures or staples are removed in 2 to 3 weeks. Although overall fertility rates are reduced in females that have had "C-sections," they may be rebred in the future.

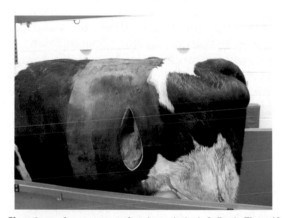

Fig. 18-35. Caesarean section through the left flank. The calf has been delivered, and the uterus has been closed and replaced in the abdomen. The incision is ready for closure. (From Fubini SL, Ducharme NG: *Farm animal surgery*, St Louis, 2004, Saunders.)

Pregnancy rates of 60% to 80% may be expected.

RETAINED PLACENTA

Retained fetal membranes are common in cattle and sheep and less common in goats. The attachments of the ruminant placenta to the uterus (placentomes) separate gradually, and the placenta is normally passed within several hours after the fetus is delivered. This delayed separation has a positive effect during dystocias, allowing the fetus to continue receiving oxygen for a prolonged time, thus increasing the chance for surviving the dystocia. The negative aspect of delayed separation is the high incidence of retained placentas after delivery and the related clinical problems that may result. Fetal membranes provide an ideal "culture medium" for bacteria, which can enter and colonize the uterus, resulting in uterine infection. In some cases bacterial toxins may enter the bloodstream, resulting in severe systemic illness (septicemia, toxemia) and possibly death.

Several risk factors have been associated with retained placentas. Retained placentas are more likely to occur following dystocias, caesarean sections, and abortions. Dietary deficiencies of selenium and vitamin A have been implicated. Hypocalcemia may be involved in some cases. Age and breed of the dam may also play a role.

The retained fetal membranes are easy to observe in cattle. They are seen protruding from the vulva and are often several feet in length (Fig. 18-36). Goats often eat all or part of the placenta once it has been expelled, leading to owner confusion about whether or not the placenta was ever passed; a vaginal examination may be necessary to confirm the status of the placenta.

The placenta in ruminants should be passed within 6 to 8 hours. If the female shows no sign of systemic illness, it is usually safe to wait until 12 to 18 hours postpartum

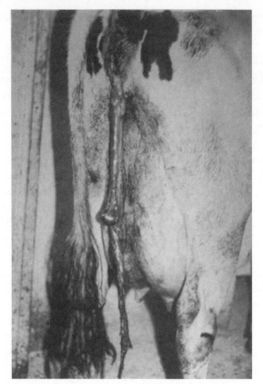

Fig. 18-36. Cow with retained fetal membranes. (Courtesy N. B. Williamson. From Noakes DE, Parkinson TJ, England GCW: *Veterinary reproduction and obstetrics*, ed 8, London, 2001, Saunders.)

for veterinary treatment. Treatment usually includes medication to stimulate contractions and involution of the uterus; oxytocin and prostaglandin (PGF2a) are most often used. Antibiotics are often given systemically and less commonly by intrauterine infusions or boluses; intrauterine treatments are currently controversial. In cattle, manual removal of the placenta may be attempted by experienced clinicians. Although manual removal may seem like an obvious choice for treatment, it is not a simple procedure, and there are many potential complications associated with it. Considerable trauma to the uterus may occur, including tearing away of the uterine lining and even prolapse of the uterus.

Small pieces of the membranes may tear off and be left in the uterus, causing uterine infection. Manual removal is typically used as a last resort when medical methods and time have failed.

Clients should never be encouraged to pull on the membranes or tie solid objects or weights to the membranes. The tetanus prophylaxis status of the animal should be determined, especially in small ruminants. Veterinary consultation is advised in all cases.

PROLAPSE OF THE VAGINA AND UTERUS

Vaginal and uterine prolapse are peripar-turient problems that are not uncommon in ruminants. Although both conditions are prolapses of reproductive organs, the risk factors, treatment, and prognosis are quite different.

Vaginal Prolapse

This condition is fairly common in ewes, less common in cows, and uncommon in goats. It usually occurs during the last 2 to 3 weeks of gestation. The etiology is unknown, though many factors have been implicated. Obesity, estrogen-containing legumes and feeds, estrogen growth implants, persistent coughing, short tail docking, multiple fetuses, hypocalcemia, hormonal imbalances, and overconsumption of low-quality forage have all been theorized to cause vaginal prolapse. In cattle, beef breeds are more commonly affected than dairy breeds.

The condition is recognized by protrusion of the vagina from the vulva. Varying degrees of prolapse from minimal protrusion to complete eversion are possible (Fig. 18-37). The cervix may be visible in cases of complete eversion. The condition is typically progressive. It often begins with mild prolapse that is seen when the animal lies down but disappears when the animal stands up. This progresses to failure to disappear when standing, with increasing swelling and irritation.

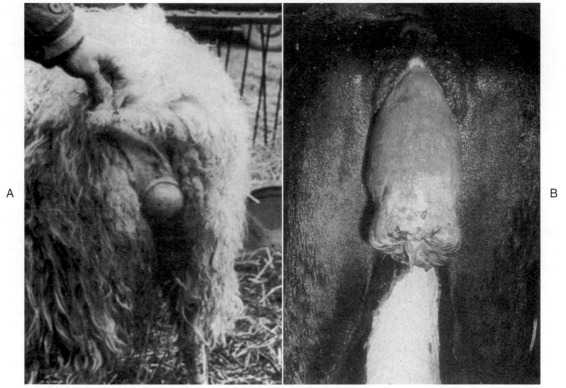

Fig. 18-37. A, Early prolapse of the vagina in a ewe. **B,** Prolapse of the vagina in a cow. (From Noakes DE, Parkinson TJ, England GCW: *Veterinary reproduction and obstetrics,* ed 8, London, 2001, Saunders.)

The animal begins to strain in response to the irritation, leading to more prolapse of the organ and creating a "vicious cycle" of progressive prolapse, inflammation, and straining. If blood supply is compromised, necrosis may begin, and absorption of toxins can cause severe systemic signs.

Treatment depends on the species and severity of the condition. The goal in most cases is replacement of the organ, followed by a method to keep it in the retained position. A caudal epidural is often used to prevent straining and desensitize the perineum. Sedation may be necessary. The prolapsed organ is gently washed with a mild antiseptic soap and thoroughly rinsed. Next, the organ

is coated with a water-soluble lubricant and carefully massaged back into its normal position. If swelling is excessive, various mixtures of salts or sugars have been used topically to "draw" water out of the exposed tissue.

Several methods can be used to retain the vagina once it has been replaced. Heavy suture material or umbilical tape has been used to suture the vulva partially closed so that the vagina cannot prolapse, but urine can be voided. Buhner's method of placing a subcutaneous purse-string suture is popular and simple to perform and gives the best results of the available suture patterns. The suture material should be removed just before parturition to prevent ripping and tearing of

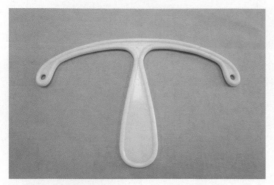

Fig. 18-38. Plastic ewe prolapse retainer.

the vulva. Buhner's suture may be used in all species. In small ruminants, plastic prolapse retainers are available (Fig. 18-38). The retainer has a large spatula arm that is inserted into the vagina and two securing arms with holes to allow them to be sutured to the skin, taped/tied to the wool, or fastened to a body harness. The retainer will not cause injury if delivery occurs while the device is in place.

Surprisingly, vaginal prolapse rarely affects pregnancy or causes dystocia. There may be an inherited predisposition for vaginal prolapse, and the condition tends to reoccur in subsequent pregnancies. Affected females are usually culled or removed from the breeding herd.

Uterine Prolapse

Prolapse of the uterus generally occurs immediately after or within a few hours of parturition. It is unusual to see the condition after 24 hours postpartum. Dairy cows and ewes are most often affected. Like vaginal prolapse, the etiology is unknown, but many factors have been associated. Many animals are hypocalcemic, which results in a flaccid, atonic uterus. During and immediately after birth, the cervix is dilated, and the flaccid uterus may be expelled by straining or any activity that causes an "abdominal press" by the female. Dystocia and traction on the

fetus or a retained placenta may increase the incidence.

The prolapse is visible as a large mass protruding from the vulva, often hanging down below the animal's hocks. It typically develops progressively, rather than being expelled in one large motion. The uterus can be distinguished from the vagina by the bumpy caruncles on the endometrial lining of the uterus; the vaginal lining is smooth (Fig. 18-39). Various degrees of additional trauma such as lacerations may occur while the organ is exposed.

Treatment is similar to that described for vaginal prolapse. A caudal epidural decreases straining and desensitizes the perineum; sedation may be indicated. The clinician decides on the position of the patient, which may be standing or recumbent. In either case, it may be helpful to have the female positioned on an incline with the hindquarters elevated so that gravity works in favor of the clinician. The exposed uterus is cleansed, and any lacerations are repaired. The organ is lubricated and gently replaced. Assistants may be necessary to elevate and support the uterus, as well as keep it clean and moist, while the clinician replaces it. A tray, towel, or surgical drape can be used like a hammock to support the uterus. Ancillary treatment with oxytocin to encourage uterine tone and involution is usually indicated after replacement. Hypocalcemia must be corrected, either orally or with parenteral calcium-containing solutions.

Once repositioned, closure of the vulva is controversial. Closure does not prevent the organ from inverting again; it merely prevents the inverted organ from being exteriorized. If the uterus is completely and fully replaced all the way to the tips of the uterine horns and uterine tone is corrected by oxytocin and calcium administration, the prolapse is unlikely to reoccur. When closure is elected, Buhner's suture is usually used.

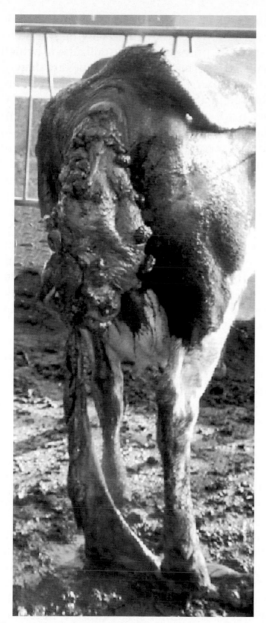

Fig. 18-39. Uterine prolapse in a cow. Note the bumpy caruncles on the uterine lining. (From McCurnin DM, Bassert JM: *Clinical textbook for veterinary technicians*, ed 5, St Louis, 2002, Saunders.)

The prognosis depends on the amount of trauma and contamination of the prolapsed tissue. Early replacement of a minimally damaged organ has a good prognosis. The condition does not tend to reoccur with subsequent deliveries, and most females are able to conceive again. However, when the organ is markedly traumatized, heavily contaminated, or necrotic, the prognosis is poor. Hemorrhage, bacterial toxemia, and septicemia may occur, leading to shock and death. A technique for surgical amputation of the uterus is sometimes used to try to salvage the animal's life in these cases. Uterine prolapse does not appear to be hereditary.

ARTIFICIAL INSEMINATION

Artificial insemination (AI) is a common procedure in ruminants, especially cattle. AI offers many benefits, including the following:
- Reduction of potential for transmission of venereal diseases
- Ability for one sire to "breed" more females than could be done with natural breeding, allowing fewer males to be used in the breeding program and allowing genetically superior males to exert more influence on a herd
- Ability to synchronize estrus in a herd of females and therefore have a shorter and better defined breeding season
- Reduction of physical injury risk to both male and female from natural mounting and penetration
- Facilitates shipping and long-term storage of semen, allowing superior genetics to be distributed more widely
- Eliminates the need to keep and care for a breeding male on the premises
- Better management of the breeding program and better planning for food, labor, and medical needs

AI is used more in dairy cattle than any other farm animal. It is used relatively widely in dairy goats and beef cattle and less often in sheep. Purebred breed associations may have regulations and constraints concerning the permissibility of AI and registration of offspring; the association should be consulted for current rules.

An AI program can be conducted in two basic ways: (1) keep breeding males on the premises and collect fresh semen as needed for prompt use or (2) store deep-frozen (cryopreserved) semen from males from any geographical location and use it when needed. Cattle spermatozoa in particular tolerate cryopreservation extremely well, allowing sperm to be kept almost indefinitely.

Frozen semen is packaged in hollow, plastic "French" straws or in ampules. Straws have largely replaced ampules; they are easily inserted into special insemination catheters or "guns" for easy use. Each straw holds 0.25 to 0.5 ml of semen. Semen straws are stored in tanks of liquid nitrogen ($-196°$ C). Multiple straws are held in the liquid nitrogen in several metal canisters with long arms that hook over the rim of the tank. In order to view the contents of a canister and retrieve the desired straw, the basket must be raised by its arm. When the liquid nitrogen tank is opened, the warmer atmospheric temperature produces a "frost line" in the neck of the tank, which is somewhat of a danger zone above which thawing may begin. Thawing and refreezing have a damaging effect on spermatozoa and must be avoided. In order to prevent accidental thawing of unused straws or ampules, they should *not* be raised above the frost line. When the desired straw or ampule is identified, it is lifted from the tank with forceps (Fig. 18-40). Care should be taken to ensure that the selected semen is identified and confirmed to be from the intended sire, since semen from several sires may be stored in a single tank. The tank should be promptly closed.

Frozen semen must be carefully handled to prevent temperature shock while thawing.

The packager of the semen provides specific instructions for thawing. Thawing should be rapid, to prevent ice crystallization, which damages sperm. Typically, ampules are thawed in ice water for 10 minutes, and straws are thawed in a warm water bath at $32°$ C to $37°$ C for 15 to 45 seconds. A standard recommendation for 0.5 ml straws is $95°$ F water bath for 40 seconds. Thawing should be done in an insulated container with a thermometer inserted to confirm the water temperature at the beginning and end of the thawing process. Importantly, once thawed, the semen should not be allowed to cool below the final water temperature of the thaw; recooling can cause significant loss of sperm. Before opening the straw or ampule, it should be dried; water kills sperm. After thawing, the semen should be used within 15 minutes for maximal viability of the sperm.

The basic insemination procedure is similar in all species. A female in heat is identified and restrained. The perineal area is cleansed and dried, and semen is deposited in the reproductive tract. However, techniques for semen deposition differ among various ruminant species.

In sheep and goats, semen may be deposited in the vagina, in the cervix, or directly into the uterus. Although conception rates tend to increase as the depth of semen deposition into the reproductive tract increases, the technical difficulty of the insemination also increases. Vaginal and cervical insemination may be done with the female standing; elevating the hindquarters facilitates the cervical procedure. A light source and vaginal speculum are necessary for visualization of the cervix. The cervix of the ewe is tortuous and has several cervical rings that make cervical entry difficult.

Depositing semen directly into the uterus may be done "naturally" through the cervix, or surgically through laparoscopy. Transcervical insemination into the uterus requires a

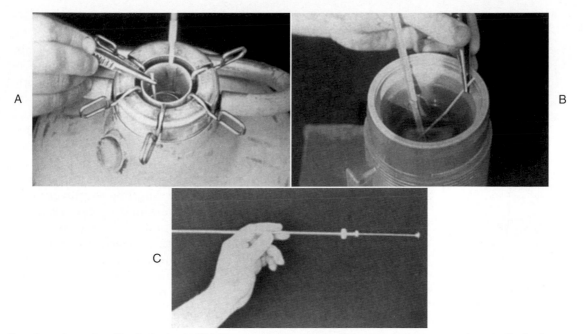

Fig. 18-40. Semen handling for bovine artificial insemination. **A,** Withdrawing a straw of frozen semen from the liquid nitrogen flask. The canister containing the semen should not be lifted above the level of the top of the neck of the flask. **B,** Thawing. After checking the identity of the sire, the straw is thawed. Water temperature is not really critical, but placing the straw in water at 37° C for 10 seconds is a typical thawing regimen. **C,** The straw is placed in an insemination catheter, which is then covered with a plastic sheath. The catheter is then ready for use, but care must be exercised not to allow the semen to become chilled again before it is inseminated. (From Noakes DE, Parkinson TJ, England GCW: *Veterinary reproduction and obstetrics*, ed 8, London, 2001, Saunders.)

light source, vaginal speculum, and special equipment for opening and penetrating the cervix. Goats may be transcervically inseminated in the standing position, but sheep are usually restrained on their backs in a V-shaped cradle. Again, the anatomy of the ewe's cervix makes this method technically challenging in sheep.

Laparoscopic insemination involves sedation of the female and restraint in dorsal recumbency; it is used primarily in sheep. The female should be held off feed and water for 24 hours before the procedure. The abdomen is clipped and sterilely prepped for surgery. The laparoscopic incisions are

performed under local anesthesia (Fig. 18-41). The surgeon places the laparoscope in the abdomen, identifies the uterus, and inserts a needle into the uterine lumen. Semen is injected with an insemination pipette or special insemination "gun." The incisions are closed with suture, and the skin is covered with antibiotic ointment. The female is placed in a quiet area for recovery and kept quiet for several hours. The surgery is quick, and complications are rare. The procedure may be repeated in subsequent years.

In cattle, semen is deposited directly into the uterus, just beyond the cervix. The cow is restrained in the standing position,

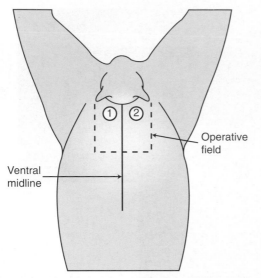

Fig. 18-41. Sites for incisions for laparoscopic insemination *(1, 2)*. The laparoscope is placed through one incision, and the insemination instruments through the other. **The surgical field is outlined.** (Modified from Pugh DG: *Sheep and goat medicine,* Philadelphia, 2002, Saunders.)

and the perineal area is cleaned and dried. The inseminator uses one hand to enter the rectum; this hand is used to locate and stabilize the cervix and extend the vagina. The other hand operates the insemination pipette, passing it through the vagina to enter the cervix, and gently manipulating it through the cervix until the tip is approximately $1/4$ inch (0.5 cm) into the uterus. The semen is slowly deposited at this location (Fig. 18-42). All insemination equipment must be kept clean and handled carefully to prevent contamination. Contamination can result in death of sperm and/or infection of the female's reproductive tract. Insemination should be performed with care, since it is possible to puncture or lacerate the reproductive tract with the equipment.

EMBRYO TRANSFER

Embryo transfer (ET) has become an increasingly valuable tool in ruminant reproduction. The process has been used mainly to obtain more progeny from genetically superior sires and dams, but more recently the potential to control certain infectious diseases has been

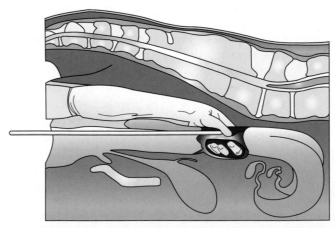

Fig. 18-42. Artificial insemination (AI) in cattle. One hand is inserted in the rectum to stabilize the cervix and confirm passage of the AI pipette into the uterus. (Modified from Noakes DE, Parkinson TJ, England GCW: *Veterinary reproduction and obstetrics,* ed 8, London, 2001, Saunders.)

recognized. By controlling the health status of the donor females and special handling of the embryos, pathogen-free embryos can be produced; it is safer to move pathogen-free embryos into a herd than young, potentially disease-carrying animals.

Most commercial interest in ET is in cattle, but the procedure is used by some purebred breeders of sheep and goats. Superovulation, the ability to cause a single female to ovulate multiple eggs, has been well-developed in cattle (unlike horses) and further increases the usefulness of ET as a production tool. Cattle embryos may be cryopreserved in liquid nitrogen, allowing them to be shipped to recipient cows anywhere in the world.

Box 18-2 shows the basic steps used in embryo transfer in cattle.

Embryo transfer in sheep and goats is handled similarly to the process for cattle, except that the hormonal manipulations and time of insemination are slightly different due to the species differences in the estrous cycle. However, both the recovery and transfer of embryos in small ruminants must usually

---

BOX 18-2 Procedure for Embryo Transfer in Cattle

1. **Superovulation of the donor cow:** Hormonal treatment is used to stimulate follicle development and control the timing of estrus and ovulation.
2. **Insemination of the donor cow:** Artificial insemination (AI) is performed, often twice (12 to 18 hours apart), when the cow displays signs of estrus.
3. **Collection of embryos:** Fertilized eggs take at least 4 days to reach the uterus; recovery of embryos is commonly done 6 to 8 days after AI. Nonsurgical methods of embryo recovery are preferred. The most common method is placement of a three-way Foley-type balloon catheter into the uterus or a uterine horn; the balloon is inflated, and the uterus is flushed with a special liquid medium (modified phosphate–buffered saline, PBS). The catheter allows simultaneous injection of the medium and backflow collection of the medium into a special container or Petri dish. The container may be fitted with a commercially available embryo filter to "strain" the embryos into a smaller volume of medium.
4. **Identification and selection of embryos:** A stereoscopic (dissecting) microscope is used to examine the medium and identify embryos. The magnification should be ×50 to ×100. The embryos are assessed for stage of development, which should be compatible with the number of days since insemination. Embryos are also rated for quality and classified as good, moderate, or poor. Degenerated or defective embryos are discarded. A micropipette is used to aspirate and transfer the embryos to holding dishes or containers filled with modified PBS solutions. They may be used fresh for up to 8 hours or may be stored cooled (4° C) for up to 3 days, or they may be cryopreserved for long-term use after special preparation for freezing.
5. **Embryo transfer:** The embryos are transferred to recipient cows that have been hormonally manipulated to prepare the reproductive tract to receive an embryo; the recipient is usually synchronized so that her estrous cycle matches that of the donor cow. The selected embryo is aspirated into a small-gauge intravenous catheter with a 1 ml syringe; the syringe is used to "inject" the embryo into the recipient. Alternatively, the embryos can be loaded into a plastic insemination straw and deposited with an insemination gun. Methods of transfer can be nonsurgical or surgical. Surgical transfer is performed in the standing cow via a flank incision or flank laparoscopy. The uterus is identified and penetrated with a blunt needle; a catheter is attached, and the embryo is injected directly into the lumen of the uterus. Nonsurgical transfer is performed similarly to the technique used for AI, but the insemination pipette is inserted more deeply into the uterus and the embryo is injected there.
6. **Pregnancy management:** Management of recipient cows is not necessarily different from cows that conceive naturally.

be via surgical methods because the anatomy of the female's cervix makes nonsurgical approaches difficult, especially in ewes. The surgical methods require general anesthesia and dorsal recumbency and use either a ventral midline incision or laparoscopy approach just cranial to the udder. Recovery of embryos is usually between 5 and 6 days after estrus, and the embryos are handled as described earlier. On average, 8 to 10 suitable embryos can be obtained from each flush of a donor female. Commonly, two embryos are transferred to each recipient female, since sheep and goats are naturally capable of supporting twin pregnancies should both of the transferred embryos survive. The necessity of surgical methods increases the risk and cost of the procedure; therefore it has not achieved the same popularity as ET in cattle.

All stages of the embryo transfer process, from collection to microscopic evaluation to storage and finally transfer, must be conducted as sterilely as possible. The embryos should be protected from temperature shock and evaporation of the liquid medium.

URINARY SYSTEM

UROLITHIASIS

Urolithiasis, the formation of urinary stones (calculi), affects cattle, sheep, and goats. Urinary stones are composed of various types and amounts of minerals and mucoproteins. Obstructive urolithiasis occurs when the urinary stones become lodged in the urinary tract and produce a partial or complete obstruction to the passage of urine. The disease is somewhat similar to that seen in felines; both males and females may form urinary stones, but females are much less likely to experience obstruction of the urinary tract because the female urethra is wider, shorter, and straighter, which facilitates passage of the stones.

Urinary tract obstruction is seen most often in male pet sheep and goats, animals being fitted for shows, and feedlot animals. There is a definite nutritional role in the development of the urinary calculi, which are composed primarily of calcium salts and phosphate compounds. The typical diet of affected animals is high in concentrates (grain), low in roughage, improperly balanced (low) in calcium-to-phosphorus ratio, and often high in magnesium. The high grain diets commonly fed to pet, show, and feedlot animals are largely responsible for the imbalances associated with the condition. Other compounds such as oxalates (from plants) or silica in the soil may play a role in some parts of the country. Limited access to water may lead to concentrated urine and therefore contribute to the problem. A hereditary predisposition may also be involved.

Uroliths may form in any part of the urinary tract. Clinical signs depend on the size and location of the stones and include most commonly stranguria and dysuria with frequent posturing to urinate. Swishing the tail indicates discomfort. Hematuria and abdominal pain may be seen. Goats commonly vocalize. Complete obstruction of the urinary tract may occur in the kidney; ureters; bladder neck; or, most commonly, the urethra. Pressure necrosis and rupture of the urinary tract may occur if complete obstructions are not relieved. Ruptures allow leakage of urine internally; bladder ruptures allow urine to empty directly into the abdominal cavity (uroperitoneum), and urethral ruptures allow subcutaneous accumulation of urine. Systemic absorption of the "leaked" urine can lead to uremia and eventually death if untreated.

The most common locations of urethral obstruction are the sigmoid flexure of the penis and the urethral process at the tip of the penis. The sigmoid flexure of the male ruminant penis provides two hairpin turns, where stones may have difficulty passing. The urethral process of sheep and goats has a small aperture that prevents passage of urinary stones. Early castration has been associated with a failure of the male urethra to reach maximal diameter, thus possibly contributing to the likelihood of urethral obstruction. However, castration (at any age) has no effect on the physiological processes that lead to stone formation.

Diagnosis usually begins with extension of the penis and palpation of the urethral process in small ruminants. Acepromazine sedation is often used to facilitate relaxation of the retractor penis muscle; xylazine is not recommended because of its diuretic effect. Abdominal palpation may be possible in small ruminants and may reveal bladder distension. Rectal examination and palpation of the bladder may be possible in larger animals. In cases of urethral rupture, subcutaneous swelling may be palpable, usually in the area of the sigmoid flexure; the swelling is typically large and fluctuant. Diagnostic ultrasound can be a valuable tool for visualizing the kidneys, ureters, bladder, and urethra. Plain-film abdominal radiographs in smaller individuals may demonstrate calcium-containing stones; contrast studies may be necessary to visualize the location and full extent of urinary stones. Blood work is important in cases of complete obstruction and may reveal elevations of blood urea nitrogen (BUN) and creatinine, as well as electrolyte abnormalities and evidence of dehydration.

Treatment depends on the location, severity, and duration of the clinical signs. In sheep and goats, the patient is usually sedated (most commonly with acepromazine intravenously) and positioned on its rump. The penis is exteriorized for examination by pulling the sheath caudally with one hand while extending the sigmoid flexure with the other hand to force the penis cranially. The glans is

grasped with dry gauze and pulled to full extension. If the obstruction is confirmed to be at the urethral process, the process can be easily amputated at its base along the glans penis. Amputation does not prevent the animal from breeding use in the future. Amputation of the urethral process is necessary to introduce a urethral catheter in these species.

Catheterization of the urethra and retrograde flushing may relieve the obstruction in some cases; however, the anatomy of the male ruminant urethra makes catheterization difficult and limits its usefulness. Also, passage of a catheter and flushing with pressure may cause ruptures if the urethral tissue has been devitalized by the calculi.

Several surgical treatments have been used for treatment and management of the condition. Surgical procedures are designed to prevent reobstruction and its associated life-threatening complications. However, the procedures do nothing to prevent the processes of stone formation; they only attempt provide better channels to eliminate the stones. Clients must understand the difference between preventing stone obstruction and preventing stone formation when considering surgery. Any attempt to prevent stone formation must involve changes in nutritional management.

Perineal urethrostomy has historically been the surgical procedure of choice. It may be performed under general anesthesia or heavy sedation with anesthesia provided by an epidural. The patient position may be standing or dorsal or lateral recumbency. The perineal area is clipped and surgically prepped. The surgeon makes a midline incision between the anus and scrotum to expose the penis. Dissection is continued to incise the penis and open the urethra. The exposed urethra is then carefully sutured to the skin to produce a permanent, new urethral opening in the perineal area (as clients frequently

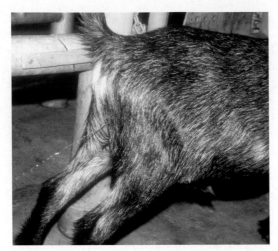

Fig. 18-43. Urination through a healed perineal urethrostomy in male goat. (From McCurnin DM, Bassert JM: *Clinical textbook for veterinary technicians*, ed 6, St Louis, 2006, Saunders.)

observe, "he pees like a girl") (Fig. 18-43). A Foley catheter is placed for several days to maintain the new opening during the initial postoperative period. Since the new opening is proximal to the sigmoid flexure and wider than the distal penile urethra, stones should theoretically void with less risk of obstruction. Unfortunately, there is a high incidence of stricture formation associated with the procedure; the procedure also prevents breeding by intact males. Urine scalding of the thighs is common after the procedure. Perineal urethrostomy is presently considered to be a salvage procedure.

Currently, cystotomy and tube cystostomy are preferred surgical procedures. Long-term survival is better, and breeding function can be preserved. General anesthesia is required; the patient is positioned in dorsal recumbency, and the ventral abdomen is clipped and surgically prepped. A right paramedian incision is made to enter the abdomen (Box 18-3). The bladder is identified and opened; this allows the surgeon to remove all bladder calculi and lavage the bladder. A catheter can then be passed through the bladder into the urethra to allow flushing of any stones in the urethra. When the bladder and urethra are cleared, the incisions in the bladder and the abdominal wall are closed. In some cases, urethral obstructions may not be cleared completely by this approach; these cases are candidates for tube cystotomy. For tube cystotomy, a Foley catheter is placed in the bladder and exited through a stab incision in the abdominal wall; this allows continual drainage of urine, giving the obstructed, inflamed urethral tissue a chance to rest and heal (Fig. 18-43). The hope is that as swelling subsides, the urethral stones will pass. The Foley catheter should be examined regularly for proper placement and patency; it should be kept clean. The skin incisions should be monitored for signs of infection and kept clean of debris and exudates. Goats may try to chew their tubes, and Elizabethan collars and belly bandages may be necessary to prevent "self-removal." The catheter is eventually clamped to force urination through the urethra, and after normal, full-stream, pain-free urination through the urethra is confirmed for 1 to 2 days, the Foley catheter is deflated and removed. The bladder generally seals and heals rapidly, without complication.

Other surgical procedures such as urethrotomy, combined perineal urethrostomy with cystotomy, bladder marsupialization (permanently attaching the bladder to the abdominal wall and creating a permanent opening for urine to void), penile amputation, and urethroscopy with laser lithotripsy have been described and used variably in different ruminant species. Some of these are only used to salvage individuals intended for slaughter.

Regardless of the treatment, clients must be educated to prevent reoccurrences. Nutritional management is *essential* for prevention. Laboratory analysis of stones from the patient can identify the principle components of the stones, allowing better nutritional management of each individual.

Likewise, nutritional analysis of the diet can be a valuable tool for the formulation of a diet that is not likely to induce stone formation.

Nutritional management generally includes free access to fresh, clean water. Sodium chloride is often added to the diet to improve water consumption, but salt also has beneficial effects on preventing the actual formation of stones. Various oral additives such as ammonium chloride may be given to acidify the urine; a urine pH less than or equal to 6.8 is desirable. Clients can be instructed to monitor voided urine one to two times weekly with pH paper or urine dipsticks. Toxicity is possible with ammonium chloride, and signs include anorexia, depression, and diarrhea. Foodstuffs high in cations, such as

---

BOX 18-3   Surgical Approaches to the Abdomen

The terminology for surgical approaches to the abdomen may seem confusing, but it is the same for all domestic species:

Celiotomy

Any incision into the abdominal cavity. Theoretically, an incision may be made anywhere, in any direction, and be of any length. However, the anatomy and biomechanics of the abdominal wall, such as the fascia, tension lines, and direction of muscle fibers, dictate the best locations and directions for incisions. When selecting a surgical approach, the surgeon must also consider the location of the organs or structures that need to be accessed.

There are three basic locations for celiotomy approaches: ventral, flank, and vaginal.

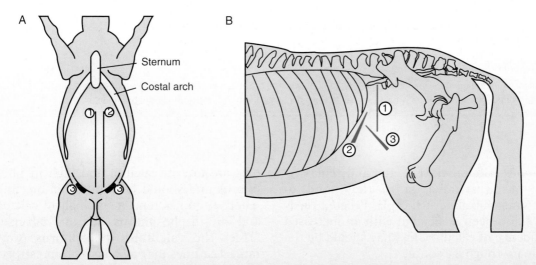

Locations for celiotomy approaches. **A**, *1*, ventral midline approach; *2*, ventral paramedian approach; *3*, inguinal approach (right and left). **B**, *1*, paralumbar fossa approach; *2*, paracostal approach; *3*, Marcenac approach.

Continued.

BOX 18-3 Surgical Approaches to the Abdomen—Cont'd

Ventral celiotomy

Ventral abdominal approaches usually require general anesthesia, with the patient in dorsal recumbency. Following are "standard" locations of ventral celiotomy incisions:

- **Ventral midline approach:** incision directly on midline, in a cranial-caudal direction, with entry into the abdominal cavity through the linea alba. The incision may be of any length or location between the xiphoid process and the pelvis. The most common ventral approach; it assists thorough exploration of the abdomen.
- **Ventral paramedian approach:** incision either to the right or the left of ventral midline and parallel to ventral midline.
- **Inguinal approach:** incision directly over an inguinal canal.
- **Transverse abdominal approach:** rarely used for entry into the pelvic cavity. Begins caudal to the umbilicus and extends transversely no farther than the fold of the flank.

Flank celiotomy

An incision through the flank into the abdomen. *Laparotomy* is a synonym for flank celiotomy. Laparotomy is performed with the patient either standing or in lateral recumbency. The incision may be made high, low, or in the middle of either flank. Following are several "standard" locations for laparotomy incisions:

- **Paralumbar fossa approach:** the most common flank approach. The paralumbar fossa is the large depression between the last rib and the tuber coxae. The skin incision is made in a dorsal-ventral direction. The deeper incisions through the muscle layers may be made either dorsal-ventral through all of the muscles, or parallel to the direction of the muscle fibers of each muscle ("grid" incision).
- **Paracostal approach:** an angled incision that parallels the last rib.
- **Marcenac approach:** a low oblique flank incision, made in a craniodorsal to caudoventral direction. Used occasionally for caesarean section.
- **Caudal rib resection:** used to approach structures that are in the dorsal abdomen that cannot be exteriorized through more ventral approaches (kidney, spleen, etc.). Portions of the caudal one or two ribs are removed with a Gigli wire saw to expose the peritoneum. The procedure opens the caudalmost aspect of the thoracic cavity en route to the abdominal cavity; entering the thoracic cavity may cause respiratory difficulty, so the anesthetist should be prepared to assist ventilation.

Vaginal celiotomy

An incision through the cranial portion of the vaginal wall into the abdomen. *Colpotomy* is a synonym for vaginal celiotomy. Colpotomy is usually performed with the patient standing. It is most often used to remove ovaries.

---

legumes (alfalfa, clover, etc.) and molasses, should be avoided, since they tend to encourage alkaline urine pH. Pelleted feeds have also been associated with an increased incidence of calculi. Grass hay should be the primary roughage source.

Balancing the calcium-to-phosphorus ratio is essential; a 2:1 ratio is recommended and may require calcium additives to achieve this balance. Cereal grains such as corn and oats are low in calcium and high in phosphorus and should be minimized or eliminated. Legumes tend to be high in calcium and low in phosphorus, and may adversely affect the calcium-to-phosphorus (Ca:P) ratio. Legumes may also be high in estrogen compounds and protein, both of which can contribute to stone formation. High protein diets should be avoided. Magnesium should not exceed 0.6% of the diet in any animal.

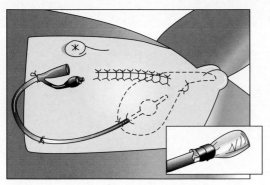

Fig. 18-44. Illustration of a tube cystostomy. Note the location of the ventral right paramedian incision and the separate incision for exiting the Foley catheter. The exposed catheter is secured to the skin with sutures at several locations. To prevent aspiration of air, the catheter opening is covered with a homemade Heimlich valve, made from the tip of a latex glove finger *(inset)*. (Modified from Pugh DG: *Sheep and goat medicine*, Philadelphia, 2002, Saunders.)

SUGGESTED READING

Cebra ML, Cebra CK: Food animal medicine and surgery. In McCurnin DM, Bassert JM, editors: *Clinical textbook for veterinary technicians*, ed 6, St Louis, 2006, Saunders.

Fubini SL, Ducharme NG: *Farm animal surgery*, St Louis, 2004, Saunders.

Hafez ESE: *Reproduction in farm animals*, ed 6, Philadelphia, 1993, Lea & Febiger.

Howard JL, Smith RA: *Current veterinary therapy: food animal practice*, ed 4, St Louis, 1999, Saunders.

Noakes DE, Parkinson RJ, England GCW: *Veterinary reproduction and obstetrics*, ed 8, London, 2001, Saunders.

Pugh DG: *Sheep and goat medicine*, St Louis, 2002, Saunders.

Smith MC, Sherman DM: *Goat medicine*, Baltimore, 1994, Williams & Wilkins.

19

Ruminant Euthanasia and Necropsy Techniques

EUTHANASIA

The euthanasia methods that are available for ruminants are similar to those for horses, and most of the same factors must be considered (see Chapter 12). However, unlike horses, most ruminants are euthanized with the intention of consumption of their body tissues by humans or animals, or both. Food consumption affects the methods for euthanasia that can be safely used, since chemical residues must be avoided. Sometimes animals must be euthanized on the farm due to emergency or severe medical conditions and will therefore not enter the human food supply. However, if these farm-euthanized animals are to be sent for rendering, the rendering company may have residue restrictions. It is advisable to investigate the local rendering operations and become familiar with their restrictions and policies.

Some owners may be emotionally attached to their ruminant animal and elect a more typical "companion animal" euthanasia and burial. The veterinary practice should be familiar with local laws and regulations concerning cremation and burial options.

According to the American Veterinary Medical Association Panel on Euthanasia (2000), the following euthanasia methods are considered acceptable for ruminants:

- Intravenous (IV) injection of barbituric acid derivatives: Tissue residues are toxic and prevent this method from being used in animals intended for animal or human consumption. Carcass disposal should prevent scavenging by other animals.
- IV injection of potassium chloride (KCl) in conjunction with general anesthesia.
- Penetrating captive bolt: This should be delivered by trained personnel. Because there are no chemical residues, this is the method most often used in slaughterhouses.

The following euthanasia methods are considered conditionally acceptable:

- IV injection of chloral hydrate, after sedation
- Gunshot: to the head only; use only when other methods are not available
- Electrocution: applied directly to the head/brain (one-step procedure) or applied after the animal is rendered unconscious by other methods (two-step procedure)

NECROPSY

Many of the same considerations must be given to performing ruminant necropsy as discussed for the horse (see Chapter 12). The importance of history-taking as part of the complete examination must not be overlooked and is especially important for herd situations. Failure to recognize or diagnose infectious diseases, toxicities, or nutritional problems can have implications for all animals in a herd and may have disastrous economic consequences.

RUMINANT NECROPSY PROCEDURE

The importance of personal protective equipment cannot be overemphasized when conducting necropsies on *any* species. The basic procedure for equine necropsy may be followed, with a few variations. Following are some of the procedural methods used for ruminants.

Position

Ruminants are usually necropsied in left lateral recumbency; this positions the rumen on the down side, where it interferes minimally with abdominal exploration and visualization.

Gastrointestinal Tract

The rumen/reticulum is often markedly distended with gas from microbial fermentation that continues after death of the animal (postmortem bloat or tympany). The distension may be severe enough to cause postmortem rectal and/or vaginal prolapse. Gas can be relieved by inserting a large-bore needle or making a small stab incision through the rumen wall directly over the gas cap. Note that incising directly over fluid contents will release them and contaminate the adjacent tissues.

The ruminant forestomachs and abomasum may be removed en bloc by first tying off the distal esophagus and the proximal duodenum with one to two string ligatures, and then transecting them. The attachments of the rumen are cut across the dorsal aspect of the abdominal cavity. The forestomachs and abomasum are then rolled out of the abdomen. Each organ should be individually opened and examined (Fig. 19-1).

The contents of the rumen/reticulum should be examined for foreign bodies, especially in the reticulum, where the honeycomb-shaped mucosa tends to trap sharp objects (Fig. 19-2). The rumen mucosa undergoes autolysis fairly rapidly and may slough easily during the necropsy examination. Submission of rumen contents for laboratory analysis may be necessary in some cases.

Ruminants, unlike horses, have gallbladders. The gallbladder is removed with the liver.

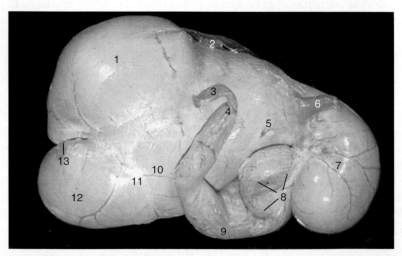

Fig. 19-1. En bloc removal of the forestomachs and abomasum of a sheep, viewed from the right side. The esophagus *(6)* and proximal duodenum *(3)* have been transected. The reticulum *(7)*, omasum *(8)*, and abomasum *(9)* are easily seen; everything else is rumen and its various compartments. (From Clayton HM, Flood PF: *Color atlas of large animal applied anatomy*, London, 1996, Mosby-Wolfe.)

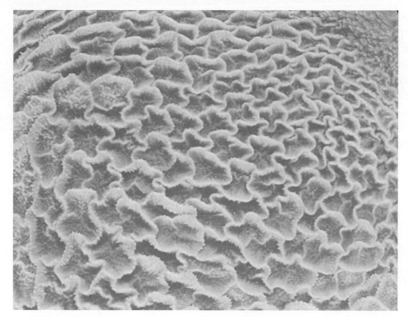

Fig. 19-2. The mucosa of the reticulum has a honeycomb shape that tends to trap foreign objects. (From Clayton HM, Flood PF: *Color atlas of large animal applied anatomy,* London, 1996, Mosby-Wolfe.)

Before removal, bile duct patency should be checked. This is done by incising into the lumen of the duodenum, applying pressure on the gallbladder, and observing bile flowing from the bile duct into the duodenum. After removal of the liver and gallbladder, the gallbladder should be opened and evaluated.

Urinary Tract

The kidneys of the cow are normally multilobulated, resembling a large bunch of grapes on the capsular surface (Fig. 19-3).

NECROPSY OF ABORTED FETUSES

Abortion diagnosis is commonly done in ruminants because of the economic impact of abortions and the need to prevent them whenever possible. A certain amount of fetal losses to stillbirth and abortion are expected in livestock production operations; the veterinarian and farm owner must decide when expected losses may be excessive and which

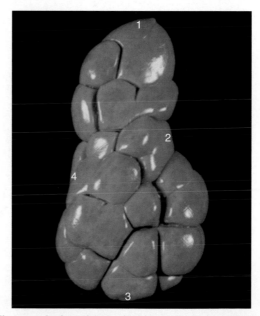

Fig. 19-3. Surface of the bovine kidney. The perirenal fat and renal capsule have been removed. *1,* Cranial pole; *2,* depression in the dorsal surface close to the hilus; *3,* caudal pole; *4,* ventral border. (From Clayton HM, Flood PF: *Color atlas of large animal applied anatomy,* London, 1996, Mosby-Wolfe.)

individual cases and circumstances may warrant a thorough diagnostic work-up. The cost of laboratory diagnostics must also be carefully considered.

The technician should be familiar with the diagnostic laboratory and its sample submission procedures so that samples are handled and shipped properly. This helps ensure valid and timely test results. The basic fetal necropsy procedure is described in Chapter 12.

SUGGESTED READING

McCurnin DM, Bassert JM: *Clinical textbook for veterinary technicians*, ed 6, St Louis, 2006, Saunders.

Smith MC, Sherman DM: *Goat medicine*, Baltimore, 1994, Williams & Wilkins.

part III

SWINE CLINICAL PROCEDURES

20

Swine Restraint and Basic Physical Examination

RESTRAINT

The principles of swine restraint are not different from other large animal species. The method used to handle swine is determined largely by the age and size of an animal and the nature of the procedure to be performed. In general, the least amount of restraint necessary to perform a procedure is best (Box 20-1).

> **BOX 20-1   Age/Sex Terminology for Swine**
>
> As with most animal terminology, terms often vary according to the geographical location and background of the people using the terms.
> - Pig: young swine, less than 120 pounds (≈4 months old), of either sex
> - Hog: large swine, more than 120 pounds, of either sex
>   (These terms are often used interchangeably, as if there are no technical differences between them. Commercial swine producers usually prefer the term "hog" when referring to their animals.)
> - Farrowing: the act of giving birth
> - Piglet: very young, small pig; generally from birth to weaning
> - Shoat: intact male, before puberty; sometimes used as a synonym for pig
> - Boar: intact male, mature
> - Gilt: immature female, before birth of first litter
> - Sow: intact female, mature
> - Barrow: castrated male; castrated before puberty
> - Stag: castrated male; castrated after puberty when secondary sex characteristics have developed

Swine have been described as stubborn but smart animals. They do not have a strong herd instinct but prefer being with other pigs rather than being alone. Pigs are very vocal animals that express fear, panic, and stress by squealing and screaming. Like many species, when one animal in a group becomes fearful or distressed, the other members of the group tend to follow suit; therefore it is wise to be calm.

Pigs are not athletic animals, but that does not mean they are slow. Smaller animals especially can be quite agile and difficult to catch. Their legs are relatively thin and somewhat easily fractured; catching them or tying them by the legs must be done carefully.

Pigs may be aggressive; biting is their only real defense. Their teeth are sharp and their jaws are powerful. It is very important to understand that an aggressive pig will not only stand its ground; it will often *go after* the object of its anger. It is a good idea to define the best "escape route" from a pen before entering it. Sows with litters are especially protective and should be approached with care, especially in an enclosed area. Boars with tusks should also be respected.

Swine are easily stressed by environmental heat. If they are further stressed by handling or other fearful situations, they can quickly become hyperthermic ("heat stroke"). Signs of heat stroke include dyspnea and open-mouth breathing, tail twitching, reluctance to move, muscle tremors and rigidity, and elevated rectal temperature. Because hyperthermia can be rapidly fatal, emergency efforts to cool swine are indicated when heat stroke is observed. Care should be taken when handling swine on hot, humid days.

Pigs dominate each other by biting the top of the neck. Handlers can take advantage of this by pressing down with the hands or tapping with a cane on the top of the neck or back. If the handler exerts this dominance before handling the pig, it often makes handling easier.

CATCHING AND MOVING SWINE

It is difficult to move and drive swine from behind in an open area; they tend to pick their own direction to move. Instead, it is best to limit their choices; pigs respect solid barriers and tend to move away from them. Handheld wooden or plastic panels, referred to as *hurdles,* are often used to separate and direct pigs in an open area (Fig. 20-1). Swine handlers usually carry lightweight canes that are used to tap on the animal when they wish to move it; tapping on the hindquarters encourages the animal to move forward, and tapping with the cane on a shoulder helps move the pig to the right or left. By using the

hurdle and cane in combination, the animal can usually be successfully moved.

The hurdle can also be used to encourage forward movement by simply walking behind the pig with the hurdle held out in front of the handler. If the pig tries to turn around, the hurdle should be placed quickly against the ground and braced with the legs to keep the pig from getting its snout under it and lifting it; adult swine are quite strong with their "rooting" motion. The hurdle can be used to direct the animal into a corner and keep it there for minor procedures.

Blindfolding a pig causes it to walk backward. A towel or bucket may be loosely placed or held over the head, and a cane used to tap and direct the pig while it walks backward to the desired location. Tugging on the tail to either side can also be used to guide the direction of the pig.

STANDING RESTRAINT

The most common form of individual restraint is the hog snare. Snares consist of a pipe sleeve and a rope or cable that runs through it; the cable is looped on one end, and the other end is held in the operator's hand. The loop is tightened or loosened by pulling on the free end, like a noose (Fig. 20-2). The loop is loosened, and the pig is approached. When the pig opens its mouth, the loop is quickly slid into the mouth and tightened to

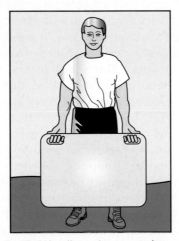

Fig. 20-1. Handheld hurdle used to move swine.

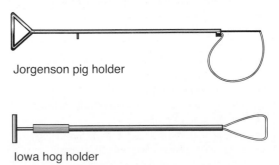

Jorgenson pig holder

Iowa hog holder

Fig. 20-2. Commercial hog snare.

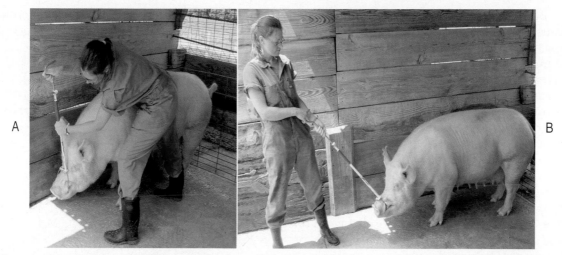

Fig. 20-3. Demonstration of the capture of an adult pig with the hog snare. **A,** The handler approaches from the side of the pig and carefully loops the snare over the upper jaw just in front of the cheek teeth. **B,** After the snare is tightened, it is obvious that the pig resents this and will resist by pulling back against the snare. This allows the handler to brace against the pig and hold it steady for examination or sample collection. (From McCurnin DM, Bassert JM: *Clinical textbook for veterinary technicians*, ed 6, St Louis, 2006, Saunders.)

form a circle around the snout and upper jaw (maxilla), with the sleeve drawn tightly down on the top of the snout. The operator should stand directly in front of the pig (Fig. 20-3). The natural response of the pig is to lean backward away from the snare; if the snare is not firmly in position, the pig can easily escape. When the hog snare is secured properly, minor procedures such as injections and blood samples can be performed. This form of restraint is for mature animals and is never to be used on piglets. It should not be kept tightened for long periods of time, generally less than 20 to 30 minutes. When used on boars with tusks, the loop should be placed behind the tusks. Snares may be obtained commercially or home-made from 1-inch pipe and a cable or rope.

A similar form of restraint is the snubbing rope (Fig. 20-4). A rope with an eye at one end is used to form a simple loop. The handler can approach the pig from behind or in front. The rope loop is dangled in front

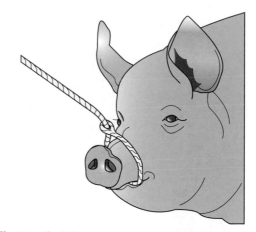

Fig. 20-4. Snubbing rope.

of the snout. When the mouth is opened, the loop is placed through the mouth and quickly tightened, and the handler stands in front of the pig for control. As with the hog snare, the natural reaction of the pig is to lean backward. The rope may be tied to a solid object if desired.

Both the hog snare and snubbing rope cause vocalization by the pig, and the squealing typically continues until the pig is released. Pigs can produce extremely loud squeals and screams when they are restrained; many pig farmers use earplugs, for good reason. Long-term exposure to this noise can damage hearing. Note also that animals that have had repeated experience with these forms of restraint can become devious in avoiding them.

A rope harness can also be made for pigs. A rope with an eye is used to form a simple loop that is passed over the neck (Fig. 20-5). The free end of the rope is loosely placed on the ground just in front of the pig, and handler stands behind the pig to encourage it to move forward (Fig. 20-6). When the pig steps forward through the loop, the handler passes the free end under the rope to form a half hitch that circles the body (Fig. 20-7). The rope is drawn tightly (Fig. 20-8). The handler

should be prepared for the pig to move quickly and unpredictably during the process of placing the harness.

CASTING RESTRAINT

Before casting a pig, the head should be controlled with some form of snout restraint

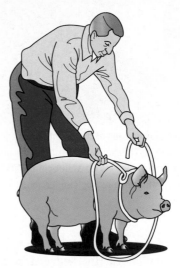

Fig. 20-6. Positioning the rope on the ground.

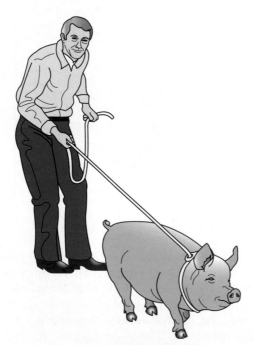

Fig. 20-5. Passing a rope loop around the neck.

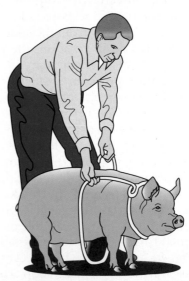

Fig. 20-7. When the pig steps through the rope, a half hitch is made in the rope.

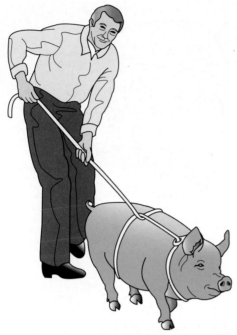

Fig. 20-8. Rope harness in position and snugged down for restraint.

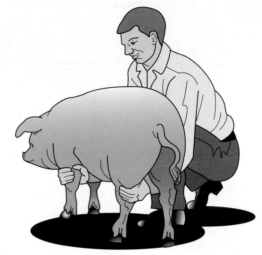

Fig. 20-9. Casting a pig by hand.

(hog snare or snubbing rope). The method used to cast the pig depends largely on the size of the animal. Smaller pigs can be manually cast by standing on the side of the pig and reaching under the pig's body to grasp the far side legs. Pulling the legs toward the handler causes the pig to fall to the ground, away from the handler (Fig. 20-9). Be sure the "landing area" is covered with something soft. Once down, the legs can be hobbled or tied.

A simple method of rope casting is to use a snubbing rope as the casting rope. The snubbing rope is placed first, and the free rope is used to circle a hind leg *above* the hock on the side opposite the desired direction of the fall (i.e., circle the left hindleg to produce right lateral recumbency) (Fig. 20-10). Pulling on the rope from behind the pig draws the nose back toward the leg, causing loss of balance and a fall to the ground (Fig. 20-11).

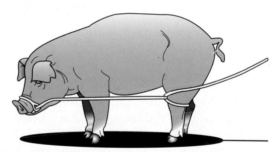

Fig. 20-10. Placing a snubbing rope around a hindleg for casting.

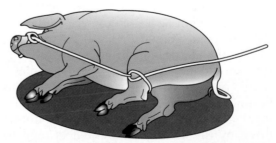

Fig. 20-11. Pulling the snubbing rope produces recumbency.

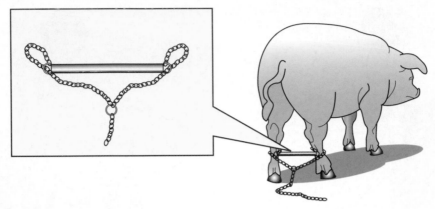

Fig. 20-12. Placement of hobbles on the rear legs.

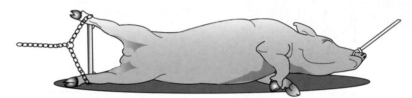

Fig. 20-13. Casting restraint using hindleg hobbles.

Hindleg hobbles can be used to cast an animal. The head is controlled with snout restraint, and the hobbles are placed around the hindlegs (Fig. 20-12). Standing behind the pig and pulling on the center rope pulls the legs backwards; the pig eventually loses balance and falls on its side. The hobbles can be left in place for the procedure (Fig. 20-13).

RESTRAINT OF PIGLETS

Baby pigs should be handled gently but firmly. They should not be chased unnecessarily and should not be caught or lifted by the ears. Neonatal piglets can be lifted by the tail, but this should be used sparingly. The piglet should never be dangled by the tail but should be quickly supported with the hands after lifting. Piglets more than 3 to 4 lb should not be lifted by the tail. Squealing piglets tend to upset the sow and other piglets, so it is usually best to take them to a separate room for procedures.

Very young piglets can be caught by grasping one or both hindlegs in one hand and lifting with the other hand under the body. Once the piglet is off the ground, release the leg and place that hand on top of the shoulders to firmly secure the body (Fig. 20-14). The piglet can also be held under the handler's arms.

Many procedures on piglets weighing up to 20 to 30 lb are done with the animal suspended by either the front or back legs and its back supported against the handler's body or thighs. This position is commonly used for castration and many injections (Fig. 20-15).

RESTRAINT FOR SPECIAL PROCEDURES

Some farms have crates, chutes, and head catches designed especially for swine. In order to encourage pigs to enter these devices, they

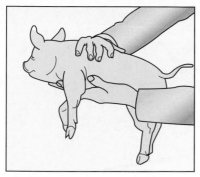

Fig. 20-14. Lifting and supporting a baby pig.

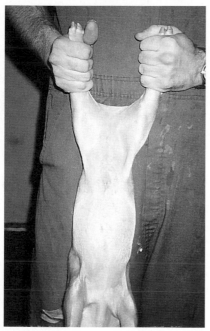

Fig. 20-15. Restraint of piglet for subcutaneous injections and castration. (From Sirois M: *Principles and practice of veterinary technology*, ed 2, St Louis, 2004, Mosby.)

should be able to see clearly through them, and the devices' openings should look large enough to fit through. Most of the head-catching devices are opened and closed by handheld levers.

Restraining V-troughs are commonrestraining devices for smaller swine. They are often portable and can be placed on tabletops or against fences or walls. The animal is lifted and placed on its back in the trough for most procedures, but the trough can be tilted from side to side to achieve more lateral positions if desired. Assistants can hold the legs for the procedure, or the legs can be easily tied by looping a rope around one leg, passing it under the trough, and looping it around the opposite leg. Both front and back legs may be tied. The trough may be inclined according to the needs of the procedure, to place the front end or hind end uppermost (Fig. 20-16).

BASIC PHYSICAL EXAMINATION

Physical examination of swine is procedurally similar to that of the other large animal species. A body system approach can be used. The following are normal values for adult swine at rest:

Temperature: 101.0° F-103.5° F
  (102.0° average)
Pulse: 60-90 per min
Respirations: 10-24 per min (16 average)

Body temperature may be taken rectally with a thermometer appropriate for the size of the animal. The pulse rate may be taken by auscultation with a stethoscope directly over the heart. Common pulse points are the auricular (ear) artery along the ear pinna and the coccygeal artery of the tail; the femoral artery may be available in recumbent animals. In small pigs, the heart rate may be felt directly over the heart by placing the hand against the chest wall just behind the left elbow. Respiratory rate is assessed by observing and counting chest or flank excursions or by auscultation of the thorax with a stethoscope; the lungs are best auscultated between ribs 6 and 11.

Note that swine are not the most cooperative animals for examination; they tend to move around and often try to escape. The methods of restraint that immobilize them,

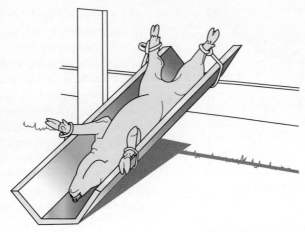

Fig. 20-16. Restraint of a small pig in a trough.

such as the hog snare, tend to produce constant, loud vocalization. Cornering the animal in a quiet area with a hurdle against a solid fence or wall may be a better approach.

SUGGESTED READING

Leahy JR, Barrow P: *Restraint of animals*, Ithaca, NY, 1953, Cornell Campus Store.

Sonsthagen TF: *Restraint of domestic animals*, St Louis, 1991, Mosby.

Sonsthagen TF: Physical restraint. In Sirois M, editor: *Principles and practice of veterinary medicine*, ed 2 , St Louis, 2004, Mosby.

21

Diagnostic Sampling and Medication Techniques in Swine

DIAGNOSTIC SAMPLING

All diagnostic procedures performed in other species, such as abdominocentesis, arthrocentesis, and transtracheal wash, can be performed in swine. Due to economic costs associated with some of these tests and the cost of treating serious medical diseases when they occur, these nonroutine diagnostic tests are more likely to be pursued in valuable breeding stock rather than in production animals. On the other hand, routine diagnostic tests such as blood sampling are commonly performed in most swine for disease screening.

VENOUS BLOOD SAMPLING

Blood is the most commonly collected material for testing in swine. Swine red blood cells are somewhat fragile; therefore using appropriately sized needles and avoiding aspirating or injecting blood through needles with unnecessary force is important. Sites for blood collection should always be cleaned before needle insertion.

Several veins are accessible for blood sampling. The site and technique for venipuncture depends on the size of the pig and the method of restraint. Locations are as follows.

Lateral Auricular Vein

The "ear" vein is useful for small samples of venous blood (≤5 mL). It is used for pigs after weaning age (4 to 5 weeks old/≈25 lb bodyweight). A 20-gauge (ga) × 1-inch needle is suitable for most animals; large adults may use an 18- to 19-ga × 1-inch needle. Butterfly catheters may be useful. Vacutainers are not recommended at this location because they tend to collapse the vein, especially in small individuals.

The vein runs near the lateral border of the ear pinna and is accessed from the dorsal (haired) side of the pinna (Fig. 21-1). It is easily visualized and can be distended with finger pressure at the base of the lateral surface of the ear, though both hands of the technician can be freed up by using a mechanical method to distend the vein. A heavy rubber band can be placed as a tourniquet around the base of the ear to distend the vein. Another method uses self-retaining forceps with long, plastic-covered jaws that can be placed across the base of the ear to distend the ear vein. This allows one hand free to stabilize the tip of the ear, while the other hand places the needle and aspirates the blood. The needle should enter the vein at a 45-degree angle to the skin, toward the tip of the ear. The ear vein may continue to bleed for several minutes after venipuncture is completed.

Coccygeal Vein

The "tail" vein is accessible in animals without docked tails but is infrequently used. It is suitable only for adult swine. A 20-ga × 1-inch needle is used. The coccygeal vein is located

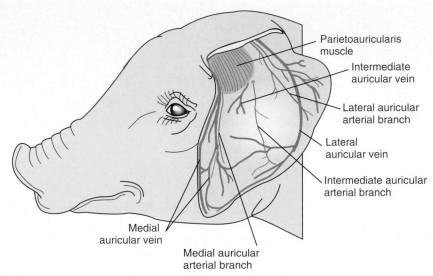

Fig. 21-1. The left ear showing blood vessels. (Modified from Dyce KM, Sack WO, Wensing CKG: *Textbook of veterinary anatomy*, ed 3, Philadelphia, 2002, Saunders.)

on the ventral midline of the tail. The tail is elevated vertically, and the needle is inserted near the base of the tail on ventral midline, perpendicular or near perpendicular to the skin. Small blood volumes (<5 ml) may be obtained.

Cranial Vena Cava

The cranial vena cava lies in the thoracic inlet between the first pair of ribs and gives rise to both the right and left jugular veins. Although it is technically more difficult to learn to draw blood from this location, it is the most satisfactory location for obtaining large blood samples. It may be performed on any size animal. The right side of the animal is always used to access the cranial vena cava, to avoid accidental damage to the phrenic nerve. The left phrenic nerve lies in a more vulnerable position, paralleling the left external jugular vein, than does the right phrenic nerve, which is more protected on the right side of the animal.

In piglets a 20-ga × 1½-inch needle may be used. Small pigs up to 50 lb require an 18- to 20-ga × 1- to 1½-inch needle. These small-sized pigs are placed in dorsal recumbency with the head held firmly still; the front legs are extended and pulled caudally for complete access to the caudal neck and shoulder area. The needle is inserted (syringe attached) on the right side, at the caudal extent of the right jugular furrow, just lateral to the manubrium of the sternum (Fig. 21-2). The needle is directed toward the *caudal aspect* of the *top* of the *opposite* (left) shoulder blade. Slight back pressure (vacuum) is kept on the syringe. The vena cava is encountered between ½ and 2 inches deep, depending on the size of the animal. Blood is easily aspirated when the needle enters the vein.

Larger animals are restrained standing, usually with a hog snare; the head should be raised slightly. Alternatively, some farms may have bleeding chutes with a head catch. Nonslip footing should be provided. If the pig sits down before or during the procedure, stop the procedure, withdraw the needle, and get the pig on all four feet. Sitting alters the anatomical landmarks for the procedure

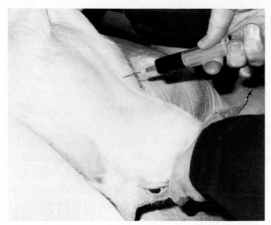

Fig. 21-2. Venipuncture of the cranial vena cava in a small pig restrained in dorsal recumbency. (From McCurnin DM, Bassert JM: *Clinical textbook for veterinary technicians*, ed 6, St Louis, 2006, Saunders.)

and makes it difficult to perform successfully. An 18- to 20-ga × 2½-inch needle is used for feeder (finisher) pigs weighing more than 50 lb; adult swine need a 16- to 17-ga × 4- to 4½-inch needle. The syringe is attached for the procedure. The technician kneels in front of the animal on its right side (facing the body of the pig) or to the side of the right shoulder (facing the neck). The needle is inserted and directed exactly as described earlier (Fig. 21-3). Once the skin has been penetrated, slight back pressure is maintained on the syringe plunger. Blood flows readily when the vein is entered. In adult pigs the vein lies quite deep, and the technician should not be surprised if a depth of 4 inches is required to reach the vein.

Several structures may accidentally be encountered during this procedure. If the needle hits a rib, pull backward slightly and try a different angle. If the trachea is penetrated, the syringe fills with air. The thoracic duct may also be entered, giving a syringe full of lymph. Punctures of these two structures are rarely life threatening and,

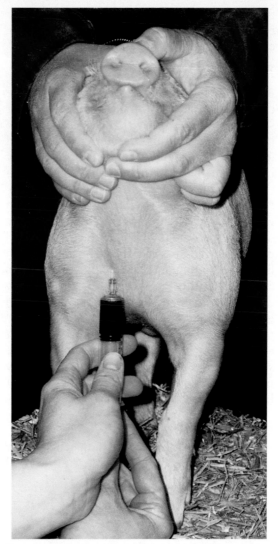

Fig. 21-3. Collecting blood from the cranial vena cava in a standing pig. The needle is inserted at the caudal extent of the right jugular furrow, lateral to the manubrium. (From McCurnin DM, Bassert JM: *Clinical textbook for veterinary technicians*, ed 6, St Louis, 2006, Saunders.)

when encountered, indicate that the needle is angled too far medially. The right vagus nerve, if hit, can damage the function of the parasympathetic nerves to the heart, and the right phrenic nerve, if hit, can alter the function of the diaphragm. Cardiac and/or respiratory signs may follow, requiring emergency treatment.

Jugular Vein

Because it is not as deep a structure as the cranial vena cava, the jugular vein is a safer structure to access with a needle. However, the jugular veins are not as large in diameter and may be quite difficult to find and hit, especially in large or heavy animals. The jugular vein can be used for sampling any age animal. Needle size ranges from 20-ga × 1½ inches in piglets to 16-ga × 3 to 3½ inches in mature pigs.

The right jugular vein is preferred, to avoid damaging the phrenic nerve. The jugular vein lies in the jugular furrow and is accessed cranially to the manubrium at the visually deepest point of the jugular furrow. The vein is not distended; this is a "blind stick" procedure. The needle (with syringe or Vacutainer attached) is inserted perpendicularly to the skin and directed dorsocaudally and slightly medially. After penetrating the skin, slight backpressure should be kept on the syringe.

Orbital Sinus (Medial Canthus of the Eye)

A venous sinus is located adjacent to the medial canthus of the eye and can be used for venous blood samples in any age pig. Approximately 5 to 10 ml of blood can be obtained. Small pigs are restrained in dorsal recumbency, inclined with the head down and firmly restrained. Larger pigs are restrained standing with a hog snare. Piglets require a 20- to 22-ga × 1-inch needle; larger pigs may use a 16- to 18-ga × 1½-inch needle. The needle is inserted deep to the nictitating membrane (third eyelid) and advanced at a 45-degree angle toward the opposite jaw. The needle will hit the lacrimal bone; rotate and slightly withdraw the needle until blood flows from the hub. The syringe is then attached; aspiration should be gentle (Fig. 21-4).

Cephalic Vein

The cephalic vein is accessible in small pigs older than 14 weeks of age but not commonly used. It runs along the cranial-medial surface of the upper forelimb. The pig is restrained by snout restraint in the standing position. The leg is not lifted off the ground. Distension of the vein is similar to small animals and may be done by hand or tourniquet. The needle is placed at a 45-degree angle to the skin, in a proximal direction. A 20-ga × 1- to 1½-inch needle is sufficient. Up to 10 ml of blood may be obtained.

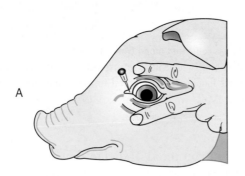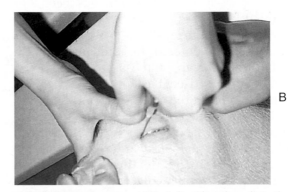

Fig. 21-4. A, Collection of blood from the medial canthus of the eye. **B,** Venipuncture of the left orbital sinus. Note the firm manual restraint of the head. (**A** modified from Sirois M: *Principles and practice of veterinary technology,* ed 2, St Louis, 2004, Mosby; **B** from McCurnin DM, Bassert JM: *Clinical textbook for veterinary technicians,* ed 5, St Louis, 2002, Saunders.)

URINE COLLECTION

Voided urine may be collected in swine, although it may be difficult to encourage urination. Males should be confined and observed; when quiet, the prepuce may be stroked with a warm, wet towel or soft brush. Titillating the vulva by stroking with the fingers, soft brush, or dry straw can be attempted in females.

Adult swine normally urinate two to three times a day.

MEDICATION TECHNIQUES

ORAL MEDICATION

Most oral medications are delivered to groups of pigs through the water or feed. Occasionally, it may be necessary to medicate individual pigs. The chief dangers to the technician are the sharp teeth and strength of the jaws, which must be respected in animals of any age. Placing the hand or fingers in the mouth should not be done unless a speculum is used to hold the mouth open. In small piglets, the corner of the mouth may be pressed inward with a finger so that the cheek tissue provides some protection for the finger.

Oral speculums are available for swine. The pig should first be restrained with a hog snare; this causes the pig to vocalize. While the mouth is open, the speculum can be placed. One type of speculum is a simple "hand paddle" style that is inserted into the mouth horizontally and, once behind the canine teeth, rotated vertically. Medications can then be given by dose syringe or pilling gun, or a stomach tube can be passed through the bars of the speculum (Fig. 21-5).

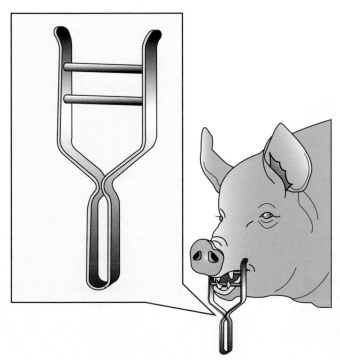

Fig. 21-5. Oral speculum for swine.

Piglets are commonly placed in a standing position for oral medications. The front legs are elevated, and the piglet's back placed against the handler's legs for support. In this position, a dose syringe or pilling gun can be used to deliver medication. If the head must be steadied, do not use the ears or throat; rather, the hands may be placed behind the ears and/or under the jaws (Fig. 21-6).

Very young piglets can be dosed orally using two methods: by mouth and by stomach tube. The piglet can be lifted by the back of the head and neck, and a syringe used to deliver small volumes (<5 ml) to the back of the tongue, being sure that the piglet swallows the medication. Injecting faster than the piglet can swallow risks aspiration of the liquid into the lungs.

Piglets can be stomach-tubed with a flexible, nonkinking rubber tube. The length of tubing to reach the stomach is estimated by measuring along the pig's body from the mouth to the last rib. The piglet is lifted by the back of the head and neck, and the tube is passed over the back of the tongue to the esophageal

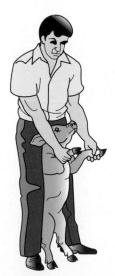

Fig. 21-6. Restraint of piglets for oral medication.

entrance. Gentle force usually passes the tube into the esophagus. Piglets usually make swallowing motions as the tube passes down the esophagus, and passage should be easy with minimal resistance. If the tube is accidentally placed in the trachea, it will pass easily but usually cannot be passed beyond the level of the base of the heart; this distance is less than the estimated distance to the stomach, which is why it is important to make this measurement before the procedure. Once the stomach is reached, up to 15 ml can be slowly delivered with a syringe connected to the tube. After injection, kink the tube for removal and remove it slowly. Observe the piglet for 10 minutes after the procedure for discomfort and regurgitation.

INJECTION TECHNIQUES

Restraint should be appropriate for the size of animal and the location of the injection. Some of the procedures in small piglets can be performed by one person, but most require two people (one to restrain, one to inject). The skin should always be cleaned before insertion of any needle.

Intravenous Injection and Intravenous Catheterization

Intravenous (IV) injections and solutions for fluid therapy are most often given in the lateral auricular (ear) vein. The cephalic vein can also be used. In small piglets, other veins such as the jugular vein may be used, since the ear vein and cephalic vein at this age are small and difficult to access. Injections should be given slowly. Butterfly catheters (19- to 21-ga) may assist delivery of larger volumes of solutions.

Indwelling IV catheters (18- to 20-ga) can also be placed in the lateral auricular vein, although they are difficult to maintain. After placing a rubber band or forceps to distend the vein, the area over the vein is clipped and aseptically prepared (prepped). The tip of the ear is held for stability, and the catheter is inserted toward the base of the ear. After insertion is completed, the tourniquet is removed and the catheter is capped and flushed. The hub is secured to the skin of the ear pinna with super glue or a similar adhesive. The pinna is supported by placing roll gauze or roll tape along the inside of the pinna, forming a "strut" for the ear. The pinna is bent around the strut to form a gentle curve. Several strips of 1-inch adhesive tape are used to encircle the ear and secure it to the strut, leaving access to the injection cap and catheter hub.

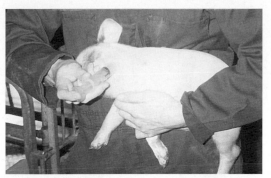

Fig. 21-7. Single handler giving an intramuscular injection to a piglet. (From Sirois M: *Principles and practice of veterinary technology,* ed 2, St Louis, 2004, Mosby.)

Intraperitoneal Injection

Fluid therapy in piglets is usually given intraperitoneally. Fluids given by this route should be isotonic and should always be warmed. The piglet is held by the hindlegs, and the area between the ventral midline and the flank fold is prepped. Sterile gloves should be worn for the injection procedure. A 16- to 18-ga × ¾- to 1-inch needle is sufficient. The needle is inserted approximately halfway between ventral midline and the flank fold, and only deep enough to enter the abdominal cavity. The needle should be manually stabilized during the infusion and not allowed to flop around, which could produce severe injury to the internal organs.

Intraperitoneal (IP) fluids may be given to larger pigs, restrained in the standing position. The injection is performed through the paralumbar fossa, after proper aseptic preparation of the skin. A 16- to 18-ga × 3-inch needle may be necessary to penetrate the body wall at this location. The needle is stabilized during the infusion.

Intramuscular Injection

As with meat-producing ruminants, concern for damaging valuable cuts of meat with injections has increased in recent years. The prime cuts of pork come from the hams, loins, and shoulder areas. Therefore intramuscular (IM) injections are preferably given in the dorsal neck muscle behind the ears. Piglets may be held in one arm and injected with the free hand (Fig. 21-7). When possible the skin-pinch injection technique is preferred, but this requires two people: one to restrain the animal and one to perform the injection. The skin adjacent to the injection site is pinched to pull the skin up, and the needle is inserted into the underlying muscle and the injection delivered. After removing the needle, the skin pinch is released. This provides a natural "Band-Aid" of skin to cover the injection site and may minimize the incidence of injection abscesses.

An 18- to 20-ga × 1-inch needle is used in small animals, and a 16- to 18-ga × 1½- to 2-inch needle is used for larger pigs. In animals with a thick layer of subcutaneous fat, the needle should be at least 2 inches in length. Injection volume at any single IM site should not exceed 2 ml in piglets or 3 ml in larger pigs.

Subcutaneous Injection

Subcutaneous injections may be given at several locations. Injections in small pigs (<50 lb) are given in the axillary area caudal to the elbow or in the inguinal region in the

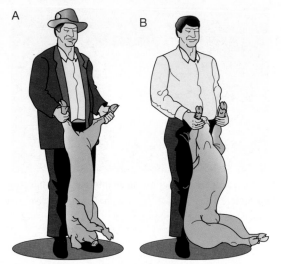

Fig. 21-8. Restraint of small swine for injection into the inguinal **(A)** or axillary **(B)** regions.

flank skin fold. The pig is restrained by the legs for this procedure, using the forelegs for access to the axillary region or the hindlegs for the inguinal region (Fig. 21-8). An 18- to 21-ga × 3/4- to 1-inch needle is suitable, and 1 to 2 ml may be injected per site.

In larger pigs, restraint is provided with a hog snare, and the area of loose skin behind the base of the ear may be used. A 16- to 19-ga × 1- to 1½-inch needle is used. Up to 3 ml may be injected per site.

Intranasal Injection

Restraint should place the head in an elevated position. This can be done by elevating the front legs and head in small pigs or with a hog snare in older pigs. The product is given with a plain syringe or with a syringe and adapter provided with the vaccine or medication. The syringe or adapter is placed inside the nostril and the contents injected, keeping the nose tilted up until the injection is complete. It may be helpful to time the injection with the inspiration of the pig. As with other species, sneezing is the usual response after the injection.

SUGGESTED READING

Jaffe TJ: Diagnostic sampling and therapeutic techniques. In McCurnin DM, Bassert JM, editors: *Clinical textbook for veterinary technicians*, ed 6, St Louis, 2006, Saunders.

Leahy JR, Barrow P: *Restraint of animals,* Ithaca, NY, 1953, Cornell Campus Store.

Teeple TN: Nursing care of food animals, camelids, and ratites. In Sirois M, editor: *Principles and practice of veterinary technology,* ed 2, St Louis, 2004, Mosby.

22

Swine Surgery and Anesthesia

Although the vast array of surgical procedures and technology available to other species is available to swine, economic considerations usually make many procedures impractical except in valuable breeding stock and valued pets.

Standing surgery is only an option for a few minor procedures. Most surgeries on swine are performed with the animal in recumbency, using either general anesthesia or a combination of local anesthesia and sedation. As in other species, whenever possible, local anesthesia and sedation are preferred to general anesthesia. Swine face the same risks associated with general anesthesia as other species but also have the additional concern of high body temperatures and possible development of malignant hyperthermia under general anesthesia. Malignant hyperthermia, part of the porcine stress syndrome, occurs rarely in swine during inhalation anesthesia (Box 22-1).

Pot-bellied pigs may be anesthetized using the techniques used for the other swine breeds. Small animal anesthesia machines and equipment may be used for pigs of this size. Malignant hyperthermia is extremely rare in pot-bellied pigs.

LOCAL ANESTHESIA

LUMBOSACRAL EPIDURAL ANESTHESIA

Epidural anesthesia in swine is performed at the lumbosacral junction; no other epidural site is readily accessible in this species. The epidural space at this location is fairly large and easy to enter with a needle. Anesthesia administered at this location is considered to be a "cranial epidural" as opposed to the "caudal epidural" frequently used in other large animal species. Epidurals are frequently performed for analgesia for caesarean section surgery; the systemic effects on the fetuses are minimal.

The proper site for the epidural must be identified. The lumbosacral junction is just caudal to a line drawn transversely through the animal to connect the crests of the wings of the ilium, where the line bisects the dorsal midline. The wings of the ilium are palpable in small swine. In large swine, anatomical landmarks must be relied upon to locate the site. Large swine are preferably injected in the standing position, standing squarely on all four legs. Looking at the pig from the side, a vertical line is drawn upwards from the patella; this line usually identifies the cranial extent of the crest of the ilium. The needle is inserted 1 to 1½ inches caudal to this line, on dorsal midline (Fig. 22-1).

The animal should be sedated for the procedure, if possible, and/or restrained with a hog snare. The hair is clipped, and the skin aseptically prepared. Up to 5 ml of 2% lidocaine is deposited subcutaneously and to a depth of 1 to 2 inches to reduce discomfort and patient movement during the actual epidural block. A final scrub is applied to the skin.

Sterile gloves should be worn for the procedure. The needle for the epidural should be

BOX   **22-1**   Porcine Stress Syndrome

Porcine stress syndrome (PSS) is an inherited disorder that primarily affects the skeletal muscles of susceptible swine. The muscle cells appear to have an impaired ability to regulate calcium flowing in and out of the cell. The responsible gene has become known as the halothane, or "Hal," gene. It is a single autosomal recessive gene, and susceptible pigs are homozygous for the gene. Three possible clinical manifestations of the genetic condition exist:

- Pale soft exudative pork (PSE): Animals with the Hal gene produce inferior quality meat that is pale (grayish), soft, and watery, which devalues the carcass. These changes occur after death of the animal, due to an abnormally rapid fall in pH in the muscle cells that damages the cell membrane and allows water to leak freely out of the cells. PSE affects a large percentage of animals that are homozygous for the Hal gene, as well as many animals that carry the gene as heterozygotes.
- Malignant hyperthermia: This is a drug-induced phenomenon characterized by muscle rigidity; tachycardia; tachypnea; metabolic acidosis; and a rapid, extreme, progressive rise in body temperature. Cardiovascular collapse and death usually occur. The condition may be triggered by halothane gas or by some of the neuromuscular blocking agents.
- PSS: This is an acute manifestation that requires a stressful "trigger" to initiate clinical signs. Physical stressors such as restraint, exertion, fighting, breeding, parturition, veterinary procedures, fighting, transportation, overcrowding, and high environmental temperatures may initiate a sudden attack of dyspnea and open-mouth breathing, elevated body temperature less than 106° F (41.1° C), tail twitching, muscle tremors, and rigidity. As the body temperature rises above 106° F, the terminal stages begin with cyanosis, collapse, and death (often within 15-20 minutes). PSS may occur at any time of year, but the incidence is much higher during hot and humid weather.

    The treatment for malignant hyperthermia and PSS is intravenous dantrolene, a muscle relaxant that is specific for skeletal muscle. However, the condition is usually observed when it is too late for the drug to be effective. Emergency measures to cool the animal should be attempted but are seldom successful. No therapy or prevention is available for PSE.

    The condition is seen primarily in heavily muscled but lean individuals. Historically there has been a higher prevalence in the Pietrain, Landrace, and Poland China breeds. A simple, highly accurate, inexpensive DNA blood test has been developed to identify the Hal gene in homozygous and heterozygous animals. By judicious planned breeding and culling, the incidence of the condition is decreasing and theoretically could be eliminated. The National Pork Producers' Council passed a resolution (1997) supporting elimination of the Hal gene from the U.S. pork population.

    Swine in general do not handle heat and humidity well. Efforts should always be made to keep pigs comfortable on hot days; providing shade, fans, and sprinklers is helpful. Caution should be used if pigs are to be placed in stressful situations on hot days. When tail-twitching, open-mouth breathing, and tremors of the rump muscles are seen, the procedure should be stopped and emergency efforts to cool the pig should be instituted.

an 18- to 20-gauge (ga) spinal needle. A 3-inch length needle is necessary in small swine, a 4-inch needle for swine weighing more than 100 kg, and 5- to 7-inch needle for swine weighing 200 kg or more. These needles are easily bent, and some clinicians prefer to use a shorter (1- to 2-inch) 14-ga needle as a protective sleeve trocar for the 18-ga needle. The 14-ga needle is placed first, and then the 18-ga needle is passed through its lumen.

Lidocaine 2% (without epinephrine) is a commonly used anesthetic drug for the block. The dose used relates to the bodyweight of the patient and the desired effects, ranging from 0.5 to 1 ml/4.5 kg bodyweight (maximum 20 ml). Lower doses provide analgesia caudal to the lumbosacral area, but higher doses can diffuse and produce analgesia as far cranially as the first lumbar vertebra. Anesthesia begins approximately 5 to 10 minutes after

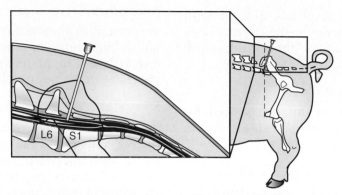

Fig. 22-1. Location of lumbosacral epidural anesthesia in the pig. L6 is the sixth lumbar vertebra, and S1 is the first sacral vertebra. Note that a vertical line from the patella indicates the crest of the wing of the ilium; the needle is placed just caudally to this line. (Modified from Muir WW et al: *Handbook of veterinary anesthesia*, ed 3, St Louis, 2000, Mosby.)

injection, maximizes at 20 minutes, and lasts as long as 2 hours.

Xylazine may also be injected into the lumbosacral epidural space. At a dose of 2 mg/kg (diluted in 5 ml sterile saline), it produces surgical anesthesia of the body caudal to the umbilicus and paralysis of the hindlegs. The analgesic effects begin within 20 to 30 minutes and may last up to 2 to 3 hours. The dose is important because doses of less than or equal to 1 mg/kg do not produce surgical anesthesia, and doses of greater than or equal to 3 mg/kg cause prolonged hindlimb paresis and ataxia that last for 36 hours or more. Lidocaine 2% may be mixed with xylazine to give a more rapid onset of analgesia (5 minutes), which may last as long as 5 hours.

Remember that epidural anesthesia does not desensitize or immobilize the head, neck, or forelimbs of an animal. The animal must be controlled with physical restraint, sedation, or both.

GENERAL ANESTHESIA

ANESTHETIC RISKS FOR SWINE

Before administering anesthesia to swine, the following risks should be considered:

Swine Are Prone to Hypoventilation

Inadequate ventilation may result in hypoxemia, which may lead to death. There are several potential sources of ventilation problems that may exist alone or in combination.

Airway obstruction

Any factor that decreases the cross-sectional area of the upper airways greatly increases the resistance to breathing.

- The larynx of swine is very sensitive to physical stimulation. Pressure and touch, even from accumulated saliva, can trigger a laryngospasm.
- The laryngeal lumen of the pig is small in relation to the size of the animal; a pig weighing 100 kg requires an endotracheal tube that would fit a large dog (≈14 mm internal diameter [ID]). Flexing the neck partially occludes the laryngeal entrance. Salivation, which is common in anesthetized pigs, can result in accumulations of saliva in the pharynx and laryngeal entrance that actually occlude the larynx.
- Laryngeal edema results readily in swine, due to their relatively fragile laryngeal mucosa. The laryngeal mucosa is quite easy to traumatize during endotracheal

intubation and responds quickly with swelling. This edema of the larynx causes further narrowing of the already small lumen diameter.

Respiratory depression

The depressant effects of drugs used for chemical restraint and anesthesia are seen in swine (as in other species).

Limited expansion of the chest wall

Recumbency and anesthetic drug depression may combine to reduce the full expansion of the chest wall. Obesity may magnify this effect.

Swine Are Prone to Hyperthermia under Anesthesia

Although swine have sweat glands in the skin, they do not function efficiently in thermoregulation of the animal. The subcutaneous accumulation of fat contributes to the development of the problem. Also, swine have a low amount of body surface area for their body size, which inhibits the dissipation of heat. Because of these factors, body temperature tends to rise when swine are anesthetized, and the effects may be increased if anesthesia is performed in a hot environment.

Occasionally, malignant hyperthermia may develop in genetically predisposed animals (see Box 22-1). This condition develops rapidly and is difficult to control; the outcome is typically fatal.

PREANESTHETIC PREPARATION AND ANESTHETIC MANAGEMENT

Preanesthetic Evaluation

History and physical examination should be performed, with an emphasis on the respiratory system. Laboratory tests should be appropriate for the length and type of surgical procedure, as well as the physical condition of the patient; a complete blood count is always advisable.

Preanesthetic Preparation

Regurgitation may occur under anesthesia but is not common. Food is withheld for 6 to 12 hours in adults and 1 to 3 hours in piglets. Water is not usually withdrawn.

Preanesthetic Drugs

Because so few superficial veins other than the ear veins can be accessed, most preanesthetic and injectable anesthetic drugs are given intramuscularly (IM). The location of intramuscular injection can affect the speed and depth of anesthesia. Intramuscular injection into the gluteal, back, or shoulder muscles provides more consistent results than injections into the neck muscles; however, gluteal injections risk damaging a valuable cut of pork (ham). The neck muscles have numerous fascial (dense connective tissue) planes; accidental injection into fascia may cause uneven, slow absorption with unreliable results. If the neck muscle is used, the safest site for injection is just caudal to the base of the ear, where there is less fascia in the muscle.

Atropine is sometimes used to control salivation in swine, which can be excessive. Atropine is given at a dosage of 0.02 mg/lb IM.

Induction Drugs

Various anesthetic induction and maintenance regimens are available for swine. Withdrawal times for meat-producing animals should be observed. A quiet induction area is preferred; restraint in a chute or crate is generally less stressful than using other forms of physical restraint (such as snout restraint). Some of the techniques in use are shown in Box 22-2.

Endotracheal Intubation

The technician should be aware of several anatomical features that are unique to swine and affect endotracheal intubation. Pigs have a small laryngeal opening and narrow

> **BOX 22-2** **Anesthetic Induction and Maintenance Regimens Available for Swine**
>
> - Telazol/Ketamine/Xylazine ("TKX"): All three drugs are mixed together in the Telazol vial and given intramuscularly (IM). This popular combination provides short-term anesthesia (20-30 minutes). It can also be used for induction to inhalant gas maintenance. Endotracheal intubation can be performed with this combination. Repeated injections of the combination may be used to extend the length of general anesthesia. Recovery from anesthesia is in 60-90 minutes.
> - Atropine/Acepromazine/Ketamine: Atropine and acepromazine are given IM and followed with ketamine IM approximately 20 minutes later. This combination is useful for minor, short procedures; anesthesia lasts approximately 10-15 minutes. Analgesia must be supplemented with local anesthetics for painful procedures.
> - Atropine/Xylazine/Ketamine: Atropine and xylazine are given IM and followed with ketamine IM approximately 10 minutes later. Anesthesia lasts about 10-15 minutes.
> - Xylazine/Telazol: Xylazine is given IM and followed with telazol IM in 5 minutes. Although analgesia and muscle relaxation are good, the depth of surgical anesthesia may be light and of short duration. Drowsiness after recovery may be prolonged (up to 24 hours).
> - Intratesticular sodium pentobarbital: A technique for anesthesia for castration of large boars has been described. Sodium pentobarbital is injected into each testicle to produce anesthesia in approximately 5 minutes. Removal of the testicles effectively removes the source of the anesthesia.
> - Inhalant gases: mask induction, with or without prior sedation, may be used in small or heavily sedated swine. Halothane, isoflurane, and sevoflurane are all suitable for use in swine, but halothane is generally avoided because of the risk of inducing malignant hyperthermia in susceptible families of swine.
> - Intravenous thiobarbiturates: An intravenous catheter or butterfly administration set may be used in the ear vein to inject thiobarbiturates. This may be the safest choice for anesthesia in pigs from family lines susceptible to malignant hyperthermia.

trachea; endotracheal tube sizes will seem small compared with the bodyweight of the animal. Pigs have a pharyngeal recess, which is a blind pouch located dorsal to the esophagus; the endotracheal tube does not advance if directed into this location. Visualization of the larynx is difficult because the mouth of the pig does not open widely and the soft palate is long.

To reduce the risk of laryngospasm and the risk of traumatizing the larynx, topical desensitization of the larynx may be done by spraying it with lidocaine. A soft, small animal urethral catheter can be used to apply the lidocaine on the larynx.

Sternal recumbency with the head and neck extended is the preferred position for intubation. The mouth is opened by an assistant, using a gauze strip placed around the mandible and another one around the maxilla to pull the mouth jaws apart. Direct visualization with a laryngoscope (long blade) is recommended for endotracheal intubation; preplacing an endotracheal tube stylet in the laryngeal entrance is helpful, similar to the technique described for small ruminants. (See Chapter 16.)

The larynx tends to angle ventrally, and the proximal trachea tends to angle dorsally. Because of the anatomy of the larynx and proximal trachea, it is suggested to begin placement of the endotracheal tube with the tube curvature angled ventrally until the tip is within the larynx (beyond the arytenoid cartilages). After the tip has cleared the larynx, it may be necessary to rotate the tube curvature 180 degrees so that the tube tip points dorsally in order to advance the tube.

Regurgitation may occur during intubation.

Maintenance of Anesthesia

Anesthesia may be maintained with injectable drugs or inhalant gases. Small animal anesthesia machines may be used on animals up to 140 kg; slightly larger animals may use a small animal machine if high oxygen gas flow rates (>4 L/min oxygen) are used.

Halothane, isoflurane, and sevoflurane may be used in swine. Halothane may cause malignant hyperthermia in susceptible individuals and is best avoided, if possible. Isoflurane and sevoflurane are not known to produce hyperthermia. The induction and maintenance concentration of the anesthetic gases is similar to that used in ruminants. (See Chapter 16.)

Nitrous oxide may be safely used in swine. It is given with oxygen at 40% to 60% of the total inspired gas concentration.

Monitoring Anesthesia

Anesthetic monitoring is similar to other large animal species. Differences are shown in Box 22-3.

Fluid Therapy

Fluid therapy with a balanced electrolyte solution may be given intravenously and is recommended in sick or dehydrated patients. The recommended administration rate for stable, anesthetized patients is 10 ml/kg/hr.

RECOVERY

Sternal recumbency is preferred for recovery from anesthesia. A cool, quiet environment is desirable. Supplemental oxygen is advisable through the endotracheal tube until the animal is extubated; smaller tubing may then be placed in a nostril to deliver oxygen until the animal attempts to rise. Extubation is performed when strong attempts to swallow are observed and should be done with the cuff deflated. Since hypoventilation is a common problem in swine, the technician should be prepared to assist ventilation if necessary. Swine are at risk for laryngeal edema and spasm, and tracheostomy materials should be readily available (scalpel handle and No. 10 scalpel blade, hemostats, and cuffed tracheostomy tube).

BOX 22-3   Anesthetic Monitoring in Swine

- The auricular artery on the dorsal aspect of the ear pinna may be used for arterial blood-gas sampling and for catheterization for direct blood pressure monitoring.
- Heart rate under anesthesia should range from 50 to 150. The auricular and femoral arteries are the best locations for pulse assessment.
- Eye signs may be difficult to interpret in swine and are highly dependent on the anesthetic drug regimen.
- Hyperthermia is a risk of inhalation anesthesia in swine and must be detected early in order to have any chance of successful treatment. Rectal temperature should be monitored for hyperthermia. Malignant hyperthermia is recognized by extremely high body temperature (>107° F); temperatures higher than 103° F are concerning, and measures to cool the animal are advisable. Other clinical signs include muscle rigidity, increased heart rate and respiratory rate, and metabolic acidosis. Note that ketamine tends to increase body temperature.

  Treatment of malignant hyperthermia begins with discontinuing anesthetic gas administration, but continuing oxygen delivery; 100% oxygen should be used to flush the anesthetic breathing circuit. Efforts to cool the body by any reasonable means should be instituted immediately. Dantrolene (1 mg/lb intravenously), a muscle relaxant, is recommended and is the only specific treatment. Fluids should be given and may include bicarbonate to treat the metabolic acidosis. Corticosteroids may be given to combat shock.

SUGGESTED READING

Cornick-Seahorn JL: Veterinary anesthesia. In McCurnin DM, Bassert JM: *Clinical textbook for veterinary technicians,* ed 5, Philadelphia, 2002, Saunders.

Fubini SL, Ducharme NG: *Farm animal surgery,* St Louis, 2004, Saunders.

Muir WW et al: *Handbook of veterinary anesthesia,* ed 3, St Louis, 2000, Mosby.

Wertz EM, Wagner AE: Anesthesia in pot-bellied pigs, *Comp Cont Ed Pract Vet* 17(3):369-381, 1995.

23

Swine Neonatal Care

Swine are polytocous animals capable of producing large litters of 8 to 14 piglets. However, not all of those born will survive until weaning, and the producer typically strives to keep losses from birth to weaning at less than 10% of the piglets born alive. Neonatal piglets are delicate beings; each lost piglet is lost income, and swine farmers go to great lengths to guarantee a healthy early environment for them.

Piglets weigh 3 to 4 lb at birth. They are generally weaned between 4 and 5 weeks of age, at a bodyweight of 20 to 25 lb. Some animals may be kept for breeding stock, but most are sold for feedlot finishing for meat (pork) production. The growth rate of this species is surprisingly rapid; the ideal slaughter weight is 220 to 240 pounds, which can be reached by 5 to 6 months of age.

GESTATION AND PARTURITION

Gestation in swine lasts an average of 114 days (range 113 to 116 days). With good management practices, it is possible to obtain two litters per year from a sow.

Moving sows to a special farrowing barn or pen within a week of the expected due date is common practice. The animal is bathed before entering the building and is introduced to the farrowing area. The farrowing area is designed to separate the sows and provide an area for their newborns that is heated and safe from being crushed by the sow when she lies down. Death by crushing is one of the most common causes of death in newborn piglets.

Within several days of farrowing, the vulva swells and the labial mucosa becomes hyperemic. Progressive enlargement of the mammary glands occurs in late gestation, but they become especially turgid and warm 1 to 2 days before parturition. The respiratory rate rises several hours before delivery, sometimes as high as 80 beats/min. Body temperature changes that signal parturition in other species have not been consistently identified in sows.

Most sows farrow at night. Signs of approaching parturition include noticeable restlessness within 24 hours of giving birth and building of a "nest" (if bedding material is available). If bedding material is not available, the female paws at the ground. Sows may lie down for variable periods of time and repeat the cycle of nesting and resting several times. Vocalization may occur, and sows may become defensive of the nesting area. Within 1 hour of parturition, sows usually lay quietly in lateral recumbency. Sows typically remain in lateral recumbency, but gilts may stand occasionally between deliveries of fetuses. Some paddling of the legs is not unusual. More visible effort is usually required to deliver the first piglet than the others.

Only small volumes of fetal fluids are expressed with the fetuses. An interval of 15 to 20 minutes is expected between each fetal delivery; intervals longer than 30 minutes should be investigated, and assistance may be necessary. The second stage of labor, the completed delivery of *all* fetuses, lasts an average of 3 to 4 hours. The delivery position of the fetus is not as problematic for swine as it is in other species. Normal delivery, without complication, commonly occurs with both anterior (head-first) and posterior (breech) presentations. The legs are typically flexed alongside the body, rather than extended as they are in other species; therefore it is usual for either a snout or a tail to appear first at the vulva. Up to 45% of fetuses may be delivered in the posterior presentation.

Stillbirths are common in this species; an average of 5% to 7% of piglets are stillborn. The time interval between the start and finish of parturition directly correlates with the number of stillborns, and it is not surprising that most stillbirths occur in the last third of the litter to be delivered. These latter-born piglets usually originate farther up in the uterine horns and have farther to travel through the birth canal. If the umbilical cord ruptures early, death may result from hypoxia.

The third stage of labor is the expulsion of the fetal membranes and is not a distinct stage of labor as defined in other species. Each piglet is encased in its own fetal membranes, but the membranes of two to three adjacent piglets may be fused together and passed as a unit. The placentas may be passed randomly between the births of piglets or after the last piglet is born. Passage of all fetal membranes should be completed within approximately 4 hours after birth of the last piglet; retained placentas are uncommon in swine. Females may attempt to eat the placentas as they are passed; it is preferable to remove the placentas as they are passed to prevent this.

Maternal behavior of the sow after giving birth is somewhat different from other species. Sows are typically fiercely protective of their young but occasionally they may kill and eat one or more piglets as they are born; this phenomenon is known as *savaging*. If savaging is observed during farrowing, all piglets should be removed as soon as they are born and kept warm. When farrowing is complete, it is usually safe to quietly return all piglets to the sow. The sow is watched to confirm that she accepts all of the piglets by allowing them to nurse. Rarely, tranquilization of the sow is necessary.

Swine are among the few species that do not practice vigorous licking of the newborns. It is common for the sow to stand and urinate after delivering all of the fetuses; she then usually lies back down and allows the piglets a prolonged time to nurse.

The most common causes of death in the neonatal period are being crushed by the sow, starvation from failure to adequately nurse, and chilling (hypothermia). Usually an attendant is present at the time of farrowing to assist in the delivery and help prevent these problems.

ROUTINE CARE OF THE NEONATAL PIGLET

Once delivery is complete, the needs of the newborn that must be addressed include the following.

OXYGENATION

The fetus is often born with its amnion, or the membranes of another fetus, around it. Because the sow does not lick and clean the newborn piglets, the membranes should be immediately removed by hand to prevent any obstruction to breathing. The fingers or a dry cloth may be used to clear the mouth and nostrils. The lungs may be cleared by holding the piglet with the head inclined downward and pumping the hindlegs several times toward the abdomen; this is a safer alternative to the traditional "slinging" maneuver. Vigorous toweling helps to stimulate breathing.

TEMPERATURE REGULATION

Piglets are born with sparse hair cover and are therefore highly susceptible to hypothermia, which can be rapidly fatal. The risk is greatest in the first 2 to 3 days after birth. Toweling dry the newborns to remove fetal fluids should be done. Farrowing barns are typically kept at an environmental temperature of 80° F to 85° F, and heat lamps or pads are used to provide each litter with a warmed area of 90° F to 95° F. Drafts must be prevented.

CARE OF THE UMBILICAL CORD AND UMBILICUS

The fetus may be born with the umbilical cord intact or broken. Intact cords are usually broken naturally as the piglet migrates toward the mammary glands to nurse. Intact cords or long cord stumps may be cut or trimmed to a length 4 to 5 cm from the umbilicus. The umbilical stump end should be dipped in 2% povidone-iodine solution or similar antiseptic solution. String or suture material may be used to ligate a bleeding cord by simply tying it around the cord.

NUTRITION (NURSING)

Newborn piglets should be active and should reach a teat within 5 minutes of birth. Attempts to nurse should follow and be successful within 30 minutes of birth. There is a preference for the more cranial teats, and piglets may begin to bite and push each other in competition for these teats. It may be necessary to place some piglets on the more caudal teats to ensure that they all have the opportunity to nurse. A "teat order" is established in the first several days after birth, with the larger, stronger piglets tending to dominate the preferred cranial teats, which are easier to access and produce greater volumes of milk.

Competition for teats may be deadly for piglets, especially in large litters where some piglets may not get enough milk to survive.

Dividing large litters by removing several piglets and placing them with sows with smaller litters is common practice; this helps ensure that all piglets have enough to eat. Sows tolerate the foster mother role well, and piglets are not particular about suckling other sows.

The sow may make a distinctive soft grunting noise that serves as a nursing call to the newborns. The piglets quickly become responsive to this noise. Most domestic sows nurse while recumbent, though standing nursing may be tolerated. On average, the litter nurses once an hour, nearly every hour, for about 6 minutes (<1 minute of actual milk ingestion). An average of 24 to 28 g of milk is consumed at each nursing.

Orphaned piglets can be raised on whole cow's milk or commercial sow milk replacer. Sow milk replacer should be mixed and fed according to the instructions. If cow's milk is used, a tablespoon of powdered skim milk can be added to each pint of milk; do not add sugar or cream. Piglets can be fed by bottle or shallow pan; pan feeding is most convenient for orphaned litters of multiple piglets. Pans, bottles, and nipples should be clean and sterilized or disinfected. Orphans should be fed every 2 to 3 hours for the first 2 to 3 days. Milk should be warmed to approximately 100° F. Prestarter or creep feed may be started at 1 week of age.

Runts have been generally defined as those weighing less than 2 lb at birth; they are often among the last pigs of the litter to be born. They seldom thrive because of competition for nursing, and as many as 60% may die without supportive care. Supplemental feeding of runts may increase their survival. Commercial sow milk replacer may be used, or a substitute mixture (1 quart whole cow's milk + ½ pint half-and-half cream + 1 raw egg) has been described. The mixture is warmed and given twice daily (15 to 20 ml per feeding), using a syringe with an attached soft plastic tube placed in the mouth. This mixture is intended to supplement nursing, not replace it.

ADEQUACY OF PASSIVE TRANSFER OF ANTIBODIES

Similar to other domestic species, colostrum ingestion is essential for transferring maternal antibodies to the young. The absorption of antibodies from the gastrointestinal tract diminishes significantly from 12 to 24 hours after birth. Colostrum should be ingested within 12 hours of birth for the best results. Orphan piglets can receive colostrum that has been milked from other sows. Testing for antibody levels in neonates is not routinely done in swine.

PROCESSING NEONATAL PIGLETS

Several management procedures are commonly performed in the first 1 to 2 days of life. These procedures can usually be performed by one person, most often by farm personnel. Veterinarians and veterinary technicians may assist in these procedures and can play an important role in teaching farm personnel to perform these procedures correctly and humanely.

Because the piglets must be temporarily removed from the sow, personnel should be prepared for possible aggression by the sow in attempts to protect her young, and also for her vocalization and that of the piglets. Some farms have a processing room where the piglets are taken for the procedures, away from the sight and sounds of the sow. Piglets should not be removed from the sow for periods longer than 1 hour.

IRON DEXTRAN INJECTION

Sow's milk is naturally low in iron, and piglets are born with little iron in their bodies. In a natural setting, pigs would acquire iron from eating soil and plants. In confinement rearing, this is not possible, and pigs of all ages are susceptible to anemia. Iron must be supplemented.

Anemia in piglets is referred to as "baby pig thumps" because of the extremely high heart rate that can be easily felt over the chest; this is accompanied by labored breathing and weakness. A source of iron should be provided to piglets, usually in the form of injectable iron dextran (150 to 200 mg) given at 1 to 3 days of age. The intramuscular injection should not be given in the ham muscles, as permanent staining of the meat may occur. The neck is the preferred site for injection.

Continued iron supplementation may be given via a second iron dextran injection in 2 to 3 weeks. Another option is to use oral iron supplements in the creep feed, which is started at 1 to 2 weeks of age. Iron status can be determined indirectly by measuring the blood hemoglobin concentration; a blood hemoglobin level of 10 mg/dl or higher is considered adequate.

CLIPPING NEEDLE TEETH

Piglets typically try to nurse almost anything that their snouts contact, including the sow's vulva and other piglets; piglets also fight each other for nursing position. Unfortunately, piglets are born with eight sharp teeth called "needle teeth." The needle teeth are actually the deciduous I3 and deciduous canine teeth of each dental arcade (Fig. 23-1). The needle teeth are cut down to reduce injuries to the sow's teats, which are painful and may become infected, and to the littermates.

Small wire cutters (side cutters) may be used to cut the teeth, or commercial "needle tooth nippers" are available (Fig. 23-2). The nippers should be sharp and not used for other procedures, and they should be disinfected between piglets. The piglet is restrained by lifting it by the neck or head. The mouth is opened by placing firm but

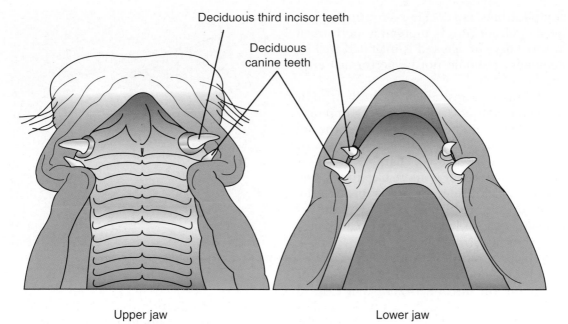

Deciduous third incisor teeth

Deciduous canine teeth

Upper jaw   Lower jaw

Fig. 23-1. Needle teeth of the piglet. (Modified from McCracken TO, Kainer RA, Spurgeon TL: *Spurgeon's color atlas of large animal anatomy,* Philadelphia, 1999, Lippincott Williams & Wilkins.)

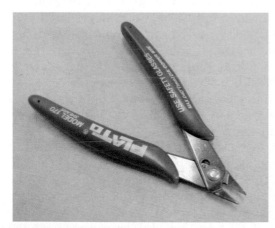

Fig. 23-2. Needle tooth nippers.

gentle pressure at the angle of the jaw, being careful not to injure the jaw. The flat side of the nippers is placed parallel to the gumline so that the distal half to two thirds of each tooth are removed. The cut should not be closer to the gumline than 1 to 2 mm; cutting too short may cut the gums or fracture the tooth roots, providing an entrance for bacteria.

The procedure is well tolerated, and no special aftercare is required.

TAIL DOCKING

Piglets tend to suck and chew on each other's tails. Tail-biting behavior continues after weaning, even into the feedlot/finishing stages. In addition to causing pain and stress, the open sores may become infected and form abscesses. It is not unusual for the infection to migrate cranially along the spinal nerves of the tail, causing ataxia and even paralysis of the hindlegs. Many feeder pig operations do not accept pigs with tails. In order to reduce tail-biting and its associated complications, tail docking is routinely practiced. Tail docking is preferably performed at 1 to 2 days of age and is tolerated well by neonates. It should not be performed after 2 weeks of age.

The piglet is restrained by supporting it under the body and holding it aloft, or it may be held between the handler's knees. The tail can be docked with wire (side) cutters or baby pig emasculators. Sharp wire cutter blades tend to result in more bleeding. Using slightly dulled blades, or briefly heating the blades to cauterize the blood vessels as the cut is made, may be helpful. Emasculators provide a crushing component as the cut is made that helps control bleeding. Emasculators used for tail docking should not be used for castration. The instrument should be cleaned and disinfected between each piglet. Piglets should be observed for several hours for excessive bleeding, and for several days for signs of infection.

The level of docking is important because the incidence of rectal prolapse increases if the tail is cut too short. The tail should be docked at about $\frac{1}{2}$ to 1 inch from its base. The freshly cut stump can be dipped or sprayed with antiseptic solution.

EAR NOTCHING/TATTOOING

The most common method of identifying swine is by ear notching. This method involves cutting out small wedge-shaped sections of ear cartilage along the margin of the ear pinna. The wedges do not grow back, leaving permanent "notches" that enlarge with the ear pinna as it grows. Special ear notching pliers, or "V-notchers," are used to remove the wedges of tissue (Fig. 23-3).

Piglets appear to tolerate the procedure well. The head should be held gently but securely. The notches should be made quickly and firmly to produce a clean cut. Piglets should be observed for excessive bleeding for several hours after the procedure and watched

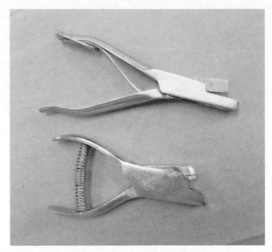

Fig. 23-3. Piglet ear notching instruments.

for signs of infection in the following days. Notching pliers should be kept sharp and should be cleaned and disinfected between each piglet.

A standard numbering system (Universal Ear Notching System) has been developed using standard locations for the ear notches. However, farmers may use any system recommended by breed associations or may design their own. The hog farmer usually numbers each litter sequentially throughout the year. Within each litter, each piglet receives an individual number. For example, a litter number of 76 indicates the 76th litter born during the farrowing season. If there are nine piglets in the litter, they are assigned an individual number from one to nine. By convention, the litter number is placed in the right ear, and the individual piglet number is placed in the left ear (Fig. 23-4).

Baby pigs can also be tattooed on the body or ear. Ear tattoos may be placed on the inside or outside of the ear pinna, using small-size ear tattoo pliers. The ear veins should be avoided if possible. Body tattoos may be placed on the shoulder or rump, where they may be easily read. Body tattoos are placed

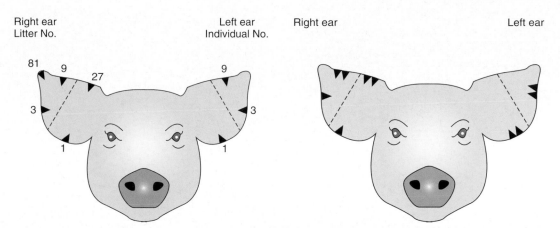

Right ear
Litter No.

Left ear
Individual No.

Right ear

Left ear

Fig. 23-4. Universal ear notching system. The litter number is placed in the right ear pinna, and the individual pig number in the left ear pinna. The pig on the right shows the litter number 76, individual pig number 8.

with a commercially available baby pig body tattooer, which is basically a short metal handle with a holder on one end for placing the interchangeable number/letter character pins. After applying tattoo ink, the pins are pressed directly into the body. Additional ink is rubbed into the holes left by the needles.

SUGGESTED READING

Ensminger ME, Parker RO: *Swine science*, ed 6, Danville, Ill, 1997, Interstate Publishers.

Hafez ESE: *Reproduction in farm animals*, ed 6, Philadelphia, 1993, Lea & Febiger.

Noakes DE, Parkinson TJ, England GCW: *Veterinary reproduction and obstetrics*, ed 8, London, 2001, Saunders.

Teeple TN: Nursing care of food animals, camelids, and ratites. In Sirois M: *Principles and practice of veterinary technology*, ed 2, St Louis, 2004, Mosby.

24

Common Clinical Procedures in Swine

GASTROINTESTINAL SYSTEM

DETUSKING

The permanent canine teeth are referred to as "tusks." In females the canine teeth are relatively small, and only occasionally do the tips protrude slightly through the lips; growth ceases after about 2 years of age in females. In males, however, the canine teeth are long and curved, and they grow continuously throughout the life of the pig. Growth of the mandibular canine teeth is pronounced, and the teeth protrude visibly from the mouth (Fig. 24-1). They are kept sharp by friction against the smaller upper (maxillary) canines. Since pigs use their teeth to fight, tusks are dangerous to humans and other pigs. Swine owners have two management options for tusks: regular trimming and complete surgical removal.

Tusk trimming, or "detusking," is performed as needed, generally every 10 to 12 months. General anesthesia or heavy sedation may be used. Sedation is combined with a hog snare or snubbing rope on the snout. Snout restraint causes the typical reaction of opening the mouth. While the mouth is open, a Gigli's (obstetrical) wire saw can be placed around the tusk and used to remove the tooth several millimeters above the gumline; at this level, the pulp cavity is not opened. Hoof nippers have also been used, but this risks shattering the tooth and exposing the pulp cavity. Trimming all four canines may be necessary in some animals.

Complete surgical removal of the mandibular canine teeth is possible. It may be done electively or to treat infections or fractures

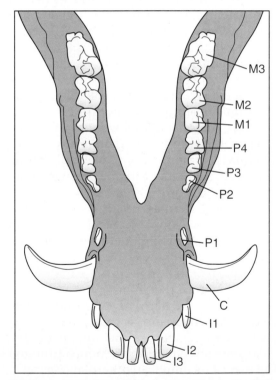

Fig. 24-1. Lower (mandibular) permanent teeth of the pig. Note the large canine teeth or "tusks" (C). (From Getty R, Sisson S, Grossman JD: *The anatomy of the domestic animals*, ed 5, Philadelphia, 1975, Saunders.)

of a canine tooth. The procedure must be done under general anesthesia and is technically difficult to perform; it is seldom done as an elective procedure. The tooth roots are long and deeply seated in the mandible. There is a risk of fracturing the mandible during elevation of the extensive tooth root and repulsion of the tooth. Owners should be warned of potential complications.

UMBILICAL HERNIAS

Umbilical herniation occurs when the natural umbilical opening in the abdominal wall fails to close completely after birth and allows contents of the abdomen to protrude through the abdominal wall. The skin and surrounding connective tissue form a "hernia sac," which is a potential space into which abdominal contents may slide in and out. The actual opening in the abdominal wall is referred to as the "hernia ring." The size of the hernia ring determines which abdominal organs or tissues can "herniate"; small defects may allow only omentum to enter the hernia sac, but larger defects may allow portions of the intestinal tract to enter. The greatest risk of a hernia is entrapment of tissue in the hernia sac, with subsequent tissue strangulation, necrosis, and death.

Umbilical hernias are not uncommon in swine. Development of the condition has a hereditary component, but umbilical infections and abscesses may contribute in some cases. Umbilical hernias are not usually recognized until the animal is 9 to 14 weeks of age, when the hernia is often noticeably large. The condition is recognized by a visible enlargement at the umbilicus; the enlargement is typically soft, nonpainful, and fluctuant (uncomplicated hernia) (Fig. 24-2). These animals are usually otherwise healthy in appearance and behavior. It may even be possible to reduce the hernia by gently massaging the hernia sac to force the contents

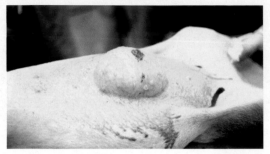

Fig. 24-2. Umbilical hernia in a pig. (From Fubini SL, Ducharme NG: *Farm animal surgery*, St Louis, 2004, Saunders.)

back into the abdomen; however, the hernia usually reappears when the massage is stopped. Hard, painful enlargements usually signal that infection and/or strangulation of the hernial contents is involved; these animals are commonly febrile, depressed, and possibly in shock if strangulation has occurred.

The condition can often be surgically corrected, but the cost of surgery usually means that other treatments must be used. These animals are often destined for slaughter, and the farmer usually strives to market the pig early, before strangulation occurs. If the hernia is large enough to touch the ground, or if the skin over the hernia is ulcerated, the pig will be declined for market; euthanasia is advised. A long-used "home remedy" for umbilical hernias is the hernia clamp. Hernia clamps may be homemade, but aluminum and disposable plastic clamps are commercially available (Fig. 24-3). To use the clamp, the contents of the hernia must be completely reduced into the abdomen. With the contents reduced, the skin of the hernia sac is pulled tautly, and the clamp is placed across the base of the sac as close to the abdominal wall as possible. The clamp is designed to prevent reherniation. If left in place long enough, the clamp causes gradual necrosis and death of the skin within its jaws; the clamp eventually

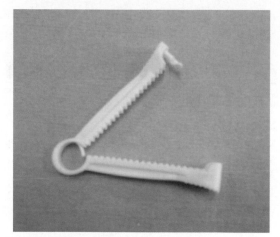

Fig. 24-3. Plastic, disposable hernia clamp.

falls off. Ideally the scar tissue that results will be firm enough to prevent reherniation of abdominal contents. However, the procedure is not without risks. The hernia clamp does nothing to close the actual hernia ring in the abdominal wall, and the hernia may reoccur. Also, the necrosis caused by the clamp provides a potential entrance for bacteria such as tetanus. The clamp also does not change the DNA of the animal and the possibility of passing the condition to offspring.

Owners of purebred breeding stock and pet animals are more likely to request surgical correction (herniorrhaphy). General anesthesia is required, and the animal is positioned in dorsal recumbency in a "V" trough. The umbilical area is clipped and aseptically prepared. The surgeon replaces the hernia contents, removes the hernia sac, and closes the hernia ring with sutures to restore the abdominal wall. If strangulated or infected tissue is present, it is usually resected (if possible). The skin and subcutaneous tissues are closed. Antibiotics are given for 3 to 5 days. Skin sutures or staples are removed 10 days after surgery.

IDENTIFICATION

The following methods are used to identify swine.

EAR NOTCHING

Ear notching of piglets is described in Chapter 23. Ear notches may be placed at any age, but it is preferable to perform the procedure in neonates. Neonates tolerate the procedure well and with minimal complications. In pigs older than 2 weeks, some form of pain relief or analgesia should be used. The incidence of hemorrhage may increase in older pigs.

TATTOOS

Pigs may be tattooed on the ear pinna or body tattooed on the shoulder or rump. Ear tattoos are placed with tattoo pliers, on either the inside or outside of the pinna. The tattoo should be placed in a thinner part of the ear, avoiding the major ear veins if possible. Tattoo ink should be rubbed thoroughly into the needle puncture holes.

Body tattoos are placed with a body tattooer. Body tattooers come in different sizes and are of two basic designs (Fig. 24-4). One design is a short handle with a holder on one end for the interchangeable tattoo characters; the characters are oriented perpendicularly to the handle. With the handle held perpendicularly to the skin, the characters are quickly but fully pressed directly into the animal and then withdrawn. This press-type design is suitable for piglets. The other design is the "slap" tattooer—a handle with a holder on one end that is offset such that the characters face 90 degrees to the long axis of the handle. With the pig confined in a chute or with snout restraint, the operator "slaps" the character end of the handle against the animal, similar to swatting a fly. The skin is

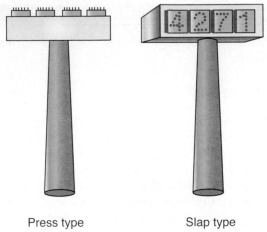

Press type   Slap type

Fig. 24-4. Body tattooer with characters on the end *(left)* of the handle (press-type tattooer) or along the side *(right)* of the handle (slap tattooer).

penetrated by the character needles, and tattoo ink is rubbed in. Slap tattooers are not suitable for young piglets.

Tattooing is well tolerated, although there is brief pain during penetration of the needles.

MICROCHIPS

As concerns for biosecurity increase, methods to permanently and uniquely identify food animals are being researched and developed. The goal is traceability through all phases of an animal's life. Government-regulated microchipping is likely to be a future solution to the growing concerns.

BRANDING

Branding is possible but infrequently practiced in swine.

EAR TAGS

Ear tags may be used for identification but are not permanent. They may fall out, be pulled out, or become difficult to read.

A permanent method of identification should be used in addition to ear tags.

REPRODUCTIVE SYSTEM

MALE REPRODUCTIVE SYSTEM

SEMEN COLLECTION

Semen is collected for evaluation as part of a breeding soundness examination or for artificial insemination (AI) of a female. The glans penis of the boar is shaped somewhat like a corkscrew; the cervix of the female has a corresponding spiral shape. During copulation, the penis enters the cervix with a slight twisting motion to form a locking fit of the two organs. Ejaculation in the boar is stimulated by the firm fit of the glans in the cervix. In order to ejaculate and collect a boar, this stimulation must be simulated. Boars are not as temperature sensitive as males of other species, but they are very pressure sensitive.

Artificial vaginas of various design have been used to collect boars, but manual stimulation is more reliable and more commonly used. Boars can be trained to mount a collection dummy, or a sow in estrus may be used. The boar is allowed to mount the sow/dummy, and as the penis is extended, the collector diverts the penis to prevent entry into the vagina. The collector wears a lubricated latex glove that has warmed to body temperature; this hand is wrapped firmly around the glans penis with the fingers in the corkscrew grooves to simulate the locking fit of the cervix. The body/shaft of the penis should not be touched. The boar will make thrusting motions, which slow somewhat as ejaculation begins. Ejaculation in this species is not rapid; 3 to 7 minutes are often required to complete the process. The ejaculate is collected in a suitable insulated container at 30° C. Semen evaluation is performed similarly to other species.

Because ejaculation releases large numbers of sperm in this species, the epididymis is quickly depleted of its reserves of sperm. Preferably, semen should be collected every other day. Daily collections, if necessary, should not be done for more than several days, and the boar should receive 2 to 3 days of rest afterward.

Electroejaculation is not recommended.

CASTRATION

In the United States and Canada, intact males cannot be marketed for meat. This is due primarily to "boar taint," a distinct, objectionable odor that is released during cooking and produces a bad flavor to the meat. Boar taint begins with the onset of puberty. Castrated males do not produce meat with this odor. If a boar is castrated after sexual maturity ("stagging"), the odor disappears about 3 to 4 weeks after the castration. Castration also may improve feed conversion and make animals easier to handle. All male pigs that are not used for breeding purposes should be castrated by 2 weeks of age. Although castration can be performed at any age, early castration is safer for the animal because of fewer surgical complications and less stress from restraint. Some farm operations castrate on day 1 or 2 after birth.

Restraint for castration depends on the age and size of the animal. Experienced personnel can hold a neonatal pig with one hand and castrate it with the other hand. Older piglets require one person to hold the animal and another to perform the castration. Piglets up to approximately 50 lb are held up by the hindlegs, with the back resting against the restrainer so that the restrainer can secure the piglet by squeezing its back and shoulders between the thighs and knees. Alternatively, the piglet can be placed in dorsal recumbency in a clean "V" trough with one person holding the front legs and another

holding the hindlegs. The surgical room or area should be clean and free of drafts.

Before beginning the surgery, the inguinal and scrotal areas are palpated to be sure that both testicles are descended and that inguinal or scrotal hernias are not present. A veterinarian should be consulted if abnormalities are detected or suspected. If the animal is palpably normal, the scrotal area is prepared for aseptic surgery with mild disinfectant solution. The use of lidocaine for local anesthesia is possible; approximately 2 to 3 ml lidocaine in a small syringe with a 25-gauge needle is used to deposit anesthetic subcutaneously and around the spermatic cord.

A Bard Parker No. 3 scalpel handle and No. 12 blade are commonly used to castrate piglets. The scrotum is tightened to force the testicles cranially toward the inguinal area (for improved ventral drainage of the incisions after surgery), and a longitudinal 1-cm incision is made directly over each testicle. The testicles are pushed out through the incisions and pulled to expose the spermatic cords. The spermatic cords must be severed to remove the testicles; the scalpel blade is used to scrape or "tease" the cord apart, which provides more hemostasis than sharply cutting the cord (Fig. 24-5). Alternatively, a piglet emasculator may be used, by applying it for approximately 1 minute. The incisions are left open to drain and may be treated with antiseptic spray. Neonatal piglets should be kept warm after the procedure and observed for hemorrhage and infection. Healing requires approximately 5 to 7 days.

Older pigs must be heavily sedated or anesthetized for castration. The animal is restrained in lateral recumbency. The scrotum is aseptically prepared for surgery. The testicles are usually removed through two incisions left open to drain, but it is possible to remove them through one incision that is closed with suture (similar to canines). If the spermatic cords are well developed, they

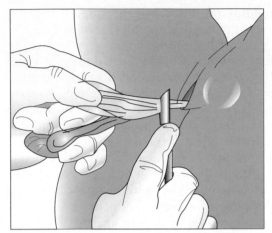

Fig. 24-5. Piglet castration. The testicle is pulled from the scrotal incision, and a scalpel blade is used to repeatedly scrape the spermatic cord until it severs. (Modified from Turner AS, McIlwraith CW: *Techniques in large animal surgery*, Philadelphia, 1982, Lea & Febiger.)

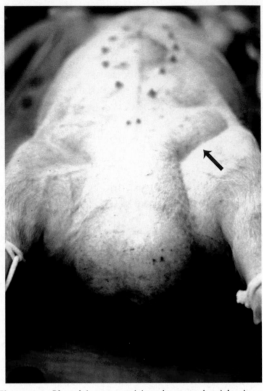

Fig. 24-6. Pig with a scrotal hernia restrained in dorsal recumbency. Note the swelling at the left inguinal area *(arrow)* that continues down into the left scrotal sac. (From Fubini SL, Ducharme NG: *Farm animal surgery*, St. Louis, 2004, Saunders.)

are ligated with suture before using an emasculator to divide the cord. Hemorrhage, infection, and seroma/hematoma are the most common complications.

Inguinal hernias are fairly common in pigs and have a hereditary etiology. The inherited anatomical defect is an abnormally large vaginal ring, which is an entrance to the inguinal canal. The typical hernia occurs when a portion of the intestinal tract enters the inguinal canal. The herniated intestine may go no farther than the inguinal canal, or it may continue into the scrotal sac to form a scrotal hernia. Scrotal hernias are larger and more often noticed, but inguinal hernias are not easily seen (Fig. 24-6). The condition may be bilateral. These hernias are often discovered at the time of castration and are problematic for two reasons. First, if castration is performed without correction of the problem, it is possible to cut into the intestines during the castration procedure. Second, if an animal with an inguinal hernia or scrotal hernia is castrated by a method that leaves the spermatic cord open (not closed with ligatures), the intestines frequently eviscerate after the castration. This is usually fatal for the animal. If an inguinal or scrotal hernia is detected, a veterinarian should be consulted. Surgery by a veterinarian to correct the hernia (inguinal herniorrhaphy) and castrate the animal is advised.

Cryptorchidism is common in pigs. Castration should never be performed unless both testicles can be palpated within their scrotal sacs. If cryptorchidism is suspected, a veterinarian should evaluate the animal and perform cryptorchidectomy, if necessary.

FEMALE REPRODUCTIVE SYSTEM

ESTROUS CYCLE DETERMINATION

Most hog producers use planned breeding programs. Planned breeding may use either "hand-mating," where one selected male is allowed to naturally breed one selected female at a time in a controlled environment, or breeding may be done via AI. Planned breeding is labor intensive, but it allows for good record keeping and better reproductive, nutritional, and veterinary management of breeding stock.

Successful breeding depends on knowledge of the estrous cycle and knowing what stage of the reproductive cycle each breeding female is in. The reproductive physiology of the female swine is reviewed in Table 24-1.

In swine the most practical method used to determine the stage of a female's estrous cycle is observation of heat. Visual signs such as enlargement and reddening of the vulva, restlessness, mounting other females, and decreased appetite may be seen. A mucoid vaginal discharge is occasionally seen. Females in standing heat respond to the sight, sound, and smell of a boar (intact or vasectomized) and seek the boar; if the boar mounts, the female assumes a characteristic motionless stance with the legs rigid and the ears stiff and erect ("popping the ears"). This stance is known as "lordosis," and a female in standing heat displays it if pressure is placed on her back. This is used to advantage by handlers; by pressing firmly down on a female's back with the hands and initiating a lordosis response, standing heat can be confirmed.

PREGNANCY DIAGNOSIS

Failure to return to estrus is a sign of possible pregnancy but is not reliable because there are other causes for failure to cycle. Rectal palpation is possible in larger females if the palpator has small arms; however, it is difficult to diagnose early pregnancy.

Transabdominal ultrasound is the primary method for diagnosing pregnancy in swine. Historically, A-mode ultrasound and Doppler ultrasound have been used most often to detect pregnancy. A-mode ultrasound is most accurate between days 30 and 90 of gestation, and Doppler is accurate from day 28 until the end of gestation. Real-time (B-mode) ultrasound is increasingly being used in swine. It can detect pregnancy

TABLE 24-1 **REPRODUCTIVE PHYSIOLOGY OF THE SOW**

Breeding season	Year-round polyestrus*
Puberty	6-7 mo[†]
Length of estrous cycle[‡]	21 days (range 19-23 days)
Length of estrus	2-3 days
Ovulation	36-42 hr after onset of estrus
Gestation	114-115 days

*Wild pigs are often seasonally polyestrous, with one season in the fall and another in the spring. Domestic sows may occasionally show decreased cycling in the summer, especially if the weather is hot and humid.
[†]Influenced by breed, level of nutrition and bodyweight, season of the year, and presence of mature boars. Females born in the fall cycle earlier than those born in spring. The presence of boars accelerates the onset of puberty, by release of pheromones that stimulate hormone release in the female.
[‡]Many sows have a nonovulatory (sterile) heat 2 days after parturition. This is followed by lactational anestrus. Regular cycles resume 4-6 days after the litter is weaned.

as early as 18 days, with best accuracy after 22 days.

The preferred patient position for ultrasound is standing. Ultrasound coupling gel or other coupling medium is necessary. The transducer is placed in the lower right flank, in an area approximately 5 cm caudal to the umbilicus and 5 cm lateral to the teat nipple line. The transducer is angled approximately 45 degrees dorsally and swept slowly from cranial to caudal to identify the uterus.

OBSTETRICAL PROCEDURES

Swine have a low incidence of dystocias, estimated at less than 1% of farrowings. The incidence is higher when litter size is small, because the fetuses are generally larger. The most common causes of dystocia are uterine inertia (failure of the myometrium to contract) and obstruction of the birth canal. During parturition, it is usual for a piglet to be born every 15 to 20 minutes. When the interval reaches 30 to 45 minutes without delivery of a piglet, the sow should be closely observed. Intervention is advisable after 45 to 60 minutes with no progress.

If the sow is having contractions, the birth canal should be checked for possible blockage. The vulva should be cleaned first. A well-lubricated, gloved hand is introduced into the reproductive tract through the vulva; the hand should be held with the fingers and thumb together in a pointed position to enter the vulva. A slight rotating motion of the hand assists passage into the pelvic inlet. The birth canal is searched for fetuses, which may be in a sideways or breech position or be large in size. Occasionally two fetuses are entangled. Once an abnormality is detected, repositioning may be necessary. Mild traction can then be placed on the head or limbs to extract the fetus. A variety of instruments are available to assist in applying traction; lambing snares, pig pullers, forceps, or nylon cord may be helpful. All manipulations should be done carefully to prevent damaging the sow.

Occasionally a full rectum may partially obstruct the sow's pelvic canal. An enema may be necessary to remove fecal material.

Uterine inertia may result from exhaustion or hypocalcemia. The sow should be kept comfortably cool and may resume labor after a brief rest. If not, veterinary consultation is advised. Oxytocin injection may help to restore uterine contractions. If not, caesarean section may be the only option to save the sow.

One common problem is determining whether a sow has delivered all of her fetuses. The end of parturition is usually signaled by the sow standing and voiding a large volume of urine, followed by lying down comfortably to allow the litter to nurse. If a question exists as to possible incomplete delivery, a manual examination of the uterus can be performed. However, it is difficult to reach the full extent of the uterine horns. Transabdominal B-mode ultrasound can be used to detect retained fetuses.

CAESAREAN SECTION

Caesarean section for treatment of dystocia should be performed as early as possible for the best chances of saving the sow and possibly obtaining live piglets. Before surgery, physical exhaustion and shock should be treated and the patient stabilized. Fluid support is best obtained by intravenous (IV) catheterization of the ear vein; lactated Ringer's solution or 0.9% saline can be given rapidly at 20 to 40 ml/kg/hr until a response is seen, and then a maintenance rate of 4 ml/kg/hr can be used. Dextrose and calcium solutions can be added to the maintenance fluids. Preoperative antibiotics are commonly given.

Various anesthetic regimens, patient positions, and incision locations are available for caesarean section. The clinician determines how best to perform the procedure. Anesthesia for caesarean section depends largely on the physical status of the sow and is selected to have minimal effects on the fetuses. Sedation with local or regional anesthesia (inverted L block or epidural) is commonly used, especially in compromised patients. General anesthesia is also an option. The procedure is usually performed with the sow in right or left lateral recumbency, with the legs tied for restraint if necessary. Dorsal recumbency is also possible. The surgery is usually performed through a vertical flank incision, although the Marcenac approach, ventral midline, and paramedian incisions are also used.

The surgical site is clipped and aseptically prepared. If local anesthesia is used, an additional scrub is performed after the anesthetic is deposited (Fig. 24-7). Materials to dry, warm, and support newborns should be available in case live fetuses are found. After surgery, the sow is moved to a clean, dry pen and the piglets are returned when she recovers. At least 2 weeks of confinement are necessary for healing and recovery.

Caesarean section is also used to deliver specific pathogen–free (SPF) piglets. Because these sows are typically healthy, general anesthesia is preferred.

PROLAPSE OF VAGINA AND UTERUS

Vaginal prolapse usually occurs before parturition (Fig. 24-8). Treatment involves sedation or anesthesia of the sow, cleansing the prolapsed tissues, and repositioning the organ. A Buhner retention suture may be used to prevent reoccurrence. The sow must be closely watched so that the suture can be removed at the onset of labor.

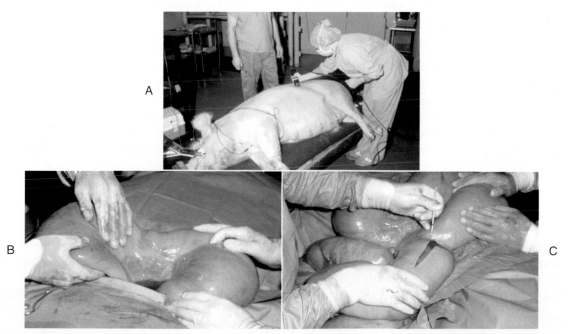

Fig. 24-7. **A,** A sow in lateral recumbency being prepared for a caesarean section. **B,** One uterine horn is exteriorized. **C,** Longitudinal uterine incision. (From Fubini SL, Ducharme NG: *Farm animal surgery,* St Louis, 2004, Saunders.)

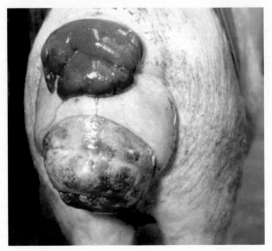

Fig. 24-8. Sow with vaginal and rectal prolapse. (From Fubini SL, Ducharme NG: *Farm animal surgery,* St. Louis, 2004, Saunders.)

Uterine prolapse occurs during or in the first several days after parturition. Excessive straining is thought to cause the prolapse. Complete prolapse is often accompanied by hemorrhage and death. Partial prolapses do occur and have a better prognosis for survival. If surgery is to be performed, the sow must first be stabilized and any profuse bleeding stopped. General anesthesia or epidural anesthesia with sedation may be used. The organ is evaluated, cleansed, and replaced if possible. Repositioning is often challenging for the surgeon. Occasionally, a laparotomy incision must be made to assist the replacement. A Buhner retention suture is recommended to prevent reoccurrence while healing progresses and is usually removed in 7 to 10 days. In extreme cases, amputation of the uterus may be required to salvage the sow for slaughter, which is typically done after the litter is weaned.

ARTIFICIAL INSEMINATION

AI is commonly and increasingly practiced in swine and can achieve farrowing rates that are comparable to natural breeding. Boars used for AI can have a profound influence on improving the performance of a swine herd, because many of the "economically important" traits (carcass traits, growth rate, feed conversion rate, etc.) are highly heritable. AI boars are readily trained to use a mounting dummy for collection. The sperm-rich fraction is filtered from the gel fraction of the ejaculate, evaluated, and diluted with semen extender according to the results of the semen evaluation. A single high-quality ejaculate can provide up to 8 to 10 insemination doses after addition of semen extender. A recommended 1 to 2 billion sperm are used for each insemination dose.

Boar semen does not survive current methods of cryopreservation well, although frozen semen can be commercially obtained. Therefore it is preferably used fresh or cooled. Fresh semen combined with extender is preferred for maximum conception rates.

Conception rates are improved if multiple inseminations are performed; the common practice is to inseminate the sow twice, 12 to 24 hours apart, in the middle of the 2 to 3 days of estrus (standing heat). In practice, this means that the first insemination is done 12 hours after detecting standing heat, followed by a second insemination 12 hours after the first. The "back pressure" test for lordosis is most commonly used to detect standing heat and is most successful if performed in the presence of a boar.

It is now fairly common practice to use semen from two boars to inseminate each female; the semen can be mixed together, or each boar can be used for a separate insemination. The rationale is to compensate for possible decreased fertility of one of the boars. Research has confirmed that conception rates are often higher if "heterospermic insemination" is practiced.

The vulva is cleaned before insemination. By applying and taking advantage of the lordosis response, sows in heat require minimal or no restraint if the procedure is performed calmly in quiet surroundings. The presence of a boar nearby is helpful. A spiral-tip insemination pipette (Melrose catheter) or a pipette with a 30-degree angled tip is used to accommodate the shape of the sow's cervix. Insemination is performed blindly, by sliding the pipette cranially along the roof of the vagina until it contacts the cervix (≈8 to 10 inches). A gentle counterclockwise twisting motion is used to "screw" the catheter in place, and the semen is injected or allowed to flow by gravity slowly into the uterus. Insemination doses average approximately 70 ml (50 to 100 ml range). The catheter is removed by twisting it clockwise.

If purebred breed registration is desired for the offspring of AI, the breed registry association should be contacted for specific regulations.

EMBRYO TRANSFER

Embryo transfer is not yet widely used in swine. Superovulation is possible, and estrous synchronization of donors and recipients can be readily achieved with oral progesterone compounds. After AI of the donor, embryos are recovered 3 to 7 days later by ventral midline celiotomy under general anesthesia. An embryo recovery solution is flushed through the oviduct into the uterine horn, and embryos are recovered through a special cannula placed in the uterine horn. Laparoscopic embryo recovery techniques have been reported.

Embryos must be kept above 15° C outside the body. Transfer to the recipient sow should be done within 24 hours. Transfer is also done surgically through a ventral midline incision, by use of a small pipette inserted directly into a uterine tube. The embryos migrate and distribute themselves throughout the uterus. Approximately 14 embryos are recommended to be transferred to the recipient. Laparoscopic transfer has been used, and a nonsurgical technique of transfer has recently been reported.

EUTHANASIA AND NECROPSY

EUTHANASIA

According to the *2000 Report of the American Veterinary Medical Association (AVMA) Panel on Euthanasia,* the following methods of euthanasia are acceptable for swine:
- Barbiturate IV injection
- Carbon dioxide gas: the only chemical used for euthanasia that does not leave tissue residues
- IV potassium chloride (KCl) in conjunction with general anesthesia: anesthesia must be induced first
- Penetrating captive bolt

The following methods are conditionally acceptable:
- Inhalant anesthetic gases (overdose)
- Carbon monoxide
- Chloral hydrate IV after sedation
- Gunshot
- Electrocution: applied to the head
- Concussion (blow) to the head: only suitable for animals younger than 3 weeks of age. Must be applied by trained personnel in order to be humane.

The reader should consult the AVMA report for descriptions and details of these methods.

NECROPSY

Necropsy is performed with the animal in left lateral recumbency. The procedure is basically the same as that described for small mammals (dogs, cats).

The technician should be familiar with the normal anatomy of the pig and be aware of several anatomical differences in this

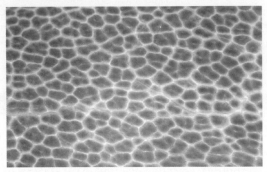

Fig. 24-9. Surface of the liver (enlarged) with clearly defined hepatic lobules. (From Dyce KM, Sack WO, Wensing CJG: *Textbook of veterinary anatomy,* ed 3, Philadelphia, 2002, Saunders.)

species. The liver of the pig has an unusual appearance that may be mistaken for a pathological condition. The liver lobules are clearly separated and defined by a high content of fibrous connective tissue (Fig. 24-9). The tonsillar tissue of the pig is diffusely scattered on the lateral pharyngeal walls, rather than being a distinct organ within a tonsillar crypt. The nasal turbinates should always be examined for distortion or atrophy, which may indicate atrophic rhinitis.

A transverse cut through the snout at the level of the premolars is used to more closely evaluate the turbinates.

SUGGESTED READING

Ensminger ME, Parker RO: *Swine science,* Danville, Ill, 1997, Interstate Publishers.

Fubini SL, Ducharme NG: *Farm animal surgery,* St Louis, 2004, Saunders.

Goswami S: Anatomy and physiology. In Sirois M, editor: *Principles and practice of veterinary technology,* ed 2, St Louis, 2004, Mosby.

Hafez ESE: *Reproduction in farm animals,* ed 6, Philadelphia, 1993, Lea & Febiger.

Noakes DE, Parkinson TJ, England GCW: *Veterinary reproduction and obstetrics,* ed 8, London, 2001, Saunders.

Pinto CRF, Eilts BE, Paccamonti DL: Animal reproduction. In McCurnin DM, Bassert JM, editors: *Clinical textbook for veterinary technicians,* ed 6, St Louis, 2006, Saunders.

Teeple TN: Nursing care of food animals, camelids, and ratites. In Sirois M, editor: *Principles and practice of veterinary technology,* ed 2, St Louis, 2004, Mosby.

Turner AS, McIlwraith CW: *Techniques in large animal surgery,* Philadelphia, 1982, Lea & Febiger.

Large Animal Instruments and Equipment

TEAT INSTRUMENTS

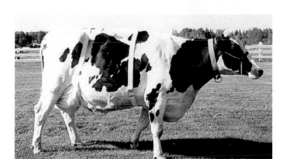

Fig. A-1. Udder support.

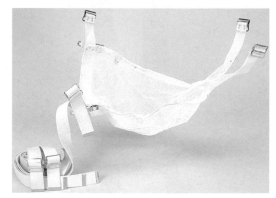

Fig. A-2. Cow with udder support.

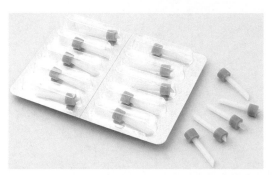

Fig. A-3. Teat dilators.

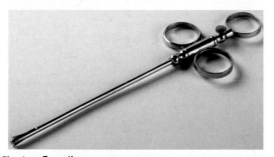

Fig. A-4. Teat slitter.

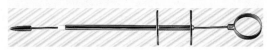

Fig. A-5. Teat tumor extractor.

The illustrations in this appendix are all from Sonsthagen T: *Veterinary instruments and equipment,* St Louis, 2006, Mosby.

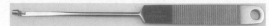

Fig. A-6. Teat curette (Cornell).

EQUINE INSTRUMENTS

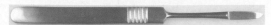

Fig. A-7. Lichty teat knife (sharp).

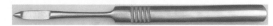

Fig. A-8. Lichty teat knife (blunt).

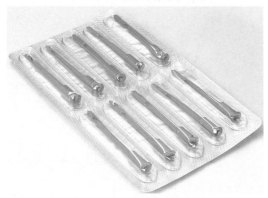

Fig. A-9. Udder infusion cannulas (disposable).

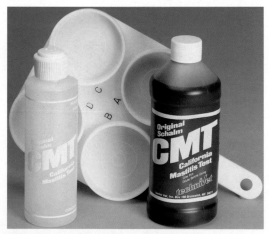

Fig. A-10. California mastitis test.

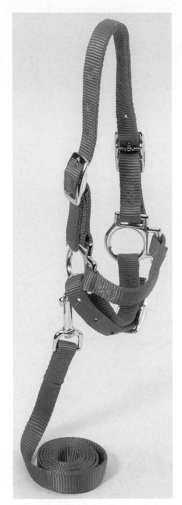

Fig. A-12. Nylon halter with nylon lead rope horse.

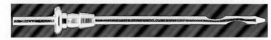

Fig. A-11. Milking tube.

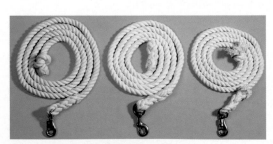

Fig. A-13. Rope-style lead rope.

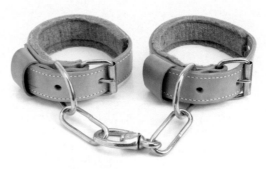

Fig. A-15. Pastern hobbles.

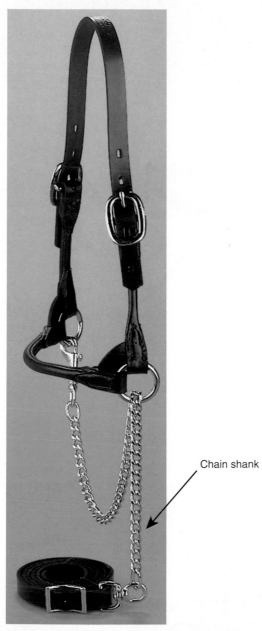

Chain shank

Fig. A-14. Halter with chain shank lead rope.

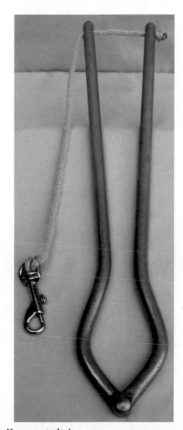

Fig. A-16. Humane twitch.

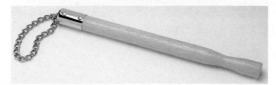

Fig. A-17. Chain twitch.

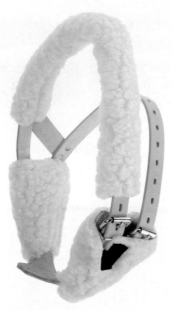

Fig. A-18. Equine neck cradle.

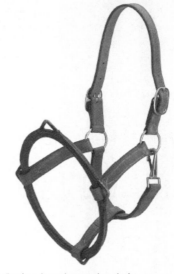

Fig. A-20. Equine dental procedure halter.

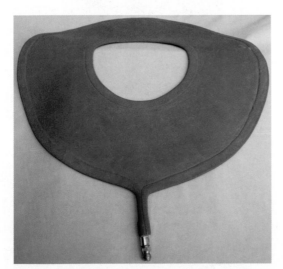

Fig. A-19. Invalid ring.

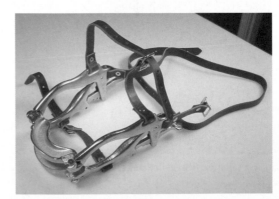

Fig. A-21. Meister oral speculum.

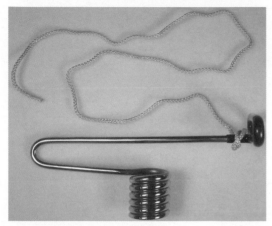

Fig. A-22. Schoupe oral speculum.

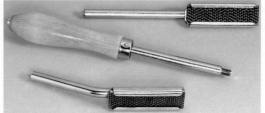

Fig. ... nt and angled bla... *Dental Floats*

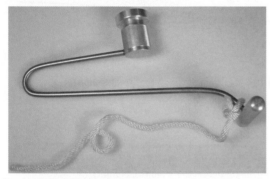

Fig. A-23. Meier's oral speculum.

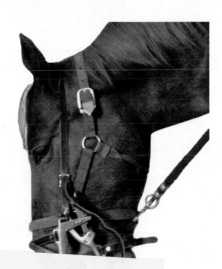

MºPerson Specium

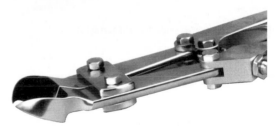

Fig. A-26. Equine double-action molar cutter (straight).

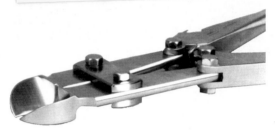

Fig. A-27. Equine double-action molar cutter (angled).

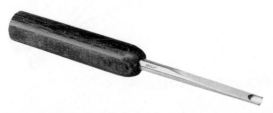

Fig. A-28. Wolf tooth elevator.

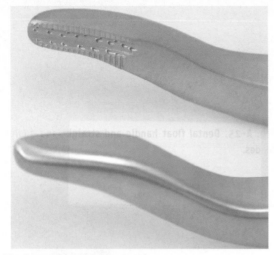

Fig. A-29. Universal extractor tip.

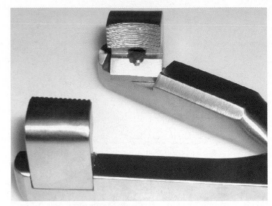

Fig. A-32. Cheek tooth tips.

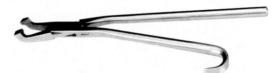

Fig. A-33. Premolar (Wolf tooth) extraction forceps.

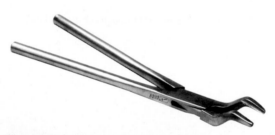

Fig. A-30. Universal smooth tooth extractor.

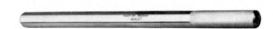

Fig. A-34. Dental tooth punch (straight).

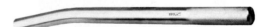

Fig. A-35. Dental tooth punch (angled).

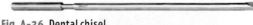

Fig. A-36. Dental chisel.

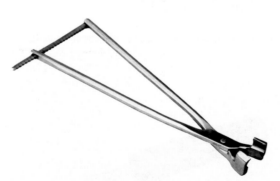

Fig. A-31. Cheek tooth extractor.

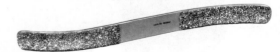

Fig. A-37. Curved dental rasp.

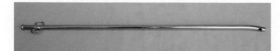

Fig. A-38. Chambers mare urinary catheter.

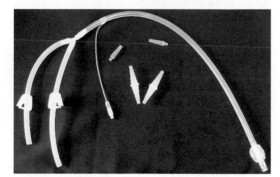

Fig. A-39. Uterine flushing catheter (dual channel).

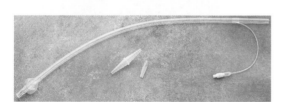

Fig. A-40. Uterine flushing catheter.

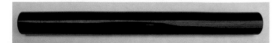

Fig. A-41. Mare vaginal speculum.

Fig. A-42. Tenotome knife.

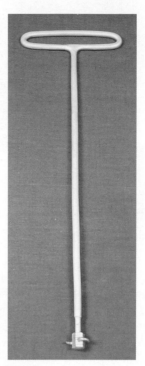

Fig. A-43. Roaring burr.

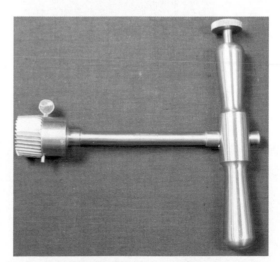

Fig. A-44. Trephine (Horsley's).

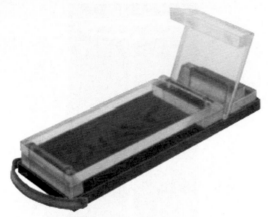

Fig. A-45. Radiographic hoof positioner.

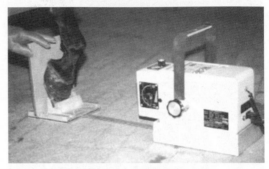

Fig. A-46. Radiographic hoof angle gauge.

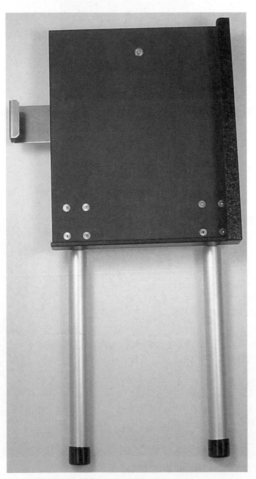

Fig. A-47. Radiographic cassette holder.

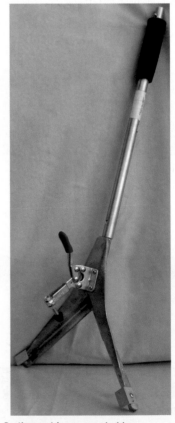

Fig. A-48. Radiographic cassette holder.

HOOF CARE INSTRUMENTS

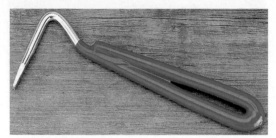

Fig. A-49. Hoof pick.

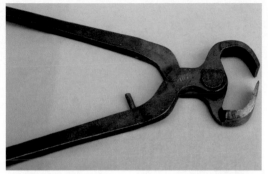

Fig. A-53. Hoof parer.

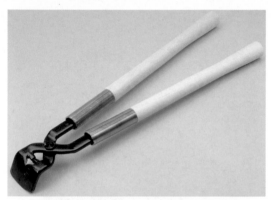

Fig. A-50. Long-handled hoof nipper.

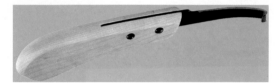

Fig. A-54. Hoof knife.

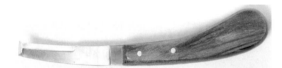

Fig. A-55. Hoof knife.

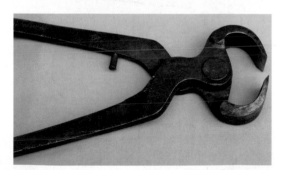

Fig. A-51. Hoof nipper.

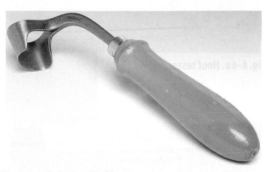

Fig. A-56. Swiss hoof knife.

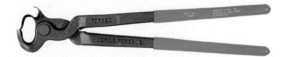

Fig. A-52. Hoof parer.

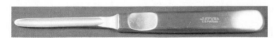

Fig. A-57. Hoof searcher.

Fig. A-58. Hughes hoof groover.

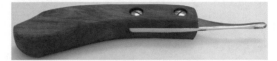

Fig. A-59. Hoof abscess knife.

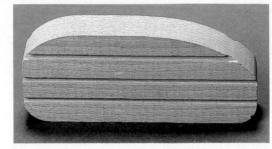

Fig. A-63. Ruminant hoof blocks (claw blocks).

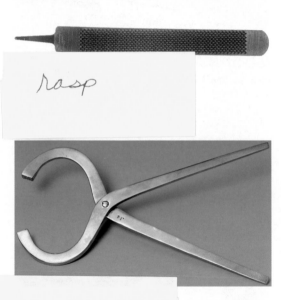

rasp

hoof tester

Fig. A-62. Clinch cutter.

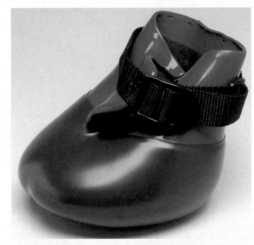

Fig. A-64. Cow boot.

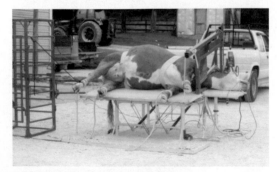

Fig. A-65. Cattle hoof trimming table.

LARGE ANIMAL CASTRATION INSTRUMENTS

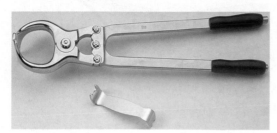

Fig. A-66. Burdizzo.

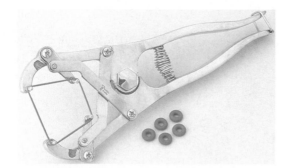

Fig. A-67. Elastrator.

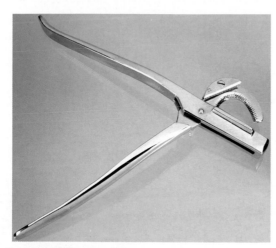

Fig. A-68. White emasculator.

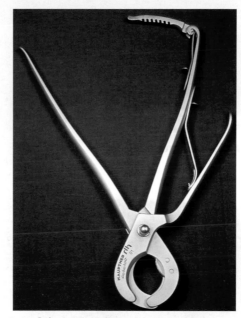

Fig. A-69. Reimer emasculator.

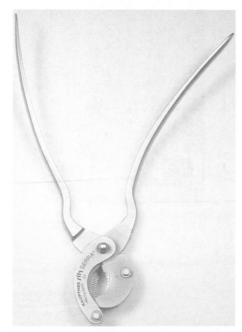

Fig. A-70. Serra emasculator.

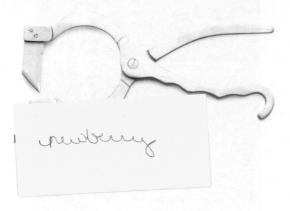

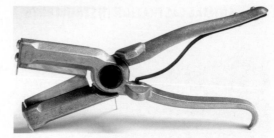

Fig. A-72. All-in-one castrator.

MISCELLANCEOUS ANESTHETIC EQUIPMENT

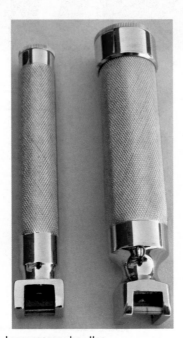

Fig. A-73. Laryngoscope handles.

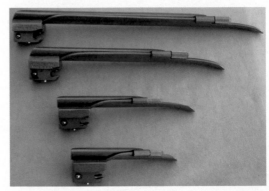

Fig. A-74. Miller laryngeal speculator (laryngoscope blades).

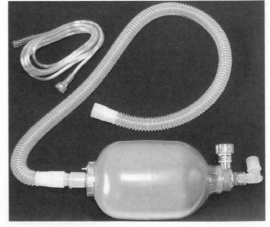

Fig. A-75. Ambu bag, large.

LARGE ANIMAL OBSTETRICAL INSTRUMENTS

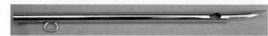

Fig. A-76. Cow urinary catheter.

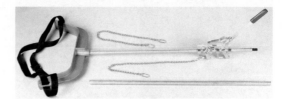

Fig. A-79. Fetal calf extractor (calf jack).

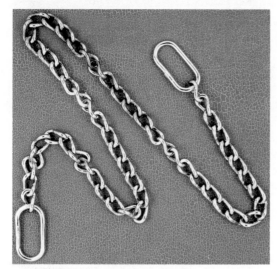

Fig. A-77. OB chains.

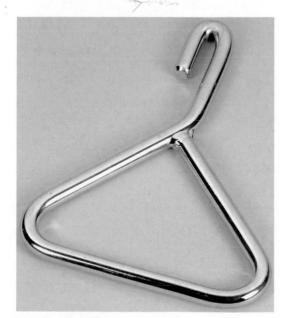

Fig. A-78. OB handles.

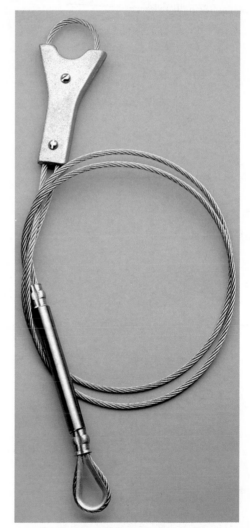

Fig. A-80. Obstetrical calf snare.

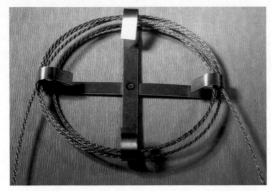

Fig. A-81. OB (Gigli's) wire.

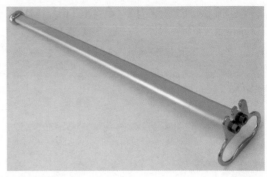

Fig. A-84. Fetatome.

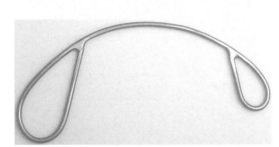

Fig. A-82. OB wire guide.

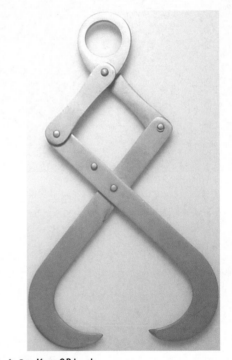

Fig. A-85. Krey OB hook.

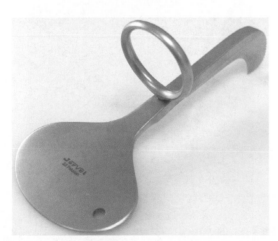

Fig. A-83. Fetotomy knife.

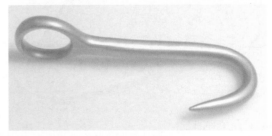

Fig. A-86. Ostertag's blunt eye hook.

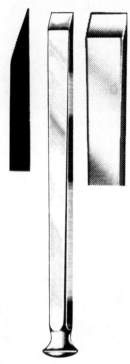

Fig. A-87. Pelvic chisel.

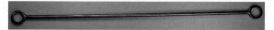

Fig. A-90. Cornell detorsion rod.

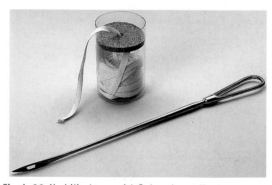

Fig. A-88. Umbilical tape with Buhner's needle.

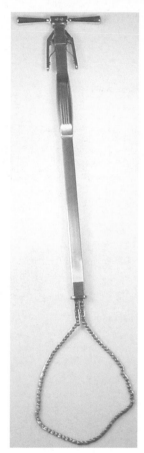

Fig. A-91. Chain écraseur.

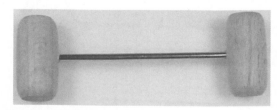

Fig. A-89. Vulva suture pins.

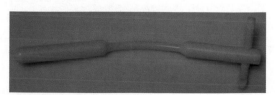

Fig. A-92. Freemartin probe.

Fig. A-93. Uterine cytology brush.

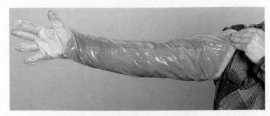

Fig. A-96. Obstetrical gloves.

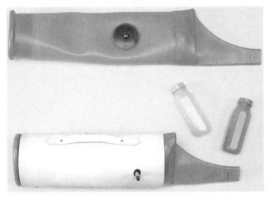

Fig. A-94. Artificial vagina.

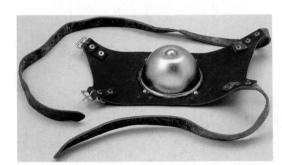

Fig. A-97. Heat mount detector (chin ball marker).

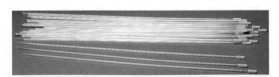

Fig. A-95. Insemination pipettes (uterine infusion pipettes).

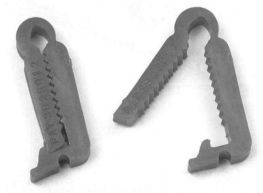

Fig. A-98. Umbilical hernia clamp.

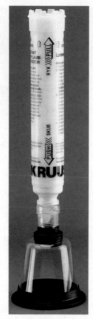

Fig. A-99. Calf, foal, lamb resuscitator.

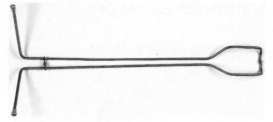

Fig. A-101. Pig OB forcep.

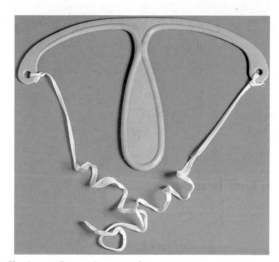

Fig. A-102. Ewe prolapse retainer.

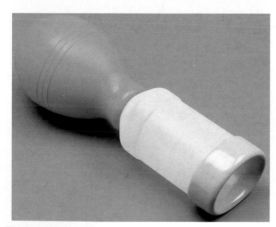

Fig. A-100. Pig resuscitator.

Fig. A-103. Lambing instrument.

IDENTIFICATION INSTRUMENTS

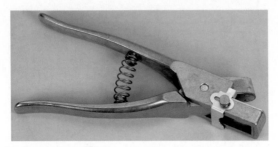

Fig. A-104. Ear notcher.

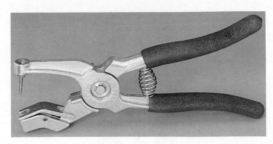

Fig. A-107. ID ear tag applicator.

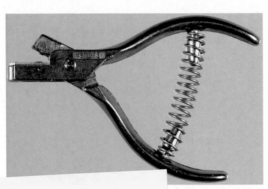

ear notcher

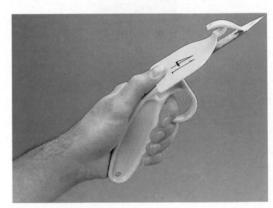

Fig. A-108. ID ear tag applicator.

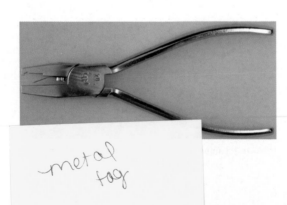

metal tag

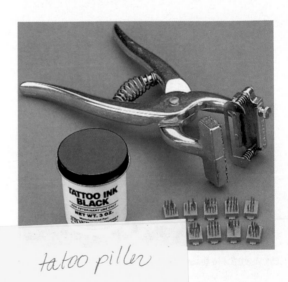

tatoo piller

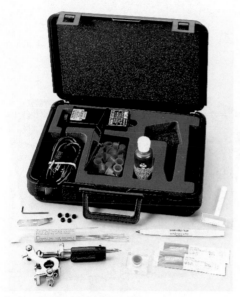

Fig. A-110. Tattoo outfit (electric).

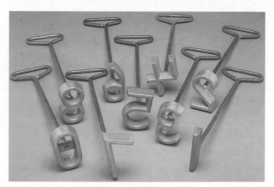

Fig. A-113. Copper freeze branding irons.

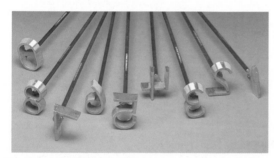

Fig. A-111. Hot branding irons.

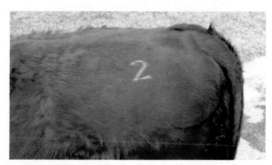

Fig. A-114. Freeze brand.

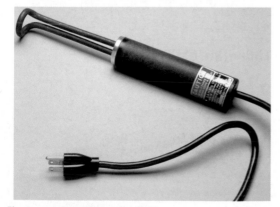

Fig. A-112. Electric branding iron.

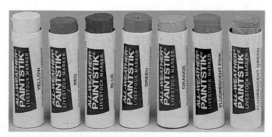

Fig. A-115. Marking chalk sticks.

DIAGNOSTIC INSTRUMENTS

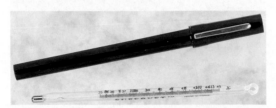

Fig. A-116. Ring-top thermometer for large animal with carrying case.

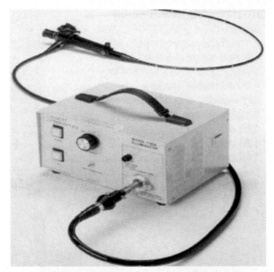

Fig. A-117. Flexible fiber endoscope and light source.

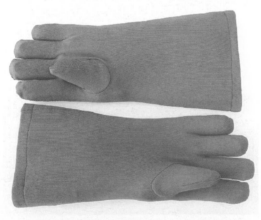

Fig. A-118. Protective lead gloves.

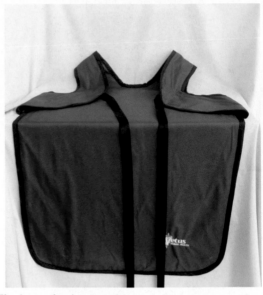

Fig. A-119. Lead x-ray apron.

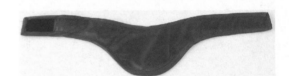

Fig. A-120. Lead thyroid collar.

DEHORNING INSTRUMENTS

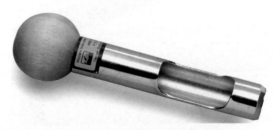

Fig. A-121. Horn gouge (tube dehorner or scoop).

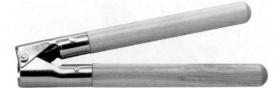

Fig. A-122. Barnes dehorner.

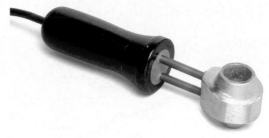

Fig. A-126. Electric dehorner.

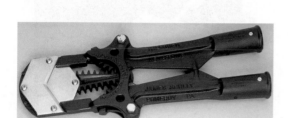

Fig. A-123. Keystone dehorner.

NEEDLE HOLDERS AND SCISSORS

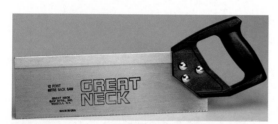

Fig. A-124. Dehorning saw.

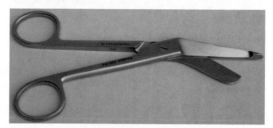

Fig. A-127. Lister bandage scissors.

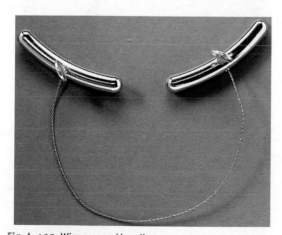

Fig. A-125. Wire saw and handles.

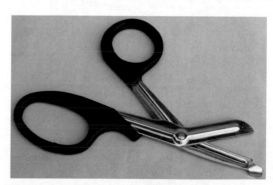

Fig. A-128. Economy utility bandage scissors.

BOVINE INSTRUMENTS

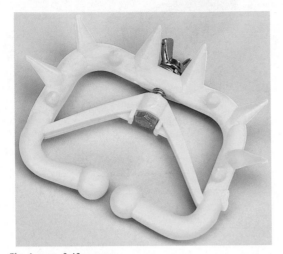

Fig. A-129. Calf weaner.

Fig. A-130. Lunge (buggy) whip.

Fig. A-131. Electric cattle prod.

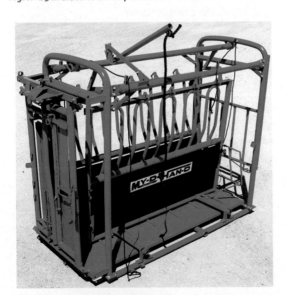

Fig. A-132. Cattle squeeze chute.

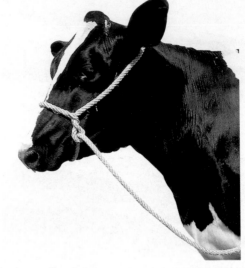

Fig. A-133. Rope halter.

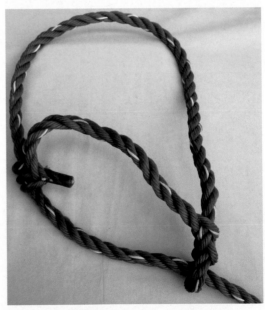

Fig. A-134. Rope halter.

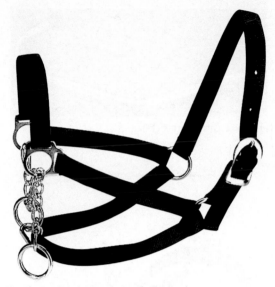

Fig. A-135. Fabric show halter (ruminant).

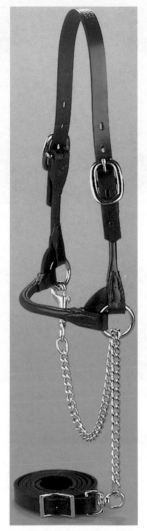

Fig. A-136. Leather show halter (ruminant).

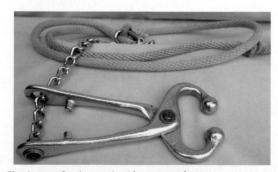

Fig. A-137. Cattle nose lead (nose tongs).

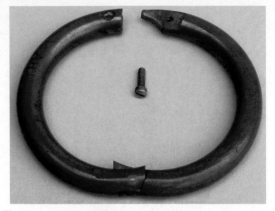

Fig. A-138. Bull nose ring.

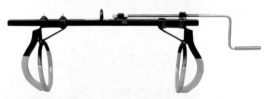

Quick release honda

Lariat

Fig. A-139. Lariet with quick release honda.

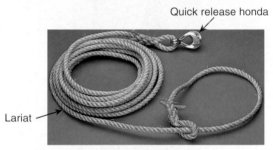

Fig. A-140. Hip lift.

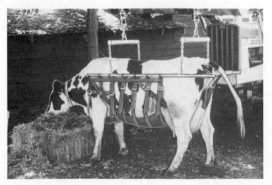

Fig. A-141. Cow sling.

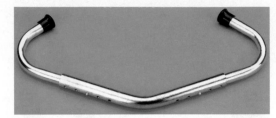

Fig. A-142. Cattle anti-kick bar.

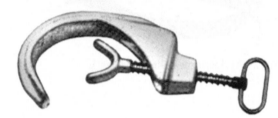

Fig. A-143. Achilles clamp (cattle).

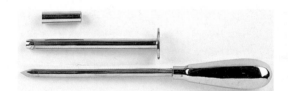

Fig. A-144. Trocar and cannula.

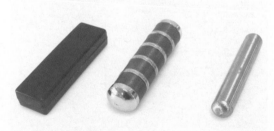

Fig. A-145. Rumen magnets.

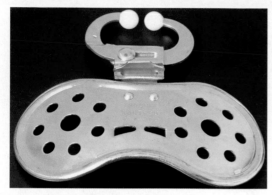

Fig. A-146. Kant suk weaner.

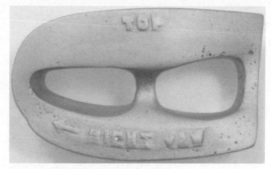

Fig. A-150. Drinkwater gag, right jaw.

INSTRUMENTS FOR ADMINISTRATION OF MEDICINE

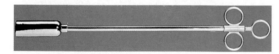

Fig. A-147. Balling gun.

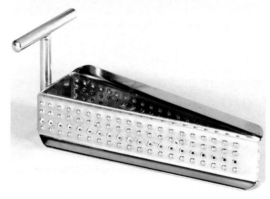

Fig. A-151. Bayer mouth wedge speculum (ramp speculum).

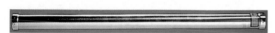

Fig. A-148. Frick speculum.

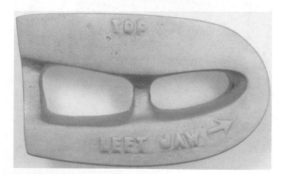

Fig. A-149. Drinkwater gag, left jaw.

Fig. A-152. 18-gauge spinal needle.

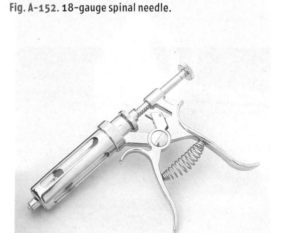

Fig. A-153. Automatic dose syringe.

Fig. A-154. 18-gauge swine bleeding needle.

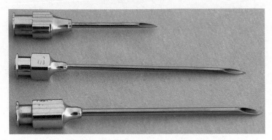

Fig. A-155. Stainless steel hypodermic needles.

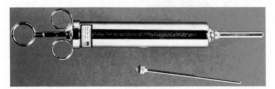

Fig. A-156. Stainless steel dose syringe and interchangeable nozzle.

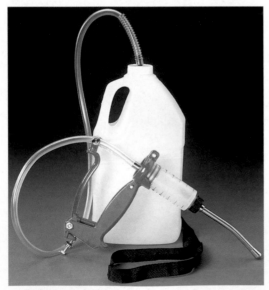

Fig. A-157. Drench matic dose syringe.

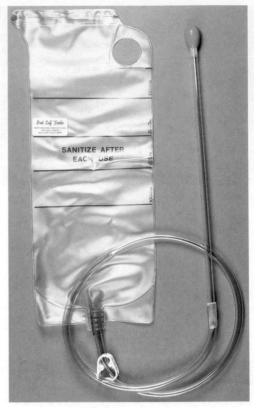

Fig. A-158. Oral calf drencher.

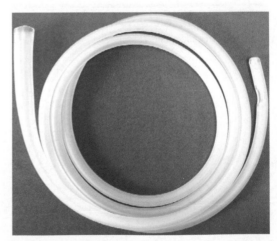

Fig. A-159. Large animal stomach tube.

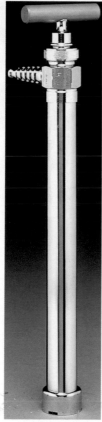

Fig. A-160. Stomach pump (drench pump).

CLIPPERS

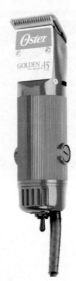

Fig. A-161. Animal clippers (electric).

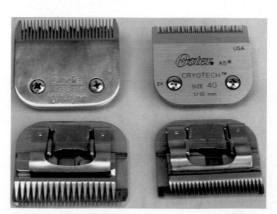

Fig. A-162. Clipper blades.

TUBES AND CATHETERS

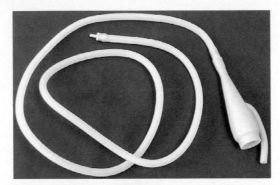

Fig. A-163. Bell IV set (simplex).

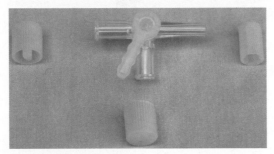

Fig. A-164. Three-way stopcock.

PIG, SHEEP, AND GOAT INSTRUMENTS

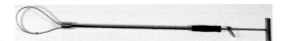

Fig. A-165. Hog snare (snout snare).

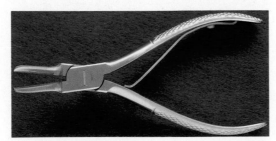

Fig. A-166. Pig tooth nipper.

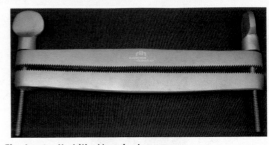

Fig. A-167. Umbilical hernia clamp.

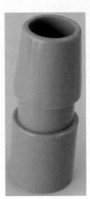

Fig. A-168. Rectal prolapse ring.

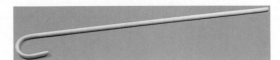

Fig. A-169. Sheep crook.

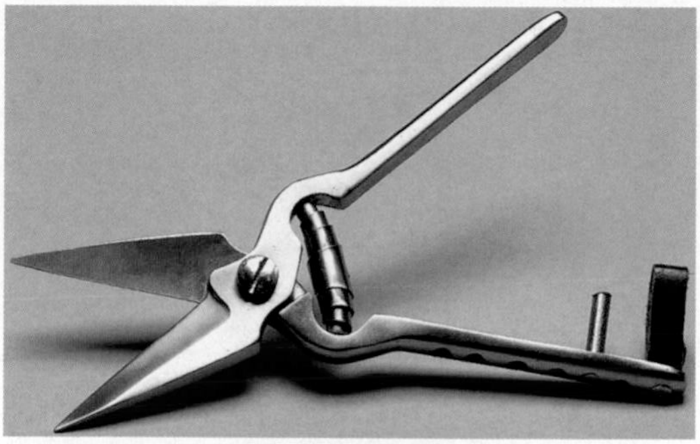

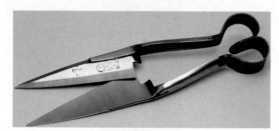

Fig. A-170. Hoof trimmer (sheep) (foot rot shears).

ORTHOPEDIC INSTRUMENTS

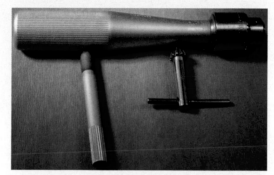

Fig. A-173. Pin chuck (Jacobs hand chuck).

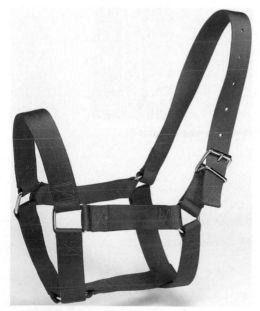

Fig. A-171. Sheep wool trimming shear.

Fig. A-172. Nylon halter (horse).

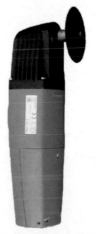

Fig. A-174. Cast cutter, electric (cast saw).

OPHTHALMIC INSTRUMENT

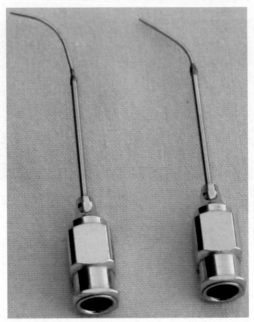

Fig. A-175. Lacrimal cannulas.

SURGICAL PACK INSTRUMENT

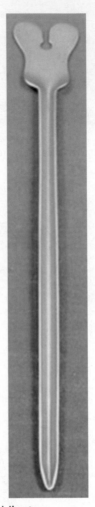

Fig. A-176. Grooved director.

Dental Formulas and Eruption Tables

EQUINE

DECIDUOUS

Dental Formula: 2(I 3/3 C 0/0 PM 3/3) = 24 Total

Eruption:		
	I1	Birth-1 wk
	I2	4-6 wk
	I3	6-9 mo
	C	—
	PM1	Birth-2 wk
	PM2	Birth-2 wk
	PM3	Birth-2 wk

PERMANENT

Dental Formula: 2(I 3/3 C 0-1/0-1* PM 3-4/3-4† M 3/3) = 36, 38, 40, or 42 Total

Eruption:		
	I1	$2\frac{1}{2}$ yr
	I2	$3\frac{1}{2}$ yr
	I3	$4\frac{1}{2}$ yr
	C*	4-5 yr
	PM1†	5-6 mo
	PM2 (first cheek tooth)	$2\frac{1}{2}$ yr
	PM3 (second cheek tooth)	3 yr (upper), $2\frac{1}{2}$-3 yr (lower)
	PM4 (third cheek tooth)	4 yr (upper), $3\frac{1}{2}$-4 yr (lower)
	M1 (fourth cheek tooth)	9-12 mo
	M2 (fifth cheek tooth)	2 yr
	M3 (sixth cheek tooth)	$3\frac{1}{2}$-4 yr

*Canines in the female are usually absent or very small and seldom erupt.
†Premolar 1 (wolf teeth) are frequently absent or fail to erupt. Lower PM1 is very unusual. Gender does not affect presence of wolf teeth.

BOVINE

DECIDUOUS

Dental Formula: 2(I 0/3 C 0/1* PM 3/3) = 20 Total

Eruption:	I1	Birth-2 wk
	I2	Birth-2 wk
	I3	Birth-2 wk
	C	Birth-2 wk
	PM2 (first cheek tooth)	Birth-2 wk
	PM3 (second cheek tooth)	Birth-1 wk
	PM4 (third cheek tooth)	Birth-1 wk

PERMANENT

Dental Formula: 2(I 0/3 C 0/1* PM 3/3 M 3/3) = 32 Total

Eruption:	I1	$1\frac{1}{2}$-2 yr
	I2	2-$2\frac{1}{2}$ yr
	I3	3-$3\frac{1}{2}$ yr
	C	$3\frac{1}{2}$-4 yr
	PM2 (first cheek tooth)	2-$2\frac{1}{2}$ yr
	PM3 (second cheek tooth)	$1\frac{1}{2}$-$2\frac{1}{2}$ yr
	PM4 (third cheek tooth)	$2\frac{1}{2}$-3 yr
	M1 (fourth cheek tooth)	5-6 mo
	M2 (fifth cheek tooth)	1-$1\frac{1}{2}$ yr
	M3 (sixth cheek tooth)	2-$2\frac{1}{2}$ yr

The canine tooth is in line with the incisors and adjacent to them and is shaped like an incisor, giving the false appearance of 4 incisors; however, it is common practice to refer to the canine tooth as the fourth incisor (I4).

PORCINE

DECIDUOUS

Dental Formula: 2(I 3/3 C 1/1 PM 3/3) = 28 Total

Eruption:	I1	1-3 wk
	I2	$1\frac{1}{2}$-2 mo lower, 2-3 mo upper
	I3	Birth
	C	Birth
	PM2	1-2 mo
	PM3	First month
	PM4	First month

PERMANENT

Dental Formula: 2(I 3/3 C 1/1 PM 4/4 M 3/3) = 44 Total

Eruption:		
	I1	12-17 mo
	I2	16-20 mo
	I3	8-10 mo
	C	8-12 mo
	PM1	5 mo
	PM2	12-16 mo
	PM3	12-16 mo
	PM4	12-16 mo
	M1	4-6 mo
	M2	8-12 mo
	M3	18-20 mo

CAPRINE AND OVINE

DECIDUOUS

Dental Formula: 2(I 0/3 C 0/1* PM 3/3) = 20 Total

Eruption:		
	I1	Birth-1 wk
	I2	Birth-1 wk
	I3	Birth-1 wk
	C	1-3 wk
	PM2	Birth-4 wk
	PM3	Birth-4 wk
	PM4	Birth-4 wk

PERMANENT

Dental Formula: 2(I 0/3 C 0/1* PM 3/3 M 3/3) = 32 Total

Eruption:		
	I1	12-18 mo
	I2	18-24 mo
	I3	30-36 mo
	C	36-48 mo
	PM2	18-24 mo
	PM3	18-24 mo
	PM4	18-24 mo
	M1	3-4 mo
	M2	8-10 mo
	M3	18-24 mo

*The canine tooth is in line with the incisors and adjacent to them and is shaped like an incisor, giving the false appearance of 4 incisors; however, it is common practice to refer to the canine tooth as the fourth incisor (I4).

Glossary: Large Animals in Layman's Terms

Terminology varies depending on geographical location, species and breed of animal, and age of the person using the term.

A

agroceryosis
Starvation; deprived of adequate food.

all-in, all-out
System of hog production in which pigs are managed by grouping them into farrowing, nursery, and growing/finishing groups. Each group is housed in a different facility, which is thoroughly cleaned and disinfected when the group moves out. Used to control many swine diseases.

angel berries
Warts.

B

bad flap
Horse with laryngeal hemiplegia.

bag
Udder.

bagging up
Enlargement of the udder with milk before parturition.

ball
Give a tablet or bolus per os.

bandage bow
Tendon or ligament damage to the distal limb from improperly fitting bandage.

bandy legged
Horse that is pigeon-toed on the hindlegs; the points of the hocks turn outward.

Bang's disease
Brucellosis (*Brucella abortus*) in cattle; named for Danish veterinarian Fredrick Bang, who discovered the bacterium in 1897.

bangtail
Horse with the tail hairs cut off horizontally at the level of the hocks.

barren mare
Mare that has never conceived or carried a foal to term.

bat
Jockey's whip.

beans
Rounded, firm accumulations of smegma in the urethral recess of the glans penis of the horse.

belly tap
Abdominocentesis.

bike
Two-wheeled cart pulled by harness racing horses.

bishoping
Altering the natural characteristics of the incisor teeth of a horse with files, drills, hot irons, or silver nitrate to make the horse appear younger than it really is. This fraudulent practice is used to pass older animals off as being younger, thus enhancing the possibility of a sale.

black teeth
Another name for the needle teeth of piglets.

bleeder
Horse with exercise-induced pulmonary hemorrhage (EIPH); bleeding occurs in the small airways of the lungs during hard exercise. In a small percentage, bleeding may be severe enough that blood from the lungs appears at the nostrils following hard exercise.

blemish
Any defect that does not affect the intended use of an animal.

blind quarter/half
A quarter or half of a mammary gland that is not producing milk when the other quarters are lactating.

blind spavin
Hock lameness in the horse, without physical or radiographic evidence. Usually considered an early stage of bone spavin. Also called "occult spavin."

blind teat
A quarter obviously full of milk that cannot be expressed from the teat orifice, and a teat cannula cannot be passed up into the teat cistern. May occur by blockage from infection, trauma, or congenital defect.

blister
A strong chemical vesicant, historically applied to the skin over a leg injury in hopes of stimulating healing and preventing reinjury. A form of counterirritation.

bog spavin
Effusion of the tibiotarsal joint of the hock.

bone spavin
A form of hock (tarsus) lameness in the horse due to arthritis of the distal intertarsal and/or tarsometatarsal joints. Also called "jack spavin."

bottom line
The dam's side of a pedigree.

bowed tendon
Inflammation of a tendon; usually refers specifically to tendinitis of the superficial and/or deep digital flexor tendons of the lower leg of the horse.

breaking water
Rupture of the chorioallantoic membrane with release of chorioallantoic fluid; signals the onset of the second stage of labor.

breeze
In racehorse training, a workout at less than maximal speed.

broken mouth
Aged ruminant that has lost some, but not all, of its incisors.

broken penis
Hematoma of the penis.

bucked shins
Inflammation of the periosteum (periostitis) on the dorsal aspect of the third metacarpal bone, often with swelling and lameness; it is a repetitive bone stress injury, most commonly seen in young horses in the early phases of race training.

buller
Nymphomaniac cow that mounts other cattle, or a steer that allows other steers to mount.

bummer lamb
Orphan lamb being raised by hand or by a foster ewe; it is "bumming" milk from other sources.

bunches
Subcutaneous abscesses.

burro
Synonym for donkey *(equus asinus)*; term used more in Western United States.

bussled pig
Pig with a scrotal hernia.

by
Referring to the male parent of an animal.

C

calf bed out
Prolapsed uterus.

capped elbow
Inflammation of the olecranon bursa, over the point of the elbow.

capped hock
Inflammation of the calcaneal bursa, over the point of the hock.

caps
Deciduous cheek teeth of the horse; they are normally shed when the permanent teeth erupt but occasionally are retained and require removal.

cast in stall
Animal that is positioned awkwardly in a stall or pen and cannot get to its feet.

catch
Indicates successful conception after breeding.

caveson
Noseband on a bridle.

chevon
Goat meat.

cheek teeth
The premolars and molars.

chest tap
Thoracocentesis.

choke
Obstruction of the esophagus.

claws
Digits on a cloven hoof.

clean up (a female)
Examine and lavage the uterus after giving birth, or treat uterine infection.

cod
Scrotum of a steer.

cold-backed
Horse that resents tightening of the girth or cinch during placement of the saddle.

coldblood
Horse without Arabian blood or other "desert breeds" in the pedigree; horses descended from the colder climate of Europe. Generally refers to the draft horse breeds and some pony breeds of European descent.

cold shoeing
Fitting and shaping a horseshoe without use of heat.

coon-footed
Horse with a long pastern, long toe, and low heel.

corded leg
Damaged tendons/ligaments of the leg, resulting from an improperly applied or maintained bandage.

corded vein
Thickened vein, often due to thrombus formation.

corded-up
Myositis of the hindquarters with stiffness of the hindlimbs; otherwise known as "tying-up" or "tied-up."

corkscrew claw
An elongated claw that grows with rotation around its long axis, producing a rolled-under appearance; usually affects the lateral claw on the hindfeet of cattle.

corns
Bruising of a horse's hoof in the area of the bars.

covering a mare
Natural breeding or "servicing" of a female horse.

cow-hocked
Horse with the points of the hocks turned inward (medially) instead of facing directly behind the horse.

cribbing
Aerophagia; vice of horses where the horse swallows air through the mouth, usually while grasping a solid object with its incisors; produces a distinct audible noise.

crippled orchid
Mispronunciation of "cryptorchid."

crutching
Shearing the wool from the perineal region of sheep.

curb
Inflammation of the plantar ligament, on the caudal aspect of the calcaneus. Horses with sickle-hocks are predisposed to developing curbs and are referred to as "curby." Cow-hocked horses are also predisposed.

cut
Castrate.

D

dancing pig disease
Congenital tremor syndrome (Myoclonia congenita) of piglets. Characterized by severe muscle tremors when awake; disappears when asleep.

diamond skin disease
Swine erysipelas *(Erysipelothrix rhusiopathiae)*; produces discolored diamond-shaped blotches of the skin over the back area.

dirty mare
Mare with a uterine infection.

distemper (equine)
Strangles in horses *(Streptococcus equi)*; an upper respiratory disease characterized by purulent nasal discharge and abscessed lymph nodes in the head and throat region.

dingleberries
Dried accumulations of feces on the hair, wool, or skin.

dishrag foal
Limp, very weak, or comatose foal.

drench
Administer liquids or liquid medications by mouth.

drops
Newborn lambs.

dry
Not lactating.

dummy
Animal with abnormal mentation or stuporous behavior; does not respond to normal stimuli.

E

easy keeper
Animal that maintains its bodyweight or gains weight on less feed than other animals in similar conditions.

eruption bumps
Firm, temporary enlargements along the ventral border of the mandible, corresponding with eruption of permanent cheek teeth in horses 2 to 4 years old. Caused by remodeling of the mandible to accommodate the developing roots of the cheek teeth; as the teeth erupt and advance, the bone remodels and removes the "bumps."

ewe-necked
Horse with a neck that has a slightly concave topline (like a ewe) when viewed from the side; the neck appears to attach low on the chest.

exciter ram
Vasectomized ram that is turned out with a flock of ewes just before breeding season, to help "bring out" females with silent estrous cycles.

F

facing
Clipping the wool from the face and eyes of a sheep, to prevent wool-blindness.

far side
Right side of a horse; also known as "off side."

farrier
Person who trims and shoes horse's hooves; preferred term to blacksmith. May complete certification courses and examinations administered by the American Farriers Association (AFA).

fistulous withers
Chronic suppurative inflammation of the supraspinous bursa in horses, due to infection.

flanking
A method of throwing a calf to the ground by reaching across its back and grabbing the skin fold of the flank, and using it to lift the animal off its feet.

flaps
Arytenoid cartilages.

fleece rot
Dermatitis of sheep caused by prolonged wetness of the skin; open sores develop, and exudates form crusts and mat the wool.

flushing
Nutritional practice of increasing a female's intake of protein and/or carbohydrates just before breeding, to improve ovulation and conception rates in ruminants and swine.

founder
Chronic laminitis, with displacement of P3 from its normal position within the hoof. Clients often use the term to refer to any case of laminitis, acute or chronic.

flounder
Common mispronunciation of "founder."

freeze firing
Practice of applying liquid nitrogen to the skin overlying an injured tendon, ligament, or bone. Used on the legs of horses with

the belief that healing of the treated injury will be faster and of better quality. A form of counterirritation.

freshening
Calving.

fresh
Recently calved.

full mouth
Ruminant or horse with all permanent teeth present.

furlong
$\frac{1}{8}$ mile = 740 ft = 201.17 m.

G

gall
Saddle or girth sore in horses.

garget
Mastitis.

gare
Long, noncrimped wool fibers that are unsuitable for spinning or dying.

gaskin
Region of a horse's hind leg between the hock and stifle.

get
The offspring of a male animal; progeny.

gill flirt
Mare with a recto-vaginal tear; usually results from laceration of the vaginal roof and rectal floor by the hoof of the fetus during delivery.

girth
Heavy rope or leather strap that holds the saddle on a horse by circling the thorax.

glass eye
Blue iris.

gomer bull
Teaser bull, surgically prepared by vasectomy and/or penile deviation to prevent impregnation of females. Gomer bulls are used to detect females in standing heat.

grass staggers
Hypomagnesemia of ruminants.

grass tetany
Hypomagnesemia of ruminants.

gravel
Purulent material or abscess in the hoof, which "migrates" proximally and ruptures and drains at the coronary band.

grease heel
Moist exudative dermatitis of the pastern/fetlock region in the horse, generally from excessive moisture. Also known as "scratches."

green
Inexperienced animal (or human).

gummer
Animal with no teeth/ruminant with no incisors; a sign of aging.

H

hand
Measurement of equine height; equal to 4 inches.

hard keeper
Animal that requires more feed to maintain its bodyweight than other animals kept under similar conditions.

hard milker
Teat with constriction at the teat orifice that makes it difficult, but not impossible, to express milk; often affects all teats.

hardware
Metallic foreign bodies in the reticulum of ruminants; they may puncture the wall of the reticulum and penetrate the diaphragm and pericardium, causing hardware disease (traumatic reticuloperitonitis).

hay flake
A small section of a hay bale. During the baling process, the baling machine divides the bale into small, regular, pressed portions. On average, one flake is 2 to 4 inches wide and weighs approximately 3 to 4 lb. Also known as a "wafer."

head shy
Animal that is sensitive to movements around the head and often tries to avoid contact in the head area.

heaves
Equine respiratory condition characterized by difficult, labored breathing with a marked abdominal component on expiration. May lead to hypertrophy of abdominal muscle (external abdominal oblique m.) and formation of a noticeable ridge of musculature ("heave line") from the flank forward to the elbow. Caused by chronic airway disease, usually from a chronic hypersensitivity response to environmental allergens such as dust, mold, and grasses. Sometimes incorrectly referred to as asthma.

high flanker
Testicle retained near the body wall, "high" in the inguinal area, and not descended into the scrotum.

high trough fever
Starvation; lack of adequate nutrition.

hinny
Hybrid resulting from crossing a stallion *(equus caballus)* with a jennet *(equus asinus)*; a rare type of mule.

hogget
Young sheep between weaning and the first shearing.

hook bone
Hip bone; tuber coxae.

hotblood
Horse with a pedigree tracing primarily to the "desert breeds" of Northern Africa and the Mediterranean. Includes the Arabian, the Barb, and breeds primarily descended from them, such as Thoroughbred, Standardbred, Quarter Horse, and Tennessee Walking Horse.

hothouse lambs
Lambs born out of season in the fall or early winter so that they can be marketed between Christmas and May, a time of peak ethnic demand for lamb meat.

J

jack
Male donkey *(Equus asinus)*.

jack
One of the two tendons of insertion of the cranial tibial muscle of the horse. The tendon inserts on the medial aspect of the hock and is sometimes cut as a treatment for bone spavin.

jack spavin
Bone spavin.

jennet
Female donkey *(Equus asinus);* also called a jenny.

jog cart
Two-wheeled exercise cart pulled by harness racing horses.

joint ill
Joint infection.

joint tap
Arthrocentesis.

jug
Lambing pen, where ewe and her lambs are kept for several days.

jugging
Administering a solution of various components (electrolytes, amino acids, vitamins, hormones, carbohydrates, etc.) intravenously via the jugular vein. Usually given to horses before a race or other sporting event in the hopes of improving performance.

K

knocked-down hip
Fracture of the point of the hip (tuber coxae), with displacement of the fractured fragment, which usually displaces ventrally.

L

lunge (longe)
Method of exercising horses in a circle. An approximately 30-foot rope or lead ("lunge line") is attached to the horse's head, and the horse is asked to walk, trot, or canter in circles around the handler. Used to train, exercise, and examine horses.

lunger
Animal with a chronic respiratory disease.

M

mad itch
Pseudorabies; a herpesvirus disease of swine with respiratory, nervous, and reproductive signs. Ruminants may occasionally be affected.

magpies
Cattle with evidence of Holstein breeding (black and white coloring).

maiden
Horse that has never won a race.

maiden mare
Female horse that has never become pregnant.

mathematician
Lame animal; "puts down 3 and carries 1."

milkshaking
Procedure of giving a solution of bicarbonate, carbohydrates, and other additives to a horse via nasogastric tube, before a race or other athletic event, to reduce fatigue and improve performance during the event. Illegal practice in most racing jurisdictions.

milk teeth
Deciduous (baby) teeth.

moon blindness
Periodic ophthalmia (recurrent anterior uveitis) in horses.

Monday morning disease
Exertional rhabdomyolysis syndrome of horses. The name originated in draft horses that were exercised Monday through Saturday and then rested on Sunday; occasionally, on the following Monday morning, the animal was stiff and reluctant to move and had palpable hardening of the rump muscles (especially the gluteals).

mother up
Process of a dam bonding with its newborn or reuniting with it after a brief separation.

mouthing
Aging an animal by its teeth.

mule
Hybrid resulting from crossing a mare *(equus caballus)* with a jack *(equus asinus)*.

muley cattle
Polled (hornless) cattle.

N

navel ill
Infection of the umbilicus in young animals.

near side
Left side of a horse, from which they are handled.

needle teeth
Deciduous upper and lower third incisors (I3) and deciduous canine teeth in the newborn piglet; they are routinely clipped to remove the sharp tips, to prevent damage to the sow's teats and to other piglets.

nerved
Horse that has had posterior digital neurectomy surgery for treatment of chronic pain in the heel region of the hoof.

nose hose
Nasogastric tube.

O

offal
The organs (viscera) removed from a carcass at slaughter.

on one line
Harness-racing horse carrying its head preferentially to one side, usually in response to lameness, especially of a hindlimb (will usually carry its head toward the side with the hindlimb lameness).

on one shaft
Hindlimb lameness in harness-racing horses often causes the horse to carry its hindquarters to the opposite side of the lameness, sometimes touching the shaft ("on the shaft") of the sulky or jog cart.

open
Not pregnant.

open knees
Incomplete ossification of the distal radial physis (growth plate), as confirmed by an x-ray. When ossification is complete (closed knees), it is an indication of skeletal maturity. Many trainers will not place a young animal in hard training until an x-ray confirms that the knees have "closed."

open up a mare
Release the scar tissue formed by Caslick's surgery, before parturition, so the mare's vulva is not torn during delivery of the foal.

original
A cryptorchid horse.

osselets
Chronic inflammation of the fetlock joint and joint capsule, noticed primarily as thickening of the dorsal aspect of the fetlock. Referred to as "green osselets" in the acute stage of inflammation, before the joint capsule has thickened.

out of
Mothered by; referring to the female parent of an animal.

out of Oklahoma, by truck
Horse of questionable breeding. Also, a stolen horse.

P

parrot mouth
Brachygnathia; overbite; the incisors fail to meet and occlude properly.

piggy
Sow due to farrow soon.

pig mouth
Prognathia; underbite of the incisors. Also known as sow mouth, monkey mouth.

pin bone
Ischiatic tuberosity.

pin firing
Thermocautery applied to the skin over an injured tendon, bone, or joint in hopes of stimulating faster and higher-quality healing. It is applied with a heated "firing iron" in a regular pattern across the skin, leaving small focal scars. Used historically. Any beneficial effects are now attributed to the period of rest that was prescribed after the firing was performed, rather than to the firing itself. A form of counterirritation.

pizzle
Penis of a male ruminant. Sometimes used to indicate only the urethral process of the ruminant penis.

pony
Horse measuring less than or equal to 14.2 hands at the withers.

pony
Method of exercising a horse or calming a nervous horse by having a calm, well-trained horse or pony accompany it closely; usually the "pony" rider has a lead rope attached to the head of the other horse, which may or may not have a rider.

popped a splint
Acute inflammation and swelling of the periosteum of a splint bone (metacarpal [MC2 or 4] or metatarsal [MT2 or 4]) in the horse, or the ligament that attaches the splint bone to the adjacent cannon bone.

popped knee
Carpitis; synovitis and capsulitis of one or more carpal joints.

pouches
Guttural pouches of the horse.

proud cut
Stallionlike behavior in a horse that has been castrated. Often (incorrectly) blamed on "incomplete" castration that failed to remove all of the epididymis or spermatic cord; however, neither of these tissues produce testosterone.

proud flesh
Exuberant granulation (scar) tissue; usually affects healing wounds on the legs of horses.

Q

quidding
Dropping feed while chewing; often indicates poor mastication from dental abnormalities.

R

ranting
Behavior of an agitated boar; nervousness, frothing at the mouth, and chomping.

red nose
Infectious bovine rhinotracheitis (IBR) of cattle; produces noticeable hyperemia of the

nasal mucosa. Highly contagious herpesvirus respiratory disease.

reefing
Circumcision, sometimes necessary to treat lesions or malignancies of the glans penis.

rig
Cryptorchid horse. Also known as "false rig."

ridgling
Cryptorchid horse or other animal.

ringing
Placing nose rings in bulls (for handling and restraint) or in swine (to prevent rooting by pigs housed on dirt or pasture).

roached mane
Practice of clipping away the entire mane, or clipping the mane so short that it stands erect.

roarer
Horse that makes a respiratory noise (stertor) during exercise; usually refers to a horse affected with laryngeal hemiplegia or paralysis that makes a characteristic "roaring" noise during inspiration.

rundowns
A type of equine leg bandage.

rupture
Hernia.

S

scissor claws
Excessive growth of one or both claws on a ruminant's foot, such that they overlap like scissors.

scope (throat, joint, etc.)
Use an endoscope or arthroscope.

scours
Diarrhea, usually refers to young animals.

scratches
Moist exudative dermatitis of the lower legs of horses, especially on the back of the pastern. Lesions (open sores, scabs, cracking of the skin) are painful and often accompanied by regional swelling and lameness. Usually due to excessive moisture conditions (mud, wet pasture, wet bedding) around the horse's lower legs and feet. Also known as grease heel, mud fever.

scur, scurl
Misshapen horn, usually from incomplete dehorning or disbudding.

seedy toe
Separation of the hoof wall and sole at the white line of the toe in horses with chronic laminitis; characterized by a widened, weak white line that often allows infection to develop in the lamina of the front of the hoof.

service
Breeding of a female by a male.

settled
Successfully bred and conceived.

sew up/stitch up a mare
Perform Caslick's surgery.

shipping fever
Acute respiratory disease that affects animals after transportation; may involve several factors, especially stress.

shoe boil
Olecranon bursitis in the horse; most often caused by repeated hitting of the elbow with the hoof during motion or trauma from

laying down in sternal recumbency (also known as "capped elbow").

shower-in, shower-out
Method of disease control on swine farms. Personnel entering the facility must remove all clothing, shower completely, and dress in clean clothing. The process is repeated before leaving the facility.

shying
Unexpected movement of an animal away from a source of pain or fear.

sickle-hocked
Conformation fault of the horse; the hocks appear to have too much angulation (flexion) when viewed from the side.

sinker
Horse with laminitis, in which distal displacement of the distal phalanx (P3) has occurred. P3 may actually protrude from the bottom of the hoof.

sitfast
Necrosis that often extends into the fatty tissue of the crest of the neck in draft horses, from trauma by the harness collar.

slipped
Aborted.

smooth mouth
Old animal with teeth worn nearly to the gumline.

snots
Nasal discharge.

sorting
Process of going through a herd and separating animals into groups.

sour
Horse with a bad attitude or apparent boredom; may resist certain circumstances or perform without enthusiasm, such as in a riding ring (ring sour) or on a racetrack (track sour). May occur when there is little variation in the animal's daily schedule.

splint
Inflammation and/or exostosis of the small metacarpal (MC2 or 4) or metatarsal (MT2 or 4) bones in the horse.

split tail
A female animal.

springer
First-calf heifer in the latter stages of gestation.

stifled
Horse with upward fixation of the patella.

stocking up
Enlargement (swelling) of the legs with subcutaneous edema; common in the distal limbs of horses.

street nail surgery
Surgery for treatment of an infected navicular bursa or bone, usually resulting from a deep puncture wound to the caudal aspect of the bottom of the hoof.

stringy
Horse with stringhalt, an involuntary hyperflexion of the hock when the horse is in motion, producing a characteristic jerking of the hindleg toward the abdomen.

suint
The perspiration of sheep; the contents are water soluble.

sulky
Two-wheeled racing cart pulled by harness racing horses.

summer sore
Open skin lesion complicated by the presence of the larvae of *Habronema* spp.; habronemiasis.

sweeney
Injury to the suprascapular nerve in horses, usually from blunt trauma to the front of the shoulder/scapula region, or chronic trauma from harness collars. Produces a characteristic gait with lateral instability of the shoulder joint.

sweet itch
Pruritic skin disease of horses, caused by hypersensitivity to the bites of *Culicoides* spp.

switch
Distal part of the bovine tail that bears longer hairs than the body of the tail.

switch
"Fake" tail used in horses by harvesting tail hairs from other horses of similar color and binding them together at one end; the switch is taped or braided into the recipient horse's natural tail to make it appear fuller and/or longer.

T

tack
The equipment worn by a horse for riding (e.g., saddle, bridle, martingale).

tagging
Shearing the wool from the perineal area and udder of a ewe, before lambing. Also, shearing the perineal area before shearing, or in animals with diarrhea.

teased in
Positive response to teasing; female is in heat.

teasing
Method of observing signs of estrus in a female horse by exposing her to limited physical or visual contact with a male horse. Used to assess readiness for breeding of the female.

teg
A 2-year-old sheep.

three-titter
Cow with a nonfunctional teat.

tie-back
Equine surgical procedure to treat laryngeal hemiplegia by suturing the affected arytenoid cartilage in an abducted position, away from the lumen of the larynx. Also known as "roaring surgery."

tongue tie
Practice of tying a horse's tongue in position by circling the tongue and mandible one to two times with roll gauze or string. Done to prevent dorsal displacement of the soft palate during a race by preventing caudal movement of the tongue during swallowing; it is placed just before a race and removed as soon as the race is over. Also called a "tie down."

traces
Long straps, usually leather, that attach a horse's harness to the shafts of a two- or four-wheeled cart, buggy, or wagon; the traces provide the connection and traction for pulling the vehicle.

trailer
Portion of the branch of a horseshoe that extends caudally behind the hoof; used to correct abnormal landing of the hind hooves in some horses. Difficult to use successfully

on front hooves because they are likely to be stepped on with the toes of the hind feet, pulling off the shoe.

trots
Diarrhea.

tucked-up
Standing with the back rounded and having a seemingly compact abdomen (greyhound-like); often indicates abdominal discomfort or, less frequently, musculoskeletal pain.

tup
Ram.

tusks
Permanent canine teeth of swine; very prominent in boars.

twin lamb disease
Pregnancy ketosis in sheep.

tying-up
General term for stiffness and reluctance to move the hindlimbs, usually with palpable hardening of the gluteal muscles. Caused by exertional rhabdomyolysis syndrome, a condition with several clinical manifestations and probably a multifactorial etiology.

U

unsoundness
Any defect that prevents an animal from achieving its intended use.

V

vernacular disease
Mispronunciation of "navicular disease."

vice
Objectionable or bad habit, often detrimental to the animal or destructive to its environment. Higher incidence in animals kept in confinement.

W

warmblood
Horse obtained by breeding a coldblood to a hotblooded horse; horses with mixed coldblood and hotblood bloodlines.

water belly
Ruptured bladder or urethra, with accumulation of urine in the subcutaneous tissues around the prepuce and ventral abdomen; seen with obstructive urolithiasis of ruminants.

wattles
Small (1- to 2-inch) fleshy masses covered with skin that hang from the mandibular region in some breeds of goats. Males and females may have wattles.

waxing
Accumulation of soft, dried colostrum at the teat ends in mares, often signaling parturition within 24 to 48 hours.

wave mouth
An undulating occlusal surface of the cheek teeth (premolars and molars).

whirl bone
Greater trochanter of the femur.

wilgil
Male pseudohermaphrodite sheep.

wind puff
Effusion of a joint, not accompanied by lameness.

windsucker
Female horse that involuntarily aspirates air through the lips of the vulva (pneumovagina); may sometimes produce a noise as air enters

and exits the vagina, especially at speeds faster than a walk.

windsucker
Horse that cribs (aerophagia).

windswept
Foal born with bilateral angular limb deformities, with a valgus deformity in limb, and varus deformity in the same joint in the opposite limb; presumed to be caused by malposition in the uterus. Seen most often in the hocks.

wobbler
Horse with ataxia of the front and/or back legs, usually due to a compressive spinal cord lesion in the neck region, though other spinal cord diseases can cause similar signs.

wolf tooth
First premolars of the horse; small, rudimentary teeth that do not always erupt in every horse. They are often removed to prevent interference with the bit. Mandibular wolf teeth are very uncommon.

wool blindness
Extreme growth of wool around the eyes, limiting or preventing vision.

wry neck
Torticollis (twisted neck); may be congenital or secondary to other conditions.

wry nose
Severe congenital defect characterized by a lateral deviation of the nasal septum; appears as a twisted nose and muzzle.

Y

yean
Give birth, in sheep and goats.

yeld mare
Mare that does not produce or raise a foal during the season.

yellowhammer
Cattle showing evidence of Jersey blood.

Index

Page numbers followed by f indicate figures; t, tables; b, boxes.